CLINICAL ELECTROMYOGRAPHY:
Nerve Conduction Studies

Second Edition

CLINICAL ELECTROMYOGRAPHY: Nerve Conduction Studies

Second Edition

SHIN J. OH, M.D.

Professor of Neurology
Medical Director, Department of Clinical Neurophysiology
Director, EMG and Evoked Potentials Laboratory and
Muscle Histopathology Laboratory,
The University of Alabama at Birmingham,
Veterans Affairs Medical Center,
Birmingham, Alabama

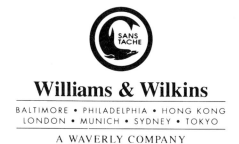

Williams & Wilkins

BALTIMORE • PHILADELPHIA • HONG KONG
LONDON • MUNICH • SYDNEY • TOKYO

A WAVERLY COMPANY

Editor: David C. Retford
Associate Editor: Molly L. Mullen
Copy Editor: Judith L. Minkove
Designer: Dan Pfisterer
Illustration Planner: Wayne Hubbel
Production Coordinator: Kim Nawrozki

Copyright © 1993
Williams & Wilkins
428 East Preston Street
Baltimore, Maryland 21202, USA

Accurate indications, adverse reactions, and dosage schedules for drugs are provided in this book, but it is possible that they may change. The reader is urged to review the package information data of the manufacturers of the medications mentioned.

Printed in the United States of America

First Edition 1984

Library of Congress Cataloging-in-Publication Data

Oh, Shin J.
    Clinical electromyography : nerve conduction studies / Shin J. Oh. — 2nd ed.
       p.   cm.
    Includes bibliographical references and index.
    ISBN 0-683-06644-7
    1. Neural conduction—Measurement.   2. Electromyography.   I. Title.
    [DNLM: 1. Electromyography.   2. Neural Conduction. WL 102.7 O36c]
RC349.N48O36   1993
616.7′4407547—dc20
DNLM/DLC
for Library of Congress   92-48896
                                                        CIP

95 96 97
3 4 5 6 7 8 9 10

This book is dedicated

to my wife, Dr. M. Kim Oh,

Associate Professor of Pediatrics, the University of Alabama at Birmingham;

to my sons, David and Michael, both MIT students; and

to the memory of my daughter, Julie.

Preface to the Second Edition

During the 8 years since the publication of the first edition of this book, I have met a number of electromyographers from every corner of the world, who have found my book an invaluable companion in their practice. If their response reflects the general sentiments of its readers, then I have achieved the goal of this book. Such success was also echoed by the unavailability of the first edition, which was "out of print" for the past 2 years.

In recent years, I have been flooded with requests for revision of this book by various colleagues, who have also shared with me their ideas for improvements of the book. To meet this challenge, I have revised the first edition.

Since 1984, there have been several developments in the field of nerve conduction. The foremost among them is the technological development of the EMG machine: e.g., automatic latency marking, automatic area calculation, and automatic testing capability of the refractory period. Another notable development is the introduction of magnetic and high-voltage low-impedance (HVLI) electrical stimulation technologies, which can stimulate the central nervous system. Nerve conduction techniques for almost all the nerves of the human body have now been described. The criteria of segmental demyelination have been better defined. AIDS, Lyme disease, and many immunologically mediated neuropathies have appeared.

To cope with these developments, I have introduced several new features in this edition: (a) descriptions of the new nerve conduction techniques; (b) refinement of the descriptions of the older techniques with more detailed anatomical and technical tips for better performance of the tests; (c) discussions of the more sophisticated tests, such as the refractory period or reflex test; (d) presentation of the magnetic and the HVLI electrical stimulation techniques; and (e) more comprehensive clinical correlation with the nerve conduction in the disease states, including neuropathies in AIDS, Lyme disease, and many immunologically mediated neuropathies. Although the magnetic and HVLI electrical stimulation tests are designed mainly for evaluation of the central nervous system, I have included them in this book because these tests are usually performed in the EMG laboratory.

It is my hope that this revised edition will continue to be an invaluable resource for electromyographers and EMG technologists in their daily service to patients in the EMG laboratory.

Preface to the First Edition, 1984

This book is written for clinician-electromyographers who aspire to provide excellent nerve conduction studies for the benefit of their patients.

Part I presents basic information on nerve conduction studies, including details of the various techniques, an anatomical guide for common nerve conductions, and normal data for adult and pediatric controls. This section may be used as a practical manual for the EMG technician who performs the more common nerve conduction tests.

Part II provides advanced information on the less common nerve conduction procedures, with attention to physiological and nonphysiological variables, anomalous innervation, and other more sophisticated details of nerve conduction studies. It also includes guides for the interpretation of nerve conduction data and information on diseased nerves. This section is written for the clinician-electromyographer who performs the rarer and more difficult nerve conduction studies and who interprets the findings in all of the nerve conduction studies.

It is hoped that this book contains sufficient encyclopedic and practical information on nerve conduction studies so that every EMG laboratory and clinician-electromyographer will find it an invaluable companion.

S. J. O.

Acknowledgments

First, I want to thank my wife, Dr. M. Kim Oh, for her steadfast support during the 2 years I spent on the revision of this book. Not only has she tolerated my irregular hours of sleeping, the untidiness of my study, and occasional neglect of my household duties, but she has also provided me with an environment at home in which I could write this revision with inspiration and scientific accuracy.

Second, I must express my appreciation to two individuals who helped me with the first edition, as well as with the second edition of this book: Dr. Mary Ward, my Administrative Assistant, who has pored over every sentence and assisted me in editing this book; and Mr. Perry Whitted, Chief of Medical Media Production Service at the VA Medical Center, Birmingham, Alabama, who drew many of the illustrations and supervised the entire illustration process with anatomical accuracy and excellence.

Third, I am grateful to three medical illustrators—Mr. David Fisher, Ms. Katharine Coleman, and Ms. Deborah Mechanik—for their superb illustrations, and to my secretary, Ms. Kathy McGhee, for her assistance with the reference search.

Lastly, I owe the production of this book to the editorial staff of Williams & Wilkins, Inc., without whose assistance and advice its completion would not have been possible.

Contents

PART I

Basic Section

Anatomical and Physiological Basis for Electromyography Studies

Motor Unit

The lower motor neuron system consists of the anterior horn cells, the peripheral nerves, neuromuscular synapses, and muscles. A motor neuron together with its axon and all the muscle fibers that it innervates is called a motor unit (Fig. 1.1).

Stimulation of a single motor neuron causes contraction of all its subservient muscle fibers. The average size of a motor unit, as measured by determination of the innervation ratio (number of muscle fibers: number of motor axons), varies in different muscles. The ratio is 2:1 to 3:1 for the laryngeal muscle and 1934:1 for the gastrocnemius. In general, muscles that control finer or smaller movements have a smaller motor unit than those that control gross movements.

There are two types of muscle fibers: type I (red) and type II (white) (Table 1.1). These types can be easily distinguished by adenosine triphosphatase (ATPase) staining: Type I is ATPase-poor and type II is ATPase-rich. Type I ("red" and "slow") muscle fibers contain more myoglobin, have less evident striations, respond more slowly, and have a longer latency than type II fibers (Fig. 1.2). They are adapted for long, slow, posture-maintaining contractions. The soleus of the cat is a typical example. Type II ("white" and "fast") muscle fibers have fewer fibers per motor unit and short, "twitch" durations. They are specialized for fine and skilled movements. The gastrocnemius of the cat belongs in this category. In human muscles, type I and II fibers are well intermixed at a ratio of 4:6. Anatomical, histochemical, and physiological differences in the properties of Type I and Type II fibers are listed in detail in Table 1.1 and Figure 1.3 (1).

It now seems that the character of the muscle is determined in part by its innerva-

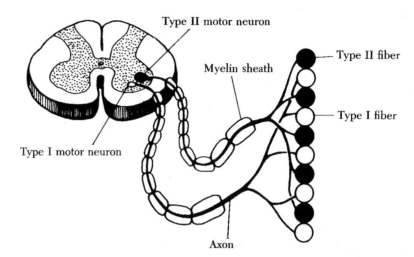

Figure 1.1. A single motor unit: motor neuron (anterior horn cell), peripheral nerve fiber (axon and myelin sheath), and all the muscle fibers innervated by the nerve fibers. *Blank circles* represent type I fibers; *solid circles* represent type II fibers.

Table 1.1.
Properties of Type I and II Fibers

	Type I Fibers	Type II Fibers
Color	Red	White
Myoglobin content	High	Low
Muscle fiber diameter	Smaller	Larger
Enzymes		
Myofibrillar ATPase	Low	High
Mitochondrial oxidative enzymes	High	Low
Glycolytic enzymes	Low	High
Energy source	Fatty acids, glucose	Glycogen
Metabolic characteristics	Aerobic oxidative phosphorylation	Anaerobic glycolysis
Twitch contraction time	Slow	Fast
Tetanus tension output	Low	High
Resistance to fatigue	High	Low
Motor units		
Size	Small	Large
Intensity required for activation	Low	High
Axon conduction velocity	Slower	Faster
Anatomical location	Deep muscle; axial portion of surface muscle	Superficial portion of surface muscle

tion. All the constituent muscle fibers of a motor unit are of the same type, indicating a strong trophic control of nerves and muscles. In a crossed innervation experiment, the nerves to fast and slow muscles were crossed and allowed to regenerate (2). When regrowth was complete and the nerve that had previously supplied the slow muscle innervated the fast muscle, the fast muscle became slow. The reverse change occurred in the previously slow muscle. It seems, therefore, that even the biochemical characteristics of muscles depend in part upon the type of innervation they receive.

Recent studies have shown that muscle fibers under the control of a single motor unit are scattered among other muscle fibers, not grouped as previously thought (3). This finding agrees with the mosaic intermixing of type I and II fibers in human muscles.

With a very weak voluntary contraction, the needle electromyography (EMG) electrode records activity from single motor units. These action potentials are called motor unit potentials (MUPs). Usually, several MUPs fire together. However, a single MUP can be isolated and recorded with good cooperation from the patient and careful manipulation of the needle electrode.

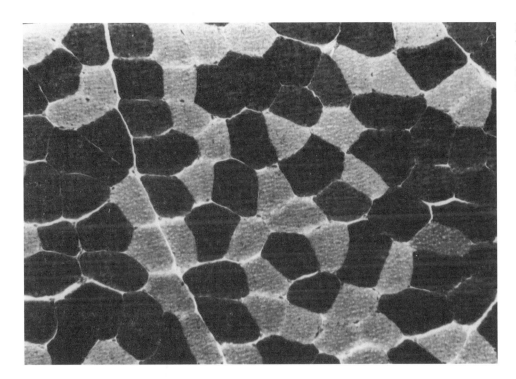

Figure 1.2. Normal muscle strained with myosine adenotriphosphatase (ATPase) at pH 9.4. Dark fibers are type II fibers; light fibers are type I fibers.

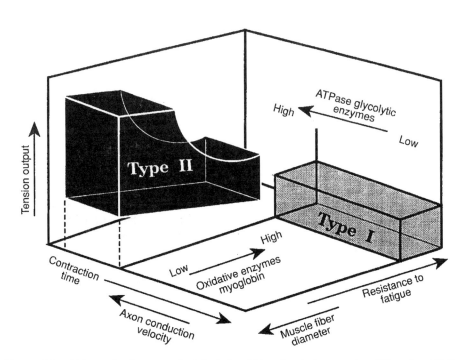

Figure 1.3. Relationship between physiological and histochemical properties of Type I and II fibers (modified from Burke(1)).

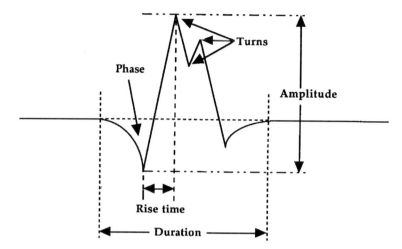

Figure 1.4.   Various components of the motor unit potential.

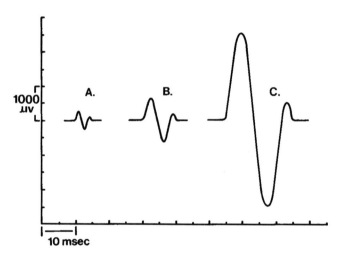

Figure 1.5.   Motor unit potential (MUP) in the various neuromuscular diseases. **A**, Small-short MUP in myopathy. **B**, Normal MUP. **C**, Large-long-duration MUP in denervation process.

The motor unit is the basic anatomical substrate for the motor unit potential. Recent studies have suggested that the spike component of MUP recorded with a concentric needle having a 150 × 580 μm recording surface is generated from five to 12 muscle fibers within a radius of 1 mm (4).

The amplitude, duration, and phase of the MUP are important in the differential diagnosis of various neuromuscular diseases (Fig. 1.4). When recorded with a concentric needle electrode, normal MUPs usually have a duration of from 3–15 msec, a peak-to-peak amplitude of 300 μV–3 mV, and a bi- or tri-phasic configuration. The small and short MUPs are characteristic in patients with myopathy, whereas in patients with denervated disorders the large and long MUPs are typical (Fig. 1.5). Giant motor unit potentials (MUPs with greater than 5 mV amplitude) are classically noted in the denervated disorders. It is likely that giant MUPs result from reinnervation of denervated muscle fibers by sprouts from intact motor axons.

Fasciculation is the short-duration spontaneous muscle twitching that is commonly seen in anterior horn cell diseases (e.g., amyotrophic lateral sclerosis). Fasciculation is thought to be a spontaneous discharge (depolarization) of the motor unit irritated by the disease process. Thus, the various parameters of fasciculation are not different from those of the MUP (Fig. 1.6).

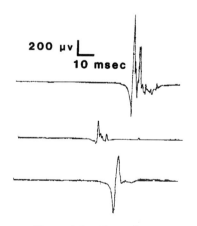

Figure 1.6.   Fasciculation.

Recently an attempt was made to record the action potential within the whole motor unit using the entire cannula as an active electrode in a modified single-fiber EMG needle (the Macro EMG needle) (4). The single fiber action potential was used to trigger a digital averager to which the signal from the larger recording surface, the cannula, was fed and averaged, usually 128–512 impulses. The shape of the Macro EMG action potential was determined by the temporal and spatial summation of the individual single-fiber potentials within the motor unit. The amplitude of the Macro EMG action potential ranged from 10–290 μV in normal individuals, was usually increased in those with neurogenic disorders, and was normal or decreased in those with myopathies.

Excitability of the Nerve and Muscle

In most cells, there is a difference in potential between the interior and the exterior of the cell. When the cell is in a resting state, the membrane potential is called the resting potential. The resting potential is always negative in nerve and muscle: negative on the inside as compared with the outside of the membrane. The resting potential is −70 mV in the nerve and −80 mV in the muscle. When the nerve and muscle work, brief positive changes in the membrane potential occur, which are called the action potential.

The terms for the various phases of the action potential are given in Figure 1.7. Action potential in a particular cell always follows a constant sequence of depolarization and repolarization of the membrane, which occurs whenever the membrane is depolarized at or beyond the threshold level. The action potential is therefore "all or none" in character and is said to obey the "all-or-none law" of excitation.

Cells in which action potentials can be triggered are called excitable. Excitability is a typical property of nerve and muscle cells. Thus, excitation occurs as a result of depolarization of the membrane to the threshold level. This depolarization is also called stimulation. When a depolarizing electrical current crosses the threshold, an excitation is triggered. The electrical current pulse that generates such a change in potential is called a stimulating current, or stimulus. Both the intensity (strength) and the duration of the stimulating current are important in the generation of excitation. The relationship between the strength and the duration of the stimulating current is called the strength-duration curve (Fig. 1.8).

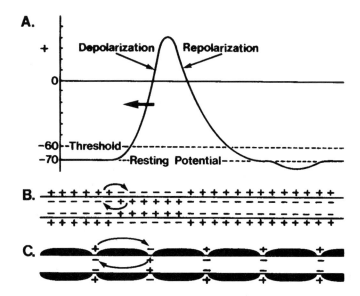

Figure 1.7. Phases of the action potential and its propagation. **A**, Terms for the various phases of the action potential. It also shows the action potential propagating from right to left. **B**, Mechanism of conduction in unmyelinated fiber: local circuit conduction. **C**, Mechanism of conduction in a myelinated fiber: saltatory conduction.

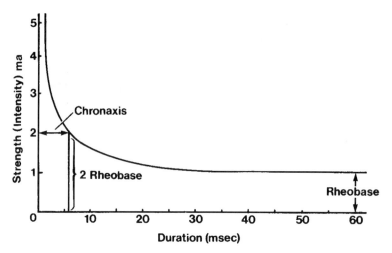

Figure 1.8. Relationship between the strength (intensity) and duration of the stimulating current and the terms for the excitability.

The rheobase is defined as the strength of a stimulating current of very long duration that is just large enough to trigger an excitation. However, chronaxie is more commonly used as a measure of the excitability of muscle or nerve. Chronaxie is defined as the necessary duration of a stimulating current of twice the rheobase strength.

The strength-duration curve on the nerve is called nerve excitability. Nerve excitability becomes abnormal 72 hr after severe nerve injury (Fig. 23.2) and is the earliest electrophysiological abnormality observed after a nerve injury. The nerve excitability test is still used in the evaluation of Bell's palsy (idiopathic facial palsy) to predict the prognosis in the early stages.

On the fifth day after severe nerve injury, the strength-duration curve of the muscle becomes abnormal. The strength-duration curve on muscle has been used extensively in the past as an electrodiagnostic test in muscle. However, because of its limited value, it has not been used in many laboratories in recent years.

Propagation of Action Potential

The actual task of the nerve and muscle is the propagation of excitation (action potential). Once initiated, the action potential is self-propagating and spreads like a wave over the membrane until it has moved along the entire cell.

The mechanism of propagation of the action potential differs in unmyelinated and myelinated nerve fibers. There is "local circuit" conduction in unmyelinated fibers and "saltatory" conduction in myelinated fibers.

For an unmyelinated axon, the mechanism of propagation occurs as diagrammed in Figure 1.7. During the peak of the action potential in a segment of nerve, the membrane potential reverses polarity, the inside becoming positive in regard to the outside. The reversal of polarity leads to a local current flow from positive to negative, as indicated by the arrows in Figure 1.7. The outward current flow through the resting membrane in front of the action potential (which is depicted as moving from right to left) depolarizes the membrane. In turn, the newly activated membrane explodes into an action potential, generates local currents, and depolarizes the next segment and so on until the action potential has moved along the full length of the axon.

The conduction speed is determined by the diameter of the unmyelinated fibers (Table 1.2). Larger fibers conduct more rapidly than small fibers because they have a lower resistance. Because of the continuous local circuit conduction, the nerve conduction velocity (NCV) of unmyelinated fibers is relatively slow. In human unmyelinated pain fibers, the NCV is 1 m/sec. The giant axon of squid, which is 0.7 mm in diameter,

Table 1.2.
Conduction Velocity in Various Nerve Fiber Types in Mammalian Nerve

Fiber Type		Function	Fiber Diameter (μm)	Conduction Velocity (m/sec)	Most Susceptibility to Conduction Block by Agents
Erland & Gasser's System	Lloyd's System for Sensory Fibers				
Myelinated fibers					
A	Ia	Proprioception; Primary muscle spindle afferents; motor to skeletal muscles	12–20	70–120	Pressure
	Ib	Afferents from Golgi tendon organ			
	II	Cutaneous touch and pressure	5–12	30–70	
		Motor to muscle spindle	3–6	15–30	
	III	Cutaneous temperature and pain	2–5	12–30	
B		Sympathetic preganglionic	3	3–15	Hypoxia
Unmyelinated fibers					
C	IV	Cutaneous pain	0.4–1.2	0.5–2	Local anesthetic
		Sympathetic postganglionic	0.3–1.3	0.7–2.3	

has a speed of conduction of 25 m/sec. In general, the NCV of unmyelinated fibers can be calculated by the following formula:

$$NCV\ of\ unmyelinated\ fibers\ (m/sec) = \sqrt{diameter\ of\ unmyelinated\ fiber\ (axon)\ (\mu m)}.$$

In myelinated fibers, the myelin sheath acts as an insulator and prevents transmembrane current flow in the internodes. The movement of the current occurs only at the nodes of Ranvier, spaced at intervals of about 2 mm in larger fibers (Fig. 1.7). The impulse hops from one node to the next. This is called saltatory conduction in myelinated fibers. In vertebrates, all the fibers that conduct at velocities of propagation in excess of 3 m/sec are myelinated. For myelinated fibers, the following formula is applied in the calculation of the NCV:

$$NCV\ of\ myelinated\ fibers\ (m/sec) = conversion\ factor \times outer\ diameter\ of\ myelinated\ fiber\ (\mu m).$$

The NCV that we measure in the human subject is predominantly contributed by the large-diameter fibers of the nerves. Thus, the NCV reflects the fastest conduction velocity of the nerve. The conversion factor varies according to the nerve and to the animal. For example, it is 4.4 for the human sural nerve (5), 5.2 for the baboon median and ulnar nerves (6), and 6.0 for the cat saphenous nerve (7).

Slowing in NCV is caused either by loss of large fibers or by segmental demyelination. When the axons are predominantly affected by the disease process, the NCVs are minimally affected. On the other hand, when the myelin is predominantly involved, marked slowing in NCV is seen because of the loss of saltatory conduction. In fact, in axonal neuropathy, the NCVs are either normal or slowed by less than 40% of normal. In contrast, in demyelinating neuropathy the NCVs are slowed by more than 40% of normal.

Neuromuscular Transmission

By nerve impulse, the action potential of the muscle is generated at the motor end-plate (neuromuscular junction) where the nerve makes contact with the muscle fibers. The structure of the motor end-plate is illustrated in Figure 1.9. The axon ends in the presynaptic terminal, which is separated from the postsynaptic membrane of muscle fibers by the synaptic cleft (200–500 Å). The presynaptic terminal contains mitochondria and many synaptic vesicles. Many experiments indicate that these vesicles contain acetylcholine (ACh). The postsynaptic membrane has repeated synaptic folding where the ACh receptors are located.

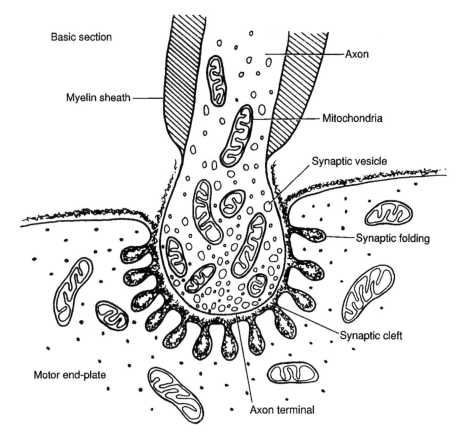

Figure 1.9.   Neuromuscular junction.

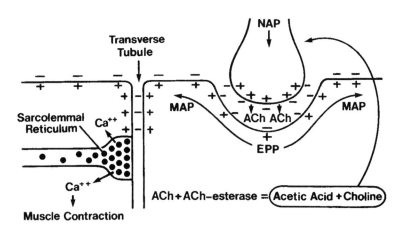

Figure 1.10.   Physiological sequences at the neuromuscular junction and muscle for muscle contraction. *Abbreviations:* NAP, nerve action potential; ACh, acetylcholine; EPP, end-plate potential; MAP, muscle action potential.

The action potential of the nerve terminal triggers the release of ACh from the vesicles into the synaptic cleft (Fig. 1.10). The released ACh diffuses across the gap and attaches to the ACh receptors on the postsynaptic membrane. This induces the depolarization, which leads to the generation of action potential of the muscle membrane.

This depolarization at the end-plate is called an end-plate potential (EPP). The EPP is nonpropagated and graded, rather than following the all-or-none law. The EPP induces a sink for current flow through the adjacent muscle cell membrane, depolarizing it to the threshold value required to initiate an action potential, which then propagates along the fiber by local circuit current flow. In healthy muscles, the EPPs are always far above the threshold. Each presynaptic action potential triggers a contraction in the muscle fibers. Thus, neuromuscular transmission is normally obligatory.

The end-plate membrane is special in containing acetylcholinesterase, which breaks down ACh into inactive choline and acetic acid. Choline and acetic acid are, for the most part, reabsorbed by the presynaptic terminal and, with the aid of acetylcholine transferase, recombined into ACh. This ACh is then stored in the synaptic vesicles of the presynaptic terminal until it is released once more.

At rest, the presynaptic terminal releases single quanta (the nearly equal-sized packets) of ACh at irregular intervals, producing the spontaneous potentials called miniature end-plate potentials (MEPPs). The MEPPs are similar in their time course to normal EPPs, but their amplitude is very much smaller than that of the EPP. The pharmacological properties of the EPP and MEPP are also identical. Studies show that the EPP is the summation of multiple MEPPs; that is, the normal EPP is generated by the simultaneous release of a large number of ACh quanta. It has been estimated that about 100–200 quanta or synaptic vesicles in amphibians and about 60 in human subjects are released per presynaptic nerve action potential (8).

When the needle electrode is inserted near the end-plate of a muscle, end-plate noise is often recorded. These potentials are the EMG equivalent of the MEPP.

The presence of Ca^{++} ions is absolutely essential for the normal course of quantal release of ACh triggered by a presynaptic action potential. The Mg^{++} ion has the opposite effect of Ca^{++} at the presynaptic membrane. Presumably, Mg^{++} ions compete with Ca^{++} ions for their site of action.

Botulinus toxin inhibits the release of ACh, producing the neuromuscular blocking that is seen with botulism. A similar mechanism is postulated in antibiotic-induced myasthenia, in which intravenous calcium gluconate is the recommended treatment because Ca^{++} ions facilitate the release of ACh.

There are two classical diseases caused by a defect in neuromuscular transmission. In myasthenia gravis (MG), the basic defect lies in the postsynaptic membrane: ACh receptor antibody-induced decrease of the functioning ACh receptors. Anticholinesterase (e.g., Mestinon) relieves myasthenic symptoms because of slowed breakdown of ACh at the postsynaptic membrane, and permits a more prolonged depolarization of the end-plate. In the Eaton-Lambert syndrome (Lambert-Eaton myasthenic syndrome), which is commonly associated with carcinoma of the lung, the main defect is the insufficient release of ACh at the presynaptic membrane induced by the antibody against voltage-dependent calcium channels (9). Guanidine and aminopyridine, which facilitate a release of ACh, are effective in relieving myasthenic symptoms in this disorder.

The MEPPs recorded in muscle of patients with MG show a greatly reduced amplitude but a normal frequency (10). A reduced amplitude of the MEPP was originally thought to be due to a reduced amount of ACh in each ACh packet. However, a recent study has shown that this was caused by the reduced number of postsynaptic ACh receptors (11). On the other hand, in the Eaton-Lambert syndrome the amplitude of the MEPP was normal, but the frequency of the MEPP did not increase as it normally does when the motor nerve terminals were depolarized by increasing the external potassium ion concentration. This observation led to the conclusion that a very low number of ACh packets are released by a nerve action potential in this disorder.

When a muscle fiber is denervated, its sensitivity to ACh increases by as much as 100-fold over a period of 1–2 weeks. This is called denervation hypersensitivity: A muscle fiber contracts in response to a smaller amount of ACh than is normally effective. This phenomenon is due to the development of multiple, highly sensitive sites in the nonjunctional membrane. Fibrillation, which is usually detectable by a needle EMG study in the muscle 2 weeks after denervation, is thought to represent denervation hypersensitivity. Thus, fibrillation is the spontaneous twitching of the hypersensitive muscle fiber in response to a small quantity of ACh in the bloodstream, which is normally ineffective. Fibrillations are usually indicative of axonal degeneration and are absent or few in number in patients with demyelination.

Muscle Contraction

A skeletal muscle consists of many thousands of muscle fibers (Fig. 1.11). Muscle fibers contain bundles of myofibrils. Each fibril is comprised of many filaments and is divided into many "sarcomeres," or units, between two Z-lines. Thin filaments (actin-troponin-tropomyosin) are anchored securely to Z-lines and extend less than half the length of the sarcomere. On the other hand, the thick filaments (myosin) in the middle part of the sarcomeres are interdigitated between the free ends of the thin filaments (actin). The various bands of the sarcomere are indicated in Figure 1.12.

During muscle contraction (shortening), the I and H bands decrease in thickness. This thinning is due to a sliding of the thin filaments (actin) between the thick filaments (myosin), thus shortening the sarcomere at the expense of the I and H bands (Fig. 1.12).

The initial event in muscle contraction is a depolarization of the muscle fiber membrane, which starts at the end-plate. The action potential is propagated by local circuit current flow along the membrane. The conduction speed is only about 5 m/sec, which is much slower than that in the axons. Through the transverse tubular system (Fig. 1.10), the depolarization is conducted into the depths of the muscle fibers. This results in a

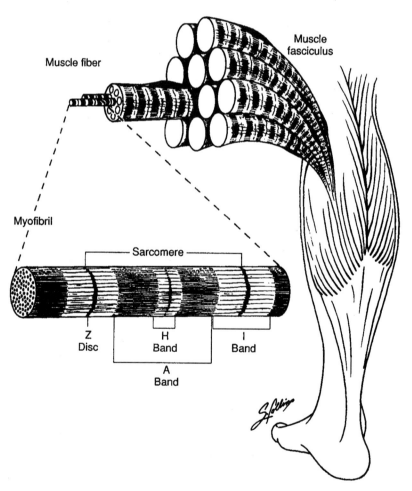

Figure 1.11.   Histological and molecular structure of skeletal muscle.

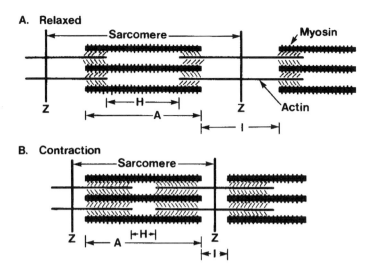

Figure 1.12. Mechanism of contraction. Note the arrangements of the myosin and actin filaments in a sarcomere and the bridges between these filaments. It is thought that changes in the configuration of the bridges produce a shear force that moves the actin filaments between the myosin filaments. **A,** Arrangement of filaments at the relaxed state. **B,** Arrangement of filaments at the time of maximal contraction. The sarcomere becomes shorter because of shortening of the H and I bands.

release of calcium from the sarcoplasmic reticulum, the ends of which abut the transverse tubules. The free calcium ions in the sarcoplasm of the muscle cell then initiate the formation of bridges between the thin and thick filaments, leading to contraction. As the action potential wanes, the sarcoplasmic reticulum rapidly resequesters the Ca^{++}, ATP breaks the bridge-coupling filaments, and the fibers relax. The energy for this movement is provided by the hydrolysis of ATP by myosin ATPase.

Myotonia is a typical example of a disorder of the muscle fiber membrane. Myotonia is characterized clinically by a difficulty of contracted muscle to relax. Myotonic response is detected very easily by a needle EMG because of the typical waxing and waning of high-frequency discharges associated with a "dive-bomber" sound. The disturbance appears to be due to an abnormally low threshold of the muscle fiber membrane, so that it fires repetitively in response to the depolarization produced by ACh release.

McArdle's disease affects the contractile mechanism due to a lack of phosphorylase, which is involved in the breakdown of muscle glycogen to glucose-6-phosphate. The most prominent symptom is painful exertional cramp. The needle EMG study in the shortened muscle in cramp shows electrical silence. Thus, this cramp fits the physiological definition of contracture. In this disorder, contracture is attributed to a critical shortage of ATP during strenuous exercise, when most of the energy for normal muscle contraction derives from glycogen. A shortage of ATP could impair muscle relaxation by inhibiting the energy-dependent calcium uptake of the sarcoplasmic reticulum. Although one study disputed this mechanism (12), it is possible that the technique used in the study was not sophisticated enough to detect a local defect in the ATP of sarcoplasmic reticulum.

The single-fiber EMG (SFEMG) electrode, having a 25-μm recording surface, records the action potential generated from one or two muscle fibers within a radius of about 300 μm (13). The single-fiber action potentials have an amplitude of 0.2–20 mV and a duration of less than 300 μsec. They give information about the individual muscle fiber (propagation velocity), its motor end-plate function (jitter), and the focal characteristics in the topography of the motor unit (fiber density). The SFEMG is used predominantly in the detection of abnormal jitter in patients with myasthenia gravis and related disorders.

REFERENCES

1. Burke R. Motor units in mammalian muscle. In: Sumner A, ed. The physiology of peripheral nerve disease. Philadelphia: WB Saunders, 1980:133–194.
2. Karpati G, Engel WK. Transformation of the histochemical profile of skeletal muscle by foreign innervation. Nature 1967; 215:1509–1510.
3. Kugelberg E. Properties of the rat hind limb motor units. In: Desmedt JE, ed. New developments in EMG and clinical neurophysiology. Basel: Karger, 1973:1:2–13.
4. Stålberg E. Macro EMG, a new recording technique. J Neurol Neurosurg Psychiatry 1980; 43:475–482.
5. Tackmann W, Spalka G, Oginszus HJ. Quantitative histometric studies and relations of number and diameter of myelinated fibres to electrophysiological parameters in normal sensory nerve of man. J Neurol 1976; 212:71–84.
6. McLeod JG, Wray SH. Conduction velocity and fiber diameter of the median and ulnar nerve of the baboon. J Neurol Neurosurg Psychiatry 1967; 30:240–247.
7. Hursh JB. Conduction velocity and diameter of nerve fibres. Am J Physiol 1939; 127:131–139.
8. Brown WF. The physiological and technical basis of electromyography. Boston: Butterworth, 1984.
9. Lennon VA, Lambert EH. Autoantibodies bind solubilized calcium channel-w-Conotoxin complexes from small cell lung carcinoma: a diagnostic aid for Lambert-Eaton myasthenic syndrome. Mayo Clin Proc 1989; 64:1498–1504.
10. Elmquist D. Neuromuscular transmission defects. In: Licht S, ed. Electrodiagnosis and electromyography. New Haven: Elizabeth Licht, 1971:376–389.
11. Engel AG, Lindstrom JM, Lambert EH, Lennon VA. Ultrastructural localization of the acetylcholine receptor in myasthenia gravis and its experimental autoimmune model. Neurology 1977; 27:307–315.
12. Rowland LP, Araki S, Carmel P. Contracture in McArdle's disease. Arch Neurol 1967; 13:541–544.
13. Stålberg E, Ekstedt J. Single fiber EMG and microphysiology of the motor unit in normal and diseased muscle. In: Desmedt JE, ed. New developments in electromyography and clinical neurophysiology. Basel: Karger, 1973:1:113–129.

2

General Concepts of Electrodiagnostic Studies in Neuromuscular Disease

Electrodiagnostic studies can be quite valuable in the diagnosis and follow-up consideration of neuromuscular diseases. They must be used, however, as an extension of the clinical evaluation and not as routine tests. After deciding which pathophysiology might explain a patient's signs and symptoms, the physician may proceed with specific electromyography (EMG) studies to shed light on diseases that might affect the anterior horn cells, nerve roots, peripheral nerves, neuromuscular junctions, or muscles.

It is important to recognize the inherent limitations of the EMG study. First, the kinds of tests and the muscles or nerves to be tested must be determined by clinical findings (Table 2.1) (1). There is no "routine" or "standard" test in the EMG laboratory. Then, the EMG findings must be interpreted in light of the clinical findings because no EMG results are pathognomonic of a specific disease entity. For these reasons, it is essential that the clinical problem be assessed thoroughly and that a careful neurological examination be performed prior to the electrophysiological study.

Three types of tests are performed in the majority of EMG laboratories: the nerve conduction study, the needle EMG study, and the repetitive nerve stimulation (RNS) test.

Nerve Conduction Study

The velocity at which an impulse is conducted along a motor or sensory nerve can be measured with great accuracy. Nerve conduction velocity (NCV) is an expression of the physiological or pathophysiological state of the nerves. There are three kinds of nerve conduction studies: (*a*) the motor nerve conduction test; (*b*) the sensory nerve conduction test; and (*c*) the mixed nerve conduction test.

Table 2.1.

Guidelines for EMG Tests for Common Entrapment Neuropathy and Neuromuscular Disorders[a]

	Most Informative Tests	Classic Abnormalities
Carpal tunnel syndrome	Sensory nerve conduction (NC) over palm-wrist and finger-wrist segment; terminal latency (median nerve)	Abnormal sensory NC over the tested segments; prolonged terminal latency
Ulnar compression neuropathy at elebow	Sensory NC over finger-wrist and mixed NC over forearm segments; motor NC across elbow	Abnormal sensory and mixed NC over finger-elbow segment; slow motor NCV across elbow
Peroneal nerve palsy	Motor NC across fibular head	Slow motor NCV across fibular head
Tarsal tunnel syndrome	Sensory NCV in the plantar nerves: terminal latency (posterior tibial N)	Abnormal sensory NC in plantar nerves; prolonged terminal latency
Radiculopathy	Paraspinal needle EMG	Abnormal spontaneous potentials
Myopathy	Needle EMG	Short-small MUPs
Peripheral neuropathy	Extensive NC studies	Slow motor and sensory NCV
Myasthenia gravis	Repetitive nerve stimulation test	Decremental response
	SFEMG	Abnormal jitter
Bell's palsy	Motor NC	Decreased amplitude
	Nerve excitability test	Abnormal nerve excitability
Myotonic disorders	Needle EMG	Myotonic potentials

[a]Modified from Oh (1).

The motor nerve conduction of a peripheral nerve is tested by stimulating the nerve with a single supramaximal stimulus at each of two proximal points along the course of the peripheral nerve and then recording the compound muscle action potential (CMAP) with a surface electrode from a muscle innervated by that nerve (Fig. 2.1). For example, the median nerve may be stimulated at the elbow and again at the wrist, with the recording electrode placed over the belly of the abductor pollicis brevis muscle. The time required for this response with distal stimulation is called the terminal latency. To obtain the conduction time, the terminal latency is subtracted from the latency at the proximal point of stimulation. The distance from the proximal to the distal point of stimulation is measured. NCV is determined by dividing this distance by the conduction time. The CMAP amplitude and shape are also analyzed. The procedure is limited to nerves that are accessible to stimulation. In the upper extremities these include the median, ulnar, and radial nerves; in the lower extremities they are the sciatic, femoral, posterior tibial, and peroneal nerves.

The sensory nerve conduction of a peripheral nerve is tested either orthodromically or antidromically (Fig. 2.2). In the orthodromic method, the sensory nerve conduction is tested by stimulating the distal part of the nerve and recording the compound nerve action potential (CNAP) directly over the proximal part of the nerve. For example, conduction along the sensory fibers of the median or ulnar nerve can be tested by stimulating the digital nerves at the fingers and recording the potential at the wrist. When the stimulating and recording electrodes are switched, this is called antidromic stimulation. Unlike motor nerve conduction, the conduction time is equal to the latency in sensory nerve conduction. Thus, conduction velocity is determined by dividing the distance by the latency. The CNAP amplitude is measured from peak to peak.

This procedure is used most often for studying the ulnar, median, sural, and radial nerves. Because a specific technique is needed to obtain CNAP in the sciatic, posterior tibial, and peroneal nerves, this procedure is usually not used for studying these nerves.

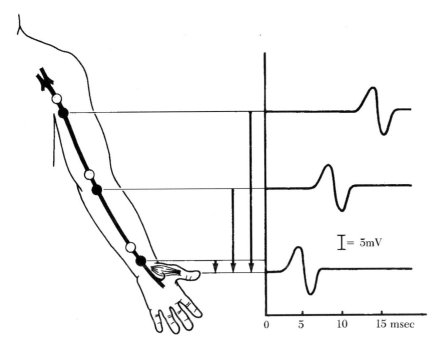

Figure 2.1.   Motor nerve conduction study in the median nerve. The recording electrodes are placed over the belly of the abductor pollicis brevis. The median nerve is stimulated at the wrist, elbow, and axilla.

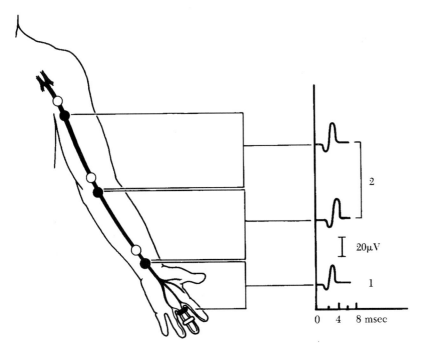

Figure 2.2.   Sensory (*1*) and mixed (*2*) nerve conduction study in the median nerve. The recording electrodes are placed over the proximal part of the nerve, and the stimulating electrodes are over the distal part of the nerve. A reference stimulating electrode is placed distal to the active stimulating electrode.

The mixed nerve conduction of a peripheral nerve is tested by stimulating the distal part of the mixed nerves (sensory and motor fibers) and recording the CNAP directly over the proximal part of the nerve (Fig. 2.2). For example, conduction along the mixed fibers of the median and ulnar nerves can be tested by stimulating the mixed nerves at the wrist and recording the CNAP at the elbow. The methods of testing, measuring amplitude, and calculating velocity are identical to the orthodromic method of sensory nerve conduction. The only difference is that mixed (motor and sensory) nerve fibers are being stimulated. The clinical significance of mixed nerve conduction studies is also identical to that of the sensory nerve conduction studies.

Theoretically, the motor, sensory, and mixed NCVs represent the maximal conduction velocities of the fastest conducting motor, sensory and mixed nerve fibers, respectively. Normally, the conduction velocity varies with age (slow under 3 years of age), skin temperature (slows about 2.0 m/sec for each degree centigrade fall), each segment of nerve (faster proximally), and different nerves (faster in the median than in the peroneal nerve). Every EMG laboratory should establish a range of normal values for each nerve according to its particular technique. Roughly, NCVs slower than 40 m/sec in the upper extremities and slower than 35 m/sec in the lower extremities are definitely abnormal. Slowing of the NCV indicates neuropathy or nerve injury. Usually, sensory nerve conduction is a more sensitive index than motor nerve conduction in the diagnosis of peripheral neuropathy or injury.

Abnormal Nerve Conduction

As stated previously, nerve conduction abnormalities are not diagnostic for any specific disease. The abnormal findings must be correlated with the clinical findings and symptoms and with other laboratory data. The nerve conduction study is most helpful in the detection of peripheral neuropathy and entrapment neuropathy, and in the assessment of peripheral nerve injuries.

With peripheral neuropathy, the nerve conduction study should be done in testable nerves in both legs and in one arm because the nerve conduction abnormalities are not observed uniformly in all peripheral nerves. Thus, the more nerves tested, the better the yield will be in detecting these abnormalities. In the majority of cases, nerve conduction abnormalities are observed in more than 50% of nerves tested. However, in a small percentage of cases, only a few nerves show abnormalities.

Nerve conduction abnormalities include slow NCV, low CMAP or CNAP amplitude, conduction block, and abnormal temporal dispersion.

It is important to remember that the NCV could be normal in a few patients with mild neuropathy of axonal degeneration. Thus, normal NCV in a patient with a definite clinical finding of peripheral neuropathy is usually indicative of peripheral neuropathy of axonal degeneration. In this case, the CMAP and/or CNAP amplitude is usually low. Sometimes the physician must rely on needle EMG of distal muscles for evidence of a denervation process.

The degree of slowing of the NCV is also helpful in assessing the main pathology of peripheral neuropathy. There are two main components in the peripheral nerves: the axon and the myelin. The axon is the least effective, and the myelin is the most effective in conduction of action potential, because of the saltatory conduction in myelinated fibers. Thus, peripheral neuropathy of axonal degeneration shows very minimal slowing in contrast to the marked slowing of NCV in peripheral neuropathy of segmental demyelination. Usually, peripheral neuropathy of axonal degeneration (e.g., alcoholic and nutritional neuropathies) has a mildly slow NCV (above 35 m/sec) (Table 22.1). In peripheral neuropathy of segmental demyelination (e.g., the Guillain-Barré syndrome), the NCV is markedly slow (less than 30 m/sec) (Fig. 2.3).

A low CMAP or CNAP amplitude is usually seen together with slow NCV. However, the CMAP or CNAP amplitude may be low in the presence of normal NCV. This is usually indicative of axonal degeneration. Absent CMAP or CNAP response is usually indicative of severe peripheral neuropathy.

Conduction block and abnormal temporal dispersion are indicative of segmental

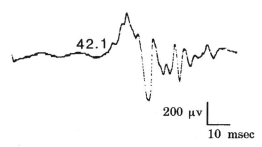

Figure 2.3. Abnormal temporal dispersion of the CMAP in the posterior tibial nerve in a case of chronic inflammatory demyelinating neuropathy. Stimulation was at the popliteal fossa; latency is 42.1 msec. The motor NCV of this nerve was 18.6 m/sec. This is typical of demyelinating neuropathy.

demyelination (Fig. 2.3). These are usually observed along with slow NCV. However, they may be present all by themselves.

Although nerve conduction findings may indicate the presence of neuropathy and may suggest the pathophysiological nature of the neuropathy, other studies must determine whether the etiology is diabetic, uremic, or secondary to metachromatic leukodystrophy.

The nerve conduction study is also of some value in the follow-up evaluation of patients recovering from neuropathies, either under specific therapies or spontaneously. In addition, they are of value in the study of families that have a neuropathy as part of a genetically determined illness. This is especially so in the detection of asymptomatic cases of Charcot-Marie-Tooth disease (2).

The nerve conduction test is very helpful in the detection of entrapment neuropathy, which is defined as a mononeuropathy resulting from mechanical irritation from some impingement by anatomical neighbors. The entrapment neuropathies present some common features: Pain is a prominent characteristic and is usually present at rest, although it may become severe at night.

Fortunately, the localized pathology of entrapment neuropathy has been segmental demyelination. Thus, there is usually segmental slowing of the NCV. The absence of the CNAP or slowing of sensory and mixed NCVs, as well as slowing of motor NCVs in the involved segment, are the classical abnormalities. The most informative tests for the various entrapment neuropathies are listed in Table 2.1. The nerve conduction study is usually normal in patients with myopathies or anterior horn cell diseases.

Needle EMG Study

The needle EMG findings are an expression of the physiological or pathophysiological state of muscles. Electrical potentials are observed after the needle electrode is inserted into the muscle. Monopolar and coaxial needles are used. In general, this procedure is well tolerated by adults, but in very young children it is usually not possible to do a completely satisfactory EMG study because of pain. This is a definite limitation in pediatric electromyography.

Three types of observations are made: (a) spontaneous electrical activity in a relaxed resting muscle, either undisturbed or induced by needle movement; (b) configuration of the motor unit potential (MUP) (phase, duration, and amplitude) with weak voluntary contraction; and (c) the pattern of MUP recruitment with maximal contraction.

No abnormal spontaneous activity is noted at rest in normal muscles. Mostly diphasic or triphasic MUPs are noted with weak muscle contraction. The duration of the MUP varies with different muscles (1–2 msec for the ocular muscles and 8–14 msec for the quadriceps) and with age (slightly increased in old age). On maximal contraction, a full interference pattern with numerous recruitments of MUPs is noted.

Abnormal EMG Findings

The needle EMG study is most helpful in differentiating between a denervation process and myopathy and in the detection of myotonia.

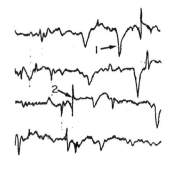

100
µv
⁺ 10 msec

Figure 2.4. Abnormal spontaneous EMG potentials. *Arrow 1* points to a positive sharp wave and *arrow 2* to fibrillation.

Denervation

In denervated muscles, fibrillation and positive sharp waves (abnormal spontaneous potentials) are noted at rest (Fig. 2.4). With total denervation the MUP is not observed at all, even on maximal attempt. With partial denervation the duration of the MUP is either normal or increased, depending on the chronicity of denervation. Usually, in association with the denervation, the collateral sprout from relatively normal axons may innervate denervated muscle fibers, resulting in the recording of larger and higher MUPs and producing a long duration of the MUPs (Fig. 2.5). Reduced patterns or discrete activity are observed on maximal contraction, depending on the severity of the denervation, as a result of the functional loss of the motor unit.

Fibrillation and positive sharp waves are usually associated with a denervation process. However, it is important to remember that they are not pathognomonic of a denervation process because they are also observed in patients with active myopathy. It is also important to remember that fibrillation and positive sharp waves are not seen during the first 10 days following injury to a nerve. Thus, if the needle EMG study is done within 10 days after an injury, often no fibrillation or positive sharp wave is observed.

Fasciculation is frequently seen when the pathological process is proximal in the anterior horn cells or nerve roots. It should be stressed that fasciculation, or spontaneous depolarization of a single motor unit, occurs in about 15% of the normal population and has no meaning except when associated with other EMG or clinical abnormalities of denervation (3). If it is seen in an otherwise normal patient, it is called "benign fasciculation."

When assessing the degree of peripheral nerve injury, the number of MUPs in the recruitment on maximal attempt is very helpful (4). With complete or severe nerve injury, the MUP is not elicited. On the other hand, with partial nerve injury some MUPs are elicitable but are reduced in number.

The EMG study is very helpful for detecting evidence of regeneration because the first EMG sign of reinnervation is observed 2 months before clinical evidence of recovery. This sign is represented by the appearance of reinnervation potentials, which are polyphasic as well as small in amplitude.

The needle EMG study is also helpful in the workup of radiculopathies. The paraspinal muscle EMG is extremely important in the detection of root diseases. Fibrillation or positive sharp waves are seen in the paraspinal muscles in 80% of patients with radiculopathy (5). We have seen many patients with positive electrophysiological evidence of radiculopathy in whom myelograms were normal. This has been especially true in patients who complain of back pain after trauma, e.g., an automobile accident. Such radiculopathy is most likely caused by a laceration of the nerve roots. EMG abnor-

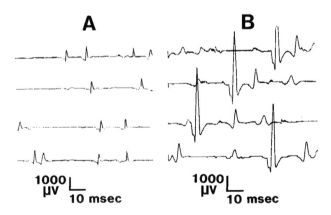

A   **B**

1000   1000
µV   µV
    10 msec   10 msec

Figure 2.5. The motor unit potential (MUP) in patients with denervation and myopathy. **A,** Small-short MUP in myopathy. **B,** Long-high-amplitude MUP in the denervation process.

malities are much more pronounced in anterior horn cell disease than in peripheral neuropathy. Fasciculation is also seen in anterior horn cell disease.

Myopathy

Muscle cells are randomly affected in patients with myopathy. Most motor units remain active, but the number of functional cells within the motor unit is diminished. Therefore, the EMG hallmark of primary myopathy is an MUP that is small in amplitude and short in duration (Fig. 2.5). Because most of the motor unit remains active, normal interference patterns will be obtained with maximal contractions. The needle EMG is the only way to detect the small MUPs seen with myopathy.

Fibrillation and positive sharp waves are often seen in the active stage of muscle fiber necrosis in patients with myopathy. This is especially noted in patients with polymyositis, alcoholic myopathy, and myotonic dystrophy. Thus, the presence of fibrillation and positive sharp waves is an expression of the degree of active necrosis in myopathy.

In patients with polymyositis, the triad of electromyographic findings is usually present: (*a*) fibrillation and positive sharp waves; (*b*) high-frequency bizarre waves (pseudomyotonia); and (*c*) many small MUPs. Two of this triad are found in over 90% of the cases of polymyositis (3).

Myotonia

Myotonia is usually present in patients with myotonia congenita, myotonic dystrophy, and hyperkalemic periodic paralysis. In the EMG examination, movement of the electrode or relaxation after contraction may result in a high-frequency burst of various motor unit discharges (Fig. 2.6). Electrical myotonia is classically fluctuating in amplitude as well as in frequency. When a loudspeaker is used as a monitoring device, the action potential creates the sound of an old-fashioned dive-bomber. Thus, myotonia is detectable only by the needle EMG study. The electrophysiological evidence of myotonia is usually associated with clinical myotonia in these diseases.

Repetitive Nerve Stimulation Test (Jolly Test)

The function of the neuromuscular junction can be assessed by repetitive stimulation of a motor nerve with a recording electrode over the appropriate muscle. In our laboratory, we stimulate, as the first-line test, the ulnar nerve at the elbow with the surface recording electrode over the abductor digiti quinti and flexor carpi ulnaris muscles (6). This test is indicated and most helpful in myasthenia gravis (MG), the Eaton-Lambert syndrome (Lambert-Eaton myasthenic syndrome), and botulism.

If the CMAPs decrease rapidly in amplitude (decremental response) at the rate of 2–50/sec, a defective neuromuscular transmission is suspected. In MG, a significant decremental response is noted in about 55% in distal muscles and in about 70% in proximal muscles (6). Normal responses are observed most often in ocular myasthenia gravis, mild generalized MG, or MG in remission. The most common type of abnormality in MG is (*a*) a normal-amplitude CMAP by single stimulation; (*b*) a decremental response at the lower rates of stimulation; and (*c*) no significant decremental response at high rates of stimulation (Fig. 2.7) (7).

In the Eaton-Lambert syndrome, the Jolly test is the only way to make a diagnosis. The classical abnormalities here are: (*a*) a low-amplitude CMAP by single stimulation; (*b*) a decremental response at the lower rates of stimulation; and (*c*) an incremental response at the higher rates of stimulation (Fig. 2.8) (6). The Eaton-Lambert syndrome is commonly seen in patients with carcinoma of the lung. Guanidine (8) and aminopyridine (9) have been found to reverse an abnormal Jolly test to normal, as well as to be clinically helpful in many cases. In botulism and drug-induced myasthenia, the Jolly test shows findings similar to those in the Eaton-Lambert syndrome with minor differences.

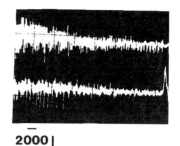

2000 μV ⌐ **200 msec**

Figure 2.6. Myotonic potentials. The waxing and waning in frequency and the amplitude of potentials are characteristic of myotonic potential.

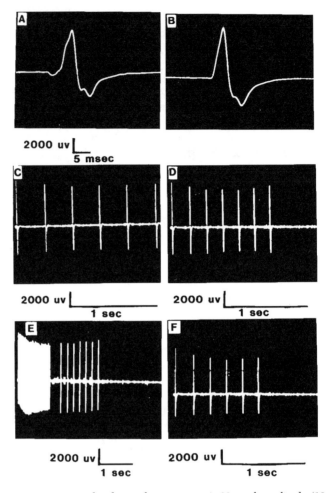

Figure 2.7. Responses in generalized myasthenia gravis. **A**, Normal amplitude (10,000 μV) of the CMAP upon single supramaximal stimulation. **B**, A 10% increment in amplitude of the CMAP after 30 sec of exercise. **C**, A 13.5% decremental response at a 3/sec stimulation. **D**, A 12.0% decremental response at a 5/sec stimulation. **E**, Normal (8% decremental) response at 50/sec stimulation and posttetanic facilitation phenomenon. **F**, Posttetanic exhaustion phenomenon: 21% decremental response at a 5/sec stimulation 4 min after a 50/sec tetanic stimulation. (From Oh SJ, Eslami N, Nishihara T, Sarala PK, et al. Electrophysiological and clinical correlation in myasthenia gravis. Ann Neurol 1982;12: 351.)

The Jolly test is also helpful in the follow-up of patients with MG as well as in the management of medications in these patients. Abnormalities usually disappear when MG is mild or in remission.

Other Studies

Nerve Excitability Test

The nerve excitability test is the quantitative measurement of the electrical excitability of the peripheral nerves. The earliest evidence of degeneration of the nerves after injury is the failure of the nerve to respond to electrical stimulation below the site of the injury. Thus, the nerve excitability test measures early evidence of nerve degeneration. This test is often used to assess the prognosis of facial palsy (Bell's palsy). If it is performed within a few days after the onset of Bell's palsy, it gives valuable information regarding the eventual prognosis of the condition (10). If the nerve excitability test reveals significant evidence of degeneration (expressed by a more than 4-mA difference between the involved and uninvolved facial nerves), it indicates a poor outlook and suggests aggressive steroid (11) or surgical therapy (12).

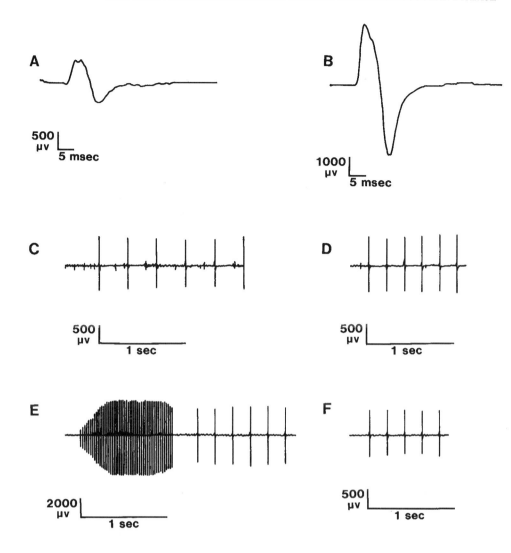

Figure 2.8. Responses in the Eaton-Lambert syndrome. **A,** Low-amplitude (1250 μV) CMAP by single stimulation. **B,** Same as A after 30 sec of exercise, showing a normalized CMAP amplitude (8000 μV). **C,** 3/sec stimulation, showing 25% decremental response. **D,** 5/sec stimulation, showing 11% decremental response. **E,** Marked facilitation (325% incremental response) during 50/sec stimulation and a normal response at 5/sec stimulation immediately after tetanic stimulation. **F,** After 5/sec stimulation 4 min after tetanic stimulation, there is a 9% decremental response.

H-Reflex

The H-reflex in the gastrocnemius-soleus muscle is the electrophysiological counterpart of the ankle reflex. The H-reflex is a late response with longer latency that has a threshold usually lower than that of direct CMAP (M-wave) in motor nerve conduction studies. In newborn infants the H-reflex can be elicited from almost every muscle. However, in adults it is obtained regularly only from the calf muscle following stimulation of the posterior tibial nerve. The H-reflex duration and amplitude are less clinically useful than the H-reflex latency. In peripheral neuropathy or S1 radiculopathy, the H-reflex in the gastrocnemius-soleus muscle is often absent or prolonged in latency because the ankle reflex is frequently absent (13). The H-reflex has been employed mainly in studies of motor neuron excitability and has only limited value in the investigation of peripheral nerve disorders.

F-Wave

Another late response is the F-wave, which is evoked by supramaximal stimulation during the motor nerve conduction study. Originally considered to be a variant of the H-reflex, the F-wave is now considered to be caused mainly by antidromic volleys in the motor fibers. The F-wave is invariably evoked in a normal individual during the motor nerve conduction study by stimulating the distal portion of the nerves. In recent years the F-wave has been used as a measure of the conduction velocity of proximal motor fibers. Recent studies have shown that F-wave latency may be the sole abnormality in some patients with peripheral neuropathy when other nerve conductions are all normal (13). This is especially true in the Guillain-Barré syndrome.

Blink Reflex

On stimulation of the supraorbital branch of the trigeminal nerve at the supraorbital foramen, the blink reflex can be recorded from the orbicularis oculi. In a normal individual, two responses (the first and second) are recorded on the ipsilateral side and one response (the second) on the contralateral side. The afferent arc of the blink reflex is provided by sensory fibers of the trigeminal nerve, whereas the efferent arc is provided by the facial nerve. Thus, a prolonged latency, or the absence of the first and second responses on the ipsilateral side and of the second response on the contralateral side, suggests a lesion in the ipsilateral trigeminal nerve. On the other hand, unilateral delay in the latency or absence of the second response, regardless of the side of stimulation, suggests a lesion of the facial nerve.

Blink reflex studies are useful in the early detection of abnormalities in disorders affecting the 5th and 7th cranial nerves, e.g., Bell's palsy, the Guillain-Barré syndrome, or cerebellopontine angle tumors (14).

Single-Fiber Electromyography (SFEMG)

Single-fiber electromyography (SFEMG), a relatively new procedure, is the most sensitive test in the diagnosis of myasthenia gravis or myasthenic syndrome. The action potential of a single muscle fiber can be obtained using a tiny needle with a recording diameter of 25 μm, which is smaller than the average normal muscle fiber diameter. When recording the single fiber action potentials from two single muscle fibers belonging to the same motor unit by inserting the electrode between two fibers, there is always a slight variability in the time interval between the two potentials in such a "potential pair." This variability, the "jitter," is normally of the order of 20 μsec. The main cause of the jitter is probably the variability in the synaptic delay in the two motor end-plates. When there is a defect of neuromuscular transmission, as noted in myasthenia gravis, the jitter is increased (Fig. 2.9). If the defect is so severe that action potentials fail to follow the nerve impulse, blocking occurs. In a survey of studies, SFEMG

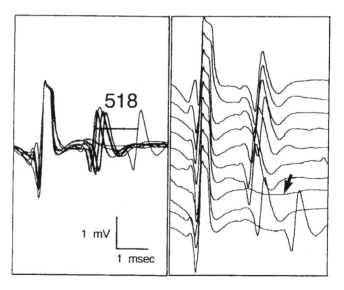

Figure 2.9. Abnormal jitter and blocking of the SFEMG in myasthenia gravis. The *horizontal line* and *number* indicate the range (R10) between the shortest and longest interpotential interval. The mean value of the consecutive interpotential interval difference (MCD) is 518 μsec. The normal MCD is 53 μsec. *Arrow* indicates blocking of one single fiber potential.

abnormalities were found in 77–100% of cases with MG (6). Stålberg and Trontelj stated that if the jitter is normal in a clinically weak muscle, the diagnosis of MG can be excluded (15).

REFERENCES

1. Oh SJ. When to ask and what to expect from EMG studies in peripheral nerve injuries. Med Times 1980; 108:94–98.
2. Dyck PJ, Lambert EH, Mulder DW. Charcot-Marie-Tooth disease: nerve conduction and clinical studies of a large kinship. Neurology 1963; 23:1–11.
3. Samaha FJ. Electrodiagnostic studies in neuromuscular disease. N Engl J Med 1971; 285:1244–1247.
4. Oh SJ. Electromyographic studies in peripheral nerve injuries. South Med J 1976; 69:177–182.
5. Knuttson B. Comparative value of electromyographic, myelographic and clinical-neurologic examinations in diagnosis of lumbar root compression syndrome. Acta Orthop Scand 1961; 49(suppl):1–135.
6. Oh SJ. Electromyography: neuromuscular transmission studies. Baltimore: Williams & Wilkins, 1988.
7. Oh SJ, Eslami N, Nishihara T, et al. Electrophysiological and clinical correlation in myasthenia gravis. Ann Neurol 1982; 12:348–354.
8. Oh SJ, Kim KW. Guanidine hydrochloride in the Eaton-Lambert syndrome: electrophysiologic improvement. Neurology 1973; 23:1084–1090.
9. Lundh H, Nilsson O, Rosen I. Treatment of Lambert-Eaton syndrome: 3,4 aminopyridine and pyridostigmine. Neurology 1984; 34:1324–1330.
10. Campbell EDR, Hickey RP, Nixon KH, Richardson AT. Value of nerve-excitability measurements in prognosis of facial palsy. Br Med J 1962; 2:7–10.
11. Devi S, Challenor Y, Duarte N, Lovelace RE. Prognostic value of minimal excitability of facial nerve in Bell's palsy. J Neurol Neurosurg Psychiatry 1978; 41:649–652.
12. Alford BR, Weber SC, Sessions RB. Neurodiagnostic studies in facial paralysis. Ann Otol Rhino Laryngol 1970; 79:227–233.
13. Lachman T, Shahani BT, Young RR. Late responses as aids to diagnosis in peripheral neuropathy. J Neurol Neurosurg Psychiatry 1980; 43:159–162.
14. Shahani BT, Young RR. Studies of reflex activity from a clinical viewpoint. In: Aminoff MJ, ed. Electrodiagnosis in clinical neurology. New York: Churchill Livingstone, 1980:290–304.
15. Stålberg E, Trontelj JV. Single fiber electromyography. Old Working, Surrey, UK: Mirvalle Press, 1979.

3

Basic Components of Electromyography Instruments

This chapter describes in detail the basic components of the electromyography (EMG) machine and provides technical tips for its utilization (Fig. 3.1). The EMG machine should be designed to respond to voltages of 0.5 μV to 10 mV in amplitude, and from 1 to 30,000 Hz in frequency. Thus, this machine is much more complex than either the electrocardiography (ECG) or the electroencephalography (EEG) machine (Table 3.1; Fig. 3.2).

Amplifier

The potentials picked up by the recording electrodes are usually very small in amplitude and consequently must be amplified by an amplifier before they can be displayed or recorded. Another role of the amplifier is to reject any unnecessary interference signals. The amplifier has control modes for sensitivity and frequency filter selection.

Sensitivity

The sensitivity control determines the amplitude of potentials, which are usually measured in microvolts per centimeter. The usual range of sensitivity in most EMG machines is from 5 to 10,000 μV (10 mV). In the sensory amplifier, which is highly specialized for the recording of sensory nerve potentials, the sensitivity is increased to 0.5 μV.

Frequency Filter Selection

An amplifier usually has low- and high-filter selection modes. This component is introduced to ensure distortion-free recording of actual potentials and to maintain the noise level as low as possible. Consequently, a high- or low-filter setting should be carefully chosen on the basis of the frequency characteristics of the EMG potentials.

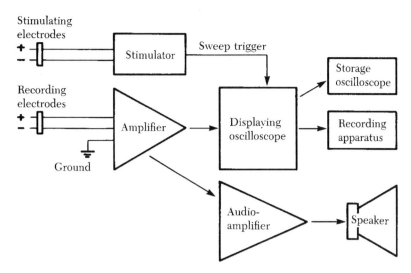

Figure 3.1. Basic components of the EMG machine.

Table 3.1.
Electrical Characteristics of the EMG, EEG, and ECG Machines

Machine	Voltage Range	Frequency Response (Hz)
EMG	0.5 μV–10 mV	1–30,000
EEG	1.0 μV–100 μV	0.1–100
ECG	1,000 μV–5 mV	0.1–30

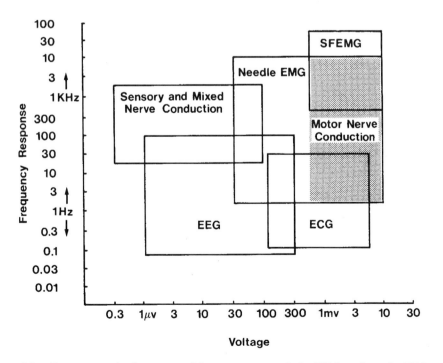

Figure 3.2. Frequency and voltage range of the various tests with the EMG machine, the EEG, and ECG machines.

Table 3.2.
Amplitude Change of the 10-KHz High Filter

Frequency of Potentials (KHz)	Amplitude of Potentials (µV)		Amplitude Change (%)
	At Electrodes	In Oscilloscope	
5	100	100	None
10	100	70	−30
20	100	35	−65

Table 3.3.
Amplitude Change of the 2-Hz Low Filter

Frequency of Potentials (Hz)	Amplitude of Potentials (µV)		Amplitude Change (%)
	At Electrodes	In Oscilloscope	
4	100	100	None
2	100	70	−30
1	100	35	−65

High-Filter Mode (Upper Frequency Limits)

The amplitude of the potentials at high-frequency settings is attenuated 30% from what the amplitude would be if the filter was not in the circuit. Potentials with frequencies faster than the setting are attenuated even more. Potentials with lower frequencies are not affected (Table 3.2).

Low-Filter Mode (Lower Frequency Limits)

The amplitude of the potentials of low-frequency settings is attenuated 30% from what the amplitude would be if the filter was not in the circuit. Potentials with frequencies slower than the setting are attenuated even more, while those with faster frequencies are not affected (Table 3.3).

For the common EMG study, a frequency range from 2 Hz (low-filter or lower frequency limit) to 10,000 Hz (high-filter or upper frequency limit) will provide sufficiently accurate reproduction of all potentials and an acceptably low noise level.

For the single-fiber EMG (SFEMG) study, the low- and high-filter settings should be 500 Hz and 30,000 Hz, respectively, to minimize the shifting of the baseline and to ensure distortion-free recording of the single-fiber action potentials.

In practice, the baseline shift, which is usually due to movement of the electrode or wire, can be minimized by increasing the low-filter setting from 2 to 20 Hz. When recording small nerve potentials, e.g., sensory or mixed compound nerve action potentials (CNAPs), the high-filter setting should be decreased to 2000 Hz to reduce the high-frequency noise. Better sensory and mixed CNAPs are obtained using these guidelines.

Oscilloscope

The cathode ray oscilloscope displays the potentials instantaneously on a linear time scale. New potentials are displayed and old potentials are erased with each sweep. In a majority of cases the electromyographer recognizes the moving potentials on the oscilloscope and interprets their clinical significance.

The storage oscilloscope is a special type of instrument that permits the potentials to be stored on the screen until the erase button is pushed. This feature is especially useful for: (*a*) detailed analysis of EMG potentials; (*b*) measurement of latency and amplitude of potentials in the nerve conduction test; (*c*) the repetitive nerve stimulation test;

Table 3.4.
Typical EMG Machine Settings for Various Procedures[a]

Setting	Needle EMG			Motor Nerve Conduction	Sensory or Mixed Nerve Conduction	H-reflex	F-wave	Repetitive Nerve Stimulation Text	SFEMG	Other Reflexes
	At Rest	Minimal Contraction	Maximal Contraction							
Sweep velocity (msec/division)	10	10	100 (5 for longer distances)	2 (2 for longer distances)	1	10	5–10	2 or 200	0.5–1.0	5–10
Sensitivity (µV)	100	500–1000	1000	2000	10	500	200	2000	500–1000	100–200
Filter										
High (KHz)	10	10	10	10	2	10	10	10	30	10
Low (Hz)	2–20	2–20	2–20	2–20	20	20	20	2–20	500	20
Audio	On	On	On	On or off	On	On or off	On or off	On or off	On	On or off
Stimulus duration (msec)	N/A	N/A	N/A	Start with 0.05–0.1; increase to obtain SMS	Start with 0.05–0.1; do not increase beyond 0.2	0.5 or 1.0	Start with 0.05–0.1; increase to SMS	Start with 0.05–0.1; increase to SMS	N/A	Start with 0.05–1.0; increase to SMS
Stimulus rate	N/A	N/A	N/A	1/sec	1/sec	every 2 or 5 sec	every 2 sec	2/sec; 3/sec; 5/sec; 50 sec	N/A	every 2 sec

[a] *Abbreviations:* SMA supramaximal stimulation; N/A, not applicable.

and (*d*) taking Polaroid pictures for permanent recordings. Because of these conveniences, many new EMG machines have storage capability in addition to the displaying oscilloscope.

There is usually a selection mode for the needle EMG study and the nerve conduction study. For the needle EMG study, the time base (triggering mode) is allowed to run freely, sweeping repetitively from left to right. In this setup, the sweep seems to be frozen because of the fast repetition of the sweep. In the nerve conduction study, the stimulus is made to trigger a single sweep on the time base. Thus, measurement of latency can be made from the onset of the sweep. There is also a selection mode for the sweep speed. The sweep speed (time base) usually ranges from 0.1 to 500 msec/cm and should be selected according to the kind of test (Table 3.4).

In modern EMG machines, there is an electronic latency indicator that automatically reads the latency of potentials when the marker is set at any particular point of the potentials, e.g., the onset of deflection of the compound muscle action potentials (CMAPs) in the motor nerve conduction test. Latency is usually read as milliseconds. This method of latency reading has replaced the old hand reading method, which was fraught with inaccuracies.

The delay line is useful in capturing the potentials on the oscilloscope. Any selected point of the potential can trigger the single sweep. Accordingly, the same potentials can be displayed on the oscilloscope repeatedly. This feature is used in the SFEMG study and in the quantitative analysis of motor unit potentials (MUPs) in the needle EMG. Details concerning the delay line are explained later.

In the majority of EMG machines, the calibration signal can be displayed easily. The calibration signal consists of a square pulse. The amplitude and duration of potentials can thus be calibrated. It is important to check the accuracy of the amplifier and oscilloscope with the calibration signal as often as possible to ensure the accuracy of the EMG studies.

Audio-Amplifier and Speaker

The audio-amplifier and speaker comprise a unique system present only in the EMG machine. In addition to the display of potentials on the oscilloscope for visual analysis, the potentials are also fed from the amplifier to an audio-amplifier and then to a loud-speaker, producing characteristic sounds. This system is especially valuable in the recognition of many EMG potentials, e.g., the dive-bomber sound of myotonic potentials. In the nerve conduction study, a single stimulus sound is heard with each stimulation.

Stimulator

In the nerve conduction study, it is necessary to stimulate the nerves electrically. As a result, the stimulator generates, for a brief period of time, a square-wave electrical current (stimulus) that stimulates the nerve at the cathode electrodes.

The stimulator has three control modes: (a) the duration of the stimulus; (b) the intensity of the stimulus; and (c) the rate of stimulation. Usually, the stimulus duration ranges from 0.05 to 1 msec. The longer the duration of the stimulus, the more pain the patient feels. It is best to start from the shortest stimulus duration in the nerve conduction study.

The intensity of stimulation can be gradually increased from 0 to 500 V or from 0 to 100 mA. In the most modern and sophisticated EMG machines, the exact intensity of the stimulus is displayed as milliamperes or volts on the stimulator. Unfortunately, however, in some small EMG machines the intensity is not displayed. Display of the stimulus intensity is helpful for the examiner to achieve the supramaximal stimulation. Again, the higher the intensity of the stimulus, the more painful it is. Therefore, a gradual increase of intensity from zero to above the maximal intensity to achieve the maximum amplitude of potentials (called supramaximal stimulation) is recommended in the nerve conduction study and in the repetitive nerve stimulation test for myasthenia gravis.

The rate of stimulation can be varied from 1/sec to 50/sec. In the nerve conduction study, one stimulation per second is often recommended because it is usually well tolerated by patients. The higher the rate of stimulation is, the more painful it is.

A low rate of stimulation (2, 3, 5/sec) is needed to test the functions of neuromuscular transmission, especially in myasthenia gravis. A high rate of stimulation (above 20/sec) is needed to document the facilitation phenomenon in myasthenic syndrome (Eaton-Lambert syndrome).

Most EMG machines have an external stimulus mode that is usually controlled by a foot pedal. This pedal regulates the single stimulation or repetitive stimulation. If the supramaximal stimulus is known, the use of the foot pedal to trigger the sweep of the oscilloscope is helpful in lessening unnecessary painful stimulation of the patient.

A "delay" in stimulation is present in some EMG machines. This means that there is a delay of the stimulus onset following the onset of the sweep. In other words, if the delay is set at 1.0 msec, the stimulus onset is visible 1.0 msec after the onset of the sweep. In some laboratories the delay feature is used in the nerve conduction study. In the past, when latency was measured by a hand ruler, delay was essential to ensure accurate measurement because the exact onset of sweep was often unclear in the recording. However, with the introduction of the electronic automatic latency indicator, the need for the delay has been lessened.

When the electronic automatic latency unit is used together with the delay, it is necessary to adjust the latency in many EMG machines. Automatic adjustment has been included in a few machines, however, so that the true latency is shown. In those in which the latency is read from the onset of the sweep, adjustment of latency is needed. The true latency of the nerve conduction equals the electronic latency minus the delay.

A train duration control unit is present in many sophisticated EMG machines. This unit controls the duration of the repetitive stimulation, and the repetitive stimulation stops automatically after the designated duration. This feature is especially useful in the repetitive nerve stimulation test for myasthenia gravis because it helps reduce the unnecessary pain associated with prolonged stimulation. Five or six potentials are needed in the majority of repetitive nerve stimulation tests. Even at a high rate of stimulation (e.g., 50/sec), 1-sec stimulation is sufficient to yield the necessary information.

For example, if the rate of stimulation is set at 3/sec and the train duration for 2 sec, the stimulation stops automatically after six stimulations, producing six potentials.

Recording Apparatus

There are three ways of recording potentials: (*a*) Polaroid photography; (*b*) paper recordings; and (*c*) tape recording. Polaroid photography was used predominantly before the time of paper recording and can still be used as the recording mode if the paper recording capacity is not available. Polaroid photographs can be made from the stored potentials in the storage oscilloscope or directly from the displaying oscilloscope by using the synchronous shutter opening with the onset of sweep. Before the introduction of the signal averager, photographic superimpositions of low-intensity trains were used to identify the small sensory CNAPs by reducing the signal/noise ratio. This technique can still be used in the laboratory where a signal averager is not available. One disadvantage of this system is that the Polaroid film is relatively expensive. Paper recording is available in most modern EMG machines.

Paper recording has simplified the recording system of the EMG potentials and is relatively inexpensive. Four modes of recording are usually available in the major EMG machines: (*a*) single shot; (*b*) superimposed shots; (*c*) continuous recording; and (*d*) raster recording (Fig. 3.3). The single shot records an actual display of potential on the oscilloscope screen. The superimposed shot records four or five tracings superimposed on a common baseline in the middle of the paper. This is especially useful in the recording of jitter in the SFEMG study. The continuous recording shows the changing potentials continuously on the paper as they occur. The raster recording mode displays several potentials in sequence from one side to the other. This mode is used mainly for recording the responses in the repetitive nerve stimulation test. In contrast to the slower speed of continuous recording, this mode has the advantage of recording the changing shape of the potential. Thus, artifacts are easily recognizable in the repetitive nerve stimulation test.

The tape recording of potentials is achieved by connecting a magnetic tape recorder to the output of the amplifier in many EMG systems. This permits the permanent recording of potentials on magnetic tape. One advantage of this system is that it simultaneously records the sounds of the potentials, making it useful for audiovisual teaching and for the later analysis of the data for research purposes.

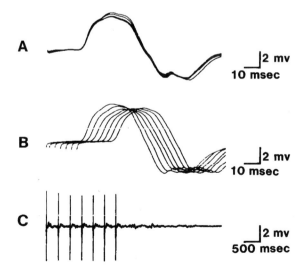

Figure 3.3. An 8% decremental response in the repetitive nerve stimulation test in a patient with myasthenia gravis recorded with varying recording modes. **A,** Superimposed mode. **B,** Raster mode. **C,** Continuous mode.

Recording Electrodes

There are two kinds of recording electrodes on the EMG machine: surface electrodes and needle electrodes.

Surface Electrodes

Surface electrodes can record the potentials from the muscles or the nerves (Fig. 3.4). These electrodes usually consist of two square or round metal (tin or silver) discs with attached lead-off wires. The most commonly used electrodes are round, flat plates 1.0 cm in diameter. Electroencephalography (EEG) electrodes can be used as EMG surface electrodes without any alteration.

When surface electrodes are used, the impedance between them and the skin must be reduced to obtain a technically satisfactory recording. This can usually be achieved by applying electrode gel under the electrodes. The electrodes are then firmly fixed to the skin with adhesive tape. When disposable "stick-up electrodes" are used, firm skin contact can easily be achieved without adhesive tape. If this method does not provide low enough impedance for the test, the skin must be washed with acetone to remove surface grease or scraped with a fine needle or sandpaper to remove the superficial scaly layer.

Surface electrodes are used predominantly in the study of nerve conduction and in repetitive nerve stimulation tests. Two electrodes are needed to record the potential from muscles or nerves: One is the active (different) electrode, and the other is the reference (indifferent) electrode. What is recorded from the muscles or nerves is, in fact, the potential differential between these two electrodes. It should be noted that there should not be any continuous conduction medium between these two electrodes (e.g., electrode gel).

Depending upon the kind of EMG machine, the active electrode is either the cathode (−) or the anode (+) (1). The cathode is an active electrode in most American-made EMG machines. However, the European-produced Dantec machine uses the anode as the active electrode. It is important to check and remember which is the active electrode in each EMG machine.

In practice, this means that when the active and reference electrodes are properly connected to the amplifier, *the upward deflection of the potential becomes negative and the downward deflection positive.* This is the conventional method of recording potential in clinical neurophysiology. If the active and reference recording electrodes are

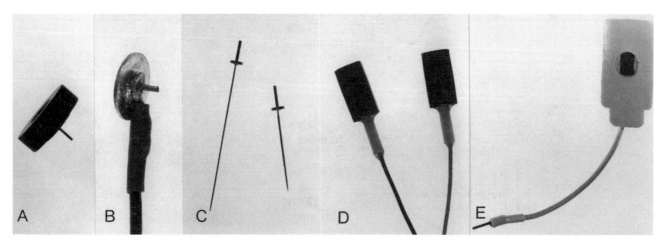

Figure 3.4.   Various recording electrodes. **A,** Dantec disc electrode. **B,** TECA surface electrode. **C,** Dantec near-nerve monopolar needle for the sensory or mixed CNAP. **D,** Dantec surface electrode. **E,** Disposable Dantec "stick-up" surface electrode.

switched when connected to the amplifier, the negative and positive deflections are reversed.

The surface electrode is attached to nearby skin as the reference electrode for the monopolar EMG study. The surface electrode is also used as the ground electrode. In this case the surface electrode is usually larger. A strap-type ground electrode is also available and should be attached to the ground connector in the amplifier.

A new type of surface electrode, the disposable "stick-up electrodes," have been marketed by Dantec Medical Inc. and TECA Corporation. These disposable electrodes minimize movement artifacts and eliminate any possibility of artifacts due to a loose electrode. Thus, these electrodes are excellent for the long-term monitoring of potentials and are ideal for the repetitive nerve stimulation test. In our laboratory, disposable "stick-up electrodes" are used routinely for all repetitive nerve stimulation tests.

Needle Electrodes

Needle electrodes are used predominantly in the needle EMG study (Fig. 3.5). The two most commonly used needles for this purpose are Teflon-coated monopolar needle electrodes and concentric needle electrodes.

The monopolar needle electrode is usually constructed from a stainless steel needle that is insulated except at its tip. The diameter of the needle averages around 0.8 mm, and the length of the needle varies from 12 to 75 mm. The Teflon-coated monopolar needle electrode is less painful, less expensive, and more sensitive in identifying fibrillation and positive sharp waves than the concentric needle electrode, making it much more popular among electromyographers. For the needle EMG study, the monopolar needle electrode is used as the active electrode and the surface electrode nearby on the same muscle as the reference electrode.

The monopolar needle electrode can be used as the stimulating electrode when the nerve is deeply located. This needle is essential in the stimulation of the sciatic nerve at the sciatic notch. The surface electrode on the sciatic notch is used as the reference electrode.

The monopolar needle electrode is sometimes used as the recording electrode for sensory or mixed CNAPs. In Europe a majority of EMG laboratories have followed Buchthal and Rosenfalck's recommendation (2) and use this method. These electrodes are specially designed for leading off potentials from sensory nerves (Dantec 13L60-13L64, Dantec Medical, Inc., Santa Clara, CA). Of stainless steel, they are coated with Teflon in such a manner that only the tip is left uninsulated. The active electrode is inserted as close to the nerve as possible, and the reference electrode is placed 3 cm laterally from the active electrode. For the best recording, the impedance of the needle

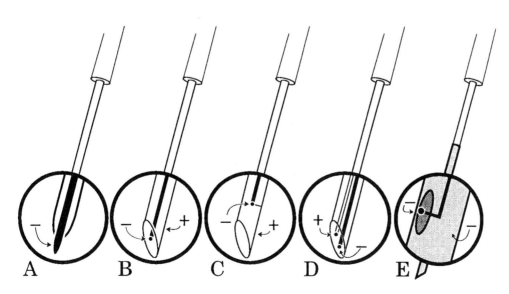

Figure 3.5. Needle electrodes. **A**, Monopolar needle electrode. **B**, Concentric needle electrode. **C**, Single-fiber needle electrode. **D**, Bipolar needle electrode. **E**, Macro EMG needle. (−) Cathode. (+) Anode.

should be as low as possible. To achieve lowest impedance, the needle should be treated electrolytically immediately before use. Fortunately, disposable sensory needle electrodes (Dantec 13R21-13R25), which are now available, do not require electrolytic treatment.

This near-nerve needle technique has several advantages over the surface electrode method. First, the noise/signal ratio can be reduced markedly by reducing the impedance. Second, very small nerve CNAPs, which are not recordable by surface electrodes, can be recorded. Third, the amplitude of the recording potential is much more reliable. Finally, the dispersion of the potential can be documented. Thus, the near-nerve needle is used in the recording of sensory and mixed CNAPs when the potentials cannot be recorded with surface electrodes even after signal averaging. More detailed discussion on this subject is found in Chapter 15.

The subcutaneous wire or monopolar needle electrode is used by some investigators as a recording electrode to record the CMAP from the belly of the muscle in the repetitive nerve stimulation test (3). In the author's laboratory a Grass steel EEG needle has been used. The needle must be inserted subcutaneously into the belly of the muscle and firmly secured.

The concentric needle electrode consists of a platinum wire located centrally inside a hollow needle but completely insulated from it. The outside diameter of the needle varies from 0.3 to 1.0 mm, with a center wire of 0.1 mm diameter. The inside wire is the active electrode and the outside cannula the reference electrode. When the concentric needle is connected to the connecting cable, caution should be used not to change the polarity of the electrodes. This needle is essential for the quantitative analysis of the motor unit potential because the normal values were derived by using a concentric needle electrode.

The concentric needle electrode is used as a recording electrode from the muscle for the motor nerve conduction studies in some EMG laboratories. Many of the studies from the Rigshospitalet EMG laboratory employed this method (4). The main disadvantage of the method is that *it does not allow for total estimation of the number of muscle fibers responding to a nerve stimulus, thus making it unsuitable for localizing a conduction block and for testing neuromuscular transmission. Another disadvantage is that the volume conduction-induced initial positive deflection of the CMAP can not be identified because the CMAP recorded with the concentric needle does not have a consistent initial negative deflection as recorded with the surface electrode from the belly of muscle.*

The bipolar needle electrode is not recommended for the needle EMG study because the MUPs that it records are smaller and shorter than the MUPs recorded by other needle electrodes. MUPs obtained by the bipolar needle electrode look like the small, short MUPs seen in patients with myopathy.

The multielectrode needle, developed by Buchthal et al. (5), is needed for the determination of motor unit territory. Fourteen platinum wires are exposed through the side of the cannula. The reference electrode is one of the outer leads of the 14.

The SFEMG needle is needed for the SFEMG study. A tiny wire is exposed through the side of the cannula. Single-fiber electrodes have a recording surface of 25 μm in contrast to the larger recording surface of 150 × 580 μm in the concentric needle electrode. Because of this small recording area, the SFEMG needle can record the electrical activity of a single muscle fiber. The outside cannula is used as the reference electrode.

The recently introduced Macro-EMG electrode is used for the Macro-EMG study (6). The Macro-EMG electrode has two active electrodes: a SFEMG electrode with a 25-μm-diameter platinum wire exposed in a side-port, which is used to trigger the sweep, and a 0.55-mm-diameter steel cannula with a 15-mm exposed surface that may record the electrical activity in the entire motor unit. The potentials obtained with the cannula are averaged to produce the averaged MUP, the Macro MUP. Owing to its large recording surface, the cannula electrode is capable of measuring the potentials from a larger portion of the motor unit than conventional EMG electrodes. Any type of electrode can be used as a separate reference electrode.

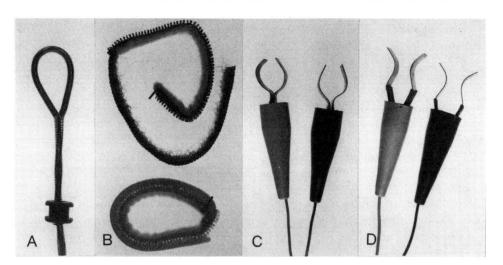

Figure 3.6. Various sensory stimulating electrodes. **A**, TECA ring electrode. **B**, Dantec Velcro strap electrode. **C**, Neurodiagnostic surface electrode. D, Oh's interdigital surface electrode.

Stimulating Electrodes

Stimulating electrodes are usually of the surface type. Surface electrodes commonly consist of two protruding metal or felt "buttons" fixed in a small plastic block. Most American-made EMG machines have the cathode as the active electrode and the anode as the reference electrode. In the old Dantec one-channel EMG machine, the anode is used as the active electrode. In more sophisticated EMG machines, there is a choice between using the cathode or the anode as the active electrode. Metal surface electrodes are lightly covered with electrode gel before use, whereas the felt types are moistened with saline solution.

Regardless of which electrode is the active electrode, it is important to remember that the active electrode should be closer to the recording electrode. If the cathode is used as the active electrode, it should be distally located in the motor NCV study and proximally located in the orthodromic sensory nerve conduction study in relation to the reference electrode. If the active electrode is located away from the recording electrode in relation to the reference electrode, the distance should be measured from the active electrode to the recording electrode. In this way, the distance and the latency become longer.

The monopolar needle electrode is used to stimulate a deeply situated nerve, e.g., the sciatic nerve. To stimulate digital nerve fibers in the fingers and toes, the ring-shaped electrode or the strap-type felt electrode is used (Fig. 3.6).

A pair of sensory needles is used for stimulating the nerve for the motor and sensory nerve conduction study. Because the active electrode is near the nerve, this method of stimulation has advantages over the surface electrodes: (*a*) it requires a lower intensity stimulus; (*b*) it can stimulate a nerve located well beneath the surface; and (*c*) it can stimulate the desired nerve without stimulating the neighboring nerves. This method is reported most often in studies from the Rigshospitalet EMG laboratory (4).

The bipolar needle may be used as a stimulating electrode for obtaining the CNAP over short segments. We have used bipolar needles as stimulating electrodes when obtaining mixed NCVs in the short segment across the elbow in the ulnar nerve (7). This method has advantages in that the stimulus artifact is almost nonexistent and the stimulation intensity is minimal.

Signal Averager

A standard item in many EMG machines, the signal averager, has the ability to record very small CNAPs. Once one has experienced the sensitivity of the signal averager, it is very hard to practice the sensory or mixed nerve conduction studies without it.

The basic aim of the signal averager is to improve the signal/noise ratio (Fig. 3.7). The amplitude of the sensory CNAP from the median nerve at the wrist in normal subjects is 20–90 μV and can be recorded with conventional EMG equipment without any difficulty. The amplitude of the sensory CNAP in the plantar or pathological nerves, however, is of the order of a few microvolts, which is about the same as or even lower than the noise level of the EMG amplifier or the electrode. Thus, it is impossible to record the very small sensory CNAPs by conventional methods. Fortunately, these extraneous noises occur randomly. With the use of the signal averager, the random noises cancel each other out, and only the time-locked sensory or mixed CNAPs are clear. *As a general rule, the signal/noise ratio improves proportionally as the square root of the number of signal averagings.* Therefore, the more averaging that is done, the better the record will be. The signal averager is used for recording sensory or mixed CNAPs when they are not clearly obtainable by conventional methods.

There are usually two control modes in the signal averager: the number of the aver-

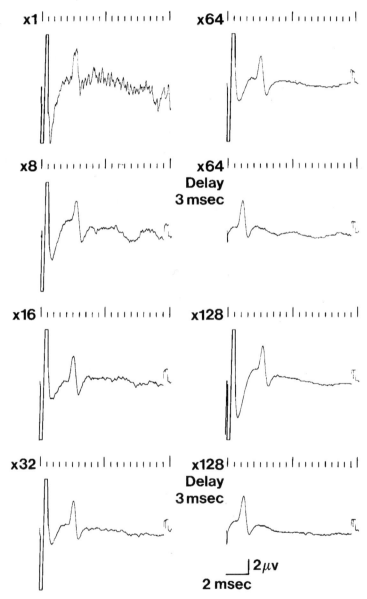

Figure 3.7. The advantage of signal averaging is shown here. Unwanted interferences are eliminated with an increasing number of averagings. A 3-msec delay eliminated the stimulus artifact.

aging sweep and the analysis time. Averaging up to 256 signals and an analysis time of 20 msec are sufficient in most nerve conduction studies.

When identifying small sensory or mixed CNAPs with "long dispersion," three repeated averagings are often needed. This is to confirm whether the averaged potentials reflect genuine potentials. If they do not, the repeated averagings do not show any consistent pattern.

Delay Line

The delay line is an essential component for the quantitative analysis of MUPs in the needle EMG and the SFEMG. Conventional methods of recording random MUPs with sufficient resolution in time consume considerable time and recording paper. When the delay line is used, the entire MUP can be recorded every time it appears and in the same position on the oscilloscope screen by delaying each MUP after it has triggered the sweep. This enables the desired number of potentials to be accumulated in a short time.

In principle, a particular level of potential triggers the sweep preceding the potentials by the interval of delay time chosen (Fig. 3.8). For example, if the delay time is set at 10 msec and the triggering level is at the negative peak, the potential appears on the oscilloscope 10 msec after the beginning of the sweep, and the interval between the start of the sweep and the negative peak of the potential is 10 msec.

In practice, owing to the brief intervals between potentials and the afterglow, each potential will appear as a stationary display on the oscilloscope. In other words, the potentials will be frozen on the screen. In the meantime, the same potentials can be repeatedly recorded on the recording paper, thereby confirming the consistency of the MUPs or the single-fiber action potentials.

In the quantitative analysis of MUPs in the needle EMG, at least 20 MUPs should be sampled for analysis by duration, amplitude, and phase. By using the delay line, this task can be completed within 30 min.

It is impossible to identify the single-fiber action potential and the jitter phenomenon without the delay line in the SFEMG. Accordingly, the SFEMG cannot be performed without the delay line.

The delay line usually has two control modes: trigger level control and delay time

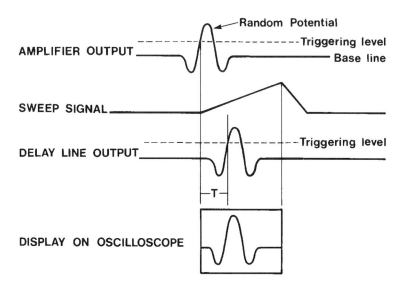

Figure 3.8. Principle of the delay line. The triggering level is set on the upward deflection of the potential with delay T msec. The triggering point will appear on oscilloscope T msec after the onset of the sweep signal. This guarantees the potential in the same position on the oscilloscope.

selection. With the trigger level control, the triggering level of the potentials can be set at any point on the downward ($+$) or upward ($-$) deflection of the potential. Ideally, the triggering level of the potentials is adjusted for the desired potential to appear entire and stationary on the display oscilloscope screen. If the trigger level is adjusted close to the baseline, even small potentials release the sweep. This can be prevented by adjusting the trigger level further away from the baseline.

The delay time should be long enough to permit determination of the beginning of the potential with certainty but short enough to catch the entire potential. A 10- to 20-msec delay time is usually used for the quantitative analysis of MUPs, whereas a shorter delay time (0.4–0.2 msec) is used for the SFEMG.

Machine Settings for the Various Procedures

When adjusting the EMG machine for specific procedures, it is important to remember that the machine should be set to record the potentials accurately without any distortion and to read the latency with the most accuracy. The recommended settings of the EMG machines in Table 3.4 are those used in the EMG Laboratory of the University of Alabama at Birmingham and are based on our own experience over the years.

REFERENCES

1. Guld C, Rosenfalck A, Willison RG. Technical factors in recording electrical activity of muscles and nerves. EEG Clin Neurophysiol 1970; 28:399–413.
2. Buchthal F, Rosenfalck A. Evoked action potentials and conduction velocity in human sensory nerves. Brain Res 1966; 3:1–122.
3. Oh SJ. Electromyography: neuromuscular transmission studies. Baltimore: Williams & Wilkins, 1988.
4. Rigshospitalet Laboratory of Clinical Neurophysiology. EMG-sensory and motor conduction: findings in normal subjects. Copenhagen: Rigshospitalet 1975:1–49.
5. Buchthal F, Guld C, Rosenfalck P. Multielectrode study of the territory of a motor unit. Acta Physiol Scand 1957; 39:83–104.
6. Stålberg E. Macro EMG, a new recording technique. J Neurol Neurosurg Psychiatry 43:475–482.
7. Nishihira T, Oh SJ. Ulnar neuropathy: an improved method of diagnosis. Arch Phys Med Rehab 1976; 57:602.

4

Nerve Conduction Techniques

General Guidelines for Performing Nerve Conduction Studies

Before attempting nerve conduction studies on patients, one must consider a number of factors. First, the patient must be aware of what to expect. In addition, the tester must prepare the limb to be tested and understand the potential problems that could arise. The following guidelines offer a step-by-step approach to performing nerve conduction studies.

1. Explain the procedure to the patient. It is important to explain to patients the nature of the procedure using the simplest language. Remember that the electrical stimulation you apply is painful. With a simple explanation, patients become less anxious and more cooperative. (I require all my electromyography (EMG) technicians and physicians to have the nerve conduction test performed on themselves so that they may know firsthand how painful it is.)

2. Place the limb to be tested in a relaxed and comfortable position both for the patient and the examiner. Nerve conduction studies are best carried out with the limb relaxed. Otherwise, movement or noise artifacts produce unnecessary interference. This is especially troublesome in sensory or mixed nerve conduction studies.

3. Measure the skin temperature. (We use the YSI Tele-thermometer, Yellow Springs Instrument Co., Yellow Springs, OH) Be sure that the limb to be tested is not cold. Motor and sensory NCVs are decreased at the rate of 1.3–2.4 m/sec for each centigrade degree drop in skin temperature [1,2]. It is important that the tested limb be warm. This is achieved in our laboratory by maintaining the room temperature at 78°F (26°C). Skin temperatures of our patients range from 31 to 34°C. Our normal nerve conduction velocity (NCV) values are obtained within this temperature range. If the tested limb feels cold, the skin temperature is usually less than 31. If this is the case, the limb should be warmed with a heater, heating pad, or electric blanket before nerve conduction studies are begun. If the normal values in the EMG laboratory are collected at the controlled temperature (e.g., 35°C), the limb should be warmed to the controlled temperature with the skin temperature controlling unit (e.g., Dantec 31B30 Regulator Unit, Dantec Medical, Inc., Santa Clara, CA).

4. Lower the electrode impedance. It is important to reduce electrode impedance as much as possible. This is usually achieved by applying electrode gel under the electrode and by affixing the electrode with adhesive tape to the skin. However, on rare occasions the impedance between

the electrodes and the skin has to be reduced further by carefully scraping the skin with a needle or sandpaper or by cleansing it with alcohol or acetone. When the electrode impedance is minimal, there is no 60-Hz interference or undue noise. Although noise interference does not produce any difficulty with the motor nerve conduction study, it becomes troublesome in sensory or mixed nerve conduction tests. This is especially true when the sensitivity is set below 5 μV.

5. A ground electrode should be attached to the limb being tested and is ideally placed between the stimulating and recording electrodes. This is recommended to avoid any possible electrocution by a transthoracic current pathway. Such a possibility exists if a ground electrode is placed on the right arm when nerve conduction velocity is being tested on the left arm. To reduce the stimulation artifact to a minimum, a ground electrode should be placed (ideally) between the stimulating and recording electrodes. However, it is inconvenient to change the ground electrode during the NCV studies over the different segments of the nerves; thus, a ground electrode should be positioned at one place on the limb being tested, as recommended in the anatomical guide. Usually, this is adequate for the nerve conduction studies. However, when there is a difficulty in obtaining the compound muscle or nerve action potentials (CMAPs or CNAPs) clearly because of stimulation artifacts, do not hesitate to place a ground electrode between the stimulating and recording electrodes.

6. Pediatric stimulating electrodes are recommended in infants. Because of the small, short extremities in infants, it is better to use the smaller pediatric stimulating electrodes. This is recommended to stimulate the tested nerve without any "stimulus spread" to other nerves and to ensure adequate distance between the two stimulated sites for the calculation of NCV.

7. Perform motor nerve conduction studies first to locate nerves for the sensory and mixed nerve conduction studies. If motor nerve conduction studies are performed first, you have the stimulation sites marked exactly for the recording electrodes for the sensory or mixed nerve conduction studies. In this way, the exact location for the recording electrodes is guaranteed.

8. Warn the patient before each stimulation is given. Let the patient be prepared for stimulation. If you warn him just before each stimulation, he can tolerate the pain quite well. An unexpected or unannounced stimulation often causes sudden movement of the limb being tested, causing the electrodes to loosen.

9. Reduce the pain of stimulation as much as possible before the next stimulation is given. To minimize discomfort, the stimulus should be of the shortest duration and lowest intensity but adequate to produce the supramaximal response of muscle or nerve potentials. A 1/sec rate of stimulation is best tolerated by patients. In normal individuals, 0.05 msec duration is long enough to produce the maximal response (no further increase of the amplitude of potential). However, because the lowest duration available is greater than 0.05 msec in some EMG equipment, the duration should be set as low as possible on those machines.

In patients with neuropathy, a longer duration of stimulus is often needed to obtain the maximal response. *For sensory or mixed nerve conduction studies, a further increase beyond 0.2 msec duration does not produce any increase in the amplitude* of CNAPs. On the other hand, for motor nerve conduction studies, the stimulus duration may have to be increased to 1.0 msec in order to obtain a response. This is indicative of the lower nerve excitability seen commonly in neuropathy, assuming that the stimulating and recording electrodes have been correctly placed.

10. Initially, follow the typical machine settings for the various nerve conductions, but be ready to change the settings if necessary. It is important to capture the response in its entirety on the oscilloscope monitor. The latency of the response and the CMAPs or CNAPs should be seen clearly in their entirety. Recommended typical settings for the nerve conduction studies are adequate for most studies (Table 3.4). However, do not hesitate to change the settings if necessary. Change is usually needed in the settings for sensitivity and sweep velocity. Suppose we have the CMAP with a latency of 40 msec, an amplitude of 1500 μV, and a duration of 40 msec: the test should then be performed with the sensitivity at 500 μV and the sweep velocity set at 10 msec.

The two most important settings on the EMG machine for the performance of nerve conduction studies are the stimulus duration and the sweep velocity. The supramaximal stimulation (higher than the stimulus which produces the maximum response) should be achieved by adjusting the duration and intensity of the stimulus. *Without the supramaximal stimulation, the amplitude of the CMAP or CNAP is meaningless.* The change of sweep velocity invites errors in the latency measurement.

Because the sensory and mixed CNAPs are small, the patient must be completely relaxed to record these potentials. To achieve this degree of relaxation, an audio monitor should be turned on. By listening to the baseline noise, the patient can relax better during the sensory and mixed nerve conduction studies.

Detailed Techniques of Nerve Conduction Studies

For routine testing, most EMG laboratories use surface electrodes as the recording electrodes. This chapter explains the techniques using these electrodes. The special techniques required when using needle electrodes are outlined in Chapter 15.

Motor Nerve Conduction Studies

Motor nerve conduction studies measure the conduction of the nerve impulse along the motor nerves. The routine method measures the conduction velocity of the large-diameter motor nerve fibers of the nerve being tested.

1. Place the recording electrodes on the distal muscle that is innervated by the tested nerve, employing the belly-tendon method. This method specifies that the active recording electrode (the cathode in most EMG machines) be placed on the midportion of the muscle belly (theoretically on the motor point) and the reference recording electrode on the tendon of the muscle. *With this method, the initial deflection of the CMAP is upward (negative).*

If the initial deflection is not negative, the following possibilities exist (Fig. 4.1):
   a. Incorrect placement of the active recording electrode on the desired muscle belly away from the motor point.
   b. Transposition of the active and reference recording electrodes.
   c. Stimulation of other neighboring nerves by misplacement of the stimulating electrodes.
   d. Stimulation of other nerves by stimulus spread when the stimulus has increased in duration and intensity.
   e. Conduction of the nerve impulse through anomalous innervation. This is observed in patients with carpal tunnel syndrome and Martin-Gruber anastomosis (see Chapter 14).

The first three possibilities can be easily checked. For confirmation of the last two possibilities, careful study by an experienced physician is needed.

2. Stimulate the various proximal locations of the motor nerve to obtain the supramaximal response. An active stimulating electrode (the cathode in most EMG machines) should be placed closer to the active recording electrode. Following the anatomical guide (see Chapter 5), place the stimulating electrode at the correct location. If no good response is obtained with reasonable stimulus intensity, move the active stimulating electrode a little to one side. This maneuver usually finds the correct location of the stimulation.

The distance between the active recording electrode and the active stimulating electrode at the most distal site of stimulation is standardized (see Chapter 5). This is necessary to interpret

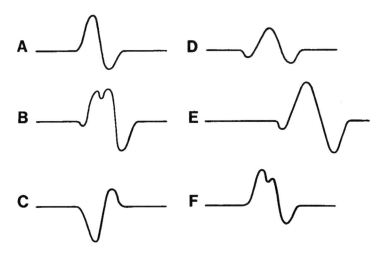

Figure 4.1. The various shapes of the CMAP. **A,** Normal CMAP is a diphasic wave with the initial negative deflection. **B,** Active recording electrode is away from the belly (motor point) and closer to the other muscle. **C,** The active and reference electrodes are reversed. **D,** Stimulation of the neighboring nerves either by misplacement of the stimulating electrodes or by stimulus spread when the stimulus is too strong. **E,** Conduction of the nerve impulse through anomalous innervation. **F,** An active recording electrode was placed on the bellies of the two muscles innervated by the same nerve.

the terminal latency in a meaningful way. Obviously, the terminal latency is proportional to the distance. Thus, it is possible to obtain prolonged terminal latency in a normal individual if an exceptionally long distance is used.

When a nerve is stimulated, watch carefully the response of the contracting muscle. If the expected response is not obtained, the correct nerve is not being stimulated. The stimulation of other neighboring nerves by misplacement of the stimulating electrode is a possibility when two nerves are situated close together. This occurs often at the axilla, where the median and ulnar nerves are separated only by the brachial artery, and at the popliteal fossa, where the posterior tibial and peroneal nerves are close together. If the wrong nerve is stimulated, the response of the contracting muscle and the shape of CMAP are both different. Usually the initial deflection of CMAP is positive.

Beware of stimulus spread when the stimulation is performed with increased duration and higher intensity. This often happens when one nerve is pathologically impaired and the other nerve is normal, as is commonly noted when stimulating the median nerve at the elbow or axilla in patients with severe carpal tunnel syndrome. Because of stimulus spread, the normal ulnar nerve is stimulated. In this case, the shape of the CMAP is different (the initial deflection is positive), and the latency is shorter compared with those obtained by stimulating at the wrist. This finding can mimic the Martin-Gruber anastomosis (see Chapter 14).

3. Measure the latency from the stimulus onset to the beginning of the initial deflection of the CMAP (Fig. 4.2). Latency is defined here as the conduction time from the onset of the stimulus to the beginning of the initial deflection of the CMAP. It is usually measured in milliseconds. The latency marker, which is available in most EMG machines, should be set at the beginning of the initial deflection of the CMAP. Then, the latency will automatically be read in milliseconds. In some sophisticated EMG machines the latency marker is automatically set by the machines and the latency is read in milliseconds. In these machines one has to check whether the automatically set latency marker is set correctly at the beginning of the initial deflection of the CMAP.

After reading the latency, we determine the NCV of the fastest conducting motor fiber of the nerve. The latency obtained by stimulating at the most distal site possible along the nerve is called the terminal (or distal) latency, and is expressed in milliseconds. We use the latency as a measure of the conduction of the motor nerve over the distal segment because the conduction velocity cannot be calculated. Conduction time from the distal point to the muscle is usually longer than what is expected from the conduction time over the proximal segment of the same nerve. This delay is caused by slowed impulses in the terminal fibers, synaptic delay, and conduction time of an action potential through muscle tissue (the residual latency). Because of this delay, we are unable to calculate the conduction velocity over the most distal segment of the motor nerves. The NCV can be calculated accurately by stimulating at two different points along the nerve and measuring the latency for each response.

4. Note the amplitude, duration, and shape of the CMAP at each stimulation site and compare them. As noted in Figure 4.2, the amplitude is measured from peak to peak and the duration

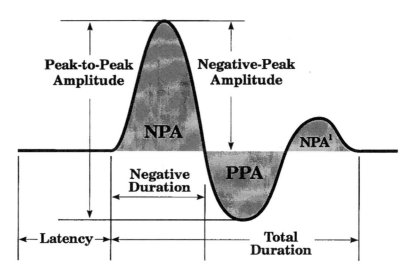

Figure 4.2. Components of the CMAP. NPA, Negative peak area; PPA, positive-peak area; NPA[1], additional negative-peak area. Total area = (NPA) + (PPA) + (NPA)[1].

from the beginning to the end of the CMAP. Normally the CMAP is biphasic. In some laboratories, the amplitude is measured from the baseline to the peak of negative deflection. This method is based on the assumption that this measurement reflects more accurately the number of muscle fibers that respond to the nerve impulse.

This assumption has been questioned by Slomic and associates, who found that the belly-tendon recording lowered CMAP amplitude by as much as 30–40% when the belly-remote recording electrode was used (3). Thus, Pickett believes that a simple, direct relationship between the proportion of active muscle fibers and negative peak-CMAP amplitude may be only a useful fiction rather than a fact (4).

The amplitude of the CMAP is roughly proportional to the number of muscle fibers that respond to the nerve impulse. The duration of the CMAP is related to the range of conduction velocities of the large-diameter motor nerve fibers.

A change in the CMAP occurs in peripheral nerve disorders. It is most prominent in entrapment neuropathies and demyelinating neuropathy, where conduction is either blocked or delayed because of segmental demyelination. In fact, the shape, amplitude, and duration of the CMAP can be diagnostic. Abnormal temporal dispersion (dispersion phenomenon) and conduction block are two such examples. Both are pathognomonic of demyelinating neuropathy. Abnormal temporal dispersion is characterized by the abnormal shape of CMAPs with multiple phases and prolonged duration (see Fig. 2.3). Conduction block is characterized by a substantial reduction of the CMAP amplitude proximal to the site of the block (see Fig. 20.6). For example, in ulnar compression neuropathy at the elbow (tardy ulnar palsy), the CMAP obtained by stimulating above the elbow may be markedly different from that obtained by stimulating below the elbow: the amplitude may be low, the duration prolonged, and the shape different (see Fig. 21.18).

When there is no evoked CMAP, even with maximal stimulation, *check first whether there is any muscle mass left on the muscle* where the recording electrode is placed. If there is muscle mass, it usually means that the nerve being tested is pathologically impaired: The nerve is either inexcitable or the conduction block is present along the nerve.

5. Measure (in millimeters) the length of the nerve between the proximal and distal sites of stimulation by surface measurement. The distance between two sites of stimulation should be obtained to calculate the conduction velocity. In most instances this distance is best measured with a measuring tape while the limb is maintained in exactly the same position as when it is stimulated. The distance to the center of the active stimulating electrode (the cathode in most EMG machines) is measured, and this point is marked on the skin with a red pencil before the electrode is removed. In the thoracic outlet segment in the ulnar or plantar nerve, the distance is best measured with an obstetrical caliper.

6. Calculate the NCV over the various segments of the motor nerves (Fig. 4.3). First, calculate the conduction time between the two stimulation sites:

$$\text{Conduction time (msec) between two stimulation sites} = \begin{array}{l}\text{latency (msec) from the proximal stimulation site}\\ -\text{ latency (msec) from the distal stimulation site.}\end{array}$$

The NCV can then be calculated:

$$\text{NCV (m/sec)} = \frac{\text{distance between two stimulation sites (mm)}}{\text{conduction time (msec) between two stimulation sites}}$$

keeping in mind that milliseconds = seconds/1000 and millimeters = meters/1000.

7. Adjust the NCV to the standard temperature, if required. Adjustment of the motor NCV is required if the skin temperature is below the desired temperature or if it has not been standardized with the skin temperature control unit.

The relationship between temperature and velocity is best expressed as a semilogarithmic plot of velocity against temperature. DeJesus et al. (5) offered the following formula that is suitable for calculators having an e^x key:

$$Y_2 = Y_1 \, e^{(M_2 \Delta T)}$$

where Y_2 is the corrected velocity of a standard temperature, Y_1 is the measured velocity at the measured temperature. ΔT is the difference in degrees centigrade between the standard and the measured temperatures, e is the base of the natural log system, and $M2$ is 0.0419.

In our laboratory, Table 4.1 is used to calculate the corrected velocity of a standard temperature using a simple calculator:

$$Y_2 = Y_1 \times K$$

where K represents $e^{(M_2 \Delta T)}$

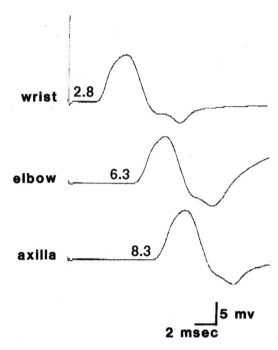

Figure 4.3. Example of the median motor nerve conduction study. The CMAP with wrist stimulation is 2.8 msec in latency, 17.5 mV in amplitude, and 11.5 msec in duration. The latency with elbow stimulation is 6.3 msec. The latency with axilla stimulation is 8.3 msec; the distance between the wrist and the elbow stimulation is 22 cm and between the elbow and axilla stimulation 14 cm. Thus, terminal latency is 2.8 msec; the motor NCV over the forearm segment is 62.8 m/sec (220 mm/[6.3 − 2.8]msec); the motor NCV over the elbow-axilla segment is 70 m/sec (140 mm/[8.3 − 6.3]msec). Skin temperature over the forearm is 32°C. No gross change in amplitude, shape, or duration of the CMAP is noted at the various stimulation sites.

Table 4.1.
Conversion Factors for the Temperature Difference in NCV

Degree Difference (DT)	K
0.5	1.021
1.0	1.043
1.5	1.065
2.0	1.087
2.5	1.117
3.0	1.134
3.5	1.157
4.0	1.183
4.5	1.207
5.0	1.233
5.5	1.259
6.0	1.286
6.5	1.313
7.0	1.341
7.5	1.369
8.0	1.398
8.5	1.428
9.0	1.458
10.0	1.520

Example:

The measured conduction velocity (Y_1) is 45.5 m/sec when the skin temperature is 29°C .
If the standard temperature is 31°C , then ΔT is 2.
K in Table 4.1 is 1.087 at the 2 difference (ΔT).
Then, the converted conduction velocity (Y2) is calculated as follows:

$$Y2 = 45.5 (Y1) \times 1.087 = 49.5 \text{ m/sec}$$

8. Compare the measured NCV with the normal values. Also compare the amplitude, duration, and shape of the CMAPs with the normals. The majority of EMG laboratories use two standard deviations (2SD) from the mean as the normal range. This means that 97.7% of the normal population will have values within 2 SD of the mean and assumes that the distribution of normal values shows the normal bell-shaped gaussian curve. This curve is applicable to the NCVs but not, however, to the amplitude of CMAP, the distribution curve of which is not bell-shaped. Therefore, the standard deviation cannot be used for the CMAP amplitude. The lowest value among normals is used as the normal limit in the majority of EMG laboratories.

Sensory Nerve Conduction Studies

The sensory nerve conduction study measures the conduction of the nerve impulse along the sensory nerves. The routine method measures the conduction velocity of the large-diameter sensory nerve fibers of the nerve being tested.

There are two methods of obtaining CNAP: orthodromic and antidromic. The orthodromic method consists of recording the CNAP proximally and stimulating the nerve distally. With the antidromic method, the location of the stimulating and recording electrodes is reversed. *The latency and conduction velocities are identical with the orthodromic and antidromic methods* if the recording and stimulating electrode positions are kept constant. One disadvantage of the antidromic method is that an accompanying motor response (because motor fibers are also stimulated) may distort the small CNAP. Ludin et al. (6) found that *the orthodromic method is far superior to the antidromic method in confirming a minimal or early polyneuropathy.* In our laboratory, the orthodromic method is used in sensory nerve conduction studies of the median and ulnar nerves, and the antidromic method is used for sural and radial nerve studies.

1. Place the recording electrodes on the correct sites following the anatomical guide (see Chapter 5). The distance between the center of the active and the center of the reference recording electrodes should be 3 cm. The location of the recording electrodes for the median and ulnar nerves was marked when the motor nerve conduction studies were performed. Even for the radial and sural nerves, there is usually no difficulty finding the correct anatomical sites for the recording electrodes because of the clear anatomical landmarks. The active recording electrode should be placed closer to the active stimulating electrode.

2. Stimulate the distal sensory nerve fibers in the orthodromic sensory conduction test and the proximal sensory nerve fibers in the antidromic sensory conduction test. The active stimulating electrode (the cathode in most EMG machines) should be placed closer to the recording electrodes.

Sometimes, a large stimulus artifact may distort the CNAP because of the baseline sway. This is especially critical when the distance is short since the CNAP is buried in the stimulus artifact. This uninvited stimulus artifact can easily be eliminated by rotating the reference stimulating electrode around the active stimulating electrode. This observation is confirmed by Kornfield et al. (7).

There is no difficulty in finding the correct location for stimulation for the median and ulnar nerves. We stimulate the fingers innervated by the respective nerves. There may be difficulty, however, in finding the correct locations for the sural and radial nerves. Move the active stimulating electrode slightly from side to side if you do not get any sensory potential with reasonable stimulus intensity. Convince yourself that you have placed the stimulating electrodes on the correct spot before concluding that there is "no potential."

3. Measure the latency. There are two methods of measuring the latency in sensory nerve conduction studies (Fig. 4.4). One method measures the latency from the onset of stimulus to the peak of the major negative deflection. Another method is to measure the latency from the onset of the stimulus to the initial positive peak or to the beginning of the major negative deflection. There is at least a 0.4-msec difference in latency between the two methods and about a 5–10

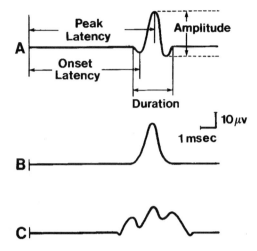

Figure 4.4. Components and shapes of the CNAP. **A,** Components of the sensory or mixed CNAP. **B,** Commonly observed CNAPs with the surface electrode. Initial positive deflection is not observed. C, CNAP with the abnormal temporal dispersion (dispersion phenomenon).

m/sec difference in the sensory NCV. We measure the latency from the onset of stimulus to the peak of the major negative deflection of the sensory CNAP in the surface electrode method. Even though our method does not measure the NCV of the fastest conduction fibers, we prefer this method because it is often difficult to identify the onset of the major negative deflection when the nerve potential is low, as noted in most pathological cases.

4. Measure the amplitude of the CNAP. The peak-to-peak amplitude of the evoked nerve potential should be measured in microvolts. In patients with neuropathy, the CNAP is either absent or small in amplitude. An amplitude of less than 10 μV in the median and ulnar nerves and less than 5 μV in the sural nerve is considered abnormal. *The CNAP is not obtainable when the sensory NCV is slower than 20 m/sec in the surface electrode method. Thus the absence of nerve potential does not necessarily mean that sensory NCV is zero.*

The detection of small CNAPs is facilitated by photographically superimposing a number of tracings on the same piece of film, so that a potential occurring at a constant time in the sweep of the oscilloscope is emphasized. The same superimposition of tracings can be achieved with the storage oscilloscope.

We can use the signal averager, needle electrode, and/or sensory amplifier to obtain small CNAPs (with an amplitude of less than 0.05 μV) which were unobtainable with the routine method. When using the signal averager, the shape and duration of the CNAP should be observed. The dispersion phenomenon (many peaks and long duration of potential) may be the sole abnormality in some neuropathies and is indicative of the broad range of NCVs among large-diameter sensory fibers (Fig. 4.4).

5. The length of the nerve is measured by surface measurement from the center of the active stimulating electrode to the center of the active recording electrode. It is expressed in millimeters. The same principles discussed in regard to the motor nerve conduction study are applied here.

6. Calculate the NCV. There are two ways of measuring the sensory NCVs.

a. In a majority of the EMG laboratories, the sensory NCV is estimated by dividing the conduction distance (millimeters) by the latency (milliseconds) (Figs. 4.5 and 4.6).

$$\text{NCV (m/sec)} = \frac{\text{distance between the active stimulating and recording electrodes (mm)}}{\text{latency over the same segment (msec)}}$$

b. In some laboratories only the latency is used. This method is based on the assumption that the latency includes the time taken to excite the nerve, thus not reflecting the genuine conduction time. If the latency is used, the distance between the stimulating and recording electrodes should be strictly standardized. In certain laboratories (8), the latency is used for the distal segment and the sensory NCV for the proximal segment, as noted in Figure 4.5.

We prefer the first method because we do not have to standardize the distance. A study by Gilliatt et al. (9) has shown that this technique does not introduce any significant error in the measurement of the NCV.

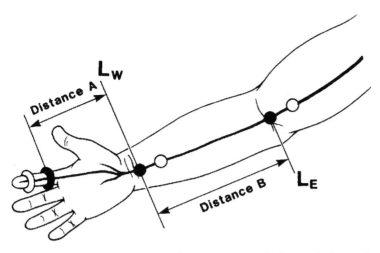

Figure 4.5.   Different methods of calculating the sensory NCV. The first method uses *distance A/Lw* (latency at wrist). The second method uses *distance B/Le* (latency at elbow) − *Lw*. *Lw* is used as the terminal latency in the second method.

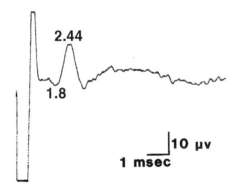

Figure 4.6.   Example of the median sensory nerve conduction over the digit II-wrist segment. The positive peak (or onset) latency is 1.80 msec, and the negative peak latency is 2.44 msec. The distance between the active stimulating and recording electrodes is 12.2 cm. The maximum sensory NCV is 67.7 m/sec. The negative peak sensory NCV is 50.0 m/sec. The amplitude and duration of the sensory CNAP are 21.5 μV and 1.05 msec, respectively. Skin temperature over the palm is 33°C.

7. Adjust the NCV to the standard temperature, if required. The same formula and table for the motor NCV adjustment are used to adjust the sensory NCV to the standard temperature.

8. Compare the measured NCV with the normal values. Also compare the amplitude, duration, and shape of the CNAPs with the normals.

Mixed Nerve Conduction Studies

The mixed nerve conduction studies measure the conduction velocity of the nerve impulse along the mixed (motor and sensory) nerves. The routine method measures the conduction velocity of the large-diameter mixed nerve fibers of the nerve being tested.

Testing method and calculation of velocity are identical to the orthodromic method of sensory nerve conduction. The clinical significance of the mixed nerve conduction is also identical to that of the sensory nerve conduction.

The mixed nerve conduction study is usually performed over the wrist-elbow and elbow-axilla segments of the ulnar and median nerves and over the axilla-Erb's point segment of the ulnar nerve, and rarely over the ankle-fibular head segment of the peroneal nerve.

1. Place the recording electrodes on the correct sites following the anatomical guide (see Chapter 5). Again, the distance between the active and reference recording electrodes should be

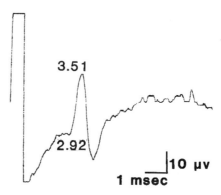

Figure 4.7. Example of the median mixed nerve conduction over the wrist-elbow segment. The onset latency is 2.92 msec, and the negative peak latency is 3.51 msec. The distance between the active stimulating and recording electrodes is 20.3 cm. The maximum mixed NCV is 69.5 m/sec, and the negative peak NCV is 57.8 m/sec. The amplitude and duration of the mixed CNAP are 40.8 μV and 1.71 msec, respectively.

3 cm. The locations of the recording electrodes are marked at the elbow and axilla in the median nerve and at the elbow, axilla, and Erb's point in the ulnar nerve. For the ulnar nerve, the location of the recording electrode is at the elbow sulcus. We prefer the elbow location simply because it is often difficult to obtain mixed CNAP below or above the elbow.

2. Stimulate the distal mixed nerve fibers following the anatomical guide (see Chapter 5). Again, the active stimulating electrode should be placed toward the recording electrodes.

For the median and ulnar nerves, the location of the stimulating electrodes was marked when the motor nerve conduction studies were performed, except at the elbow for the ulnar nerve. For the latter, the stimulating electrode should be at the elbow sulcus. When stimulating the ulnar nerve at the axilla, one should be careful not to stimulate the median nerve. Remember that the ulnar nerve is situated below the brachial artery and that you should look for the appropriate motor response of the hand.

To the inexperienced examiner, it is not easy to obtain mixed CNAPs over the elbow-axilla segment in the median or ulnar nerves. This difficulty is overcome by maximal lengthening of the segment being tested and by pressing the recording surface electrode closer to the nerve. We usually use an adhesive tape roll for this purpose because it is electrically nonconductive. This pressing measure is also helpful for obtaining mixed CNAPs over the Erb's point in many individuals.

3. Measure the latency from the start of stimulation to the peak of the major negative deflection or to the peak of the initial positive deflection of the mixed CNAP, whichever method is required.

4. Note the amplitude of the mixed CNAP. Amplitude of less than 10 μV in the median and ulnar nerves is considered abnormal even in mixed nerve conduction. When the CNAP is too small to be detected by the routine method, photographic superimposition or use of the signal averager helps in obtaining the small mixed CNAP.

5. Measure (in millimeters) the length of the nerve by surface measurement from the active stimulating electrode to the active recording electrode.

6. Calculate the NCV (Fig. 4.7).

$$\text{NCV (m/sec)} = \frac{\text{distance between the active stimulating and recording electrodes (mm)}}{\text{latency over the same segment (msec)}}$$

7. Adjust the NCV to the standard temperature, if required. The formula and table for the motor NCV are used to make this adjustment.

8. Compare the measured NCV with the normal values. Also compare the amplitude, duration, and shape of the mixed CNAPs with the normals.

H-Reflex Study

The H-reflex study on the gastrocnemius-soleus muscle measures the latency over the monosynaptic reflex arc through the afferent Ia fibers and efferent alpha motor fibers of the S1 root (Fig. 4.8). The H-reflex is normally present at birth in the intrinsic hand and

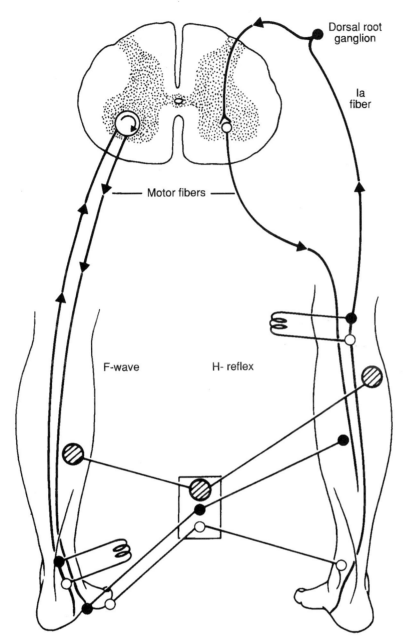

Figure 4.8.   Anatomical pathways for the H-reflex and F-wave. For the H-reflex, the Ia fiber is the afferent pathway and the α-motor fiber is the efferent pathway. For the F-wave, the α-motor fiber is the afferent as well as the efferent pathway. Note also the monosynaptic reflex arc in the H-reflex pathway.

foot muscles but is present consistently only in the gastrocnemius-soleus muscle after 12 months of age. In other muscles the facilitation technique is needed to obtain the H-reflex with some reliability (Chapter 17).

The H-reflex on the gastrocnemius-soleus muscle is best obtained when the patient is placed prone, with the feet suspended over the edge of the table or with a pillow placed under the ankles. It is easily obtained from the motor conduction setups by changing the sweep velocity to 10 msec and the sensitivity to 500 μV.

1. Place the recording electrodes on the gastrocnemius muscle, as shown in the anatomical guide (see Chapter 5).
2. Stimulate the posterior tibial nerve at the popliteal fossa following the anatomical guide

(see Chapter 5). *The stimulus duration should be 0.5 or 1.0 msec*, which makes it more selective for the afferent Ia fibers (10). Shorter durations would favor the activation of motor axons. *An active stimulating electrode should be placed closer to the spine (away from the recording electrodes)*. This location is marked when the motor conduction is performed.

3. Stimulate manually at the rate of once every 2 sec (or longer) to avoid the blocking

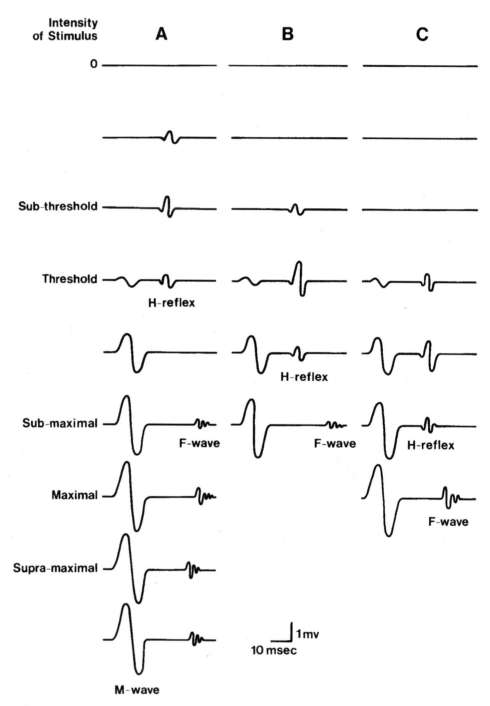

Figure 4.9.   Differentiation between the H-reflex and F-wave. **A**, Any subthreshold late response is the H-reflex. The highest amplitude is noted with the subthreshold stimulus. **B**, Any subthreshold late response which becomes higher than the M-wave is the H-reflex. **C**, Any late response that is higher than M-wave in amplitude at a given stimulus is the H-reflex. Any supramaximal late response is the F-wave.

Table 4.2.
Differentiation Between H-reflex and F Response

Measurement	H-Reflex	F-Wave
Nature of response	Monosynaptic reflex; e.g. H-reflex on the gastrocnemius-soleus muscle is an electrophysiological counterpart of ankle reflex	Not a reflex; antidromic motor neuron discharge
Pathways		
Afferent arc	Ia sensory fibers	α-motor fibers
Efferent arc	α-motor fibers	α-motor fibers
Best stimulus to evoke the response relative to the M response	Subthreshold; absent with the supramaximal stimulation	Supramaximal; absent with the subthreshold stimulation
Appearance and persistence of the response	Rather constant at low rates of stimulation ($^{1}/_{2}$–30 secs)	Variable
Latency	Rather constant	Variable
	Latency shorter than the F response latency	
Highest amplitude	Can be up to 50–100% of the maximum M-wave; much bigger than the F-wave	Usually small, less than 5% of the maximum M-wave
The muscles to be tested without any facilitation[a]	Gastrocnemius-soleus muscle in adult; intrinsic hand and foot muscles in infants up to 1 yr	Almost every distal muscle

[a]In other muscles, H-reflex can be obtained with facilitation (see Chapter 17).

response. Increase the intensity gradually and observe the H-reflex and M-wave (CMAP from the gastrocnemius).

The H-reflex is classically obtainable with an intensity usually too low to produce the M-wave. Thus maximal amplitude of the H-reflex is often obtained with low intensity. With a gradual increase of intensity, the M-response increases its amplitude while the H-reflex amplitude is decreasing. With supramaximal stimulation, the H-reflex is no longer obtainable and is sometimes replaced by an F-wave.

Differentiation between the H-reflex and F-wave is not always easy. The following guidelines are helpful in recognizing the H-reflex (Fig. 4.9). *A late response is always the H-reflex when it meets one of the following criteria:*

1. It is elicited by a subthreshold stimulus;

2. Its amplitude is higher than the M-wave at a given stimulus; and

3. Its amplitude is more than 50% higher than the maximum M-wave amplitude.

Conversely, the late response is always the F-wave when it is elicited with the supramaximal stimulus (Fig. 4.9).

When the criteria are not met, the H-reflex should be differentiated from the F-wave by the classical change of amplitude of the H-wave in relation to the M-wave with a change in stimulus intensity and by the shape and latency of the late responses (Table 4.2).

The H-wave is classically triphasic with an initial positive deflection and a large negative deflection in the gastrocnemius-soleus muscle. H-reflex latency is shorter than the F-wave latency. The latency classically varies with each F-wave, while the latency of the H-reflex is relatively constant.

The H-reflex recording is helped by the trace contraction of plantar flexors and by the Jendrassik maneuver (the patient hooks his hands together by the flexed fingers and pulls apart as hard as he can).

4. Measure the latency from the start of stimulation to the onset of the initial deflection of the H-reflex (Fig. 4.10). The latency of the H-reflex is usually in the range of 25–35 msec in normal individuals.

5. Measure the body height (Table 4.3) or the length of the lower leg (both in centimeters) between the stimulating site and the medial malleolus. Because the H-reflex latency is dependent on the traveling pathway, the body height must be considered in judging the latency normal or abnormal. In some laboratories the length of the lower leg is used to adjust the H-reflex latency, in which case the length of the lower leg must be measured (11).

6. Compare the patient's H-reflex latency with the normal values. The easiest comparison to make in the study of unilateral lumbosacral radiculopathy is to compare the involved and uninvolved sides. A difference of 1.5 msec in the H-reflex latency in both legs of the same patient has been considered objective evidence of S1 radiculopathy (11). Careful technique and absence of marked leg length discrepancy are prerequisites for this comparison to be meaningful.

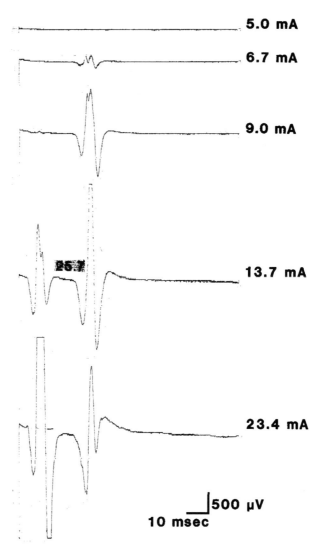

5.0 mA

6.7 mA

9.0 mA

13.7 mA

23.4 mA

500 μV

10 msec

Figure 4.10.   Example of the H-reflex from the medial gastrocnemius muscle. The numbers at the left show the stimulus intensities. The stimulus duration used for this test is 0.5 msec. The H-reflex shows the classical triphasic shape with 25.7-msec latency. The H-reflex amplitude is higher than the M-wave at 13.7 mA stimulus intensity. The 25.7 msec H-reflex latency is normal for a 45-year-old man with 167 cm height.

F-Wave Study

The F-wave study measures the latency over the afferent and efferent arcs of motor fibers from the stimulating site and anterior horn cells (Fig. 4.8; Table 4.2). This response is evoked by supramaximal stimulation during the motor nerve conduction study.

The F-wave is easily obtained by stimulating the distal portion of the median, ulnar, peroneal, and posterior tibial nerves using motor nerve conduction setups and changing the sweep velocity to 10 msec and the sensitivity to 200 μv.

If the F-wave is difficult to elicit, slight voluntary muscle contraction often enhances the response. The F-wave is easily obtained from the distal muscles after distal stimulation but is difficult to obtain after proximal stimulation because the latter yields an F-wave with a shorter latency, and the response is hidden in the CMAP (M-wave).

1. Place the recording electrodes on the distal muscle that is innervated by the testing nerve, employing the belly-tendon method.
2. Stimulate the nerve in the distal portion: the wrist for ulnar and median nerves and the

Table 4.3.
Height Conversion Table[a]

Feet	Inches	Inches	Cm	Feet	Inches	Inches	Cm
3	0	36	91.4	5	0	60	152.4
3	1	37	94.0	5	1	61	154.9
3	2	38	96.5	5	2	62	157.5
3	3	39	99.1	5	3	63	160.0
3	4	40	101.6	5	4	64	162.6
3	5	41	104.1	5	5	65	165.1
3	6	42	106.7	5	6	66	167.6
3	7	43	109.2	5	7	67	170.2
3	8	44	111.8	5	8	68	172.7
3	9	45	114.3	5	9	69	175.3
3	10	46	116.8	5	10	70	177.8
3	11	47	119.4	5	11	71	180.3
4	0	48	121.9	6	0	72	182.9
4	1	49	124.5	6	1	73	185.4
4	2	50	127.0	6	2	74	188.0
4	3	51	129.5	6	3	75	190.5
4	4	52	132.1	6	4	76	193.0
4	5	53	134.6	6	5	77	195.6
4	6	54	137.2	6	6	78	198.1
4	7	55	139.7	6	7	79	200.7
4	8	56	142.2	6	8	80	203.2
4	9	57	144.8	6	9	81	205.7
4	10	58	147.3	6	10	82	208.3
4	11	59	149.9	6	11	83	210.8

[a]Conversion formula: 1 foot = 12 inches = 30.48 cm. 1 inch = 2.54 cm.

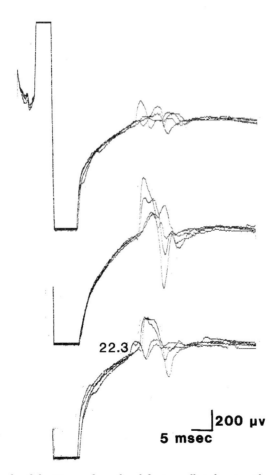

Figure 4.11. Example of the F-wave from the abductor pollicis brevis with wrist stimulation. The shortest latency among 12 F-waves is 22.3 msec, normal for a 45-year-old man with 167 cm height.

ankle for peroneal and posterior tibial nerves. *An active stimulating electrode (the cathode in most EMG machines) should be placed closer to the spine (away from the recording electrodes).*

3. Stimulate manually at the rate of once every 2 sec (or more) to avoid the blocking response. Stimulate the nerve with the supramaximal intensity and observe the M-wave and the late F-wave.

4. Obtain F-waves at least 10 times and measure the latency from the start of the stimulus to the onset of initial deflection of the F-wave with the shortest latency. The latency of the F-wave after distal stimulation is usually in the range of 23–33 msec for median and ulnar nerves and 50–60 msec for peroneal and posterior tibial nerves in normal individuals (Fig. 4.11).

5. Measure the body height in centimeters (Table 4.3). Because the F-wave is dependent on the traveling pathway of afferent and efferent motor fibers, body height is a major factor in judging the latency normal or abnormal. In some laboratories the length of a leg or arm is used to obtain the F-wave NCVs, in which case the patient's arm or leg length must be measured.

6. Compare the patient's F-wave latency with normal values. The easiest comparison to make is the F-wave latencies between the right and left sides. If greater than 2 msec, the difference is considered significant (12). The F-wave latency is prolonged in patients with proximal peripheral neuropathy.

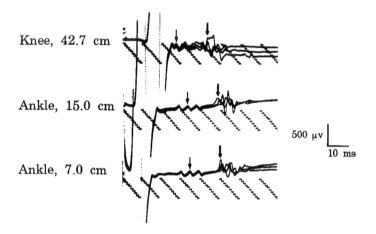

Figure 4.12.   Late responses in abductor hallucis muscle to posterior tibial nerve stimulation. *Broad arrow* indicates F waves: *narrow arrow* indicates axon reflex. (From Daube J. Nerve conduction studies. In: Aminoff MJ, ed, Electrodiagnosis in clinical neurology. 2nd ed. New York: Churchill Livingstone, 1986:277.)

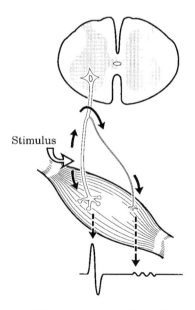

Figure 4.13.   Anatomical pathways for axon "reflex."

In some individuals an axon "reflex" may be present between the M-wave and F-wave (Fig. 4.12) (13). This should not be mistaken for the F-wave. An axon "reflex" is usually smaller in amplitude and more consistent in shape than the F-wave. Stimulation distal to the site of axon branching produces a late response via the axon branches (Fig. 4.13) (13). This axon branching occurs in some disease processes. However, at this time the clinical significance of the axon reflex is not clear.

REFERENCES

1. Henriksen JD. Conduction velocity of motor nerves in normal subjects and patients with neuromuscular disorders. (Thesis) Minneapolis: University of Minnesota, 1956.
2. Lowitzsch K, Hopf HC, Gallard J. Changes of sensory conduction velocity and refractory periods with decreasing tissue temperature in man. J. Neurol 1977; 216:181–188.
3. Slomic A, Rosenfalck A, Buchthal F: Electrical and mechanical responses of normal and myasthenic muscle. Brain Res 1968; 10:1–74.
4. Pickett JB. Neuromuscular transmission. In: Summer A, ed. The physiology of peripheral nerve disease. Philadelphia: WB Saunders, 1980:238–264.
5. DeJesus PV, Hausmanowa-Petrusewicz I, Barchi RL. The effect of cold on nerve conduction. Neurology 1973; 23:1182–1189.
6. Ludin HP, Lutschg J, Valsangracomo F. Vergleichende Untersuchung: orthodromer und antidromer sensibler Nervenleitgeschwindigkeiten. Z EEG EMG 1977; 8:180–186.
7. Kornfield MJ, Cerra J, Simons DG. Stimulus artifact reduction in nerve conduction. Arch Phys Med Rehabil 1985; 66:232–234.
8. Hammer K. Nerve conduction studies. Springfield: Charles C Thomas, 1982.
9. Gilliatt RW, Melvik ID, Velate AS, Willison RG. A study of normal nerve action potentials using an averaging technique (barrier grid storage tube). J Neurol Neurosurg Psychiatry 1965; 28:191–200.
10. Hugon M. Methodology of the Hoffman reflex in man. New developments in EMG and clinical neurophysiology. Basel: Karger, 1973; 3:277–293.
11. Braddom RL, Johnson EW. Standardization of H reflex and diagnostic use in S1 radiculopathy. Arch Phys Med Rehabil 1974; 55:161–166.
12. Fisher MA, Shrivole AJ, Terxera C, Grainer LS. The F-Response{md}A clinically useful physiological parameter for the evaluation of radicular injury. Electromyogr Clin Neurophysiol 1979; 19:65–75.
13. Daube J. Nerve conduction studies. In: Aminoff MJ, ed. Electrodiagnosis in clinical neurology. 2nd ed. New York: Churchill Livingstone, 1986:265–306.

Anatomical Guide for Common Nerve Conduction Studies

In this chapter we describe the anatomical guidelines for nerve conduction studies of the commonly tested nerves. The well-trained electromyography (EMG) technician can perform these tests without any difficulty. The methods described in this chapter are used daily by the EMG technicians and physicians at the Medical Center of the University of Alabama at Birmingham. We have found these methods to be practical and sensitive in the diagnosis of neuropathy, although obviously some of our methods are different from those used in other EMG laboratories. When our methods are used, the results should be compared with our normal values. If other methods are used, the results should be compared with normal values obtained by those methods.

A majority of American-made EMG machines have the cathode as the active electrode and the anode as the reference electrode. In a few EMG machines (Dantec, for example), the reverse is true, while in more sophisticated EMG machines one has a choice between using the cathode or the anode as the active stimulating electrode. Thus, it is important to check and remember which is the active electrode in the recording electrodes as well as in the stimulating electrodes in each EMG machine. In any case, *the positivity of the potentials should be deflected downward in the obtained potentials.* The symbols used in the figures in this chapter are shown in Figure 5.1.

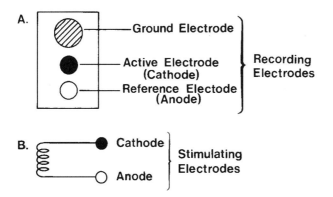

Figure 5.1. Symbols for electrodes.

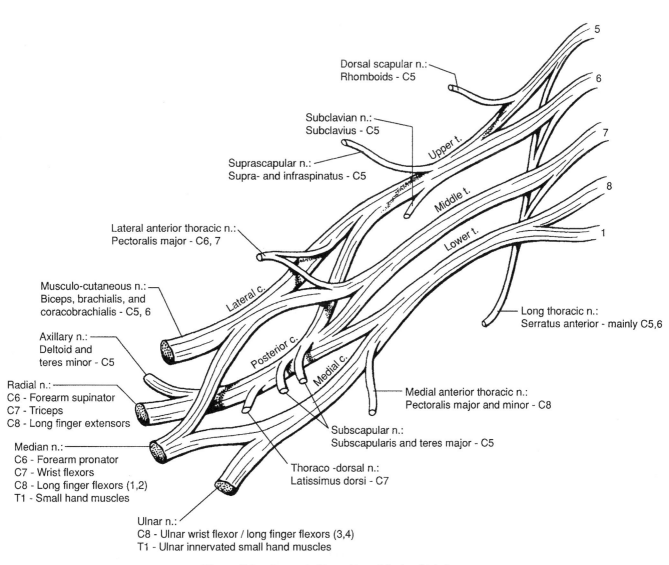

Figure 5.2. Anatomical branching of the brachial plexus.

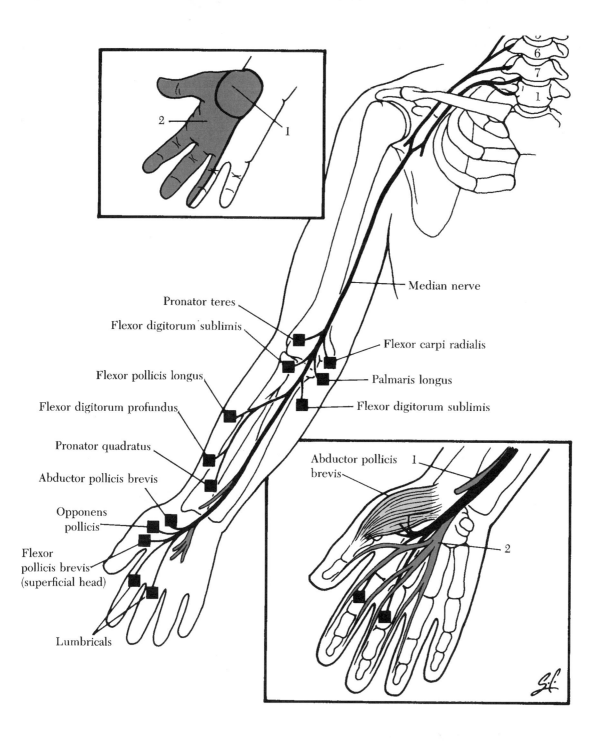

Figure 5.3. Anatomical course and innervation of the median nerve. Sensory branches are indicated by (*1*) and (*2*): (*1*) palmar branch; (*2*) main median sensory branch.

Figure 5.5. Sensory nerve conduction study for the median nerve. **A**, Finger-wrist segment. *Position:* Palm up; *Ground:* Palm; *Instrument setting:* Sensory Nerve Conduction; *Response:* No motor response; *Recording electrodes:* At the wrist, between the two prominent middle tendons (site marked during motor nerve conduction study); *Stimulating electrodes:* Ring electrodes. **B**, Palm-wrist (carpal tunnel) segment. *Active stimulating electrode:* Base of the index finger; *Reference electrode:* About 3 cm distal to active electrode; *Recording electrodes:* Same as above; *Stimulating electrodes:* 6 cm distal from the active recording electrode, or at the midpoint between the base of the index finger and the active recording electrode, whichever is longer, along the line connecting the active recording electrode, and the digit II-III interspace.

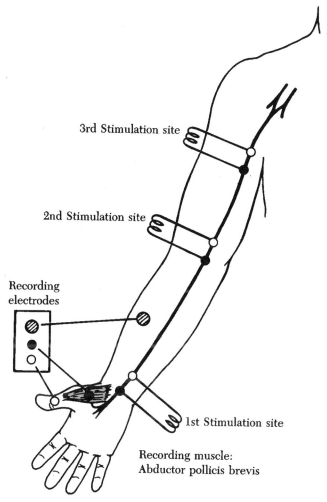

Figure 5.4. Motor nerve conduction study for the median nerve.

Position: Arm extended, palm up; *Active electrode:* Midportion of the hyperthenar muscle (abductor pollicis brevis): *Reference electrode:* Thumb; *Ground electrode:* Flexor surface of forearm; *Instrument setting:* Motor Nerve Conduction; *Response:* Brisk movement of the thumb, index, and middle fingers.

1st stimulation site: At the wrist, 5 cm proximal to the active electrode, between the two prominent middle tendons or on the midline along the crease between the hyper- and hypothenar muscles.

2nd stimulation site: At the elbow crease, on the ulnar side of the pulsating brachial artery.

3rd stimulation site: At the axilla, just forward of brachial artery.

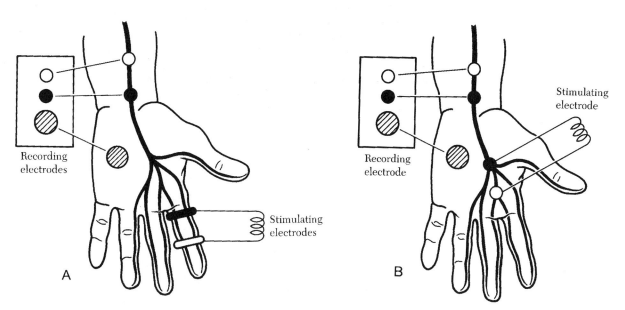

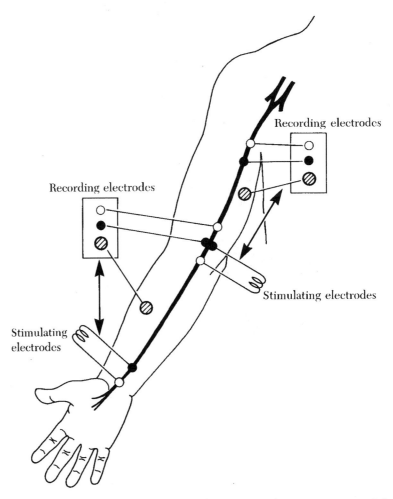

Figure 5.6.   Mixed nerve conduction study for the median nerve. *Position:* Arm extended, palm up; *Ground electrode:* Forearm; *Instrument setting:* Mixed Nerve Conduction; *Response:* Brisk movement of the thumb, index, and middle fingers. (Sites for the recording and stimulating electrodes were marked at the wrist, elbow, and axilla during the motor conduction study.) *Over the wrist-elbow segment—recording electrodes:* Between the two prominent middle tendons at the wrist; *Over the elbow-axilla segment—recording electrodes:* Just forward of the pulsating brachial artery; *Stimulating electrodes:* Just to the ulnar side of the pulsating brachial artery at the elbow.

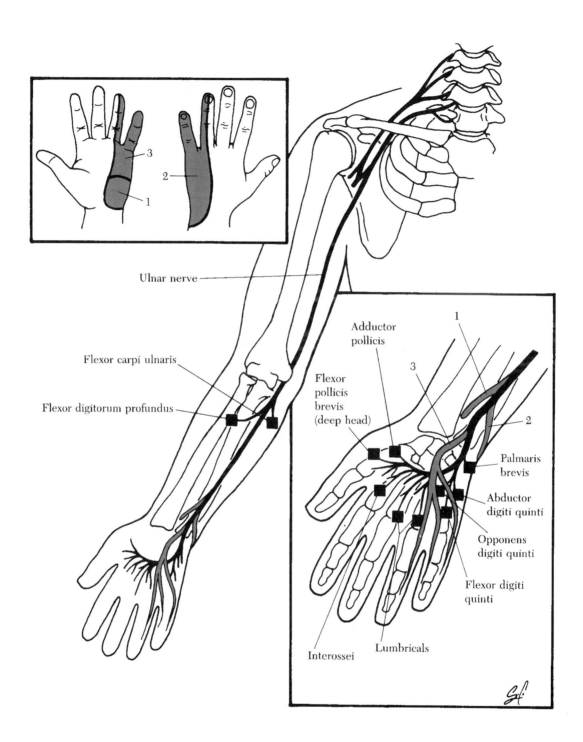

Figure 5.7. Anatomical course and innervation of the ulnar nerve. Sensory branches are indicated by (*1*), (*2*), and (*3*): (*1*) palmar branch; (*2*) dorsal cutaneous branch; (*3*) superficial sensory branch.

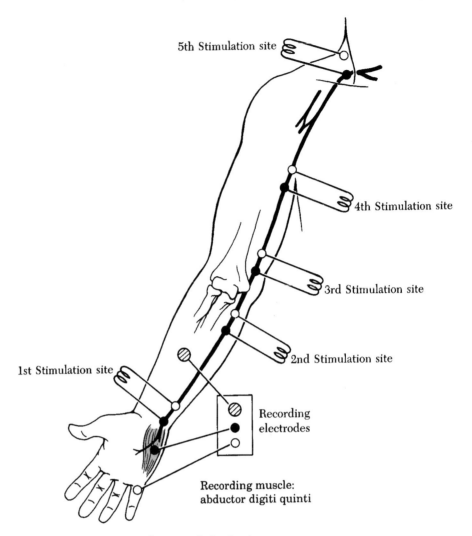

5th Stimulation site

4th Stimulation site

3rd Stimulation site

2nd Stimulation site

1st Stimulation site

Recording electrodes

Recording muscle: abductor digiti quinti

Figure 5.8.   Motor nerve conduction study for the ulnar nerve.

5th stimulation site: At the supraclavicular fossa, lateral to the posterior border of the sternocleido-mastoid and the superior margin of the clavicle; *4th stimulation site:* At the axilla, posterior to the pulsating brachial artery; *3rd stimulation site:* At 5–6 cm above the elbow sulcus, between the biceps and triceps muscles; *2nd stimulation site:* At 4 cm below the elbow sulcus; *1st stimulation site:* At the wrist, 5 cm proximal to the active recording electrode, the radial side of the prominent tendon on the ulnar aspect (flexor carpi ulnaris tendon); *Position:* Arm extended, palm up; *Active electrode:* Midportion of the hypothenar muscle (abductor digiti quinti); *Reference electrode:* Little finger; *Ground electrode:* Flexor surface of the forearm; *Instrument setting:* Motor Nerve Conduction; *Response:* Brisk movement of the little finger; The distance across the elbow should be 9–10 cm.; The distance between the Erb's point and axilla was measured with an obstetrical caliper with the arm 45° from the side.

Figure 5.10.   Mixed nerve conduction study for the ulnar nerve.

Position: Arm extended, palm up; *Ground electrode:* Forearm; *Instrument setting:* Mixed Nerve Conduction; *Response:* Brisk movement of the little finger. (Sites for the recording and stimulating electrodes were marked at Erb's point, axilla, and wrist during the motor nerve conduction study.) *Over the axilla-Erb's point segment (thoracic outlet segment)—recording electrodes:* Lateral to the posterior border of sternocleidomastoid and the superior margin of the clavicle; *Stimulating electrodes:* Just behind the pulsating brachial artery; *Over the elbow-axilla segment—recording electrodes:* At the axilla, posterior to the pulsating brachial artery; *Stimulating electrodes:* At the groove of the elbow; *Over the wrist-elbow segment—Recording electrodes:* At the ulnar sulcus between two bony prominences; *Stimulating electrodes:* Just radial to the prominent tendon on the ulnar side of the wrist.

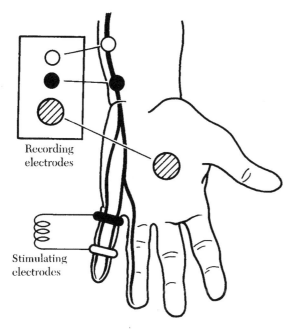

Figure 5.9. Sensory nerve conduction study for the ulnar nerve.

Recording electrodes: At the wrist, radial side of the prominent tendon on the ulnar side (already marked during the motor conduction study); *Stimulating electrodes:* Ring electrodes: *Active electrode:* At the base of the little finger; *Reference electrode:* About 3 cm distal to the active electrode; *Position:* Palm up; *Ground electrode:* Palm; *Instrument setting:* Sensory Nerve Conduction; *Response:* No motor response.

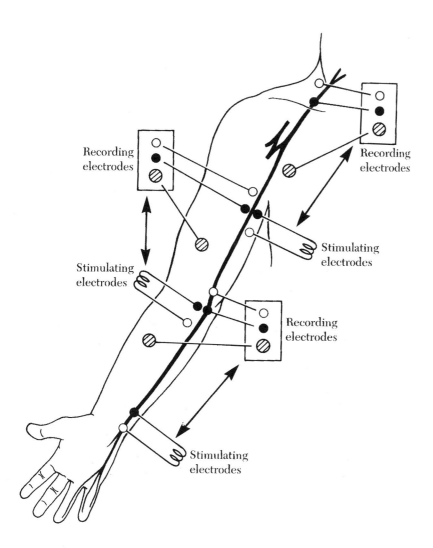

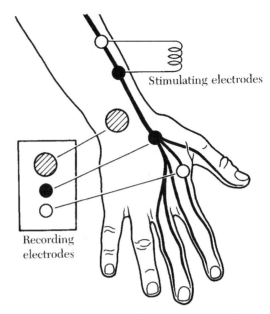

Stimulating electrodes

Recording
electrodes

Figure 5.11. Sensory nerve conduction study for the radial nerve (antidromic method).
  Position: Palm down, hand extended; *Ground electrode:* Dorsum of the hand; *Instrument setting:* Sensory Nerve Conduction; *Response:* Pain radiating toward the thumb and index finger; *Stimulating electrodes:* On the ridge of the radius, 10–14 cm from the recording electrodes; *Recording electrodes:* At the base of the web between the thumb and index finger.

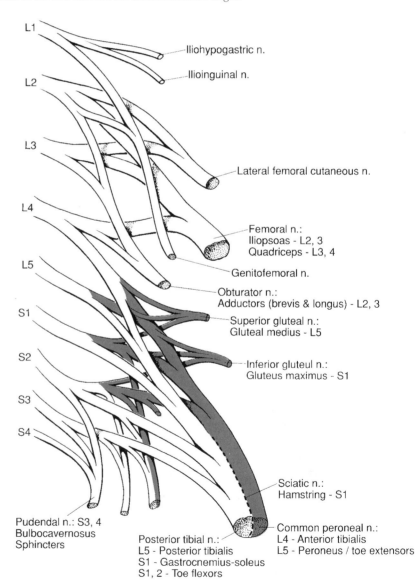

L1

L2

L3

L4

L5

S1

S2

S3

S4

Iliohypogastric n.

Ilioinguinal n.

Lateral femoral cutaneous n.

Femoral n.:
Iliopsoas - L2, 3
Quadriceps - L3, 4

Genitofemoral n.

Obturator n.:
Adductors (brevis & longus) - L2, 3

Superior gluteal n.:
Gluteal medius - L5

Inferior gluteul n.:
Gluteus maximus - S1

Sciatic n.:
Hamstring - S1

Common peroneal n.:
L4 - Anterior tibialis
L5 - Peroneus / toe extensors

Posterior tibial n.:
L5 - Posterior tibialis
S1 - Gastrocnemius-soleus
S1, 2 - Toe flexors

Pudendal n.: S3, 4
Bulbocavernosus
Sphincters

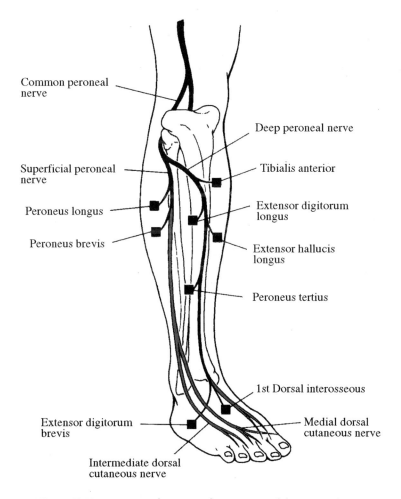

Figure 5.13. Anatomical course and innervation of the peroneal nerve.

Figure 5.12. Anatomical branching of the lumbosacral plexus.

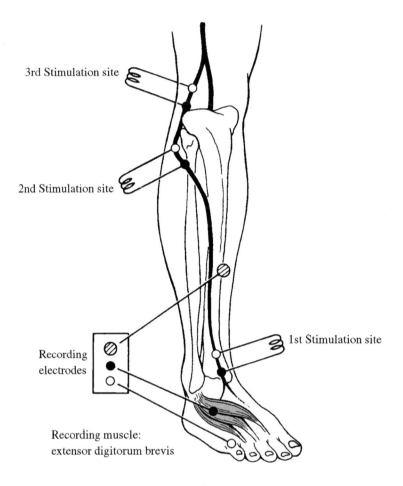

3rd Stimulation site

2nd Stimulation site

1st Stimulation site

Recording
electrodes

Recording muscle:
extensor digitorum brevis

Figure 5.14.   Motor nerve conduction study for the peroneal nerve. *Position:* Patient lying on back; *Active electrode:* extensor digitorum brevis; *Reference electrode:* base of the little toe; *Ground electrode:* anterior tibialis; *Instrument setting:* Motor Nerve Conduction; *Response:* upward movement of the great toe (toward the head); *3rd stimulation site:* Just inside the lateral half of the popliteal space at the level of the midpatella; *2nd stimulation site:* At the knee, just under the fibular head (posterior to the fibular head); *1st stimulation site:* At the ankle, 8 cm proximal to the active recording electrode, at the midpoint between the medial and lateral malleoli at the top of the ankle.

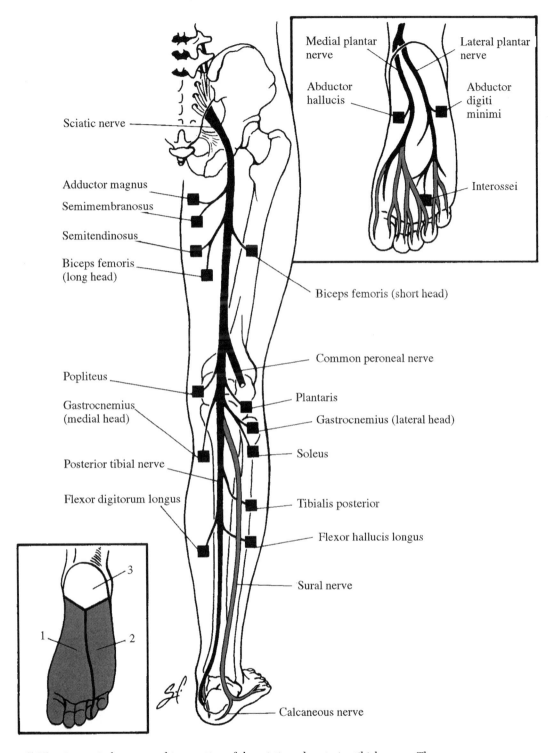

Figure 5.15. Anatomical course and innervation of the sciatic and posterior tibial nerves. The sensory branches of the posterior tibial nerve are indicated by (1), (2), and (3): (1) medial plantar nerve; (2) lateral plantar nerve; (3) calcaneal branch.

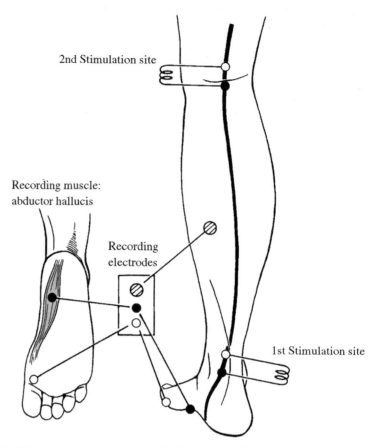

Figure 5.16. Motor nerve conduction study for the posterior tibial nerve.

Position: Patient lying on back; *Active electrode:* Abductor hallucis; *Reference electrode:* Base of the great toe; *Ground electrode:* Calf muscle; *Instrument setting:* Motor Nerve Conduction; *Response:* Downward movement of the great toe (away from the head).

2nd stimulation site: At the knee, just medial to the midpoint of the knee crease.

1st stimulation site: At the ankle, just behind the medial malleolus, 10 cm proximal to the active recording electrode.

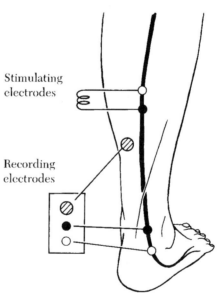

Figure 5.17. Sensory nerve conduction study for the sural nerve (antidromic sensory nerve conduction).

Stimulating electrodes: about 14 cm proximal to the recording electrode, just lateral to the midline of the width of the calf muscle; *Recording electrodes:* just behind the lateral malleolus; *Position:* patient lying on side, knee resting on opposite knee, foot flexed back at a 45° angle; *Ground electrode:* calf muscle; *Instrument setting:* Sensory Nerve Conduction; *Response:* pain radiating toward the little toe.

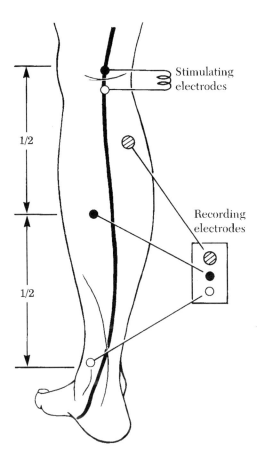

Figure 5.18. H-reflex study in the gastrocnemius-soleus muscle.

Position: Patient lying on belly; a towel or pillow under the ankle is helpful; *Ground electrode:* Calf muscle; *Instrument setting:* H-Reflex; *Response:* Downward movement of the great toe (away from the head); *Stimulating electrode:* Just medial to the midpoint of the knee crease in the popliteal fossa. (Note that the active stimulating electrode is proximally located.) *Recording electrode:* Halfway between the popliteal crease and the proximal medial malleolus over the medial gastrocnemius.

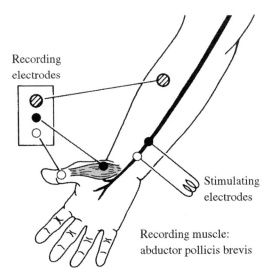

Figure 5.19. F-wave study for the median nerve.

Position: Arm extended, palm up; *Active electrode:* Midportion of the hyperthenar muscle (abductor pollicis brevis): *Reference electrode:* Thumb; *Ground electrode:* Flexor surface of the forearm; *Instrument setting:* F-Wave Study; *Response:* Brisk movement of the thumb; *Stimulation site:* At the wrist; *Active stimulating electrode:* 5 cm proximal to the active recording electrode between the two prominent tendons or on midline following the crease between the hyper- and hypothenar muscles (note that the active stimulating electrode is proximally located); *Reference stimulating electrodes:* Placed distally.

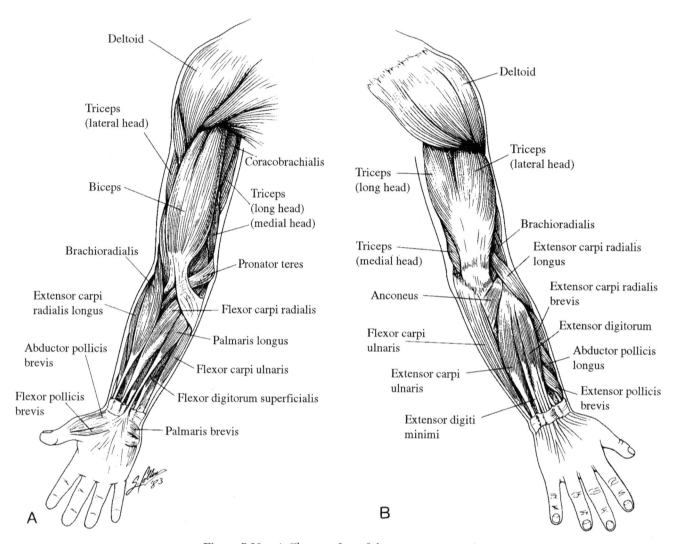

Figure 5.20.   **A**, Flexor surface of the upper extremity showing the various superficial muscles. **B**, Extensor surface of the upper extremity showing the various superficial muscles.

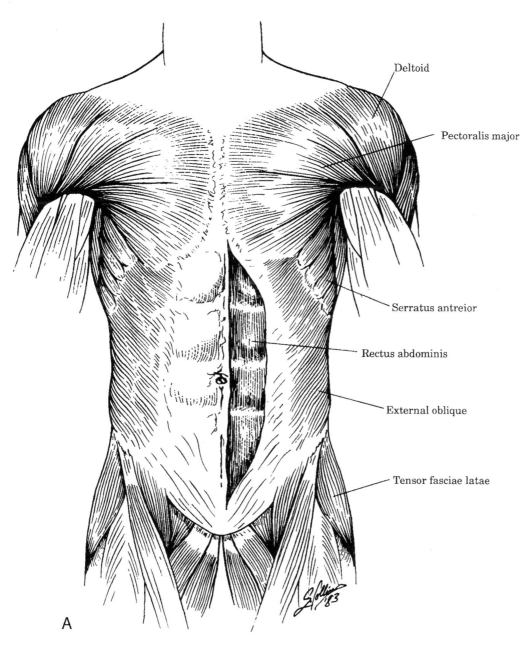

Figure 5.21. **A**, Anterior view of the trunk showing the superficial muscles. **B**, Posterior view of the trunk showing the superficial muscles.

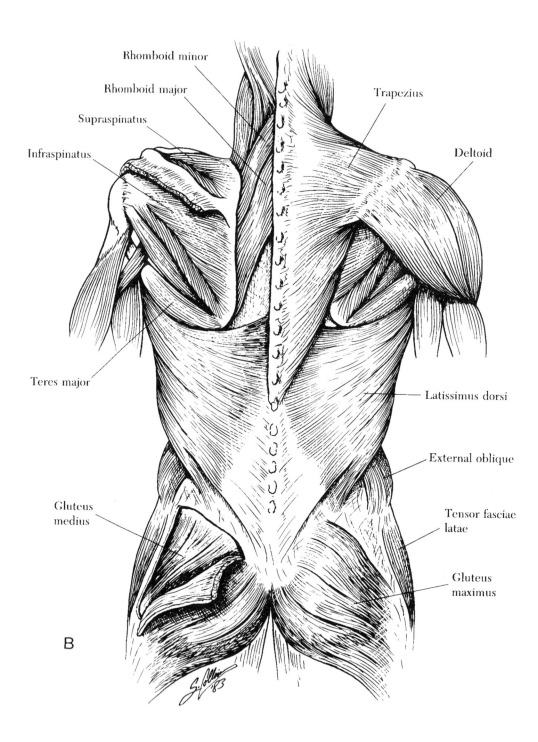

Rhomboid minor

Rhomboid major

Supraspinatus

Infraspinatus

Trapezius

Deltoid

Teres major

Latissimus dorsi

External oblique

Tensor fasciae latae

Gluteus medius

Gluteus maximus

B

Figure 5.21—*continued*

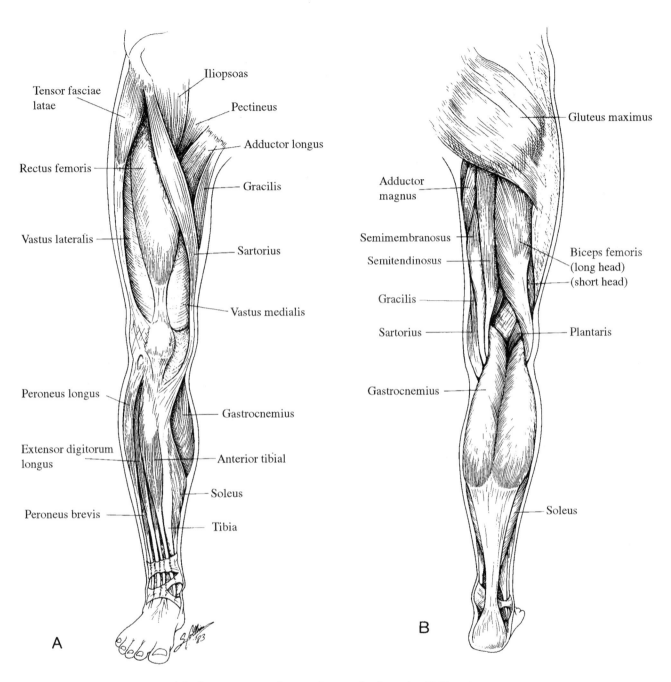

Figure 5.22. **A**, Anterior view of the lower extremity showing the superficial muscles. **B**, Posterior view of the lower extremity showing the superficial muscles.

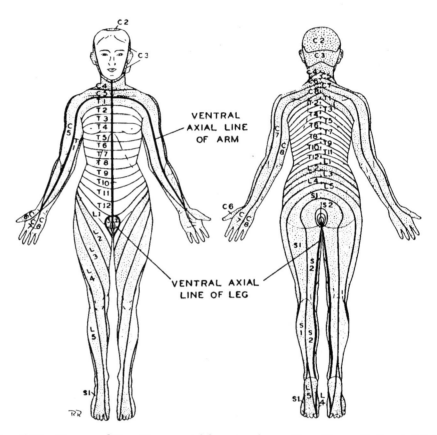

Figure 5.23.   Keegan and Garrett's segmental dermatomal map. (From Keegan JJ, Garrett FD. The segmental distribution of the cutaneous nerves in the limbs of man. Anat Record 1948;102:411).

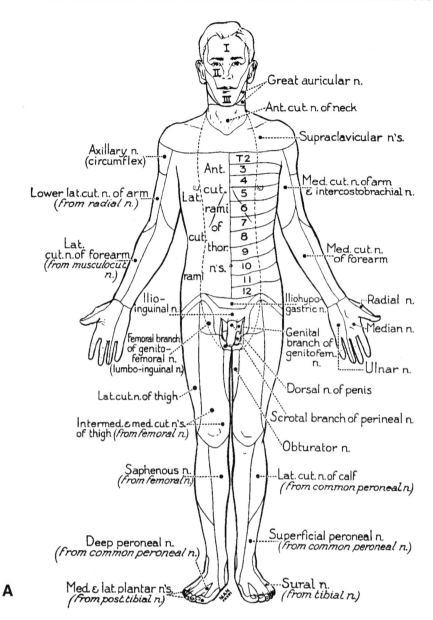

Figure 5.24. **A**, Sensory territory of the peripheral nerves from the anterior aspect. The numbers on the left side of the trunk refer to the intercostal nerves. On the right side are the sensory territories of the lateral and medial branches of the anterior primary rami. The asterisk just beneath the scrotum is in the field of the posterior cutaneous nerve of the thigh. (From Haymaker W, Woodhall B. Peripheral nerve injuries: principles of diagnosis. Philadelphia: WB Saunders, 1953:43.) **B**, Sensory territory of the peripheral nerves from the lateral aspect. The face and anterior half of the head are innervated by the three divisions of the trigeminal: I, ophthalmic; II, maxillary; III, mandibular. The territory of the intercostal nerves are indicated by numerals. The unlabeled territory between great and second toe is supplied by the deep peroneal nerve. (From Haymaker W, Woodhall B. Peripheral nerve injuries: principles of diagnosis. Philadelphia: WB Saunders, 1953:42.) **C**, Sensory territory of the peripheral nerves from the posterior aspect. The boundaries of the sensory territory of the posterior primary rami are indicated by *broken lines.* The designations *Post. cuta. rami of thora. n's* refer to the cutaneous branches of the posterior primary rami; *Lat cut. rami* indicates the distribution from the lateral branches of the anterior primary rami. For purposes of orientation the spinous processes of the first thoracic (T1), the first lumbar (L1) and the first sacral (S1) vertebrae are indicated by *arrows.* (From Haymaker W, Woodhall B. Peripheral nerve injuries: principles of diagnosis. Philadelphia: WB Saunders, 1953:40.)

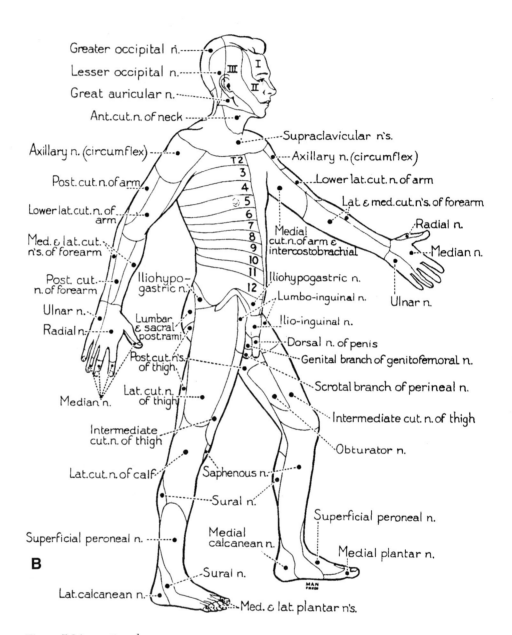

Greater occipital n.

Lesser occipital n.

Great auricular n.

Ant. cut. n. of neck

Axillary n. (circumflex)

Post. cut. n. of arm

Lower lat. cut. n. of arm

Med. & lat. cut. n's. of forearm

Post. cut. n. of forearm

Iliohypogastric n.

Ulnar n.

Radial n.

Lumbar & sacral post. rami.

Post. cut. n's. of thigh

Median n.

Lat. cut. n. of thigh

Intermediate cut. n. of thigh

Lat. cut. n. of calf

Superficial peroneal n.

Lat. calcanean n.

Supraclavicular n's.

Axillary n. (circumflex)

Lower lat. cut. n. of arm

Lat. & med. cut. n's. of forearm

Radial n.

Medial cut. n. of arm & intercostobrachial

Median n.

Iliohypogastric n.

Ulnar n.

Lumbo-inguinal n.

Ilio-inguinal n.

Dorsal n. of penis

Genital branch of genitofemoral n.

Scrotal branch of perineal n.

Intermediate cut. n. of thigh

Obturator n.

Saphenous n.

Sural n.

Superficial peroneal n.

Medial calcanean n.

Medial plantar n.

Sural n.

Med. & lat. plantar n's.

T2
3
4
5
6
7
8
9
10
11
12

III
I
II

B

Figure 5.24—*continued*

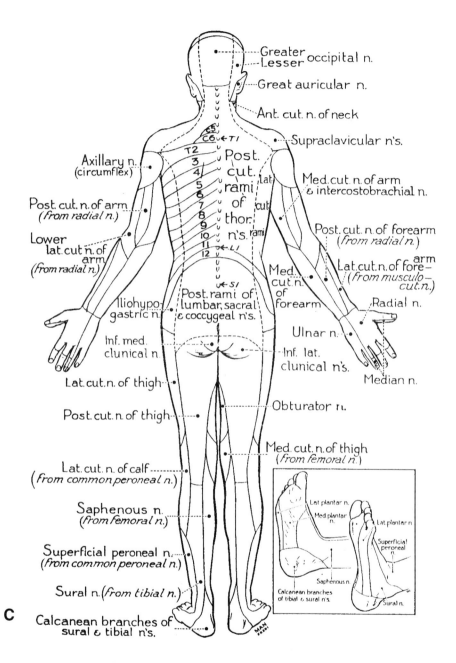

C

Figure 5.24—*continued*

Required Tests for Specific Problems

The following guidelines are offered for the workup of specific problems. In our laboratory, electromyography (EMG) technicians automatically use these instructions for the specific problems listed whenever the physician decides that the workups for such problems are needed. Nerve conduction tests are selected for their maximal yield and should be considered minimal workups. Additional tests are performed depending on the findings and needs of individual patients. For other conditions, the physician-electromyographer usually is involved in the actual testing because the procedures are too complex for the EMG technician to perform.

When a needle EMG study is indicated for specific problems, the physician-electromyographer should perform this test following specified guidelines. The needle EMG study will further clarify the nature and severity of the neuropathy.

Recently, the American Association of Electrodiagnostic Medicine (AAEM) published its guidelines for electrodiagnostic medical consultations (1). Its guidelines are somewhat different from ours.

Peripheral Neuropathy (Polyneuropathy or Polyneuritis)

Nerve conduction studies in one upper extremity and both lower extremities are required in patients with peripheral neuropathy. The test should include: (*a*) motor, sensory, and mixed nerve conduction in one ulnar and one median nerve; (*b*) sensory nerve conduction in bilateral sural nerves; (*c*) motor nerve conduction in bilateral peroneal and posterior tibial nerves; and (*d*) F-waves in median, ulnar, peroneal, and posterior tibial nerves.

The needle EMG is recommended in at least two distal muscles and one proximal leg muscle to document a distal-proximal involvement. If polyneuroradiculopathy is suspected, the needle EMG in the paraspinal muscles is mandatory to confirm root involvement.

Findings. Because peripheral neuropathy is diffuse and predominantly involves the distal portion of the nerves, the abnormality is also diffuse and more prominent in the distal segments. Usually more than 50% of the nerves tested show abnormal nerve conduction findings. In some cases only a few nerves tested show abnormalities. When the proximal segment of peripheral nerves is affected, the F-wave may show the sole abnormalities.

AAEM Guidelines. The nerve conduction study should include motor conduction in a distal nerve in a leg and a distal nerve in an arm, sensory nerve conduction of two distal nerves, and H-reflex and/or F-wave studies in one leg. The needle EMG should be performed in at least one distal muscle in each leg and in a distal muscle in one arm.

Carpal Tunnel Syndrome

The test for carpal tunnel syndrome should include motor, sensory, and mixed nerve conduction in the median and ulnar nerves in the symptomatic arm. If carpal tunnel syndrome is confirmed in the symptomatic arm, the terminal latency and sensory nerve conduction should be checked over the finger-wrist and palm-wrist segments in the opposite arm. Special attention should be paid to the terminal latency and to the sensory nerve conduction over finger-wrist and palm-wrist segments of the median nerves. *It is very important to standardize the distance (5 cm)* between the active recording electrode and the stimulating electrode at the wrist in the terminal latency study.

If the sensory nerve conduction studies in the II digit-wrist and palm-wrist segments are normal, the sensory nerve conduction should also be tested in the I digit-wrist and III digit-wrist segments before concluding that there is no electrophysiological evidence of carpal tunnel syndrome. The needle EMG test in the abductor pollicis brevis or opponens pollicis muscle is recommended to document whether there is any secondary axonal degeneration.

Findings. Since carpal tunnel syndrome is due to compression of the median nerve at the carpal tunnel (the wrist), typical findings are: (*a*) absent sensory nerve potentials or slow sensory nerve conduction velocity (NCV) over the finger-wrist segment; and (*b*) prolonged terminal latency. In mild cases the abnormalities in sensory NCV over the finger-wrist and palm-wrist (carpal tunnel) segments are the sole abnormalities; the terminal latency is usually normal. Carpal tunnel syndrome is bilateral in 32% of the cases (2). For this reason, the opposite median nerve must be tested when carpal tunnel syndrome is confirmed on one side.

AAEM Guidelines. The nerve conduction study should include motor nerve conduction in the median nerve (below the elbow) and sensory nerve conduction in the digit-wrist segments of the median and ulnar nerves. If the sensory nerve conduction in the digit-wrist segment of the median nerve is normal, the palm-wrist segment should be included. If the median distal motor latency is prolonged, the distal motor latency of at least the ulnar nerve should be tested. For the needle EMG the test in a median-innervated hand and forearm muscle is recommended. If there are EMG abnormalities in median innervated hand muscle, an ulnar-innervated intrinsic hand muscle should also be examined.

Ulnar Compression Neuropathy at the Elbow (Tardy Ulnar Nerve Palsy or Cubital Tunnel Syndrome)

The tests for ulnar compression neuropathy at the elbow should include motor, sensory, and mixed nerve conduction in the median and ulnar nerves in the symptomatic arm. Special attention should be paid to the motor NCV across the elbow. *The distance across the elbow in the extended arm should be 9–10 cm.* In some EMG laboratories, a distance of 10 cm with the arm flexed is recommended. If the latter method is used, the values obtained must be compared with the normal NCV values for that method. If an ulnar neuropathy is confirmed on one side, the opposite extremity must be tested because ulnar neuropathy is bilateral in 39% of cases (3).

To distinguish tardy ulnar nerve palsy (trans-sulcal compression) from cubital tunnel syndrome, the ulnar nerve across the elbow segment should be studied by the short-segmental incremental method (inching technique). For the needle EMG, the test in the abductor digiti quinti or first dorsal interosseous muscle and the flexor carpi ulnar muscle is recommended to document whether there is any secondary axonal degeneration.

Findings. Tardy ulnar nerve palsy is caused by compression of the ulnar nerve at the elbow sulcus. Typical findings are: (*a*) slow motor NCV across the elbow; and (*b*) slow NCV or absent nerve potential in mixed nerve conduction over the elbow-wrist segment and in sensory nerve conduction over the finger-wrist segment. In milder cases, the abnormalities in the mixed and sensory NCV studies may be the sole findings.

In cubital tunnel syndrome the most prominent nerve conduction abnormalities are noted in the segment 2–4 cm distal to the epicondyline line, while in tardy ulnar nerve palsy, the most prominent nerve conduction abnormalities are noted in the segment 2 cm distal or proximal to the epicondyline line.

Thoracic Outlet Syndrome

The tests for thoracic outlet syndrome should include (*a*) motor, sensory, and mixed nerve conduction; and (*b*) F-waves in the ulnar and median nerves in the symptomatic arm. Motor and mixed nerve conduction across the thoracic outlet (the axilla to Erb's point) in the ulnar nerve should be tested. Special attention should be paid to measuring the distance between these two points. We recommend that this measurement be performed with a sharpened obstetrical caliper with the arm in an extended position and at an angle of 45° from the side of the chest. We have found the mixed nerve conduction across the thoracic outlet segment to be more reliable than the motor nerve conduction because of the many technical difficulties encountered in stimulating the nerve over the Erb's point with the surface electrode. If the motor nerve conduction shows slowing and the mixed NCV is normal, the test should be repeated; these results are most likely caused by technical difficulties that result from the inability to stimulate the nerve because of the profuse subcutaneous fat deposits over this area in obese individuals. The needle EMG test in the abductor digiti quinti, flexor carpi ulnaris, and abductor pollicis brevis or opponens pollicis muscles is recommended to document the extent of denervation.

Findings. Considering the number of patients who are referred to the EMG laboratory to rule out this disorder, positive nerve conduction abnormalities are rare and are seen only in patients with neurological abnormalities (neurogenic thoracic outlet syndrome). In patients with neurogenic abnormalities the classical findings are sensory and mixed nerve conduction abnormalities over the entire segment including the Erb's point-axilla segment, prolonged F-wave latency in the ulnar nerve, and low CMAP amplitude in the median nerve. In nonneurogenic cases, nerve conduction tests are more helpful in ruling out carpal tunnel syndrome and ulnar compression neuropathy at the elbow.

Peroneal Nerve Palsy

The tests for peroneal nerve palsy should include motor nerve conduction in the peroneal and posterior tibial nerves in the symptomatic leg and sensory nerve conduction in the superficial peroneal nerve. *The segmental nerve conduction across the fibular head (below the fibular head-popliteal fossa) should also be included.* The needle EMG test in the anterior tibialis, peroneus longus, and extensor digitorum brevis muscles is recommended to document the extent of denervation and the presence of a secondary axonal degeneration.

Findings. Because the compression is usually across the fibular head, slow motor NCV across the fibular head and abnormal sensory nerve conduction in the superficial peroneal nerve are typical findings. *When stimulating the peroneal nerve at the popliteal fossa, the movement of the great toe should be observed.* If it moves toward the head, the peroneal nerve is being stimulated. When the posterior tibial nerve is being stimulated, the toe moves away from the head.

Bell's Palsy

The tests for Bell's palsy should include: (*a*) motor nerve conduction; and (*b*) nerve excitability tests of bilateral facial nerves. In the latter tests, special attention should be given to minimal twitching of the distal facial muscles, e.g., the orbicularis oculi or orbicularis oris. When this occurs, the intensity (strength) of the stimulus should be recorded in milliamperes. We recommend three tests on each side. The mean value of the three tests should be the intensity reading. In motor nerve conduction tests, special attention should be given to the distance between the stimulating and recording electrodes so that this distance is equal on both sides.

Findings. If there is a 4 mA or greater difference in the nerve excitability test between the symptomatic and asymptomatic sides, it usually means that partial nerve degeneration is present in the symptomatic facial nerve. The absence of any response beyond 20 mA indicates complete nerve degeneration. Terminal latency is rarely prolonged in facial nerve palsy, although the amplitude of the compound muscle action potential (CMAP) is usually lower in the paralyzed facial muscle. A reduction of the amplitude of the CMAP to 5% or less of normal is indicative of poor prognosis in Bell's palsy.

Plexopathy

For brachial plexopathy, the tests should include motor, sensory, and mixed nerve conduction in the median and ulnar nerves and sensory nerve conduction in the musculocutaneous and radial nerves in the symptomatic arm. For proximal brachial plexopathy, the latency test to the shoulder girdle muscles is required. For lumbo sacral plexopathy, the tests should include motor nerve conduction in the peroneal and posterior tibial nerves and sensory nerve conduction in the sural and superficial peroneal nerves. If proximal lumbar plexopathy is suspected, the motor nerve conduction in the femoral nerve and the sensory nerve conduction in the saphenous nerve are required. For the needle EMG, an extensive test in muscles innervated by the various nerves and the paraspinal muscles is recommended to localize the lesion clearly.

Findings. With distal plexopathy, nerve conduction findings in many commonly tested nerves are abnormal. _Abnormal sensory nerve conduction is the most important finding indicative of a plexus neuropathy_ in contrast to normal sensory nerve conduction in radiculopathy. With proximal brachial plexopathy, the latency to the shoulder girdle muscles is often prolonged and sensory nerve conduction in the musculocutaneous nerve is often abnormal. However, the needle EMG study is usually more fruitful in localizing the plexopathy than is the nerve conduction study.

Nerve Conduction Studies for Hemodialysis Patients or Renal Transplantation Patients

Testing for nerve conduction in chronic renal failure patients on hemodialysis or with renal transplantation should include: (_a_) motor, sensory and mixed nerve conduction in the median and ulnar nerves in one arm; (_b_) sensory nerve conduction in the sural nerve; and (_c_) motor nerve conduction in the peroneal and posterior tibial nerves in one leg. The same side should be tested each time the patient is seen because it is important to compare the nerve conduction results. It is usually a good idea to check the arm opposite the arteriovenous fistula. It is important to standardize the skin temperature when doing serial tests.

Findings. Peripheral neuropathy is very common in patients with renal failure who are on chronic hemodialysis or undergoing renal transplantation, and so many nerves show nerve conduction abnormalities including slowing of the NCV. With improvement of renal function, the nerve conduction also improves.

Radiculopathy

For cervical radiculopathy, the tests should include motor, sensory, and mixed nerve conduction in the median and ulnar nerves in the symptomatic arm. For lumbosacral radiculopathy, the tests should include motor conduction in the peroneal, posterior tibial, and sensory nerve conductions in the sural nerve of the symptomatic leg. The H-reflex on gastrocnemius-soleus muscle in both legs is also included in the workup for lumbosacral radiculopathy. The F-wave study in the tested motor nerves should also be performed. The needle EMG test for cervical radiculopathy should include cervical paraspinal, supraspinatus, deltoid, biceps, triceps, pronator teres, abductor pollicis brevis, and first dorsal interosseus muscles. For lumbar radiculopathy, the EMG test should include lumbar paraspinal, gluteus, vastus lateralis, anterior tibialis, peroneus longus, and gastrocnemius muscles. *The paraspinal EMG study is most important since an abnormal test can definitely localize the lesion to the roots.* The needle EMG study in the limb muscles is designed to test two muscles innervated by one root but by two different peripheral nerves so that it can better localize the lesion to the root.

Findings. With classical radiculopathy, the nerve conduction findings are usually normal. However, a low CMAP amplitude or prolonged F-wave latency may be observed in radiculopathy when it is severe or when multiple roots are involved. These tests are performed to rule out any neuropathy that may mimic radiculopathy. The H-reflex on the gastrocnemius-soleus muscle may be absent or prolonged in latency on the involved side in S1 radiculopathy.

AAEM Guidelines. At least one motor and sensory conduction study, preferably of a symptomatic area, should be performed in a clinically involved limb. The needle EMG should include the testing of sufficient muscles such that a radiculopathy can either be defined or would be most likely from the electrodiagnostic information.

Anterior Horn Cell Diseases

The tests for anterior horn cell diseases should include: (*a*) motor, sensory, and mixed nerve conduction in the median and ulnar nerves in one arm; (*b*) sensory nerve conduction in the sural nerve; and (*c*) motor nerve conduction in the peroneal and posterior tibial nerves in one leg. The F-wave study in the tested motor nerves should also be included. The needle EMG is recommended in three muscles innervated by different nerves and roots in at least three limbs (cranial muscles count as one limb). This is to document *the widespread denervation process* that is typical of anterior horn cell disease.

Findings. In classical cases of anterior horn cell diseases, nerve conductions are relatively normal. Sensory and mixed nerve conductions should be normal. The amplitude of the CMAP is often low, and the F-wave latency is often prolonged. This test is performed to rule out demyelinating neuropathy, which can mimic anterior horn cell diseases, e.g., amyotrophic lateral sclerosis.

AAEM Guidelines. At least one motor and one sensory conduction study should be performed in at least two clinically involved limbs. If possible, motor conduction studies should be in the distribution of nerves innervating clinically weak muscles and/or muscles with EMG abnormalities. The needle EMG should be performed in at least two muscles innervated by different nerves and roots in at least three limbs, or two limbs and cranial muscles, as well as a paraspinal muscle in at least one limb. These studies should focus on clinically involved limbs and muscles and sample distal and proximal muscles.

Floppy Infant Syndrome

The tests for floppy infant syndrome should include: (*a*) motor, sensory, and mixed nerve conduction in the median nerve in one arm; (*b*) sensory nerve conduction in the sural nerve; and (*c*) motor nerve conduction in the peroneal and posterior tibial nerves in one leg. The needle EMG test in anterior tibialis and vastus lateralis or iliopsoas muscles is recommended. In our experience, if the nature of floppy infant syndrome cannot be determined with a needle EMG in these muscles, further study is usually unfruitful.

Findings. One cause of floppy infant syndrome is peripheral neuropathy. This can be confirmed or ruled out by the nerve conduction tests. If peripheral neuropathy is diagnosed by these tests, the more painful EMG test can often be omitted in children.

Myopathy

The tests for myopathy should include: (*a*) motor, sensory, and mixed nerve conduction in one median nerve; (*b*) sensory nerve conduction in one sural nerve; and (*c*) motor nerve conduction in one peroneal nerve. The needle EMG test is recommended in deltoid, biceps, iliopsoas, and vastus lateralis muscles since myopathy preferentially involves proximal muscles.

Findings. Nerve conduction should be normal in patients with pure myopathy. However, with many myopathies—including myotonic dystrophy, hypothyroidism, carcinomatous neuromyopathy, sarcoidosis, and polymyositis associated with systemic necrotizing vasculitis—peripheral neuropathy is present concomitantly. If any of these tests is abnormal, a peripheral neuropathy workup should be performed.

AAEM Guidelines. At least one motor conduction velocity and one sensory conduction study in a clinically involved limb should be performed. An adequate study would require EMG examination of muscles in at least two limbs, including a proximal and distal muscle in a clinically involved limb.

Other Disorders

For all other disorders, the EMG technicians must follow detailed instructions from the physician.

REFERENCES

1. American Association of Electrodiagnostic Medicine. Guidelines in electrodiagnostic medicine. Muscle Nerve 1992;15:229–253.
2. Thomas JE, Lambert EH, Dseuz KA. Motor nerve conduction in the carpal tunnel syndrome. Neurology 1967;10:1045–1050.
3. Harmon RL. Bilaterality of ulnar neuropathy at the elbow. EMG Clin Neurophysiol 1991;31:195–198.

7

Normal Values for Common Nerve Conduction Tests

EMG Laboratory, Medical Center of the University of Alabama at Birmingham: Normal Nerve Conduction Data

The data in this part of the chapter were collected with surface recording and stimulating electrodes from 40 normal controls between the ages of 20 and 60 years, following the technical and anatomical guidelines discussed in Chapters 4 and 5. The skin temperature was above 31° C in all controls and was usually between 31° and 34° C.

When the values obtained varied by more than 2 standard deviations (SD) from the mean values, they were considered abnormal in the studies of latency, nerve conduction velocity (NCV), and duration of the compound muscle and nerve action potentials (CMAPs, CNAPs). For the amplitude of the CMAP and CNAP, values below the lowest normal value were considered to be abnormal.

These normal data are applicable to patients between the ages of 20 and 60 years. Above age 60, 1 m/sec per decade for the motor NCV and 2 m/sec per decade for the sensory NCV should be allowed when interpreting the results (Tables 7.1–7.10).

Table 7.1.
Median Motor Nerve Conduction

| Parameter | Terminal Latency (msec) | NCV (M/sec) | | CMAP | |
		Elbow–Wrist	Axilla–Elbow	Duration (msec)	Amplitude (mV)
Mean ± SD	2.78 ± 0.41	58.78 ± 4.41	65.76 ± 4.90	12.58 ± 1.68	14.62 ± 8.45
Normal limit	3.60	49.96	55.96	15.94	5.00

Table 7.2.
Median Sensory Nerve Conduction

Segment	NCV (m/sec)		CNAP	
	Onset	Peak	Duration (msec)	Amplitude (µV)
Digit II–wrist				
Mean ± SD	60.88 ± 5.07	49.54 ± 4.14	1.57 ± 0.39	30.93 ± 12.07
Normal limit	50.74	41.26	2.35	10.00
Palm–wrist				
Mean ± SD	58.60 ± 6.00	41.85 ± 3.90	1.16 ± 0.33	71.38 ± 37.92
Normal limit	46.60	34.05	1.82	10.00

Table 7.3.
Median Mixed Nerve Conduction

Segment	NCV (m/sec)		CNAP	
	Onset	Peak	Duration (msec)	Amplitude (µV)
Wrist–elbow				
Mean ± SD	64.47 ± 4.28	55.99 ± 3.30	1.58 ± 0.38	32.05 ± 16.28
Normal limit	55.91	49.39	2.34	10.00
Elbow–axilla				
Mean ± SD	74.83 ± 4.78	63.47 ± 4.76	1.48 ± 0.39	44.53 ± 18.96
Normal limit	65.27	53.95	2.26	10.00

Table 7.4.
Ulnar Motor Nerve Conduction

Parameter	NCV (m/sec)					CMAP	
	Terminal Latency (msec)	Elbow–Wrist	Elbow	Axilla–Elbow	Erb's Point–Axilla	Duration (msec)	Amplitude (mV)
Mean ± SD	2.03 ± 0.24	61.15 ± 5.27	51.31 ± 5.25	63.33 ± 5.47	68.36 ± 5.07	13.43 ± 1.61	11.49 ± 2.51
Normal limit	2.52	50.61	42.81	52.69	58.22	16.63	5

Table 7.5.
Ulnar Sensory Nerve (Digit V-Wrist Segment)

Parameter	NCV (m/sec)		CNAP	
	Onset	Peak	Duration (msec)	Amplitude (µV)
Mean ± SD	60.93 ± 5.17	47.48 ± 4.11	1.23 ± 0.38	22.74 ± 14.43
Normal limit	50.59	39.26	1.99	8.00

Table 7.6.
Ulnar Mixed Nerve Conduction

Segment	NCV (m/sec)		CNAP	
	Onset	Peak	Duration (msec)	Amplitude (µV)
Wrist–elbow				
Mean ± SD	68.35 ± 4.55	55.44 ± 3.99	1.77 ± 0.38	33.20 ± 14.83
Normal limit	59.25	47.46	2.53	10.00
Elbow–Axilla				
Mean ± SD	73.07 ± 5.76	57.15 ± 4.48	1.43 ± 0.39	34.83 ± 18.11
Normal limit	61.55	48.18	2.21	10.00
Axilla–Erb's point				
Mean ± SD		64.09 ± 5.64		27.56 ± 14.16
Normal limit		52.81		10.00

Table 7.7.
Radial Sensory Nerve Conduction (Distal Segment)

| Parameter | NCV (m/sec) | | CNAP | |
	Onset	Peak	Duration (msec)	Amplitude (μV)
Mean ± SD	67.08 ± 5.35	50.87 ± 3.28	1.19 ± 0.14	31.06 ± 8.66
Normal limit	56.38	44.31	1.47	10.00

Table 7.8.
Peroneal Motor Nerve Conduction[a]

| Parameter | Terminal Latency (msec) | NCV (m/sec) | | CNAP | |
		FibH-Ank	PopF-FibH	Duration (msec)	Amplitude (mV)
Mean ± SD	3.72 ± 0.53	49.51 ± 3.93	53.93 ± 7.11	11.84 ± 2.22	10.09 ± 4.81
Normal limit	4.78	41.65	39.11	16.28	4.00

[a]*Abbreviations:* FibH-Ank, fibular head-ankle; PopF-FibH, popliteal fossa-fibular head.

Table 7.9.
Posterior Tibial Motor Nerve Conduction

| Parameter | Terminal Latency (msec) | NCV: Popliteal Fossa–Ankle (m/sec) | CMAP | |
			Duration (msec)	Amplitude (mV)
Mean ± SD	3.85 ± 0.63	49.83 ± 4.60	12.30 ± 3.26	19.06 ± 7.23
Normal limit	5.11	40.63	18.82	5.00

Table 7.10.
Sural Sensory Nerve Conduction (Mid-calf–Lateral Malleolus Segment)

| NCV (m/sec) | | CNAP | | Latency (msec)[a] | |
Onset	Peak	Duration (msec)	Amplitude (μV)	Onset	Peak
54.48 ± 5.16[b]	43.26 ± 4.29	1.72 ± 0.52	18.12 ± 8.27	2.46 ± 0.32	3.17 ± 0.32
44.16[c]	34.68	2.76	6.00	3.10	3.81

[a]Distance is set at 14 cm.
[b]Mean ± SD.
[c]Normal limit.

Normal F-Wave Latencies

The F-wave latencies are proportional to the patient's height. Therefore the values in patients should be compared with the height-adjusted normal values (Table 7.11; Figs. 7.1–7.4).

The predicted values of the F-wave latencies from distal stimulation can be calculated by using the following formulas:

$$\text{Median F-wave latency (msec)} = 0.183 \times \text{height (cm)} - 4.81$$
$$2\,\text{SD} = 3.10$$
$$\text{Ulnar F-wave latency (msec)} = 0.202 \times \text{height (cm)} - 8.51$$
$$2\,\text{SD} = 3.82$$
$$\text{Peroneal F-wave latency (msec)} = 0.323 \times \text{height (cm)} - 8.61$$
$$2\,\text{SD} = 4.70$$
$$\text{Posterior tibial F-wave latency (msec)} = 0.436 \times \text{height (cm)} - 27.01$$
$$2\,\text{SD} = 6.22$$

The upper normal limit of the F-wave latency is 2 SD above the predicted value.

Table 7.11.
Normal Values of F-wave Latency and H-reflex

Nerves	Mean ± SD (msec)	Normal Limit (msec)
Median nerve	25.32 ± 2.19	29.70
Ulnar nerve	25.68 ± 2.29	30.26
Peroneal nerve	46.88 ± 4.25	55.38
Posterior tibial nerve	48.89 ± 4.19	57.27
H-reflex on the gastrocnemius-soleus muscle	28.02 ± 1.95	31.93

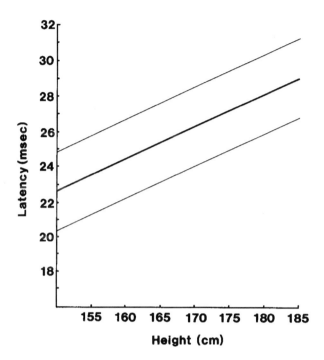

Figure 7.1. F-wave latencies in median nerves with distal stimulation. The *thick line* is the regression line; the *thin lines* indicate the normal limits (2 SD from the regression line).

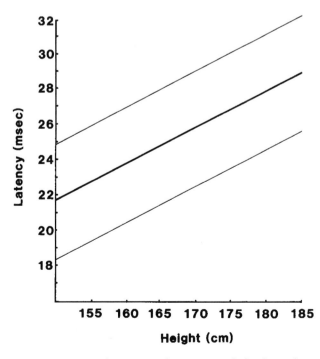

Figure 7.2. F-wave latencies in ulnar nerves with distal stimulation.

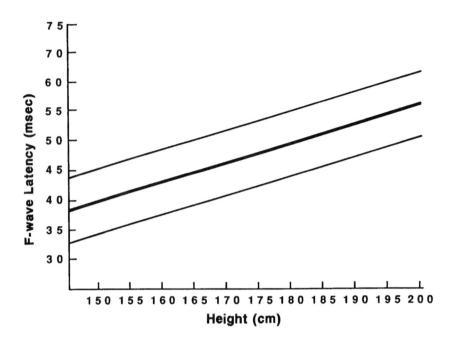

Figure 7.3.   F-wave latencies in peroneal nerves with distal stimulation.

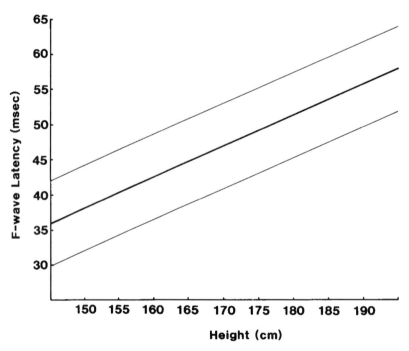

Figure 7.4.   F-wave latencies in posterior tibial nerves with distal stimulation.

Normal H-Reflex Latencies in the Gastrocnemius-Soleus Muscle

H-reflex latencies are dependent on height. The values in patients should be compared with the height-adjusted normal values (Table 7.11; Fig. 7.5). The predicted normal values can be calculated by using the following formula:

$$\text{H-reflex latency (msec)} = 3.013 + (0.146 \times \text{height in cm})$$
$$2\,SD = 3.1$$

The normal upper limit of the H-reflex latency is 2 SD above the predicted value.

Normal Values for Difference Between the Distal and Proximal Motor Nerve Conduction Parameters

Conduction block and abnormal temporal dispersion are two electrophysiological hallmarks of demyelination. To define the conduction block, an amplitude or area in the distal CMAP has to be compared with those in the proximal CMAP. To define the abnormal temporal dispersion, the duration of the CMAP has to be compared either with that of normal CMAP or the duration of the proximal CMAP has to be compared with the distal CMAP.

Normal limits of the difference in the amplitude, area, and duration are shown in Table 7.12. These values are the summary of data obtained in the motor nerve conduction in the median, ulnar, peroneal, and posterior tibial nerves in 40 normal controls between the ages of 20 and 60 years. The skin temperature was above 31° C in all controls and was usually between 31° C and 34° C.

Amplitude, duration and area of the CMAP were measured by the automated computerized program (Fig. 4.2). In amplitude, the negative-peak, positive-peak, and peak-to-peak amplitudes were measured. In duration, the negative duration, positive duration, and total duration were measured. In area, the negative area, positive area, and total area were measured.

Conduction block is defined to be present, when the distal-proximal amplitude or area difference are outside of the normal limits (> normal mean + 2 SD) (Table 7.12).

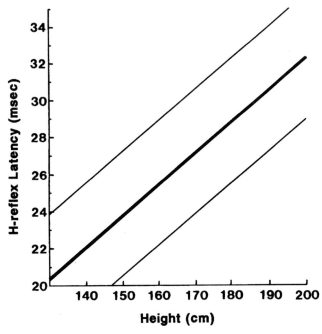

Figure 7.5. H-reflex latencies from the gastrocnemius-soleus muscle.

Table 7.12.
Normal Values for "Conduction Block" and "Temporal Dispersion"

Parameters	Mean	Standard Deviation	Normal Limit
Area (criteria for conduction block)			
Median, ulnar, peroneal nerves			
Total area	1.5	11.4	24%
Negative area	3.0	11.1	25%
Positive area	11.2	10.7	33%
Posterior tibial nerve			
Total area	10.8	9.1	29%
Negative area	4.3	10.3	25%
Positive area	13.8	12.1	38%
Amplitude (criteria for conduction block)			
Median, ulnar, peroneal nerves			
Peak-peak amplitude	10.2	7.3	25%
Negative-peak amplitude	10.9	9.8	30%
Positive-peak amplitude	7.9	12.9	34%
Posterior tibial nerve			
Peak-peak amplitude	22.6	6.7	36%
Negative-peak amplitude	24.5	8.4	41%
Positive-peak amplitude	17.8	10.2	38%
Duration (criteria for temporal dispersion compared with the normal CMAP duration)			
Distal CMAP			
Total duration	20.7	5.0	31 msec
Negative duration	5.8	0.7	7 msec
Positive duration	15.18	4.3	24 msec
Proximal CMAP			
Total duration	24.2	5.4	35 msec
Negative duration	6.0	0.9	8 msec
Positive duration	18.1	5.3	29 msec
Proximal-distal difference of duration (criteria for temporal dispersion compared with proximal segment)			
Median, ulnar and peroneal nerves			
Total duration	5.0	10.8	27%
Negative duration	2.4	8.7	20%
Positive duration	5.6	15.0	36%
Posterior tibial nerve			
Total duration	4.3	14.2	33%
Negative duration	10.5	9.6	30%
Positive duration	3.0	21.6	46%

Abnormal temporal dispersion is defined to be present when the distal-proximal duration difference are outside of the normal limits (> normal mean + 2 SD) or when the duration of the CMAP duration is longer than the normal limits (> normal mean + 2 SD) (Table 7.12).

Laboratory of Clinical Neurophysiology, Rigshospitalet, Copenhagen: Normal Nerve Conduction Data

The data from the Laboratory of Clinical Neurophysiology, Rigshospitalet, in Copenhagen, presented here, have been summarized from their book (1). Their motor and sensory nerve conduction studies are different from ours in three respects. In their studies:

1. Needles were used as stimulating and recording electrodes.
2. Temperature was controlled to 36–38°C.
3. Values obtained were compared with age-adjusted normal values.

The materials and methods used are described in their book (1).

Two factors are important when conduction along an abnormal nerve is compared with normal values: (*a*) control for age: findings in patients must be compared with those for normal subjects in the same age group; and (*b*) standardized recording conditions: temperature, type and position of electrodes, resolution of the potential in time and signal/noise ratio, and measurement of the distance of conduction, the conduction time, and the action potential parameters.

Subjects

Normal volunteer subjects without a history or signs or symptoms of involvement of the nerves examined were chosen. Data from the ulnar nerve distal to the wrist were obtained from 100 controls and 96 patients with carpal tunnel syndrome. Because there was no difference between patients and controls, the two groups were pooled.

Standardized Recording Conditions

The procedures for recording sensory and motor conduction have been described in Chapter 11 (2–13).

Temperature Near the Nerves

The temperature of the surface of the limb was kept within 36–38° C, corresponding to 35–37° C near the nerve. An infrared heating element (45 cm long, 500 W, controlled by a thermo-couple on the limb) was placed 20–30 cm above the extremity.

Electrode Type and Position

Sensory Nerve

Stimulation. At distal sites the nerves were stimulated percutaneously. The anode was placed around the distal phalanx of the finger or toe, and the cathode 20 mm proximal to it (median nerve at digit I or III, ulnar nerve at digit V, radial nerve at digit I, sural nerve at the dorsum pedis). When recording at the palm, fine platinum needles (0.3 mm in diameter) were used as cathodes placed subcutaneously at digit III. Similarly fine platinum needle electrodes were used as cathodes when stimulating the big toe and recording from the superficial peroneal or posterior tibial nerve.

At more proximal sites the nerves were stimulated by needle electrodes of the same dimensions as those used for recording. They were placed near the nerve (radial nerve at the wrist, musculocutaneous nerve at the elbow, axillary nerve at the regio deltoidei, sural nerve at the lateral malleolus, peroneal nerve at the retinaculum superior, posterior tibial nerve at the medial malleolus and saphenous nerve at the medial epicondyle).

To stimulate sensory fibers maximally via surface electrodes, the current pulse was 20–80 mA (0.2 msec in duration); the current pulse via needle electrodes was 5–10 mA. A further increase in stimulus current increased neither the amplitude nor the number of slow components in the response.

Recording. The recordings were done via needle electrodes (stainless steel, 0.7 mm in diameter). One electrode (bared tip 3 mm) was placed near the nerve such that the motor threshold was 0.5–1 mA (4). The remote electrode (bared tip 5 mm) was placed at the same level as the near-nerve electrode at a transverse distance of 3–4 cm. The impedance of the electrodes was reduced by passing an alternating current of 40 mA for 30 sec through the near-nerve electrode and of 80 mA for 30 sec through the remote electrode with the electrodes placed in a 0.9% NaCl solution at 90°C. The electrodes were kept in airtight plastic bags and sterilized by irradiation with neutrons because boiling or dry heat increased the impedance; they were discarded after being used once.

Motor Nerve

Stimulation. This was performed via the same needle electrodes as those used for recording the sensory potentials. The maximal stimulus current was 5–7 mA, or 10 times the weakest current which just evoked a muscle action potential.

Recording. This was by a concentric electrode (0.07 mm^2 tip area) placed in the end-plate zone or via an 80 μm stainless steel wire placed transversely near the center of the belly of the muscle.

Resolution in Time and in the Signal/Noise Ratio

The potentials were recorded at 2.5 or 5 msec/cm. At longer distances of conduction a delay of 4–20 msec was used between the stimulus and the recording to ascertain the same resolution in time.

Sensory potentials of less than 4 μV in amplitude and slow components were recorded by electronic averaging of 250, 500, 1000, 2000 or 4000 traces (1/sec). The interval between sampling points was 20 or 40 μsec.

Measurement

Sensory Nerve

The maximum sensory conduction velocity was determined from the latency of the initial positive peak of the potential. The minimum velocity along the sensory nerve was not determined unless the resolution of the recording was high enough to distinguish potentials 0.02 μV in amplitude.

To distinguish the late components in the sensory potential, the responses to 500–4000 stimuli were averaged and recorded. The criterion of identification was that a potential similar in shape and increased in amplitude with the number of responses roughly to the same extent was a calibration signal averaged together with the response. Isolated components or bursts following the main components of the potential was not considered.

The amplitude was measured peak to peak.

Motor Nerve

Motor Conduction Time. This was measured to the initial deflection from the baseline of the muscle action potential. The latencies measured (t_m) were corrected to a standard conduction distance (d_s) by means of the velocity recorded in the proximal segment of the nerve (v).

$$\text{Corrected latency} = t_m - \frac{(d - ds)}{v}$$

where d is the distance between the stimulating cathode and the recording electrode.

Amplitude of Action Potentials. This was recorded by concentric electrodes and was measured peak to peak. With wire electrodes placed in the end-plate zone, the shape of the potentials was usually diphasic with negative onset. The amplitude of the negative peak and the peak-to-peak amplitude were measured. Action potentials with positive onset or with negative onset and irregular shape were excluded from the material (15–30%).

Confidence Limits

For each segment of nerve, the data are presented in a table and a figure. The thick line in each figure is the regression line calculated by the method of least squares; the thin lines represent the 95%, and the dashed lines the 99% upper and lower confidence limits. The upper and lower limits in tables represent the 95% upper and lower confidence respectively (See Figures 7.6–7.9 and Tables 7.13–7.41).

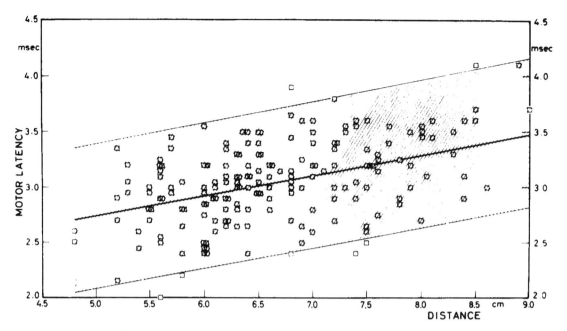

Figure 7.6. Terminal latencies of median nerves in relation to distance. Latencies are corrected to 50 years of age. The hatched area represents the 95% confidence range. From Buchthal F, Rosenfalck A, Trojaborg W. Electrophysiological findings in entrapment of the median nerve at wrist and elbow. J. Neurol Neurosurg Psychiatry 1974;37:342.

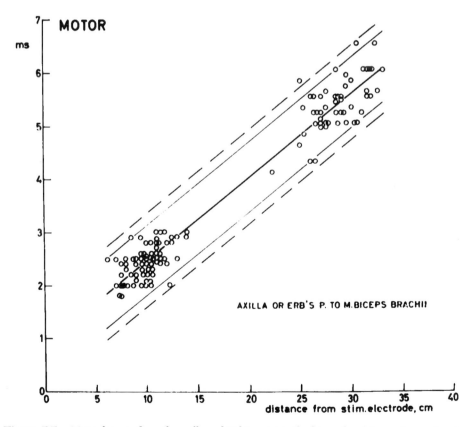

Figure 7.7. Motor latency from the axilla and Erb's point to the biceps brachii muscle as a function of distance. N =   121. From Laboratory of Clinical Neurophysiology, Rigshospitalet, Copenhagen. Electromyography: sensory and motor conduction. Findings in normal subjects; 1975:34.

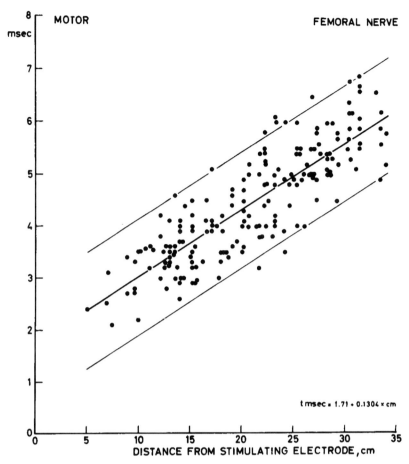

Figure 7.8. Motor latency of the femoral nerve as a function of distance. From Laboratory of Clinical Neurophysiology. Rigshospitalet, Copenhagen. Electromyography: sensory and motor conduction. Findings in normal subjects; 1975:43.

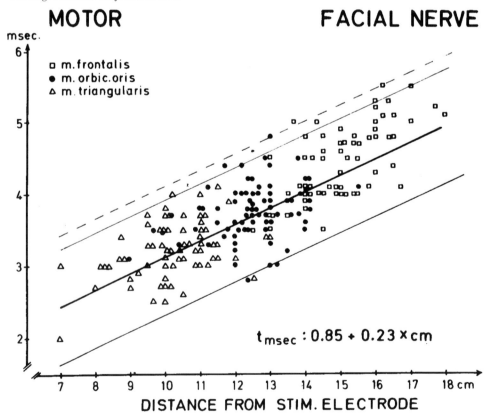

Figure 7.9. Motor latency of the facial nerve as a function of distance. From Laboratory of Clinical Neurophysiology. Rigshospitalet, Copenhagen. Electromyography: sensory and motor conduction. Findings in normal subjects; 1975:26.

Table 7.13.
Median Nerve: Motor Nerve Conduction[a]

Age Years	Terminal Latency (msec)[b]			Amplitude of CMAP (mV)		NCV Elbow–Wrist (msec)		
	Mean	Upper Limit	N	Mean	Lower Limit	Mean	Lower Limit	N
15–24	3.0	3.7	15	22	9	65	56	16
25–34	3.1	3.8	18	20	9	64	55	17
35–44	3.2	3.9	32	19	8	63	54	23
45–54	3.3	4.0	40	17	7	62	52	25
55–64	3.4	4.1	34	16	7	61	51	11
65–74	3.5	4.2	15	15	6	60	50	7
75–89	3.6	4.3	7	14	6	59	50	18

[a]The recording concentric needle is in the abductor pollicis brevis muscle.
N = number of controls.
[b]Latencies are corrected to a distance of 6.5 cm.

Table 7.14.
Median Nerve: Sensory NCV

Age Years	Digit I–Wrist (msec)			Digit III–Wrist (msec)			Wrist–Elbow (Digit III Stimulation) (msec)			Palm–Wrist (msec)			Digit III–Palm (msec)		
	Mean	Lower Limit	N	Mean	Lower Limit	N	Mean	Lower Limit	N	Mean	Lower Limit	N	Mean	Lower Limit	N
15–24	57	47	25	64	55	34	71	62	14						
25–34	55	46	18	62	53	21	68	60	14	64	54	3	63	56	3
35–44	54	44	35	60	51	35	66	57	15	62	52	3	61	54	3
45–54	52	43	45	58	49	46	64	55	22	60	51	9	59	53	9
55–64	51	41	38	57	48	40	62	53	9	58	49	5	58	51	5
65–74	49	40	16	55	46	16	60	51	6						
75–84	48	38	7	53	44	7	57	49	5						

Table 7.15.
Amplitude of Median Sensory CNAP

Age Years	Digit I–Wrist (µV)		Digit III–Wrist (µV)		Digit II–Elbow (µV)		Digit III–Palm (µV)	
	Mean	Lower Limit	Mean	Lower Limit	Mean	Lower Limit	Mean	Lower Limit
15–24	43	17	16	7	7.5	3		
25–34	37	15	14	6.5	7	2.5	25	13
35–44	33	13	13	6	6	2.5	24	14
45–54	29	12	11	5	5	2	22	11
55–64	25	10	10	4.5	4.5	2	21	10
65–74	22	9	9	4	4	1.5		
75–84	19	8	8	3.5	3.5	1.5		

Table 7.16.
Ulnar Nerve: Motor Nerve Conduction[a]

Age Years	Terminal Latency (msec)[b] Mean	Terminal Latency (msec)[b] Upper Limit	N	Amplitude of CMAP (mV) Mean	Amplitude of CMAP (mV) Lower Limit	5 cm Distal to Sulcus N. Ulnaris–Wrist (m/sec) Mean	5 cm Distal to Sulcus N. Ulnaris–Wrist (m/sec) Lower Limit	"Across" Sulcus n. Ulnaris (m/sec)[c] Mean	"Across" Sulcus n. Ulnaris (m/sec)[c] Lower Limit	5 cm Proximal to Sulcus n. Ulnaris–Wrist (m/sec) Mean	5 cm Proximal to Sulcus n. Ulnaris–Wrist (m/sec) Lower Limit	N
15–24	2.4	2.9	19	19	8	67	61	61	50	65	58	10
25–34	2.4	3.0	18	19	8	67	61	60	50	65	58	12
35–44	2.5	3.1	18	18	8	67	61	58	50	64	57	14
45–54	2.6	3.1	38	18	7	67	61	57	50	64	57	15
55–64	2.6	3.2	48	17	7	67	58	54	43	61	53	15
65–74	2.7	3.2	15	17	7	61	52	49	43	58	50	11
75–82	2.7	3.3	9	17						55	47	7

[a]The recording concentric needle is in the abductor digiti V.
[b]Latencies are corrected to a distance of 7 cm.
[c]From 5 cm proximal to 5 cm distal to the sulcus n. ulnaris.

Table 7.17.
Ulnar Motor Latency: To the Flexor Carpi Ulnaris from 5 cm Proximal to the Sulcus n. Ulnaris (Age 15–74)[a]

Distance (cm)	Latency (msec) Mean	Latency (msec) Upper Limit	N
9	2.6	3.2	2
10	2.8	3.4	3
11	2.9	3.5	15
12	3.0	3.6	10
13	3.2	3.8	15
14	3.3	3.9	15
15	3.4	4.0	8

[a]Amplitude: mean 14 mV, lower limit 6 mV

Table 7.18.
Ulnar Motor Latency to the Adductor Pollicis Muscle from the Wrist

Age Years	N	Latency[a] (msec) Mean	Latency[a] (msec) Upper Limit	Amplitude to CMAP (mV) Mean	Amplitude to CMAP (mV) Lower Limit
15–24	4	3.1	3.8	20	8
25–34	10	3.2	3.9	20	7
35–44	12	3.3	3.9	19	7
45–54	12	3.3	4.0	19	7
55–64	15	3.4	4.0	18	7
65–74	10	3.4	4.1	17	7

[a]Latencies are corrected to a distance of 10 cm.

Table 7.19.
Ulnar Nerve: Sensory NCV

Age Years	Digit V–Wrist (m/sec) Mean	Digit V–Wrist (m/sec) Lower Limit	N	Wrist–5 cm distal to Sulcus n. Ulnaris (m/sec) Mean	Wrist–5 cm distal to Sulcus n. Ulnaris (m/sec) Lower Limit	"Across" Sulcus[a] n. Ulnaris (m/sec) Mean	"Across" Sulcus[a] n. Ulnaris (m/sec) Lower Limit	Wrist–5 cm Proximal to Sulcus n. Ulnaris (m/sec) Mean	Wrist–5 cm Proximal to Sulcus n. Ulnaris (m/sec) Lower Limit	N
15–24	59	48	21	72	63	63	49	67	58	10
25–34	58	47	15	70	61	61	49	66	57	12
35–44	57	46	23	69	60	60	49	65	56	14
45–54	55	44	54	67	58	58	49	64	54	15
55–64	56	47	56	67	57	57	44	62	55	18
65–74	52	43	25	63	54	52	44	58	51	11
75–84	49	40	8					53	46	6

[a]From 5 cm distal to sulcus n. ulnaris to 5 cm proximal to sulcus n. ulnaris in the extended position of the elbow.

Table 7.20.
Amplitude of the Ulnar Sensory CNAP

Age Years	Digit V–Wrist (μV)		Digit V–5 cm Distal to Sulcus n. Ulnaris (μV)		Digit V–5 cm Proximal to Sulcus n. Ulnaris (μV)	
	Mean	Lower Limit	Mean	Lower Limit	Mean	Lower Limit
15–24	17	7	9	4	5.5	2
25–34	16	6	8	3.5	5.5	2
35–44	14	5.5	7.5	3.5	5.5	2
45–54	13	5	7	3	5.5	2
55–64	10	4	4.5	2	3.5	1.5
65–74	7	2.5	3	1.5	3	1
75–84	5	2			2.5	1

Table 7.21.
Radial Nerve: Motor Conduction (Stimulus at the Elbow)

Age Years	Latency to Extensor Digitorum Communis (m/sec)[a]		Amplitude of CMAP (m/sec)			Motor NCV Axilla-Elbow (m/sec)		
	Mean	Lower Limit	Mean	Lower Limit	N	Mean	Lower Limit	N
15–24	3.0	3.5			28	68	58	15
25–34	3.0	3.5			11	67	58	3
35–44	3.0	3.6	14	7	7	67	57	2
45–54	3.1	3.6			17	66	57	8
55–64	3.1	3.6			8	66	56	3

[a]Latencies are corrected to a distance of 11 cm.

Table 7.22.
Radial Nerve: Latencies from Axillary Stimulation

Parameter	Brachioradialis[a] (msec)		Triceps[b] (msec)	
	Mean	Lower Limit	Mean	Lower Limit
Latency	2.6	3.1	2.5	3.2
Amplitude	15	7	20	11
Stimulation	At elbow		At axilla	
N	60		28	

[a]Latencies are corrected to a distance of 9 cm.
[b]Distance = 11 cm.

Table 7.23.
Radial Nerve: Sensory NCV

Age Years	NCV after Digit I Stimulation (msec)									NCV after Wrist Stimulation (m/sec)					
	Digit I–Wrist			Wrist–Elbow			Elbow–Axilla			Wrist–Elbow			Wrist–Axilla		
	Mean	Lower Limit	N	Mean	Lower Limit	N	Mean	Lower Limit	N	Mean	Lower Limit	N	Mean	Lower Limit	N
15–24	58	48	34	67	59	27				65	57	22	69	62	8
25–34	58	48	14	66	58	9				64	57	15	67	60	5
35–44	57	48	12	64	56	7	70	61	25	63	56	12	66	59	4
45–54	57	47	14	63	55	7				63	55	21	65	58	11
55-64	57	47	12	61	54	5				62	54	12	64	57	3
65–74	56	46	5	60	52	2				61	54	4			

Table 7.24.
Amplitude of Radial Sensory CNAP

Age Years	Digit I–Wrist (μV) Mean	Digit I–Wrist (μV) Lower Limit	Digit I–Elbow (μV) Mean	Digit I–Elbow (μV) Lower Limit	Digit I–Axilla (μV) Mean	Digit I–Axilla (μV) Lower Limit	Wrist–Elbow (μV) Mean	Wrist–Elbow (μV) Lower Limit	Wrist–Axilla (μV) Mean	Wrist–Axilla (μV) Lower Limit	N
15–24	14	5.5	5.5	2.5			35	13			
25–34	13	5	5	2			34	12			
35–44	13	5	5	2	3	1.5	33	12	10	4.5	24
45–54	12	5	5	2			31	12			
55–64	12	4.5	4.5	2			30	11			
65–74	11	4.5	4.5	2			29	11			
75–84			4	2							

Table 7.25.
Musculocutaneous Nerve: Motor Nerve Conduction

Age Years	NCV from Erb's Point to Axilla (m/sec) Mean	NCV from Erb's Point to Axilla (m/sec) Lower Limit	Amplitude of CMAP (μV) Mean	Amplitude of CMAP (μV) Lower Limit	N
15–24	70	63	17	9	14
25–34	68	60	16	8	16
35–44	65	58	15	8	8
45–54	63	55	13	7	10
55–64	60	53	13	7	9
65–74	58	50	12	6	4

Table 7.26.
Musculocutaneous Nerve: Motor Latency to Biceps Brachii Muscle (Age 15–74)

Distance (cm)[a]	Mean	Latency (msec) Upper Limit	N
From the axilla			
7	2.0	2.6	9
9	2.3	3.0	21
11	2.6	3.3	31
13	2.9	3.6	9
From Erb's point			
25	4.8	5.5	5
27	5.1	5.8	17
29	5.4	6.1	13
31	5.7	6.4	12
33	6.0	6.7	4

[a]Measured with obstetrical clippers.

Table 7.27.
Musculocutaneous Nerve: Sensory NCV

Age Years	Nerve Conduction Velocity (m/sec) Elbow–Axilla Mean	Elbow–Axilla Lower Limit	N	Axilla–Erb's Point Mean	Axilla–Erb's Point Lower Limit	N	Amplitude of CNAP (μV) Elbow–Axilla Mean	Elbow–Axilla Lower Limit	Axilla–Erb's Point Mean	Axilla–Erb's Point Lower Limit
15–24	68	61	15	68	59	14	36	17	11	3.5
25–34	66	59	8	65	57	6	34	16	9	3
35–44	64	57	8	63	54	7	33	16	7	2.5
45–54	62	55	13	60	52	10	31	15	6	2
55–64	60	53	10	58	49	9	29	14	5	2
65–74	58	51	6	55	47	4	28	13	4	1.5

Table 7.28.
Motor Latency from Erb's Point to the Shoulder Girdle Muscles (Age 15–62)

Anatomical Sites	Distance (cm)	Latency (msec)		N
		Mean	Upper Limit	
Suprascapular n.				
Supraspinatus m.	8–9	2.6	3.2	19
	10–11	2.7	3.2	16
Infraspinatus m.	13–15	3.4	4.2	20
	16–18	3.4	4.4	15
Axillary n.				
Deltoid m.	15–16	4.3	5.3	20
	18–19	4.4	5.1	17
Musculocutaneous n.				
Biceps brachii m.	19–21	4.6	5.8	19
	23–25	4.7	5.9	15
	27–29	5.0	6.0	14
Radial n.				
Triceps brachii m.	20–23	4.5	5.3	16
	25–28	4.9	5.8	23
	30–33	5.3	6.3	16

Table 7.29.
Peroneal Nerve: Motor Nerve Conduction to Extensor Digitorum Brevis

Age Years	Latency[a] (msec)			Amplitude of CMAP (mV)		NCV (m/sec)						N
						2 cm Distal to Fibular Head to Ankle		"Across"[b] Fibular Head		9 cm Proximal to Fibular Head–Ankle		
	Mean	Lower Limit	N	Mean	Lower Limit	Mean	Lower Limit	Mean	Lower Limit	Mean	Lower Limit	
15–24						52	44	52	43	51	45	14
25–34						51	44	51	43	51	44	2
35–44						51	44	51	42	51	44	6
45–54	4.1	5.0	41	10	3	50	43	50	42	51	44	5
55–64						50	43	50	41	51	44	3
65–74						50	43	49	41	51	44	1

[a]Latency is corrected to a distance of 9 cm.
[b]From 9 cm proximal to the fibular head to 2 cm distal to it.

Table 7.30.
Peroneal Nerve: Motor Nerve Conduction: to Peroneus Longus and Anterior Tibialis Muscles (Age 15–74)

Distance (cm)	Latency (msec)			Amplitude of CAMP (mV)		NCV "Across" Fibular Head (m/sec)	
	Mean	Upper Limit	N	Mean	Lower Limit	Mean	Lower Limit
6	2.2	2.9	2				
7	2.4	3.1	2				
8	2.6	3.3	12				
9	2.8	3.5	10	15	6	58	50
10	3.0	3.7	18				
11	3.2	3.9	12				
12	3.4	4.1	6				
13	3.6	4.3	2				
14	3.8	4.5	1				

Table 7.31.
Peroneal Nerve: Sensory NCV

Age Years	Toe I–Ankle (m/sec) Mean	Toe I–Ankle (m/sec) Lower Limit	Toe I–Ankle (m/sec) N	Ankle–2 cm Distal to Fibular Head (m/sec) Mean	Ankle–2 cm Distal to Fibular Head (m/sec) Lower Limit	Ankle–2 cm Distal to Fibular Head (m/sec) N	"Across" Fibular Head Mean	"Across" Fibular Head Lower Limit
15–24	46	37	18	57	49	20	56	49
25–34	45	36	3	56	48	9	56	49
35–44	44	35	9	55	48	16	55	48
45–54	43	34	9	54	47	13	55	47
55–64	42	33	5	54	46	13	54	47
65–74	41	32	3	53	45	6		

[a]From 2 cm distal to the fibular head to 9 cm proximal to it.

Table 7.32.
Peroneal Nerve: Amplitude of Sensory CNAP

Age Years	Toe I–Ankle (m/sec) Mean	Toe I–Ankle (m/sec) Lower Limit	Ankle–2 cm Distal to Fibular Head (m/sec) Mean	Ankle–2 cm Distal to Fibular Head (m/sec) Lower Limit	"Across" Fibular Head (m/sec) Mean	"Across" Fibular Head (m/sec) Lower Limit
15–24	8	2	4.5	1.2		
25–34	6	1.5	4	1		
35–44	4.5	1.1	3.5	0.9	3.5	1.2
45–54	4	0.8	3	0.8		
55–64	2.5	0.6	2.5	0.7		
65–74	2	0.5	2	0.6		

Table 7.33.
Posterior Tibial Nerve: Motor Nerve Conduction

Age Years	Latency (msec) Mean	Latency (msec) Upper Limit	Amplitude of CMAP (mV) Mean	Amplitude of CMAP (mV) Lower Limit	NCV of Popliteal Fossa–Medial Malleolus (m/sec) Mean	NCV of Popliteal Fossa–Medial Malleolus (m/sec) Lower Limit	N
Recording electrodes on abductor hallucis muscle							
15–25	3.9[a]	4.8	19	6	52	45	21
40–65	3.9	5.1	13	4	49	43	10
Recording electrode on gastrocnemius muscle							
15–18	4.8[b]	5.3	22	6			13
40–52	4.7	5.3	27	7			7

[a]Latencies are corrected to 10 cm.
[b]Latencies are corrected to 18 cm.

Table 7.34.
Posterior Tibial Nerve: Sensory NCV

Age Years	NCV (m/sec) Toe I–Medial Malleolus Mean	NCV (m/sec) Toe I–Medial Malleolus Lower Limit	NCV (m/sec) Toe I–Medial Malleolus N	NCV (m/sec) Medial Malleolus–Popliteal Fossa Mean	NCV (m/sec) Medial Malleolus–Popliteal Fossa Lower Limit	NCV (m/sec) Medial Malleolus–Popliteal Fossa N	Amplitude (μV) Toe I–Medial Melleolus Mean	Amplitude (μV) Toe I–Medial Melleolus Lower Limit	Amplitude (μV) Toe I–Popliteal Fossa Mean	Amplitude (μV) Toe I–Popliteal Fossa Lower Limit
15–24	46	39	22	56	50	20	3	0.5	0.8	0.2
25–34	45	38	3	56	49	2	2	0.3	0.8	0.2
35–44	44	38	4	55	49	4	1.5	0.2	0.6	0.1
45–54	44	37	6	55	48	3	1	0.2	0.5	0.1
55–64	43	36	3				0.7	0.1		

Table 7.35.
Sural Nerve

Age Years	Sensory NCV (m/sec)						Amplitude of CNAP (µV)			
	Dorsum Pedis–Lateral Malleolus			Lateral Malleolus–"Sura"			Dorsum Pedis–Lateral Malleolus		Lateral Meleolus–"Sura"	
	Mean	Lower Limit	N	Mean	Lower Limit	N	Mean	Lower Limit	Mean	Lower Limit
15–24	51	41	16	55	48	28	5	1.1	14	5.5
25–34	50	41	1	55	48	11	4.5	1	13	5.0
35–44	49	40	7	54	47	14	4	0.9	12	4.5
45–54	49	40	8	54	47	22	3.5	0.8	10	4.0
55–64	48	39	3	53	46	9	3	0.7	9	3.5
65–74	48	38	2	53	46	9	2.5	0.6	8	3.5

Table 7.36.
Saphenous Nerve: Medial Epicondyle at Knee–Inguinal Ligament

Age Years	Sensory NCV (m/sec)		Amplitude of CNAP (µV)		
	Mean	Lower Limit	Mean	Lower Limit	N
15–24	60	54	1.5	0.4	15
25–34	58	52	1.3	0.3	7
35–44	57	50	1.1	0.3	3
45–54	55	48	0.9	0.2	3
55–64	53	47	0.8	0.2	5
65–74	51	58	0.7	0.2	1

Table 7.37.
Minimum NCV Sensory of Potential in Normal Nerve

Segment	Mean (m/sec)	Lower Limit (m/sec)	Distance (cm)	N
Median nerve				
Digit III to wrist	16	11	18	38
Digit I to wrist	16	10	13	6
Ulnar nerve				
Digit V to wrist	16	10	14	18
Digit V to 5 cm distal to sulcus n. ulnaris	23	15	30	18
Digit V to 5 cm proximal to sulcus n. ulnaris	26	15	40	19
Sural nerve				
Lateral malleolus to "sura"	15	11	15	22
Dorsum pedis to lateral malleolus	18	9	11	11
Dorsum pedis to "sura"	22	12	26	15
Posterior tibial nerve				
Toe I to medial malleolus	20	12	21	17
Toe I to retinaculum superior				
Saphenous nerve				
Medial epicondyle to inguinal ligament	25	14	41	17
Peroneal nerve				
Retinaculum superior to 2 cm distal to capitulum fibulae	21	12	29	12
Toe I to popliteal fossa	25	17	66	13

Table 7.38.
Femoral Nerve: Motor Latency to the Rectus Femoris Muscle (Age 15–72)

Distance (cm)	Latency (msec)		N
	Mean	Upper Limit	
7.5	2.7	3.8	4
10.0	3.0	4.1	11
12.5	3.4	4.5	21
15.0	3.7	4.8	24
17.5	4.0	5.1	17
20.0	4.3	5.4	17
22.5	4.6	5.7	26
25.0	5.0	6.1	18
27.5	5.3	6.4	23
30.0	5.6	6.7	14
32.5	6.0	7.1	14

Table 7.39.
Motor Latency to Frontalis, Triangularis, and Orbicularis Oris Muscles (Age 15–70)

Distance (cm)	Latency (msec)		N
	Mean	Upper Limit	
7.5	2.5	3.3	2
8.5	2.8	3.6	7
9.5	3.0	3.8	15
10.5	3.2	4.0	28
11.5	3.5	4.3	26
12.5	3.7	4.5	38
13.5	3.9	4.7	27
14.5	4.1	4.9	26
15.5	4.4	5.2	18
16.5	4.6	5.4	14
17.5	4.8	5.6	4

Table 7.40.
Amplitude of the CMAP in the Facial Nerve

Muscle	Amplitude of CMAP (mV)		N
	Mean	Lower Limit	
Frontalis	2.2	0.5	55
Triangularis	9.0	1.0	59
Orbicularis oris	3.5	1.0	62

Table 7.41.

Normal Nerve Conduction Data:[a] Electromyography Laboratory, The University of Alabama at Birmingham, May 1983

Anatomical Site	Terminal Latency (msec), and NCV (m/sec)[b]		Amplitude, Normal Limit
	Mean ± SD	Normal Limit	
Upper Extremities			
Median nerve			
Sensory Conduction			
Palm–wrist	41.85 ± 3.90	34.05	10 µV
Finger–wrist	49.54 ± 4.14	41.26	10 µV
Mixed conduction			
Wrist–elbow	55.99 ± 3.30	49.39	10 µV
Elbow–axilla	63.47 ± 4.76	53.95	10 µV
Motor conduction			
Terminal latency	2.78 ± 0.41	3.60	5 mV
Wrist–elbow	58.78 ± 4.41	49.96	
Elbow–axilla	65.76 ± 4.90	55.96	
F-wave latency	25.32 ± 2.19	29.70	
Ulnar nerve			
Sensory conduction			
Finger–wrist	47.48 ± 4.11	39.26	8 µV
Mixed conduction			
Wrist–elbow	55.44 ± 3.99	47.46	10 µV
Elbow–axilla	57.14 ± 4.48	48.18	10 µV
Erb's point–axilla	64.09 ± 5.64	52.81	10 µV
Motor conduction			
Terminal latency	2.03 ± 0.24	2.51	5 mV
Wrist–elbow	61.15 ± 5.27	50.61	
Across elbow	51.31 ± 4.25	42.81	
Elbow–axilla	63.33 ± 5.47	52.69	
Erb's point–axilla	68.36 ± 5.07	58.22	
F-wave latency	25.68 ± 2.29	30.26	
Radial nerve			
Sensory conduction (distal)	50.87 ± 3.28	44.31	10µV
Lower Extremities			
Peroneal nerve (motor)			
Terminal latency	3.72 ± 0.53	4.78	4 mV
Knee–ankle	49.51 ± 3.93	41.85	
Knee–popliteal fossa	53.93 ± 7.11	39.11	
F–wave latency	46.88 ± 4.25	55.38	
Posterior tibial nerve (motor)			
Terminal latency	3.85 ± 0.63	5.11	5 mV
Knee–ankle	49.83 ± 4.60	40.63	
F-wave latency	48.89 ± 4.19	57.27	
H-reflex on the calf muscle	28.02 ± 1.95	31.93	
Sural nerve (sensory)			
Mid-calf–lateral malleolus	43.26 ± 4.29	34.68	6 µV

[a]Skin temperature: above 31°C. Age range 20–60. Number of controls: 40.

[b]Terminal latency, F-wave latency, and H-reflex are expressed as msec. All other values represent NCV (m/sec).

REFERENCES

1. Righospitalet Laboratory of Clinical Neurophysiology. 1975. Electromyography: sensory and motor conduction. Findings in normal subjects. Rigshospitalet, Copenhagen.
2. Behse F, Buchthal F. Normal sensory conduction in the nerves of the leg in man. J Neurol Neurosurg Psychiatry 1971;34:404–414.
3. Buchthal F, Rosenfalck A. Evoked action potentials and conduction velocity in human sensory nerves. Brain Res 1966;3:1–122.
4. Buchthal F, Rosenfalck A. Sensory potentials in polyneuropathy. Brain 1971;94:241–262.
5. Buchthal F, Rosenfalck A. Sensory conduction from digit to palm and from palm to wrist in the carpal tunnel syndrome. J Neurol Neurosurg Psychiatry 1971;34:243–252.
6. Buchthal F, Rosenfalck A, Trojaborg W. Electrophysiological findings in entrapment of the median nerve at wrist and elbow. J Neurol Neurosurg Psychiatry 1974;37:340–360.
7. Gassel MM. A study of femoral nerve conduction time. Arch Neurol 1963;9:607–614.

8. Gassel MM. A test of nerve conduction to muscles of the shoulder girdle as an aid in the diagnosis of proximal neurogenic and muscular disease. J Neurol Neurosurg Psychiatry 1964;27:200–205.

9. Payan J. Electrophysiological localization of ulnar nerve lesions. J Neurol Neurosurg Psychiatry 1969;32:208–220.

10. Singh N, Behse F, Buchthal F. Electrophysiological study of peroneal palsy. J Neurol Neurosurg Psychiatry 1974;37:1202–1213.

11. Trojaborg W, Sindrup EH. Motor and sensory conduction in different segments of the radial nerve in normal subjects. J Neurol Neurosurg Psychiatry 1969;32:354–359.

12. Wagner AL, Buchthal F. Motor and sensory conduction in infancy and childhood: reappraisal. Develop Med Child Neurol 1972;14:82–216.

13. Zander Olsen, P. Prediction of recovery in Bell's palsy. Acta Neurol Scand 1975(Suppl 61);52:1–121.

8

Pediatric Nerve Conduction Studies

Needle electromyography (EMG) has a definite limitation in the pediatric population because of the poor cooperation from patients. The examiner is often forced to draw a conclusion based on a small amount of information. In spite of this, however, the nerve conduction study can be performed without difficulty in a majority of pediatric patients, and the results are as accurate as for adults.

In the workup of suspected neuromuscular disorders in pediatric patients, we recommend that the nerve conduction test be performed first. It often provides a definite diagnosis if the patient has peripheral neuropathy (Table 8.1). Moreover, the nerve conduction test can be performed without much difficulty in most older children. The presence of the parents is usually helpful. However, this has to be individualized since some parents cannot stand to watch their children having the nerve conduction test. In occasional small children who are not cooperative for the nerve conduction test, chloral hydrate 50 mg/kg is recommended for sedation (1). When testing infants, we recommend the following guidelines:

1. A pediatric simulator should be used because the distance between the active and reference electrodes is shorter.
2. The posterior tibial nerve should be tested first because it shows the most reliable and technically satisfactory response.
3. Often the response from the extensor digitorum brevis is difficult to record after stimulation of the peroneal nerve at the ankle in infants. This is again due to the proximity of the stimulating electrode to the recording electrode. In this situation, the latency from the knee may be the only objective finding in the peroneal nerve.
4. In motor conduction studies of the median and ulnar nerves, the nerve conduction velocity (NCV) can be calculated over the elbow-axilla segment if the response with wrist stimulation is unrecordable.
5. Sensory nerve conduction is easier to study in the median and ulnar nerves. If there is difficulty in obtaining the compound nerve action potential (CNAP) from the wrist after stimulation at the fingers, the recording electrodes should be placed on the elbow. Usually no difficulty is encountered when obtaining the sensory CNAP at the elbow.

Table 8.1.
Diagnostic Possibilities in Peripheral Neuropathy at Varying Ages of Onset[a]

Infancy
    Congenital sensory neuropathy
    Hypomyelinative neuropathy, Dejerine-Sottas neuropathy
    Riley-Day syndrome
    Infantile axonal dystrophy
    Krabbe's disease
Early childhood (1–3 years of age)
    Giant axonal neuropathy
    Metachromatic leukodystrophy
    Ataxia telangiectasia
    Bassenkornzweig disease
Late childhood (5–15 years of age)
    Friedreich's ataxia
    Refsum's disease
    Charcot-Marie-Tooth disease
    Roussy-Levy syndrome
All ages
    Guillain-Barré syndrome
    Chronic inflammatory demyelinating neuropathy (CIDP)
    Toxic neuropathies
    Tick paralysis
    Metabolic neuropathies

[a]The most common form of peripheral neuropathy is the Guillian-Barré syndrome, followed by the Charcot-Marie-Tooth disease and Friedreich's ataxia (28).

Normal Nerve Conduction in the Premature Baby

For premature infants at 23–24 weeks of gestational life, motor NCVs are about one-third and the terminal latencies about twice those of full-term newborns (2). For premature infants from a gestational age of 30 weeks, the following findings are noted in the nerve conduction study:

1. The motor and sensory NCVs are slower than in full-term newborns.
2. There is a statistically significant linear correlation between the motor and sensory NCVs and the gestational and conceptual ages (Tables 8.2 and 8.3; Figs. 8.1–8.4, 8.6–8.9).
3. The motor NCVs in the upper extremities are usually faster than those in the lower extremities (3). No such data are available for the sensory NCV.
4. There is no correlation between the amplitude of CMAP and the gestational age (4).
5. There is an inverse correlation between gestational age and motor latency when the latency is corrected to a standard distance (4) (Fig. 8.5).

These findings indicate that *the NCV is a function of gestational and conceptual age*, independent of the birth weight (4–7) and that it can be used to estimate the gestational age. It appears that, at least from a gestational age of 30 weeks, maturation of myelinated nerve fibers seems to be equally fast, whether the fetus is intra- or extrauterine.

Thus, the motor and sensory NCVs can be used as additional differential parameters between "small-for-date" infants and premature infants. The NCV in the former is within the range of that in mature full-term infants. For premature infants the NCV is slower than that in mature full-term infants.

According to Moosa and Dubowitz (8), the conduction velocity of a peripheral nerve can be used to assess gestational age within 2–3 weeks. In addition, these authors maintained that the accuracy of prediction increases when more than one nerve is examined. The 95% confidence limit for assessing gestational age according to a mean velocity was 2.7 weeks for the combined velocities of the ulnar and posterior tibial nerves (Fig. 8.9). The H-reflex latency in calf muscles of the premature baby is longer than that of newborns (9). There is an inverse linear relationship between the H-reflex latency and conceptional age (Fig. 8.10). The regression of H-latency/cm leg length against conceptional age showed an even stronger relationship (Fig. 8.11).

Table 8.2.
Correlation of Nerve Conduction and Gestational or Conceptional Age

Investigators	Nerve Conduction Performed	Significant Correlation with[a]
Blom and Finnstrom (30)	Median and ulnar sensory NCV	Gestational and conceptional ages
Ruppert et al. (31)	Median, ulnar, and peroneal motor NCV	Gestational age
Dubowitz et al. (6)	Ulnar and posterior tibial motor NCV	Gestational age
Moosa and Dubowitz (8)	Ulnar and posterior tibial motor NCV	Gestational age
Blom and Finnstrom (3)	Ulnar and peroneal motor NCV	Gestational age
Cruz Martinez et al. (19)	Median and posterior tibial NCV	Gestational age
Schulte et al. (7, 32)	Ulnar and posterior tibial NCV	Conceptional age
Littman (29)	Ulnar motor NCV	Conceptional age

[a]Gestational age is the time from the first day of the mother's last menstrual period to birth. Conceptional age is gestational age plus age from birth.

Table 8.3.
Normal Motor Nerve Conduction in Premature Babies

Nerve	Mean Gestational or Conceptional Age (Week)	Mean Body Weight (g)	No.	Latency, Mean ± SD (msec)	NCV, Mean ± SD (m/sec)	Investigator
Median	35.8 (G)	2566	30	2.8 ± 0.46[a]	22.4 ± 2.60	Cruz Martinez et al. (19)
Ulnar	35.8 (C)	2129	17		25.9 ± 4.08	Schulte et al. (32)
Peroneal	35.5 (C)	2006	18		16.6 ± 1.72	Cerra and Johnson (33)/Blom and Finnstrom (3)[b]
Posterior tibial	35.8 (G)	2566	30	3.6 ± 0.53[a]	19.0 ± 2.73	Cruz Martinez et al. (19)
H-reflex	35.8 (G)	2566	30	19.5 ± 1.46		Cruz Martinez et al. (19)
	31.0–34.0 (C)		30	19.2 ± 2.2 (1.21 ± 0.23)[c]		Bryant et al. (9)
	35.0–39.0 (C)		26	16.7 ± 1.5 (0.87 ± 0.09)		
	40.0–45.0 (C)		27	16.0 ± 1.5 (0.78 ± 0.09)		

Note: Sensory nerve conduction data are not available because the number of premature babies was too small (3). Definition of premature: infants born less than 37 weeks after the beginning of the mother's last menstrual period.
[a]Terminal latency.
[b]Data from two sources were compiled. Cerra used surface electrodes, and Blom and Finnstrom used the concentric needle as the recording electrode.
[c]H-latency per cm leg length. Leg length is measured from a dimple at the lumbosacral junction or from the anterior iliac crest to the medial malleolus.

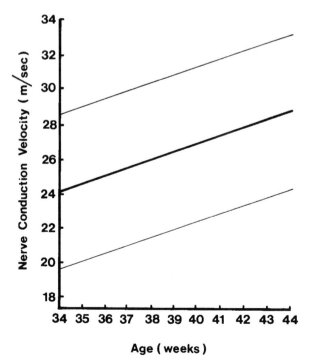

Figure 8.1. Motor NCV in the median nerve as a function of gestational age in preterm and full-term infants (19). The *thick line* indicates the regression line (mean NCV), and the *thin lines* the 95% confidence limits.

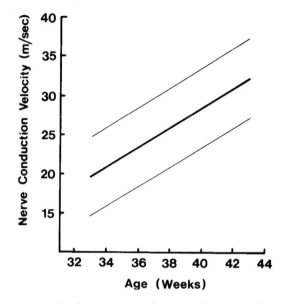

Figure 8.2. Motor NCV in the ulnar nerve as a function of conceptional age in preterm and full-term infants (23). The *thick line* indicates regression line (mean NCV), and the *thin lines* twice the standard deviation around the mean NCV.

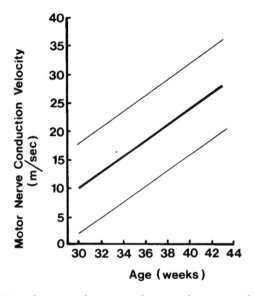

Figure 8.3. Motor NCV in the peroneal nerve as a function of conceptional age in preterm and full-term infants (23). (See the legend for Fig. 8.2.)

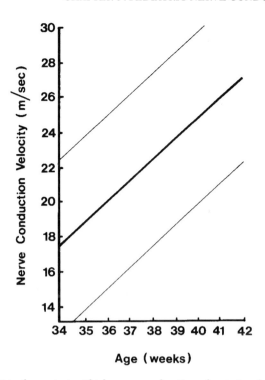

Figure 8.4. Motor NCV in the posterior tibial nerve as a function of gestational age in preterm and full-term infants (13). (See the legend for Fig. 8.1.)

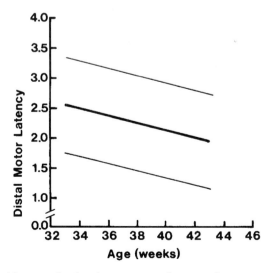

Figure 8.5. Terminal latencies for the ulnar nerve as a function of conceptional age in preterm and full-term infants (23). The latency is corrected to a standard distance of 2.5 cm. (See the legend for Fig. 8.2.)

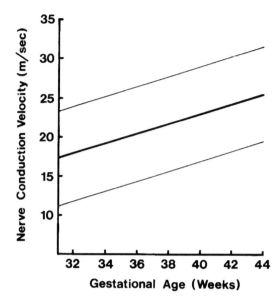

Figure 8.6.   Sensory NCV in the median nerve as a function of gestational age in preterm and full-term infants. (See the legend for Fig. 8.2.) Drawn from Blom and Finnstrom's data (30).

Figure 8.7.   Sensory NCV in the finger-wrist segment of the ulnar nerve as a function of conceptional age in preterm and full-term infants (23). (See the legend for Fig. 8.2.)

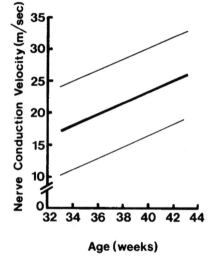

Figure 8.8.   Sensory NCV in the wrist-elbow segment of the ulnar nerve as a function of conceptional age in preterm and full-term infants (23). (See the legend for Fig. 8.2.)

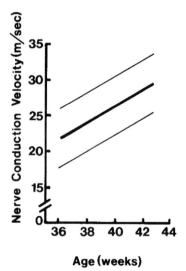

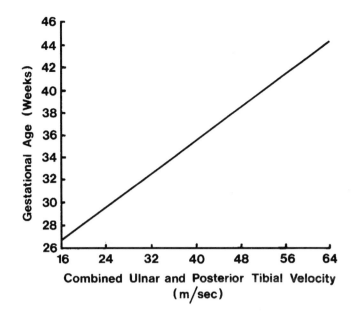

Figure 8.9. Graph for reading gestational age from combined ulnar and posterior tibial motor NCVs (27).

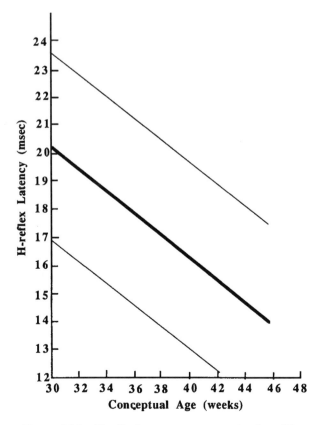

Figure 8.10. H-reflex latency versus conceptional age (9).

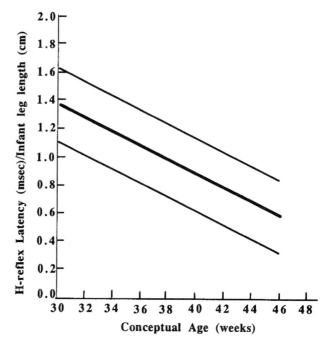

Figure 8.11.   H-reflex latency per infant leg length vs. conceptional age (9).

Normal Nerve Conduction in Infants and Children

Motor Nerve Conduction

Normal motor nerve conduction values are seen in Tables 8.5–8.7 and Figures 8.12, 8.14–8.21).

For Full-Term Newborns

The following findings are observed in the full-term newborn:

1. The motor NCV is about 50% that of the normal adult value.
2. The motor NCV is faster in the upper limbs than in the lower limbs.
3. The amplitude of the compound muscle action potential (CMAP) is about one-third that of the normal adult value in the upper extremities and about one-half that of the normal adult value in the lower extremities.
4. The terminal latency values are always below the adult values, but the distances are shorter in newborns (the mean value in the median nerve in newborns is 1.5 cm vs. 3 cm in children 6–11 years old). If the latencies are corrected to a standard distance, they are longer than the normal adult values (Fig. 8.10).

For Infants and Children

The following observations have been documented for infants and children:

1. The motor NCV reaches 75% of the adult value at 1 year of age and 100% at 4 years, increasing in a logarithmic function (10). No further increase is noted between 4 and 16 years of age.
2. The normal adult values for the motor NCV are reached earlier in the lower limbs than in the upper limbs, indicating that the maturation of the motor nerves is faster in the lower limbs than in the upper limbs (11).
3. The amplitude of the CMAP increases three-fold in the upper limbs and two-fold in the lower limbs by the time the child reaches 6–11 years old (11).
4. The terminal latency values are below adult values, partly as a result of the shorter distances involved (11). They gradually fall from the full-term newborn values during the first 6 months, remain stationary during the next 18 months, and rise after 2 years of age. This change is

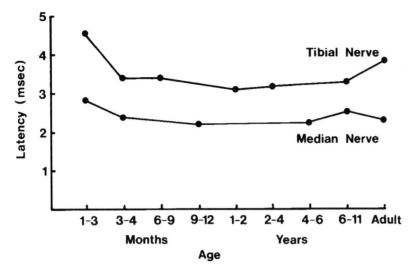

Figure 8.12. Normal terminal latencies for median and posterior tibial nerves. Terminal latencies are corrected to 3 cm in the median nerve and to 10 cm in the posterior tibial nerve. This is drawn from Cruz Martinez et al.'s data for infants and chidren (11) and from Oh's data for adults.

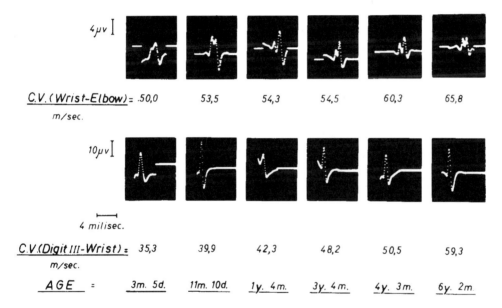

Figure 8.13. Two separate peaks of the sensory CNAP recorded from the median nerve at the elbow with stimulation of digit III. From Cruz Martinez et al. (13), with permission.

noted despite increasing distances with growth (12). If the terminal latencies are corrected to a standard distance, they fall rapidly to the adult values in the first 6 months. This is especially true of the motor nerves of the lower limbs, indicating an earlier maturation of these nerves. In fact, the corrected terminal latencies are slightly below the adult values between the ages of 6 months and 2 years (Fig. 8.12).

Sensory Nerve Conduction

Normal values for sensory nerve conduction are seen in Tables 8.8 and 8.9 and in Figures 8.22–8.25.

For the Full-Term Newborn:

The following findings are observed in the full-term newborn (13, 14):

1. The sensory NCV is slightly below 50% of the normal adult values.
2. The sensory NCV is faster in the upper limbs than in the lower limbs.
3. The amplitude of the sensory CNAP is slightly below the normal adult values.

For Infants and Children

The following findings have been observed in infants and children (13, 14)

1. The sensory NCV reaches 50% of the adult value around 3 months of age, 75% at 1 year, and 100% at 4 years, the distal and proximal sensory NCVs increasing in a logarithmic function.

2. The normal adult values of the sensory NCV are reached earlier in the lower limbs than in the upper limbs, indicating that maturation of sensory fibers of the legs occurs earlier than in the arms.

3. One striking feature of the sensory CMAP in children is the two peaks in proximal recording sites (Figure 8.13). The double peaks are rare in newborns but are common in the ulnar nerves in children between 3 months and 4 years old, and in the median nerve between the ages of 3 months and 6 years. The finding has also been described in the sural nerve (15). The presence of double peaks suggests that two groups of sensory fibers are in different stages of maturation.

4. The amplitude of sensory CNAPs increases 100% or more during the first 6 months of life, reaches the adult value usually at the age of 1 year, and becomes higher than adult values between 1 and 5 years of age.

Comments

Without the help of a signal averager, Gamstorp and Shelburne (16) found that recording of sensory CNAPs is often difficult in infants younger than 3 months because of the low amplitude. They therefore considered that the absence of sensory CNAPs is significant in children only after the age of 3 months. However, Cruz Martinez et al. (13) were able to obtain sensory CNAPs in all patients, regardless of their age, with the help of the signal averager.

Mixed Nerve Conduction

Normal values for mixed nerve conduction are shown in Table 8.10 and Figures 8.26 and 8.27. Mixed nerve conduction shows patterns similar to those noted in sensory nerve conduction. The mixed NCV is a logarithmic function of the patient's age. *A double peak is a conspicuous finding at the elbow.* Amplitude of the mixed CNAP increases three-fold during the first 6 months and soon reaches the normal values of the young adult.

H-Reflex

The H-reflex latency in calf muscles of newborns is approximately half that of adults (Tables 8.11–8.12) (17, 18). The overall latency decreases slightly during the first year as the NCV in peripheral nerves increases. Thereafter, the latency increases with age and growth in length of the nerves and does not reach adult values until after puberty and cessation of growth of the extremity.

In adults and children older than 1 year, the H-reflex is normally obtainable in the calf muscle by stimulating the posterior tibial nerve. It can be readily obtained in other nerves in premature and full-term infants (19). The percentage of infants with an H-reflex in the arm decreases progressively during the first year (Table 8.4), until by

Table 8.4.
Frequency of the H-Reflex in Infants

Age	Thomas and Lambert (23) Ulnar Nerve (%)	Cruz Martinez et al. (11) Median Nerve (%)	Gamstorp (22) Ulnar Nerve (%)
Premature	67	96.6	
Newborn	87	86.0	22
0–1 month	62	86.0	
1–2 months		76.0	31
3–5 months	17	68.0	
6–12 months	0	31.0	0.4

approximately the age of 1 year it can no longer be found. The latency of the H-reflex for the median nerve at the wrist decreases from that of premature and newborn infants to that of children over 1 year of age. The NCV of afferent Ia fibers, which is calculated by the H-reflexes at two points in the median nerve, increases during the same period. The NCV of afferent fibers is faster than the motor NCV over the same segment by 3–11% (11).

F-Wave

During the first 2.5 years when the NCV and arm length increase rapidly, *the F-wave latency remains constant at around 15 msec (Tables 8.19–8.21) (20).* Then the F-wave latency increases gradually and reaches 95% of the adult value between the ages of 19 and 20 years (Figs. 8.29 and 8.30). However, the F-wave amplitude and F/M-wave amplitude ratio show no significant difference among the various age groups. According to yet another study, the F-wave latency remains at 15–17 msec during the first 12 years of life regardless of age or height (21).

Normal Values for Nerve Conduction in Infants and Children

Motor Nerve Conduction

Extensive studies of motor nerve conduction were performed by Gamstorp (22), Cruz Martinez et al. (11), and Radtke (10) in normal infants and children. Their data are included in the following discussion. Wagner and Buchthal (4) pooled data from various sources and provided values for normal NCVs.

Radtke's Method

Radtke (10) studied motor NCVs for the ulnar, median, posterior tibial, and peroneal nerves in 120 normal children between 2 weeks and 15 years of age.

RECORDING: Surface electrodes are used for recording the CMAP, with conventional placement for the ulnar, median, and peroneal nerves. For the posterior tibial nerve, the electrodes are placed over the abductor digiti quinti.

STIMULATION: Surface electrodes are used for stimulation, with the following sites being stimulated for each nerve:

- Median nerve: at the wrist and above the elbow (sulcus medialis bicipitis);
- Ulnar nerve: at the wrist and elbow;
- Peroneal nerve: at the ankle and fibular head; and
- Posterior tibial nerve: at the ankle and popliteal fossa.

MEASUREMENT: The conventional methods are used for measuring latency and distance.

TEMPERATURE: Not controlled.

NORMAL DATA: Approximate values for the NCV of each nerve are shown in Figures 8.14–8.17. These values were obtained from 115 measurements in ulnar nerves, 112 in median nerves, 111 in posterior tibial nerves, and 105 in peroneal nerves. The quantitative values for the NCV of each nerve are given in Table 8.5.

COMMENT: A logarithmic increase in the NCV is noted between birth and the age of 4 years, at which time the values are approximately twice the original ones. No further increase is reported between the ages of 4 and 16 years.

Wagner and Buchthal's Data

Wagner and Buchthal (4) pooled data from Thomas and Lambert (23), Gamstorp and Shelburne (16), Baer and Johnson (24), and Radtke (10), and provided the values shown in Figures 8.18–8.21 for normal motor NCVs for ulnar, median, peroneal, and posterior tibial nerves.

Conventional methods are used for the motor nerve conduction tests on the ulnar, median, and peroneal nerves. For the posterior tibial nerve, the recording electrodes are placed on the abductor digiti quinti muscle (10, 24).

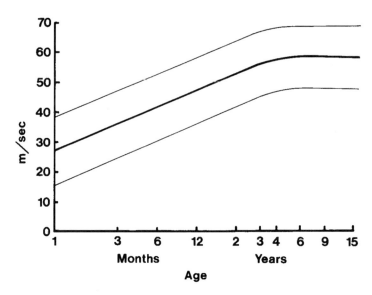

Figure 8.14. Normal motor NCV in median nerve infants and children (10). The *thick line* indicates the regression line, and the *thin lines* twice the standard deviations around the regression line.

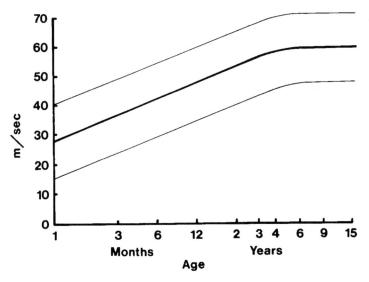

Figure 8.15. Normal motor NCV in ulnar nerve in normal infants and children (10). (see the legend for Fig. 8.14.)

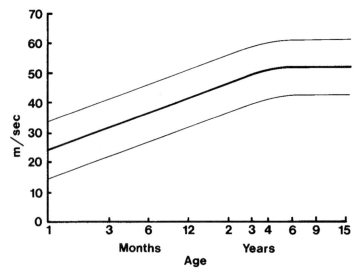

Figure 8.16. Normal motor NCV in peroneal nerve in normal infants and children (10). (See the legend for Fig. 8.14.)

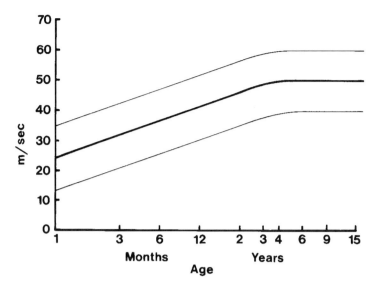

Figure 8.17. Normal motor NCV in posterior tibial nerve in normal infants and chidren (10). (See the legend for Fig. 8.15.)

Table 8.5.
Normal Motor NCVs in Children 4–15 Years of Age[a]

Nerve	Mean ± SD (m/sec)	Normal Limit (m/sec)
Median	59.2 ± 6.3	46.6
Ulnar	59.8 ± 5.0	49.8
Peroneal	51.4 ± 5.8	39.8
Posterior tibial	50.1 ± 5.1	39.9

[a]From Radtke (10)

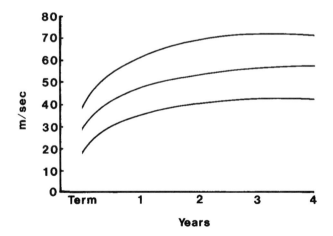

Figure 8.18. Normal motor NCV as a function of age in years in 236 median nerves in infants and children (4). The *upper* and *lower lines* indicate twice the standard deviation around the mean value.

The values in Figures 8.18–8.21 are approximate values obtained from 306 ulnar and 236 median nerves (wrist to elbow) and from 229 peroneal and 164 posterior tibial nerves (ankle to popliteal fossa).

Cruz Martinez et al.'s Method

RECORDING: The CMAP is recorded with surface electrodes placed on the following muscles using the belly-tendon method (11).

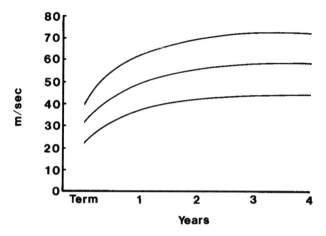

Figure 8.19. Normal motor NCV as a function of age in years for 306 ulnar nerves in infants and children (4). (See the legend for Fig. 8.18.)

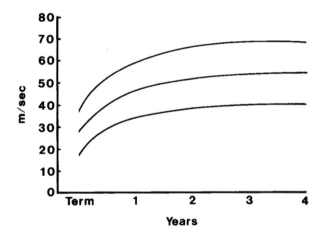

Figure 8.20. Normal motor NCV as a function of age in 229 peroneal nerves in infants and children (4). (See the legend for Fig. 8.18.)

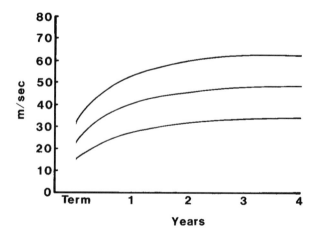

Figure 8.21. Normal motor NCV as a function of age in years in 164 posterior tibial nerves (4). (See the legend for Fig. 8.18).

- Median nerve: on the thenar muscle; and
- Posterior tibial nerve: on the abductor digiti quinti muscle.

STIMULATION: Stimulation of the nerves is performed with surface electrodes, with an interelectrode distance of 15 mm. The nerves are stimulated at the following points:

- Median nerve: at the wrist and proximal to the elbow; and
- Posterior tibial nerve: close to the medial malleolus and popliteal fossa.

MEASUREMENT: The latency and distance are measured following the conventional method. The peak-to-peak amplitude is also measured.

TEMPERATURE: The skin temperature is recorded. When necessary, the skin is warmed with an infrared lamp. No other information is given.

NORMAL DATA: See Table 8.6.

Gamstorp and Shelburne's Method

RECORDING: Surface electrodes are placed on the following muscles using the belly-tendon method (16).

- Ulnar nerve: on the hypothenar muscle;
- Median nerve: on the thenar muscle; and
- Peroneal nerve: on the extensor digitorum brevis muscle.

STIMULATION: The active stimulating surface electrode (8 mm in diameter) is placed at the following points:

- Ulnar nerve: above the elbow and at the wrist;
- Median nerve: at the elbow and the wrist; and
- Peroneal nerve: at the lateral border of the popliteal fossa and at the ankle.

Table 8.6.
Normal Motor NCVs in Children[a]

	Median Nerve		Posterior Tibial Nerve	
Age	Terminal Latency (msec)	NCV (m/sec)	Terminal Latency (msec)	NCV (m/sec)
Newborn (38–42 weeks)	2.50 ± 0.31	26.9 ± 2.60	3.35 ± 0.41	24.5 ± 2.35
0–1 month	2.60 ± 0.26	28.5 ± 2.04	3.20 ± 0.61	25.3 ± 1.96
1–3 months	2.30 ± 0.31	30.8 ± 2.61	2.85 ± 0.45	27.8 ± 3.89
3–6 months	2.10 ± 0.26	39.4 ± 3.64	2.20 ± 0.24	36.3 ± 4.98
6–12 months	2.12 ± 0.34	42.5 ± 4.65	2.46 ± 0.34	39.9 ± 3.89
1–2 years	2.0 ± 0.23	47.0 ± 2.89	2.40 ± 0.27	42.6 ± 3.80
2–4 years	2.17 ± 0.14	53.4 ± 3.84	2.81 ± 0.47	49.8 ± 5.79
4–6 years	2.23 ± 0.20	56.4 ± 4.22	3.20 ± 0.55	50.0 ± 4.26
6–11 years	2.50 ± 0.20	59.5 ± 2.71	3.60 ± 0.57	52.4 ± 4.19
25–60 years	3.20 ± 0.40	55.0 ± 3.80	5.90 ± 0.44	45.1 ± 3.80

[a]From Cruz Martinez et al. (11). Results are given as the mean ± standard deviation.

Table 8.7.
Normal Motor NCVs in Ulnar, Median, and Peroneal Nerves in Children[a]

	NCV (m/sec)		
Age	Ulnar Nerve	Median Nerve	Peroneal Nerve
At birth	32.3 ± 4.4 (N = 30)[b]	29.0 ± 3.7 (N = 30)	29.0 ± 4.3 (N = 29)
1 week–4 months	42.6 ± 8.5 (N = 18)	33.9 ± 8.7 (N = 18)	36.7 ± 7.3 (N = 18)
4–12 months	49.9 ± 6.8 (N = 25)	40.0 ± 5.3 (N = 24)	48.2 ± 8.3 (N = 25)
1–3 years	59.8 ± 8.1 (N = 21)	49.5 ± 5.9 (N = 21)	53.7 ± 8.1 (N = 21)
4–8 years	65.4 ± 8.5 (N = 26)	58.3 ± 5.4 (N = 25)	57.5 ± 6.9 (N = 26)
8–16 years	67.6 ± 6.0 (N = 26)	63.6 ± 5.7 (N = 20)	57.6 ± 7.3 (N = 20)

[a]From Gamstorp et al. (16). Results are the mean ± standard deviation.
[b]Number of controls.

The reference stimulating electrode is a plate, 15 × 20 cm, which is placed on the chest of the child or under his back.

MEASUREMENT: Latency and distance are measured following the conventional methods.

TEMPERATURE: Not controlled.

NORMAL DATA: See Table 8.7.

Sensory and Mixed Nerve Conduction

There are only two papers reporting studies of sensory and mixed nerve conduction in infants and children. Cruz Martinez et al. (13) recently conducted an extensive study of sensory and mixed nerve conduction, and Gamstorp and Shelburne (16) studied sensory nerve conduction in children.

Cruz Martinez et al.'s Method

RECORDING: The CNAP is recorded with surface electrodes with a 20-mm interelectrode distance. Sensory CNAP is recorded at the following sites (13):

- Ulnar sensory nerve conduction at the wrist and elbow;
- Median sensory nerve conduction at the wrist and elbow;
- Sural nerve conduction at the sura (midcalf) and popliteal fossa; and
- Median and ulnar mixed nerve conduction at the elbow.

An average of 100 responses is used to record the sensory and mixed CNAPs.

STIMULATION: The following sites are percutaneously stimulated for each nerve:

- Ulnar sensory nerve: V finger is stimulated with ring electrodes;
- Median sensory nerve: I, II, and III fingers are stimulated with ring electrodes;
- Sural nerve: near the lateral malleolus; and
- Median and ulnar mixed nerves: at the wrist.

MEASUREMENT: Latency is measured from the stimulus onset to *the positive peak*. NCV is calculated by dividing the distance by the latency. Sensory NCVs are determined over the fingers I-, II-, and III-wrist segments and over the wrist-elbow segment following stimulation of finger III for the median nerve, over the finger V-wrist and wrist-elbow segments for the ulnar nerve, and over the lateral malleolus-sura and sura-popliteal fossa for the sural nerve. Mixed NCV is determined for the wrist-elbow segment in the median and ulnar nerves. The amplitude, shape, and duration of the CNAP are measured according to conventional methods.

TEMPERATURE: The temperature of the skin over the nerves is 34–34.5°C in both hands. The temperature of the room in 25–26°C.

NORMAL DATA: See Tables 8.8–8.10 and Figures 8.22–8.27.

H-Reflexes in Infancy

Gamstorp (22), Thomas and Lambert (23), and Cruz Martinez et al. (11) studied the H-reflex in children. Cruz Martinez et al. provided normal values for the median nerve, and Thomas and Lambert (23) for the ulnar nerve.

RECORDING: Conventional methods for motor nerve conduction are used.

STIMULATION: Conventional methods of stimulation are applied at the wrist and elbow. The only difference is that the active stimulating electrode is placed proximally. The H-reflex is evoked with a submaximal stimulus.

MEASUREMENT: Latency is measured using the conventional method. When the H-reflex is evoked at the wrist and at the point proximal to the elbow, the conduction velocity of afferent fibers (Ia) of the median and ulnar nerves is calculated by using the conventional motor NCV calculation method.

TEMPERATURE: Not controlled.

NORMAL VALUES: For the median nerve, see Table 8.11.

For the ulnar nerve, mean ± SE (23):

Table 8.8.
Normal Sensory Nerve Conduction in the Finger–Wrist Segment of the Median and Ulnar Nerves in Children[a]

| | Median Nerve | | | | | | | | | Ulnar Nerve | | |
| | Digit 1 | | | Digit II | | | Digit III | | | Digit V | | |
Age	NCV (m/sec)	Amplitude (µV)	Duration (msec)	NCV (m/sec)	Amplitude (µV)	Duration (msec)	NCV (m/sec)	Amplitude (µV)	Duration (msec)	NCV (m/sec)	Amplitude (µV)	Duration (msec)
Newborn	19.4 ± 2.0	10.3 ± 4.4	1.7 ± 0.2	19.7 ± 3.3	7.0 ± 2.6	1.9 ± 0.6	20.8 ± 2.2	7.2 ± 2.1	1.8 ± 0.3	18.4 ± 3.4	5.5 ± 3.1	1.7 ± 0.2
1–3 months	21.2 ± 2.3	16.2 ± 3.6	1.6 ± 0.3	26.7 ± 5.2	12.4 ± 4.8	1.6 ± 0.2	29.0 ± 5.2	12.2 ± 4.7	1.6 ± 0.3	27.7 ± 6.4	9.4 ± 3.2	1.4 ± 0.1
3–6 months	29.2 ± 4.9	23.8 ± 4.2	1.3 ± 0.2	34.9 ± 4.6	17.8 ± 5.1	1.4 ± 0.2	37.1 ± 4.7	17.7 ± 3.8	1.4 ± 0.2	37.1 ± 5.3	13.2 ± 3.2	1.2 ± 0.1
6–12 months	31.8 ± 4.4	27.3 ± 7.8	1.2 ± 0.2	36.5 ± 3.8	16.7 ± 6.0	1.27 ± 0.1	38.7 ± 4.5	18.0 ± 7.2	1.2 ± 0.2	40.0 ± 5.1	13.0 ± 5.6	1.2 ± 0.2
1–2 years	35.5 ± 5.8	35.2 ± 10.3	1.2 ± 0.1	43.3 ± 7.4	22.6 ± 3.8	1.3 ± 0.2	44.0 ± 6.3	22.1 ± 4.2	1.3 ± 0.2	44.2 ± 7.8	16.3 ± 2.4	1.28 ± 0.2
2–4 years	38.8 ± 5.3	38.3 ± 8.6	1.1 ± 0.1	46.4 ± 4.6	22.8 ± 4.2	1.27 ± 1.3	47.5 ± 4.3	22.0 ± 3.1	1.27 ± 0.2	48.8 ± 3.0	16.0 ± 3.6	1.17 ± 0.1
4–6 years	38.9 ± 3.5	36.6 ± 6.4	1.1 ± 0.2	46.1 ± 4.4	19.2 ± 5.4	1.24 ± 0.2	46.5 ± 4.8	19.2 ± 6.6	1.22 ± 0.1	47.7 ± 6.8	14.2 ± 2.7	1.14 ± 0.1
6–14 years	42.9 ± 3.8	36.1 ± 6.4	1.06 ± 0.1	49.3 ± 4.7	16.8 ± 4.6	1.19 ± 0.1	48.9 ± 4.2	19.0 ± 4.7	1.13 ± 0.2	46.6 ± 5.6	13.4 ± 4.2	1.06 ± 0.2
20–29 years	44.2 ± 3.3	40.3 ± 9.3	0.9 ± 0.1	54.6 ± 4.1	16.3 ± 4.4	1.06 ± 0.1	53.4 ± 3.0	22.2 ± 7.3	1.05 ± 0.1	53.1 ± 2.4	11.5 ± 0.7	1.01 ± 0.1

[a]From Cruz Martinez et al. (13). Results are the mean ± standard deviation.

Table 8.9.
Normal Sensory NCVs in the Wrist-Elbow Segment of the Median and Ulnar Nerves in Children[a]

Age	Median Nerve				Ulnar Nerve			
	NCV (m/sec)	Amplitude (µV)		Duration (msec)	NCV (m/sec)	Amplitude (µV)		Duration (msec)
		Comp.1[b]	Comp. 2[b]			Comp. 1	Comp. 2	
Newborn	30.6 ± 2.9	2.9 ± 1.0		2.3 ± 0.4	25.2 ± 3.6	2.2 ± 0.9		2.7 ± 0.5
1–3 months	31.4 ± 1.0	2.22 ± 1.3		2.4 ± 0.3	28.9 ± 1.5	2.62 ± 0.9		2.3 ± 0.3
3–6 months	44.9 ± 4.9	3.5 ± 1.5	5.2 ± 1.8	2.3 ± 0.3	41.9 ± 3.0	3.1 ± 1.5	4.5 ± 1.0	2.2 ± 0.2
6–12 months	51.4 ± 6.9	2.78 ± 1.5	6.7 ± 1.8	2.0 ± 0.2	51.6 ± 6.6	2.8 ± 1.1	6.0 ± 1.7	1.8 ± 0.2
1–2 years	57.1 ± 5.7	3.37 ± 1.4	8.1 ± 1.7	2.1 ± 0.3	55.0 ± 5.2	3.5 ± 1.4	6.8 ± 1.2	2.1 ± 0.3
2–4 years	61.7 ± 5.0	2.6 ± 0.7	5.9 ± 1.8	2.2 ± 0.4	60.3 ± 5.3	3.0 ± 1.3	6.2 ± 1.2	1.3 ± 0.2
4–6 years	63.1 ± 6.3	2.7 ± 0.9	4.75 ± 1.5	2.0 ± 0.3	58.4 ± 2.6	2.9 ± 1.0	4.1 ± 1.2	2.0 ± 0.3
6–14 years	64.9 ± 5.4	1.7 ± 0.8	3.1 ± 1.4	2.0 ± 0.4	60.5 ± 5.4	2.4 ± 1.2	4.7 ± 1.5	1.7 ± 0.2
20–29 years	67.9 ± 5.0	3.1 ± 1.4		1.4 ± 0.2	61.4 ± 4.3	3.9 ± 1.5		1.5 ± 0.2

[a]From Cruz Martinez et al. (13). Results are the mean ± standard deviation.
[b]Component: Peak in nerve potential.

Table 8.10.
Normal Mixed NCVs in the Wrist–Elbow Segment of Median and Ulnar Nerves in Children[a]

Age	Median Nerve			Ulnar Nerve		
	NCV (m/sec)	Amplitude (µV)	Duration (msec)	NCV (m/sec)	Amplitude (µV)	Duration (msec)
Newborn	30.6 ± 3.8	7.75 ± 3.1	2.2 ± 0.6	30.5 ± 2.3	7.4 ± 2.2	1.4 ± 0.5
1–3 months	34.0 ± 4.6	10.8 ± 6.3	2.0 ± 0.3	37.1 ± 3.7	11.3 ± 5.0	1.18 ± 0.2
3–6 months	47.6 ± 7.2	21.6 ± 4.2	2.0 ± 0.3	45.3 ± 6.4	23.4 ± 7.7	1.5 ± 0.2
6–12 months	54.9 ± 9.6	37.9 ± 16.2	1.7 ± 0.2	56.2 ± 4.1	31.0 ± 13.7	1.4 ± 0.2
1–2 years	59.7 ± 6.1	43.5 ± 18.5	1.6 ± 0.2	60.0 ± 7.7	48.6 ± 13.7	1.4 ± 0.2
2–4 years	66.4 ± 5.0	44.1 ± 14.2	1.6 ± 0.2	62.5 ± 3.5	41.8 ± 15.4	1.3 ± 0.1
4–6 years	63.4 ± 4.2	33.4 ± 12.4	1.6 ± 0.2	62.3 ± 2.6	40.3 ± 19.5	1.4 ± 0.1
6–14 years	66.2 ± 3.9	32.3 ± 13.3	1.6 ± 0.2	62.7 ± 4.6	45.8 ± 16.7	1.4 ± 0.2
20–29 years	71.0 ± 3.4	33.1 ± 12.3	1.4 ± 0.2	63.2 ± 3.6	36.6 ± 10.7	1.37 ± 0.2

[a]From Cruz Martinez et al. (13).

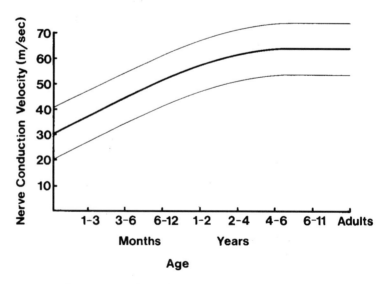

Figure 8.22.   Normal sensory NCV for median nerve in infants and children. (See the legend for Fig. 8.14). This figure is drawn from Cruz Martinez et al.'s data (13).

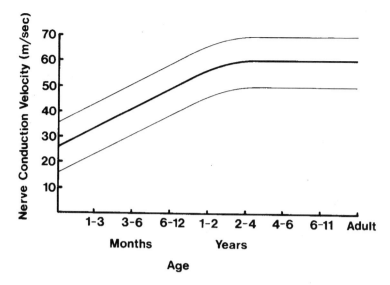

Figure 8.23. Normal sensory NCV for ulnar nerve in infants and children. (See the legend for Fig. 8.14). This figure is drawn from Cruz Martinez et al.'s data (13).

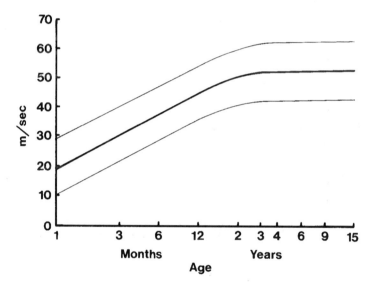

Figure 8.24. Normal sensory NCV for sural nerve in infants and children (13). (See the legend for Fig. 8.14.)

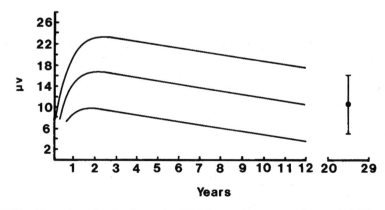

Figure 8.25. Normal amplitude of sensory CNAP for sural nerve in infants and children (13). (See the legend for Fig. 8.18.)

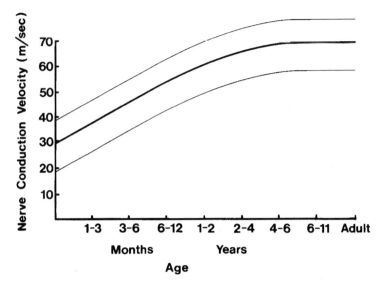

Figure 8.26. Normal mixed NCV for median nerve in infants and children. (See the legend for Fig. 8.14.) This figure is drawn from Cruz Martinez et al.'s data (13).

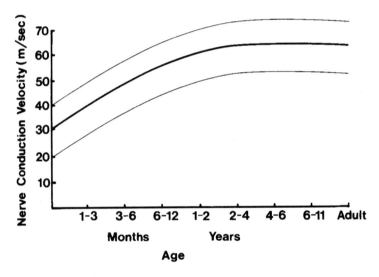

Figure 8.27. Normal mixed NCV for ulnar nerve in infants and children. (See the legend for Fig. 8.14.) This figure is drawn from Cruz Martinez et al.'s data (13).

Table 8.11.
Normal Latency and H-Reflex Conduction Velocity of the Median Nerve in Children[a]

Age	Latency (msec)		NCV (m/sec)
	Mean ± SD	Normal Limits	
Premature[b]	19.5 ± 1.5	22.5	24.4 ± 3.9
Newborn (38–42 weeks)	18.1 ± 1.1	20.3	29.8 ± 3.8
0–1 month	17.7 ± 1.0	19.7	31.3 ± 2.0
1–3 months	17.0 ± 1.0	19.7	34.2 ± 3.2
3–6 months	15.9 ± 1.1	18.1	40.5 ± 2.3
6–12 months	15.9 ± 0.9	17.7	46.9 ± 5.6

[a]From Cruz Martinez et al. (13).
[b]Premature from 30 weeks of gestational life. For the premature infant at 23–24 weeks of gestational life, the H-reflex latencies are twice the value for the full-term newborn (2).

Latency at wrist: 18.7 ± 0.32 msec (mean ± SE) (N = 34)
Latency at elbow: 15.7 ± 0.21 msec (N = 34)
NCV of afferent fibers: 30.1 ± 1.13 m/sec (N = 12)

H-Reflexes in the Gastrocnemius-Soleus Muscle in Infants and Children

Mayer and Mosser studied the H-reflex in the gastrocnemius-soleus muscle in infants and children (17, 18).

RECORDING: An active surface electrode is placed at the distal edge of the calf muscle at a point where the three components of the gastrocnemius-soleus muscle are close together. A reference electrode is placed on the Achilles tendon.

STIMULATION: The posterior tibial nerve is stimulated at the popliteal fossa using the conventional method of stimulation for the H-reflex.

MEASUREMENT: Latency is measured using the conventional method.

NORMAL DATA: See Table 8.12.

COMMENTS: An H-reflex latency above 17 msec is abnormal for newborns and infants, and an H-reflex latency above 20 msec is abnormal for children.

Blink Reflex

Newborn Infants

Kimura et al. (25) studied the blink reflex in neonates using the same stimulating and recording electrodes as for adult subjects.

RECORDING: An active surface electrode is placed on the lateral aspect of the orbicularis oculi muscle with a reference electrode on the lateral surface of the nose. The reflex responses are recorded on both sides simultaneously. A ground electrode is placed around the arm.

STIMULATION: The supraorbital nerve is stimulated with the active surface electrode placed over the supraorbital foramen on one side.

MEASUREMENT: The latencies of R1 and R2 responses are measured from the stimulus onset to the initial deflection of the evoked response. At least four responses of R1 and R2 are recorded for each subject, and the shortest latency is measured.

TEMPERATURE: Not controlled.

NORMAL DATA: See Table 8.13.

COMMENTS: According to Kimura et al. (25), the R1 response can be recorded in a majority (90%) of infants. Its latency is significantly greater than that in adults despite a considerably shorter length of the reflex arc in infants. Unlike in adults, the R2 response is elicited in only two-thirds of infants, mostly on the side ipsilateral to the stimulus. Thus, *the R1 measurement is valuable in assessing the blink reflex pathway.* In contrast, the R2 response is so variable and inconsistent in newborn infants that not much clinical significance can be attached to its absence or asymmetry at this age.

Table 8.12.
H-Reflex Latency and Amplitude in the Gastrocnemius-Soleus Muscle in Infants and Children

Age	Latency (msec)			Amplitude (mV)		No. of Subjects
	Mean	Range	Normal Limit	Mean	Range	
1–3 days	15.7	13–17	17	5.8	2.2–8.2	25
4–30 days	14.8	13–17	17	7.2	4.1–8.4	9
1–5 months	14.3	14–15	15	5.4	2.3–9.4	17
6–12 months	14.9	13.5–16.5	16.5	6.4	2.8–12.2	17
1–3 years	15.8	14–18.5	18.5	9.4	4.3–13.9	10
3–7 years	17.7	16–19.5	19.5	13.8	8.4–20.0	5

Table 8.13.
Normal Values of the Blink Reflex in 30 Neonates

Measurement	Mean ± SD	Normal Limit	Side Difference (Normal Limit)
Latency (msec)			
R1	12.10 ± 0.96	14.02	0.82
Ipsilateral R2[a]	35.85 ± 2.45	40.75	4.51
Amplitude (mV)			
R1	0.51 ± 0.18		
Ipsilateral R2	0.39 ± 0.19		

[a]Ipsilateral to stimulus.

Table 8.14.
Normal Values of the Latency of the R1 Components of the Blink Reflex in 76 Children

Age	Mean ± SD (msec)	Normal Limit (msec)	Side Difference (msec)
1–24 months	11.1 ± 1.2	13.5	1.7
2–9 years	10.3 ± 0.9	12.1	1.25

Children

Clay and Ramseyer (26) studied blink reflexes in 38 normal children ranging in age from 1 month to 9 years.

RECORDING: An active surface electrode is placed on the orbicularis oculi muscle and a reference electrode over the malar eminence. Ground electrodes are placed under the chin.

STIMULATION: The supraorbital nerve is stimulated using surface electrodes following the conventional method.

MEASUREMENT: Latency is measured from the onset of the stimulus to the beginning of the initial deflection of the evoked response.

TEMPERATURE: Not controlled.

NORMAL DATA: See Table 8.14.

COMMENT: The early component (R1) attains normal adult values by the age of 24 months. Both ipsilateral and contralateral late components (R2) are absent until the age of 20 months, are widely variable between 21 and 56 months, and attain normal adult values at the age of 6 years. It seems unlikely that the determination of late responses in children can be helpful.

Facial Motor Nerve Conduction

Newborns

Kimura et al. (25) studied the facial motor nerve conduction in neonates.

RECORDING: An active surface electrode is placed on the lateral aspect of the orbicularis oculi muscle with a reference electrode on the lateral surface of the nose. A ground electrode is around the arm.

STIMULATION: The facial nerve is stimulated with the active surface electrode placed just anterior to the mastoid process.

MEASUREMENT: Latency and amplitude measurements are conventional.

TEMPERATURE: Not controlled.

NORMAL DATA: See Table 8.15.

Children

Clay and Ramseyer (26) studied facial nerve latency in 38 normal children ranging in age from 1 month to 9 years.

RECORDING: An active electrode is placed on the orbicularis oculi muscle and a reference electrode over the malar eminence. A ground electrode is placed under the chin.

STIMULATION: The facial nerve is stimulated at the angle of the jaw.

MEASUREMENT: Latency is measured from the onset of stimulus to the beginning of the initial deflection of the CMAP.

TEMPERATURE: Not controlled.

NORMAL DATA: See Table 8.16.

COMMENT: The slightly prolonged direct facial response in children under 24 months of age compared with that in the slightly older child probably reflects a degree of delayed myelination of the peripheral nerve because the length of the nerve tested is shorter in the younger child.

Phrenic Nerve Conduction

Moosa (27) studied phrenic nerve conduction in 63 normal children ranging in age from 8 weeks to 11 years.

RECORDING: An active surface electrode is placed on the 5th or 6th intercostal space in the anterior axillary line, and a reference electrode is placed 2 cm posterior to the active electrode. A ground electrode is placed on the lower portion of the manubrium sterni.

STIMULATION: The phrenic nerve is stimulated using surface electrodes at the posterior border of the sternocleidomastoid muscle at the level of the upper border of the thyroid cartilage. A reference electrode is placed on the manubrium sterni.

MEASUREMENT: Latency is measured by the conventional method.

TEMPERATURE: Skin temperature is not controlled. Room temperature is 28°C.

NORMAL DATA: See Table 8.17 and Figure 8.28.

COMMENTS: The measurement of phrenic latency is a simple and safe procedure even in children. The phrenic nerve-diaphragm unit appears to mature fully by about 6–8 months after birth.

F-Waves

Kwast et al. (20) and Misra et al. (21) studied the F-waves in infants and children.

Kwast's Method

Kwast et al. used the concentric needle electrode to record F-waves from the muscles.

RECORDING: The CMAP is recorded with a concentric needle electrode from the abductor pollicis brevis muscle for the median nerve and from the abductor ditigi quinti muscle for the ulnar nerve.

Table 8.15.
Normal Values for Facial Motor Nerve Conduction in 30 Neonates

Measurement	Mean ± SD	Normal Limit	Side Difference (Mean ± SD)
Latency (msec)	3.30 ± 0.44	4.18	0.32 ± 0.33
Amplitude (mV)	0.48 ± 0.30		0.95 ± 0.56

Table 8.16.
Normal Values for Facial Nerve Latency in 76 Children

Age	Mean ± SD (msec)	Normal Limit (msec)	Side Difference (msec)
1–24 months	3.1 ± 0.31	3.72	0.8
2–9 months	2.5 ± 0.31	3.12	0.8

Table 8.17.
Normal Values of the Phrenic Nerve Latency in Children

Age	Mean ± SD (msec)	Normal Limit (msec)	Number of Subjects
Preterm (37 wks)	2.6 ± 0.3	3.2	20
Full term	2.5 ± 0.4	3.3	10
0–5 months	2.2 ± 0.4	3.0	24
6–11 months	2.6 ± 0.7	4.0	18
12–23 months	2.8 ± 0.7	4.2	16
2–5 years	2.9 ± 0.5	3.9	13
5–11 years	4.2 ± 0.7	5.6	24

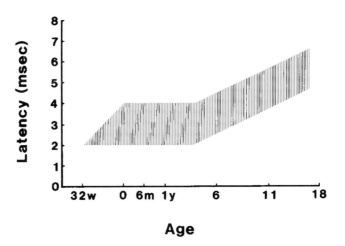

Figure 8.28.   Normal latency for phrenic nerve in infants and children. Hatched area represents mean ±2 SD. This figure is modified from Moosa (27).

STIMULATION: The conventional method of stimulation for the motor nerve conduction with a surface electrode is applied at the wrist. The only difference is that the active stimulating electrode is placed proximally.

MEASUREMENT: Latency (the shortest latency) is measured using the conventional method. The amplitude of the F-wave is measured from peak to peak. The F-dispersion is measured from the shortest F-wave latency to the longest latency.

NORMAL VALUES: Tables 8.18 and 8.19; Figures 8.29 and 8.30.

COMMENTS: During the first 2.5 years of life when the NCV and arm length increase rapidly, the F-wave latency remains constant at around 15 msec. After that, the F-wave latency increases gradually and attains 95% of the adult value between the ages of 19 and 20 years. The F-wave amplitude and F/M-wave amplitude ratio show no significant differences among the various age groups.

Misra's Method

Misra et al. used the surface electrode to record F-waves from the muscles (21).

RECORDING: The CMAP is recorded with surface electrodes from the abductor pollicis brevis muscle for the median nerve.

STIMULATION: The conventional method of stimulation for the motor nerve conduction with a surface electrode is applied at the wrist. The only difference is that the active stimulating electrode is placed proximally.

MEASUREMENT: Latency (the minimal latency; F-min) is measured using the conventional method. The amplitude of the F-wave (F-amp) is measured from peak to peak,

Table 8.18.
F Wave Latency, F Chronodispersion, and F Amplitude in the Median Nerve in Infants and Children

Age (years)	Latency (msec)		Fch (msec)[a]	Fa (mV)[a]	No. of Subjects
	Mean ± SD	Normal Limit	Mean ± SD	Mean ± SD	
0–1.5	15.4 ± 0.9	17.2	3.0 ± 1.1	1.6 ± 0.8	20
1.5–3	15.3 ± 0.7	16.7	2.9 ± 1.1		14
3–5	17.0 ± 1.1	19.2	3.6 ± 1.4	2.0 ± 1.0	23
5–7	18.2 ± 1.0	20.2	4.1 ± 1.4		13
7–12	19.5 ± 1.1	21.7	3.8 ± 1.2		20

[a]Fch-F chronodispersion. Fa-F wave amplitude.

Table 8.19.
F Wave Latency, F Chronodispersion, and F Amplitude in the Ulnar Nerve in Infants and Children

Age (years)	Latency (msec)		Fch (msec)[a]	Fa (mV)[a]	No. of Subjects
	Mean ± SD	Normal Limit	Mean ± SD	Mean ± SD	
0–1.5	14.6 ± 0.7	16.0	2.5 ± 0.9	2.4 ± 1.1	19
1.5–3	14.7 ± 0.4	15.5	3.6 ± 1.3		12
3–5	15.9 ± 0.8	17.5	3.1 ± 1.0	1.9 ± 0.9	25
5–7	17.6 ± 0.9	19.4	3.6 ± 1.2		15
7–12	19.1 ± 1.0	21.1	3.6 ± 1.5		15

[a]Fch-F chronodispersion. Fa-F wave amplitude.

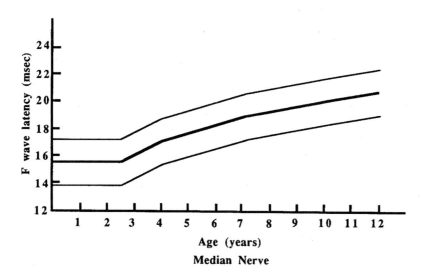

Figure 8.29.   F wave latency for the median nerve.

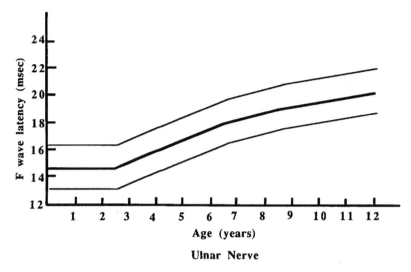

Figure 8.30. F wave latency for the ulnar nerve.

and the minimal-maximal latency difference (FΔ) is measured from the minimal F-wave latency to the maximal latency. The F-wave duration is measured from the onset of the initial deflection to the end of the last deflection.

TEMPERATURE: Skin temperature is not controlled.

NORMAL VALUES: See Table 8.20.

COMMENTS: According to Misra et al.'s data, *an F-wave latency longer than 20 msec is clearly abnormal for all children (up to the age of 12 years), regardless of height and age.* The F-wave latency shows a biphasic pattern: in neonates, 17 msec; in infants, 15 msec; in children, 16 msec.

The Mayo Clinic Method

No details about this method were given. It is obvious from the article that surface electrodes were used to record F-waves from the muscles and that conventional methods

Table 8.20.
F Wave Latency, F Chronodispersion, and F Amplitude in the Median Nerve in Neonates, Infants

	Latency (msec)		FΔ (msec)[a]	Famp (mV)[a]	Fdur (msec)
Age (years)	Mean ± SD	Normal Limit	Mean ± SD	Mean ± SD	Mean ± SD
Neonates (1–28 days)	17.0 ± 1.3	19.6	1.9 ± 1.0	1.1 ± 0.5	8.5 ± 1.5
Infants (1 month–1 yr)	14.9 ± 1.5	17.9	0.2 ± 0.1	0.2 ± 0.1	7.4 ± 2.7
Children (2–12 yr)	16.3 ± 1.9	20.1	0.2 ± 0.1	0.2 ± 0.1	7.8 ± 1.4

[a]FΔ, Minimal maximal latency difference; Famp-F, wave amplitude; Fdur-F, wave duration.

Table 8.21.
Normal F-Wave Latencies in Infants

Age (months)	Nerve	Normal Range (msec)	Normal Limit (msec)	Distance (cm)	No.
1–6	Peroneal	22–25		35–36	2
7–12	Peroneal	19–23		20–47	3
	Posterior tibial	19–24		43–47	2
12–24	Peroneal	21–26	26	30–53	10
	Posterior tibial	22–26	26	42–52	9

for F-wave testing were utilized (1). This is the only article that reported normal values of the F-wave latencies for the peroneal and posterior tibial nerves in infants and children even though the number of subjects was small (Table 8.21).

REFERENCES

1. Miller RG, Kuntz NL. Nerve conduction studies in infants and children. J Child Neurol 1986;1:19–26.
2. Cruz Martinez A, Ferrer MT, Martin MJ. Motor conduction velocity and H-reflex in prematures with very short gestational age. Electromyogr Clin Neurophysiol 1983;23:13–19.
3. Blom S, Finnstrom O. Motor conduction velocities in newborn infants of various gestational ages. Acta Paediatr Scand 1968;57:377–384.
4. Wagner AL, Buchthal F. Motor and sensory conduction in infancy and childhood: reappraisal. Dev Med Child Neurol 1972;14:189–216.
5. Dubowitz V. Nerve conduction velocities in premature and full-term infants. Dev Med Child Neurol 1965;7:426–427.
6. Dubowitz V, Whittaker GF, Brown BH, Robinson A. Nerve conduction velocity{md}an index of neurological maturity of the newborn infant. Dev Med Child Neurol 1968;10:741–749.
7. Schulte FJ, Michaelis R, Linke L, Nolte R. Motor nerve conduction velocity in term, preterm, and small-for-date newborn infants. Pediatrics 1968;42:17–26.
8. Moosa A, Dubowitz V. Assessment of gestational age in newborn infants: nerve conduction velocity versus maturity score. Develop Med Child Neurol 1972;14:290–295.
9. Bryant PR, Eng GD: Normal values for the soleus H-reflex in newborn infants 31–45 weeks post conceptional age. Arch Phys Med Rehabil 1991;72:28–30.
10. Radtke HW. Motorische Nervenleitgeschwindigkeit bei normalen Sauglingen and Kindern. Helv Paediatr Acta 1969;24:390–398.
11. Cruz Martinez A, Ferrer MT, Perez Conde MC, Bernacer M. Motor conduction velocity and H-reflex in infancy and childhood. II. Intra- and extrauterine maturation of the nerve fibers; development of the peripheral nerve from 1 month to 11 years of age. Electromyogr Clin Neurophysiol 1978; 8:11–27.
12. Dunn HG, Buckler WStJ, Morrison GCE, Emery AW. Conduction velocity of motor nerves in infants and children. Pediatrics 1964;34:708–727.
13. Cruz Martinez A, Perez Conde MC, del Campo F, Barrio M, Gutierrez AM, Lopez E. Sensory and mixed conduction velocity in infancy and childhood. 1. Normal parameters in median, ulnar and sural nerves. Electromyogr Clin Neurophysiol 1978;18:487–504.
14. Mortier W. Die sensible nervenleitgeschwindigkeit bei fruhgeborenen neugeborenen und alteren kindern. Monattsschr Kinderheikd 1971;119:282–284.
15. Buchthal F, Rosenfalck A, Behse F. Sensory potentials of normal and diseased nerves. In: Dyck PJ, Thomas PK, Lambert EH, eds. Peripheral neuropathy. Philadelphia: WB Saunders, 1975:442–464.
16. Gamstorp I, Shelburne SA. 1965. Peripheral sensory conduction in ulnar and median nerves of normal infants, children, and adolescents. Acta Paediatr Scand 1965;54:309–313.
17. Mayer RF, Mosser RS. Maturation of human reflexes. In: Desmedt JE, ed. New developments in electromyography and clinical neurophysiology, vol 3. Basel: Karger, 1973:294–307.
18. Mayer RF, Mosser RS. Excitability of motoneurons in infants. Neurology 1969;19:932–945.
19. Cruz Martinez A, Perez Conde MC, Ferrer MT. 1977. Motor conduction velocity and H-reflex in infancy and childhood. I. Study in newborns, twins and small-for-dates. Electromyogr Clin Neurophysiol 1977;17:492–505.
20. Kwast O, Rajewska GK, Kozlowski K: Analysis of F wave parameters in median and ulnar nerves in healthy infants and children. Age related changes. Electromyogr Clin Neurophysiol 1984;24:439–456.
21. Misra UK, Tiwari S, Shukla N, Nishith SD, Malik GK, Nag D. F-response studies in neonates, infants and children. Electromyogr Clin Neurophysiol 1989;29:251–254.
22. Gamstorp I. Normal conduction velocity of ulnar, median and peroneal nerves in infancy, childhood and adolescence. Acta Paediatr Scand (Suppl) 1963;146:68–76.
23. Thomas JE, Lambert EH. Ulnar nerve conduction velocity and H-reflex in infants and children. J Appl Physiol 1960;15:1–9.
24. Baer RD, Johnson EW. Motor nerve conduction velocities in normal children. Arch Phys Med Rehab 1965;46:698–704.
25. Kimura J, Bodensteiner J, Yamada T 1977. Electrically elicited blink reflex in normal neonates. Arch Neurol 1977;34:246–249.
26. Clay SA, Ramseyer JC. The orbicularis oculi reflex in infancy and childhood. Neurology 1976;26:521–524.
27. Moosa A. Phrenic nerve conduction in children. Develop Med Child Neurol 1981;23:434–448.
28. Evans OB. Polyneuropathy in childhood. Pediatrics 1979;64:96–105.
29. Littman B. Peripheral nerve maturation in premature infants. Neuropadiatrie 1975;3:284–291.
30. Blom S, Finnstrom O. 1971. Sensible nervenleitgewindigkeit bei neugeborenen kindern. Z EEG EMG 1971;2:6–21.

31. Ruppert ES, Robertson AF, Johnson EW. Motor nerve conduction velocities in infants of low birth weight. J Pediatr 1967;70:693–694.

32. Schulte FJ, Albert G, Michaelis R. Gestationsalter under nervenleitgeschwindigkeit bei normalen und abnormalen neugeborenen. Dtsch Med Wonchenschr 1969;94:599–601.

33. Cerra D, Johnson E. Motor nerve conduction velocity in premature infants. Arch Phys Med Rehab 1962;43:60–164.

9

Artifacts

"Artifacts" are defined as any waves not originating from nerves or muscles. Fortunately, many of the artifacts found in the electromyography (EMG) laboratory are easily identifiable and correctable. The real hazard exists when artifacts are mistaken for genuine responses or when they distort or obliterate the genuine response, causing an erroneous interpretation of results.

Power Line Artifact

The most common artifact is the power line artifact (60 Hz waves in North America or 50 Hz waves in Great Britain). This appears on the oscilloscope as a cyclic pattern that may have a distorted sinusoidal wave form with variable superimposed peaks. The time between the repetitive portions of the wave form for 60-Hz waves will be 16.7 msec (1/60th of a second), or one-half this value, 8.4 msec (Fig. 9.1). The amplitude of the interference always appears larger at higher sensitivity settings. It is often difficult to study abnormal spontaneous potentials in the needle EMG as well as sensory or mixed nerve conduction in the presence of 60-Hz artifacts.

Proper attention to instrument, electrodes, electrode placement, patient grounding, and the elimination of controllable sources of interference permit the interference rejection properties of the modern EMG machine to provide an EMG study that is essentially free of power line artifact. This means that an entirely satisfactory EMG study can be performed in the physician's office or the hospital without any additional shielding. There are a few basic steps to take that will minimize unwanted artifacts:

EMG Laboratory

1. Fluorescent lamps should not be installed in the EMG examining room. If fluorescent lamps are present, they should be turned off during the examination because they are a notorious source of 60-Hz artifact. An ordinary ceiling lamp with a dimming device is ideal for lighting the EMG laboratory, and it does not produce any electrical interference. If normal room illumination proves to be a source of interference, a special shielded examining lamp should be obtained.

2. The circuit to the EMG machine should be isolated from circuits that are connected to other electrical appliances. Electrical interference is common during the operation of electrical appliances if the EMG machine and the appliances share a common circuit.

3. Power cords and extension cords for appliances and lamps that pass in the vicinity of the patient should be unplugged from the outlet, not merely turned off. These are the greatest source of interference. Most modern wiring is carried in grounded metallic conduits that mini-

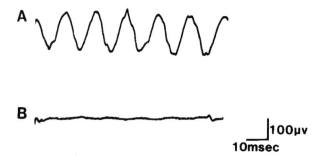

Figure 9.1. 60-Hz artifact. Note the constant time interval (about 16 msec) between the peaks. *A*, The 60-Hz artifact is produced by poor contact between the ground electrode and the skin. *B*, The artifact is eliminated by putting more electrode gel beneath the ground electrode.

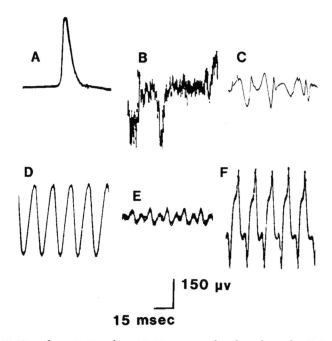

Figure 9.2. EMG artifacts. *A*, Heartbeat. *B*, Movement of surface electrode. *C*, Loose contact. *D*, 60-Hz artifact. *E*, Diathermy interference. *F*, Interference from adjacent electric generator. Modified from Rodriguez and Oester (3), with permission.

mize interference, but any wiring not in a metallic conduit is a potentially serious source of interference if it passes anywhere near the patient.

4. The operation of a diathermy apparatus on the same power line as the EMG machine or near it causes strong interference that is often hard to eliminate even with complete screening of the input electrodes and filtering of the house current (Fig. 9.2). Because the extraneous potentials produced make an accurate EMG study difficult to obtain, a diathermy apparatus should not be near the EMG laboratory or on the same power line as the EMG machine. Certainly, diathermy machines should not be used during the EMG examination if they are connected with the same circuit as the EMG machine.

5. The modern EMG machine has various interference rejection properties, e.g., a high common rejection mode and a high input impedance compared with the electrode impedance. These properties diminish 60-Hz artifacts. Therefore, when the EMG machine is well grounded by plugging its power cable into a properly wired grounded outlet, it is itself rarely a source of a 60-Hz artifact.

Patients

In practice, the major source of 60-Hz artifacts are the electrodes themselves, which may make poor contact with the patient or be defective (Fig. 9.2). Thus, the electrodes are the first item to check when there are 60-Hz artifacts.

1. The electromyographer must check for good contact between the ground and recording electrodes and the patient. A generous application of electrode gel may be enough to eliminate 60-Hz artifacts. The electrode should also be firmly affixed to the skin with tape, which does not adhere well if the patient is perspiring. In some cases the skin must be cleaned with acetone or alcohol to remove surface oil or scraped with a fine needle or sandpaper to remove the superficial scaly layer. Skin lotion and powder also cause poor contact of electrodes with the patient, and these must be removed by acetone or alcohol. A hairy surface may also result in poor electrode contact.

2. Any defective electrodes can easily be checked by a battery-operated ohmeter and replaced.

3. The patient should be grounded only by means of the ground electrode via the EMG machine, and should not touch any other grounded metallic object or electrically operated machine. These measures not only eliminate the sources of annoying artifact but are also essential for the safety of the patients.

4. Unless necessary, a second electrically operated apparatus should not be used with a patient connected to the EMG machine. Such an arrangement is unavoidable if a skin temperature control unit is required during the nerve conduction study, but often this unit must be turned off or disconnected to eliminate a 60-Hz artifact. This artifact is more annoying during the sensory nerve conduction study, but it can usually be canceled out by signal averaging.

5. Under some conditions, merely moving a patient away from a wall to the center of the room or to some other wall of the room can reduce the amount of 60-Hz artifact picked up by the patient.

Examiner or Observer

The ungrounded examiner is often an excellent source of 60-Hz interference to the patient, as are observers who are standing close to the patient. When the examiner touches the patient or the pick-up electrode, an increase in 60-Hz interference is sometimes noted. To avoid this, the examiner should touch the ground electrode or otherwise ground himself with a ground wire.

Artifacts from the Cardiac Pacemaker

In patients with a cardiac pacemaker, tiny regular artifacts mimicking fibrillation or positive sharp wave can be seen during the needle EMG study (Figs. 9.3–9.5). Because there is continuous regular firing at the rate of the pulse and the amplitude of artifact increases as the EMG needle is placed closer to the heart, this artifact can be differentiated from fibrillations or positive sharp waves. A high index of suspicion is needed to recognize this artifact, which may otherwise be interpreted as fibrillation.

We have observed a few instances in which the compound nerve action potentials (CNAPs) were not obtainable in the upper extremity due to the regular pacing of the cardiac pacemaker. This should not be interpreted as abnormal.

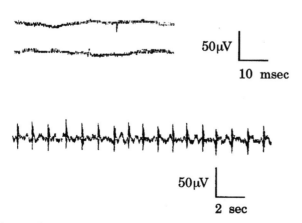

Figure 9.3. Artifacts in the vastus lateralis muscle from a cardiac pacemaker. The lower recording is from a point closer to the heart in the same muscle.

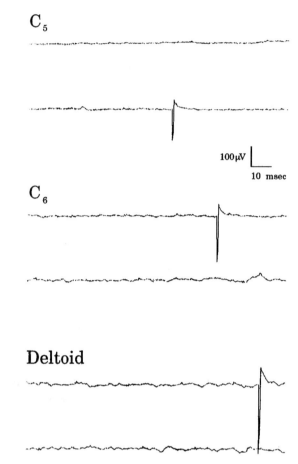

Figure 9.4. Artifacts in the cervical paraspinal and deltoid muscles, mimicking positive sharp waves. Notice that the amplitude of artifact increases as the EMG needle is placed closer to the heart.

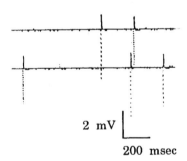

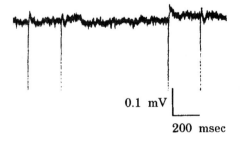

Figure 9.5. Artifacts from a dual pacemaker.

Artifacts from the Transcutaneous Nerve Stimulator

In recent years there has been an increasing number of patients who use the transcutaneous nerve stimulator (TNS) for relief of pain. The frequency of stimulation ranges from 1 to 120 per second and can be adjusted. Depending on the frequency of stimulation, the TNS unit can be a source of tiny regular artifacts in the needle EMG study (Fig. 9.6). This is especially true when the stimulator is placed near the area where the needle EMG is performed. To avoid this unnecessary but avoidable source of artifacts, *it is our policy to turn off the TNS unit* while performing the nerve conduction study as well as the needle EMG study.

Artifacts from the Spinal Cord Epidural Stimulator

In some patients epidural electrode stimulation on the spinal cord has been used to relieve pain. The epidural electrode is connected to a subcutaneous implanted stimulator. Unlike the TNS, which is visible to the examiner, this device is not easily visible or palpable. It can be an annoying source of tiny regular artifacts during the paraspinal needle EMG test (Fig. 9.7). When confronted with unexplainable tiny regular artifacts, *it is wise to ask the patient whether he/she has any such implanted pacing device.*

Radiofrequency Interference

Radiofrequency energy from AM and FM radios, television, police and taxi radios, citizens' band (CB) radios, and some hospital paging systems may be of sufficient intensity to be picked up by the electromyography amplifier (1). These signals cause trouble because their modulation, speech, or music lies within the spectrum of sensitivity of the

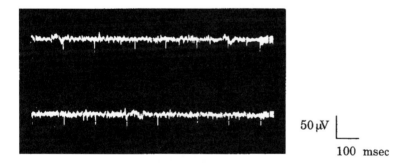

Figure 9.6.   Artifacts from a TNS unit, mimicking fibrillations.

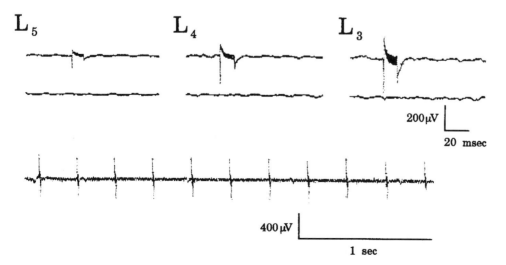

Figure 9.7.   Artifacts from a spinal cord epidural stimulator.

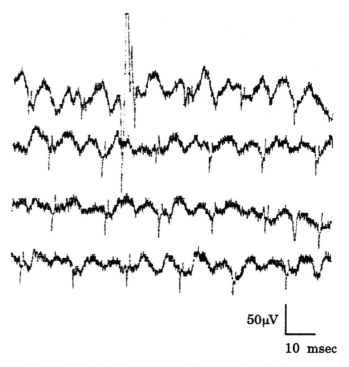

50μV

10 msec

Figure 9.8. Radiofrequency artifacts mimicking fibrillations.

EMG amplifiers. The radiofrequency signals may be heard over the loudspeaker of the EMG machine and may be seen as interfering potentials on the screen mimicking abnormal spontaneous potentials (Fig. 9.8). A radiofrequency rejection circuit built into the modern EMG machine usually eliminates all common interference with the exception of radio transmitters. Fortunately, in practice, radiofrequency interference is usually short-lived. If the radiofrequency interference is persistent, it is sometimes difficult to eliminate. The following recommendations may help to eliminate radiofrequency interference:

1. The EMG laboratory should be located on the far side of the building from any transmitting antennae and on the lowest floor of the building.

2. Because the radiofrequencies that cause most EMG artifacts are of the shorter wavelengths, this interference can often be reduced merely by moving a metallic or screened partition between the patient and the offending source of radiation. In more persistent cases, the screening can be extended to enclose two or three sides of the patient.

3. Where the radiofrequency energy enters the EMG apparatus through the power line, special power line filters may be employed to some advantage. Care should be exercised in using these filters, so as not to break the normal connection between the apparatus and a proper electrical ground.

4. The greatest freedom from all environmental artifacts can be obtained by means of a six-sided screened enclosure surrounding the patient and the apparatus.

Large-Stimulus Artifacts

The shorter the stimulus duration, the smaller is the stimulus artifact. No major problem arises because of the stimulus artifact in routine studies. With sensory or mixed nerve conduction, however, the stimulus artifact may distort the nerve potential because of the baseline sway. In some EMG stimulators, a suppressor of the stimulus artifact is available. The following basic steps should be followed before resorting to an electronic artifact compensator:

1. Avoid placing the electrode above superficial veins.
2. Place the ground electrode between the stimulating and recording electrodes.

3. Cover the stimulated finger or toe with hydrophobic cotton to prevent contact with other fingers or toes.

4. Keep the surface of the skin dry between the stimulating and recording electrodes. An excessively large stimulus artifact is observed when electrode gel or perspiration bridges from the stimulator to the recording or ground electrodes, or when the stimulator lead wires are near the recording electrodes. Stimulator leads cannot be shielded and can cause a large stimulus artifact.

5. *Sometimes a slight rotation of the stimulating reference electrode around the active stimulating electrode reduces the stimulus artifact.* This has also been confirmed by Kornfield et al. (2).

When the CNAP is small or absent, a strong stimulus is often used to stimulate the nerve supramaximally. A strong stimulus can introduce a motor artifact that can be mistaken for a CNAP. This is especially true for the antidromic sensory nerve conduction test. Differentiation between a sensory CNAP and a motor artifact can usually be made by recording orthodromically.

Needle Artifacts

Defective insulation of the needle causes bizarre artifacts. The needle insulation should be tested when it is suspected of being defective. For the monopolar needle, one terminal from the ohmeter is connected to the needle, and the other terminal to a pledget of moist cotton. The shaft of the needle is explored with the cotton, which makes firm contact as it slides from one end to the other. If the ohmeter registers any current flow except at the exposed tip of the needle, the insulation is defective. Such needles should be discarded. After long use, coaxial needles may become short-circuited at their tips. The two leads should be tested with a constant current ohmeter. Each lead is connected to a separate terminal. When the needle is immersed in a conducting solution, the ohmeter will register the passage of current; when the tip is dry, no current will pass through the ohmeter unless the electrode is shorted.

Artifact Caused by Muscle Action Potentials

When a patient has difficulty relaxing, artifacts caused by muscle action potentials can give rise to serious problems because they often have a greater amplitude than the CNAPs themselves. The patient should be encouraged to relax completely. To achieve this, an audio monitor should be turned on during the sensory and mixed nerve conduction studies. By listening to the baseline noise, the patient can relax better. Usually complete relaxation can be achieved by changing the position of the extremity under examination. Signal averaging can only partially offset artifacts such as these. A great advantage is afforded by an automatic or a manual artifact rejection device that enables the examiner to reject an artifact so that only potentials with very few visible artifacts or none at all are fed into the averager.

Movement artifacts caused by painful stimuli may distort the CNAP or displace the needle electrode. This can be eliminated by reducing the stimulus intensity or by the examiner's firmly holding the extremity in position.

It cannot be emphasized too strongly that every possible measure should be taken to abolish or minimize undesirable artifacts in order to observe and record the potentials without any distortion. In checking the sources of artifacts, the most common should be considered first, after which other possibilities are ruled out one by one.

REFERENCES

1. TECA Corporation. Artifact and interference. In: EMG—operating notes. White Plains, NY: TECA Corp, 1973.
2. Kornfield MJ, Cerra J, Simons DG. Stimulus artifact reduction in nerve conduction. Arch Phys Med Rehabil 1985;66:232–234.
3. Rodriguez AA, Oester YT. Fundamentals of electromyography. In: Licht S, ed. Electrodiagnosis and electromyography. 3rd ed. Baltimore: Williams & Wilkins, 1971:303.

10

Electrical Safety and Risks in Electrodiagnostic Practice

Guidelines for Electrical Safety

It is important to understand that there is a potential hazard during the performance of electromyography (EMG) procedures. The electricity can kill an individual if the equipment is not properly maintained and grounded and if adequate precautions are not taken. The degree of danger is a direct function of the amount of current that flows through the patient's body. When current flows through the body, it may result in a tingling sensation, a perceptible shock, muscle paralysis, respiratory failure, or fibrillation of the heart (Table 10.1), depending on the amount of current flow.

The electrical hazards are generally caused by faults in the grounding system that cause a leak through the cardiac region, usually producing ventricular fibrillation. If the grounding system is properly installed, leakage of current from an EMG system is minimal; with adequate grounding, any leakage caused by defective equipment is shunted harmlessly to the ground. Electrical equipment is generally designed so that the outer frame is solidly grounded via a third ground wire included in the power cable, which in turn is grounded by a third ground terminal in the power receptacle. This ground connection provides a safe path to the ground for leaked current, rather than permitting it to flow through the patient.

The following guidelines, provided by the TECA Corporation (1), are recommended for electrical safety in the EMG laboratory.

EMG Laboratory

1. The power receptacle should have three holes, not two. If you find a two-holer to be the only receptacle available, refuse to run the test on the basis that you would be endangering the safety of the patient and yourself.

2. The integrity of the ground at the outlet is very important. The power receptacle should be

Table 10.1.
Effects of 60 Hz Electrical Shock Current Through the Body Trunk on an Average Individual

Current Intensity (mA)	Effect
1	Sensation threshold
5	Accepted as maximum harmless current intensity
10–20	"Let-go" current before sustained muscular contraction
50	Pain. Possible fainting, exhaustion, mechanical injury. Heart and respiratory functions continue.
100–300	Ventricular fibrillation starts, but respiratory center remains intact. Usually results in death.

promptly repaired or replaced if damaged or if it shows signs of wear. Consult a qualified biomedical engineer if in doubt about your power outlet.

3. Unnecessary electrical equipment should be kept away from the EMG examining room.

Equipment

1. Whenever a new EMG machine is installed for use on patients, it should first be thoroughly checked for safety by a qualified person in the laboratory in which it is to be used.

2. The EMG machine must be properly grounded. This is usually accomplished by plugging the power cable plug into a properly wired grounded outlet.

3. There should be a periodic check by a biomedical engineer to see that there is no excessive electrical leakage from the EMG machines.

4. When the equipment exhibits any of the following symptoms or when abuse of the equipment is suspected, it should be taken out of service immediately, repaired, and checked by a competent technician:

- Equipment that is wet or has been subjected to spillage of liquids;
- Equipment that has been dropped or subjected to physical abuse or that contains loose internal or external parts.
- Equipment which gives a "tingling sensation" when touched;
- Equipment that gets unusually hot or gives off unusual odors or sounds;
- Equipment that has been modified or that has had power-line-operated accessories or attachments added. This should not be used until a properly qualified technical person has investigated and approved electrical leakage and patient electrical safety considerations; and
- Damaged or cracked insulation in the power cable, especially at its entry to the equipment, at the power plug, and at all other connectors. This includes connectors and/or plugs that have been subjected to crushing or other mechanical abuse. The path from the ground pin in the power cable plug to the frame of the equipment must always be electrically continuous.

Patient Precautions

To ensure that the patient is grounded at one point via the EMG machine, the following precautions should be taken:

1. Use a wooden examining table. Do not use a metal bed.

2. The patient should never make any contact with the following objects to avoid any potential leaking or current through the body:
   a. Any metal object, grounded or ungrounded, e.g., plumbing, structural parts, decorative architectural trim.
   b. Any part of the EMG equipment cabinet or panel.

Failure to observe the above precautions will not cause injury to the patient in a properly wired and grounded environment when modern, properly functioning EMG equipment is used. However, prudence and the avoidance of annoying artifact dictate careful adherence to them.

3. Because the patient is grounded when connected to the EMG machine, patient contact with nearby power-line-operated appliances that are ungrounded, poorly grounded, or defective presents a special hazard and can cause electrical injury to the patient by the leakage of current

through the body. Therefore, all power-line-operated devices should be kept well away from the operator and the patient, and should be given the same electrical safety considerations as the EMG equipment. Patient proximity to power-line-operated devices and their power cables also results in power line frequency artifact.

4. Never connect a second power-line-operated apparatus to a patient connected to the EMG machine without first carefully considering the resulting electrical safety problems. Artifact problems are also usually present in this situation.

5. Do not apply stimulating electrodes in such a way that the cardiac area is included between them. Ground, recording, and stimulating electrodes should be on the same side of the body and on the same extremity to minimize the path of any leakage through the body.

6. Use great care and vigilance when testing patients with an impaired skin sensory response, patients who are not alert, or patients otherwise not able to report discomfort or pain.

Risks in Electrodiagnostic Practice

Several special problems presented by patients with underlying medical diseases must be addressed here. If they are not recognized, serious untoward effects to the patients as well as to the EMG technicians or the electromyographers could result. This issue has become more acute with the outbreak of AIDS in recent years and is especially important in the case of electromyographers who perform the needle EMG test. There are no special problems associated with the performance of nerve conduction studies with surface electrodes as long as *they are not placed on open wounds or the skin is not scraped with a needle or sandpaper or by cleansing it with alcohol or acetone.*

Because of the concern about transmission of AIDS and other blood-borne illnesses to patients, as well as for the safety of health care workers, stricter measures have been adopted in recent years in many laboratories including our own: (*a*) *disposable needles are used whenever possible for the needle EMG test;* (*b*) protective barriers such as gowns, masks, and protective eyewear may be worn by health care providers during the testing of all patients following "Universal Precautions" recommended by the Centers for Disease Control (CDC) (2). *As a rule, EMG technicians and electromyographers wear gloves for the performance of all procedures in our laboratory.*

The following guidelines are used in the EMG and Evoked Potentials Laboratory at the University of Alabama at Birmingham for the management of some of the more common problems. Our guidelines are similar to those recommended by the AAEM (2).

Bleeding Disorders

Patients with a variety of bleeding disorders may be referred for needle EMG. The referring physician and the electromyographer must examine each case individually, carefully weighing the potential risks and benefits. An increased potential for bleeding may be expected in patients with thrombocytopenia who have a platelet count of less than $50,000/cu^3$, with a prothrombin time of more than 1½ to 2 times the control values, or with a partial thromboplastin time greater than 1½ to 2 times the control values. However, *additionally prolonged local pressure will usually be sufficient to induce hemostasis.* This is also the case with patients who have other coagulopathies or are receiving anticoagulants. Needle examinations should be avoided in patients with hemophilia and other hereditary coagulation disorders unless clotting functions have first been appropriately corrected (4).

There has been one report of a complication of subcutaneous bleeding secondary to the needle EMG in a patient receiving anticoagulants and with a partial thromboplastin time greater than twice the control value (5).

Cardiac Valvular Diseases

Patients with rheumatic or other types of valvular disease and those with prosthetic valves are at risk of developing endocarditis as a result of transient bacteremias. However, the risk from needle electromyography is similar to the risk from repeated venipunctures in whom prophylactic antibiotics are not used. Thus, in agreement with the 1979 AAEE guidelines, we do not recommend prophylactic antibiotics for patients undergoing needle EMG (6). However, more recent AAEM guidelines recommend that consideration be given to prescribing antibiotic coverage similar to that prescribed for dental procedures (7). The basis of this recommendation is not clear. *Among the listed dental or surgical procedures that are very likely to initiate the bacteremia that results in endocarditis, the needle EMG or venipuncture is not listed (8).*

Cardiac Pacemakers

Do not stimulate patients who are wearing a cardiac pacemaker or other cardiac or diagnostic probes unless the test is mandatory for the patient's management. *Needle EMG and nerve conduction studies utilizing percutaneous nerve stimulation may be performed with little risk in patients who have cardiac pacemakers (9).* LaBan's study did not show any ECG abnormality or clinical side-effects in five patients with "demand pacemakers" during nerve conduction study of nerves in arms and legs. The study found that untoward responses appear unlikely if current paths are confined within the standard clinical parameters (9). We have not personally observed any untoward side effects due to the nerve conduction study in patients with cardiac packmakers as long as the precautions outlined below were followed.

Special care should be given to proper grounding. In general, the closer the stimulation is to the pacemaker and pacing leads, the greater is the chance for inducing a voltage of sufficient amplitude to inhibit the pacemaker. Therefore, *a stimulator should be used only with extreme caution if it is necessary to stimulate areas near the pacemaker implantation site, the pacemaker lead, or other cardiac probes.* There can be electrical contact inside the body between electrodes placed within it. There may be electrodes placed on the heart, e.g., pacemaker leads. A catheter that carries fluids to or from the body can function as a conductive pathway. Under those circumstances resistance can be as low as 500 ohm, because these contacts bypass the skin and enter the body (10). Therefore, the impedance drops by 10– to 20–fold, and the patient is much more susceptible. With such a low contact resistance, the same voltage causes 10 times more current flow in the susceptible patient with internal leads. This means that extreme care should be taken when performing the nerve conduction study in these patients, especially when stimulating the brachial plexus ipsilateral to the pacemaker implantation site (11). *In patients with external cardiac pacemakers, the conductive lead that is inserted into the heart (usually transvenously) and connected to the external cardiac pacemaker presents a serious potential hazard of electric injury to the heart.* AAEM guidelines do not recommend nerve conduction studies in such patients (3).

Chest Wall EMG

Pneumothorax was reported with needle nerve stimulation of the intercostal nerves in 8.8% of cases (12). Pneumothorax was also reported with the needle EMG study in the supraspinatus and paracervical muscles in a single case each (13, 14). Considering the number of needle EMGs performed in the supraspinatus and paracervical muscles, such complications are extremely rare. In my opinion, there should not be any pneumothorax if the needle EMG study is properly performed in the supraspinatus or paracervical muscles. Nevertheless, the physician must use clinical judgment to decide if the value of the information to be obtained is greater than the risks of producing a pneumothorax. This is especially so when requesting the needle EMG study in the intercostal muscles or needle stimulation of the intercostal nerves.

Use of Needle Electrodes in Patients with Possible Jakob-Creutzfeldt Disease

Because of the infectious nature and resistance to conventional sterilization procedures of the transmissible agent responsible for Jakob-Creutzfeldt disease, *it is essential that needle electrodes be discarded after use in any patient who is clinically suspected of having Jakob-Creutzfeldt disease, regardless of whether the needles are disposable or not.* Furthermore, before being discarded all needles and blood-contaminated materials from demented patients undergoing electromyography should be incinerated or *autoclaved for 1 hr at 121℃ (15).* When autoclaving is not available, *1-hr exposure to 0.5% sodium hypochlorite* (10-fold dilution of household bleach) can provide excellent disinfection. Such needles should never be reused. So far, no case of Jakob-Creutzfeldt disease transmitted via an EMG needle has been reported.

Hepatitis

The CDC has estimated that 12,000 healthcare workers become infected with hepatitis B each year (16). Even though the risk of contracting hepatitis B in the EMG laboratory is small, *it is medically prudent for the electromyographer to have a hepatitis B vaccination* since the needle EMG test occasionally involves contact with blood, and this disease is preventable by vaccination (16, 17).

Universal precautions for blood and body fluids should be carefully followed by technicians and physicians in the EMG laboratory in dealing with patients with known or suspected infectious hepatitis (18). This includes the appropriate use of handwashing, protective barriers (gloves, gown, mask, and eyewear), and care in the use and disposal of needles and other sharp instruments. *Disposable EMG needles are preferred for the needle EMG examination in patients with known or suspected infectious hepatitis.* If reusable needles are used, they must be autoclaved for 15 minutes at 121°C before reusing (17, 19).

Human Immunodeficiency Virus and AIDS

Human immunodeficiency virus (HIV) is known to be transmitted through blood or body fluids. Thus, HIV is a definite risk to the electromyographer who performs the needle EMG study. EMG testing is not contraindicated, however, in patients who have HIV. *Universal precautions for blood and body fluids* should be carefully followed by EMG technicians and electromyographers in dealing with patients who are known or suspected to have HIV or AIDS (20). *EMG needles, disposable and nondisposable, should be discarded* in a prominently labeled container and disposed of according to hospital policy after use in such patients. Great care must be taken to avoid any accidental wounds from EMG needles contaminated with blood. Double-gloving and the wearing of a gown over the uniform are preferred.

Even when surface electrodes are used for the nerve conduction study, disposable surface electrodes are preferred for such patients. According to the AAEM guidelines (3), needles may routinely be reused without risk of transmission of the HIV virus to subsequent patients if standard disinfection protocols are followed after chemical treatment. For example, viral infectivity is undetectable within *1 minute with 0.5% sodium hypochlorite (10-fold dilution of household bleach), 70% alcohol, or 0.5% nonidet-P40,* and within 10 minutes with 0.08% quaternary ammonium chloride or with a 1:1 mixture of acetone-alcohol (21, 22). Surface electrodes should also be chemically treated before reusing.

There is no doubt that these precautions, however tedious they may be, will insure the maximal safety of patients and EMG laboratory staff. In many years of working with EMG equipment, I have not yet experienced or heard of any major accidents associated with EMG testing.

REFERENCES

1. TECA Corporation. Electrical Safety. In: EMG–Operating notes. White Plains, NY: TECA Corp, 1973.
2. Centers for Disease Control. Update: universal precautions for prevention of transmission of human immunodeficiency virus, hepatitis B virus, and other bloodborne pathogens in health-care settings. MMWR 1988;37:24.
3. AAEM: Guidelines in Electrodiagnostic Medicine. Muscle Nerve 1991;15:229–253.

4. Wintrobes M. The hereditary coagulation disorders, In: Wintrobes M et al., eds: Clinical hematology. Philadelphia: Lea & Febiger, 1981;1158–1205.

5. Butler ML, Dewan RW. Subcutaneous hemorrhage in a patient receiving anticoagulant therapy: an unusual EMG complication. Arch Phys Med Rehabil 1984;65:733–734.

6. AAEE. Guidelines in EMG. Rochester, Minnesota, 1979.

7. AAEE: Guidelines in electrodiagnostic medicine. Rochester, Minnesota, 1988.

8. American Heart Association. Prevention of bacterial endocarditis. JAMA 1990;264:2919–2922.

9. LaBan MM, Petty D, Hauser AM, Taylor RS. Peripheral nerve conduction stimulation: its effect on cardiac pacemakers. Arch Phys Med Rehabil 1988;69:358–362.

10. Grass ER. Electrical safety specially related to EEG. Quincy, MA: Grass Instrument Co., 1978; Bulletin No. 757078.

11. Youmans CR Jr, Bourianoff G, Allensworth DC, et al. Cardiovascular alterations during electroconvulsive therapy in patients with cardiac pacemakers. South Med J 1972;65:361–365.

12. Johnson ER, Powell J, Caldwell J, Crane C. Intercostal nerve conduction and posterior rhizotomy in the diagnosis and treatment of thoracic radiculopathy. J Neurol Neurosurg Psychiatry 1974;37:330–332.

13. Honet J, Honet JC, Cascade P. Pneumothorax after electromyographic electrode insertion in the paracervical muscles: case report and radiographic analysis. Arch Phys Med Rehabil 1986;67:601–603.

14. Reinstein L, Twardzik FC, Mech KF Jr. Pneumothorax: a complication of needle electromyography of the supraspinatus muscle. Arch Phys Med Rehabil 1987;68:561–563.

15. Brown P, Gibbs CJ, Amyx HL, Kingsbury DT, Rohwer RG, Sulima MP, Gajdusek DC. Chemical disinfection of Creutzfeldt-Jakob disease virus. NEJM 1982;306:1279–1282.

16. Centers for Disease Control. Guidelines for prevention of transmission of human immunodeficiency virus and hepatitis B virus to health-care and public-safety workers. MMWR 1989;38:S-6.

17. Centers for Disease Control. Protection against viral hepatitis: recommendations of the Immunization Practices Advisory Committee. MMWR 1990;39:5.

18. Centers for Disease Control: Update: universal precautions for prevention of transmission of human immunodeficiency virus, hepatitis B virus, and other bloodborne pathogens in health-care settings. MMWR 1988;24:37.

19. Centers for Disease Control. Perspectives on the control of viral hepatitis, type B. MMWR 1976;(suppl. 17):25.

20. Centers for Disease Control: Update: Universal precautions for prevention of transmission of human immunodeficiency virus, hepatitis B virus, and other bloodborne pathogens in health-care settings. MMWR 1988;24:37.

21. Martin LS, McDougal JS, Loskoski SL. Disinfection and inactivation of the human T lymphotropic virus type III/lymphoadenopathy-associated virus. J Infect Dis 1985;152:400–403.

22. Resnick L, Veren K, Salahuddin Z, Tondreau S, Marklam PD. Stability and inactivation of HTLV-III/LAV under clinical and laboratory environments. JAMA 1986;255:1887–1891.

PART II

ADVANCED SECTION

11

Uncommon Nerve Conduction Studies: Techniques and Normal Values

It has been repeatedly stressed that each electromyography (EMG) laboratory should establish normal nerve conduction values using its own techniques. In practice, however, it is almost impossible for each laboratory to establish normal nerve conduction values for each of the various nerves. Therefore, the best alternative is to compare results with normal values in the literature. To make this meaningful, the individual laboratory must carefully follow the instructions for the measurement and the nerve conduction technique. In this chapter we describe various techniques used to study nerve conduction and give normal values for many nerves that are tested infrequently. Clinicians will find it useful to compare their patients' values with the normal values listed here. Because we cannot summarize all of the techniques described in the literature, we have selected those that meet the following requirements:

1. The details of recording, stimulation, and measurement are well described;
2. Normal values are presented in the statistical terms; and
3. There is a major difference in technique, e.g., needle versus surface electrodes or a different site of stimulation.

If there is only one method published for the nerve and that method does not meet the criteria, we still include the technique simply because it is still useful. When many methods using essentially the same techniques are available, we have chosen the one that best meets the aforementioned criteria.

For the convenience of readers, we have italicized the methods we prefer in the EMG Laboratory of the University of Alabama at Birmingham (UAB) when similar methods of testing are described.

The symbols used in the figures in this chapter are shown in Fig. 11.1.

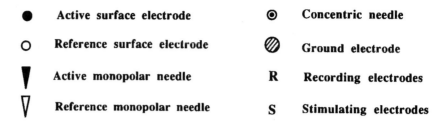

Figure 11.1. Symbols for electrodes.

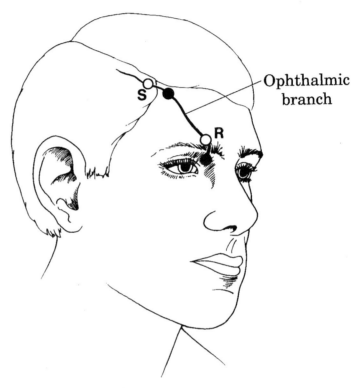

Figure 11.2. Sensory nerve conduction of the ophthalmic branch of the trigeminal nerve.

Trigeminal Nerve

Ophthalmic Nerve Sensory Conduction

Raffaele et al. (1) described a method of sensory nerve conduction of the ophthalmic branch of the trigeminal nerve (Fig. 11.2).

RECORDING: An active recording surface electrode is placed on the supraorbital foramen. The reference electrode is placed on the upper eyelid.

STIMULATION: Bipolar surface electrodes are placed at the upper lateral corner of the forehead. Stimulus duration is 0.05 msec.

MEASUREMENT: Latency is measured from the stimulus onset to the negative peak of the CNAP. The NCV is calculated by dividing the distance by the latency. Amplitude is measured by the conventional method.

TEMPERATURE: Skin temperature is controlled between 32–34°C.

NORMAL DATA: Number of subjects: 10. Age range: 18–54 yr.

Measurement	Mean ± SD	Normal Limit
Latency (msec)	0.81 ± 0.11	1.03
Amplitude (μV)	32.8 ± 2.8	
NCV (m/sec)	59.1 ± 8.9	41.3

Facial Nerve

Motor Nerve Conduction

Zander Olsen's Method

Zander Olsen (2) described motor nerve conduction in the facial nerve (Fig. 11.3) with the needle at both the stimulating and the recording electrode (Fig. 11.4).

RECORDING: The compound muscle action potentials (CMAPs) are recorded with a concentric or wire electrode from the frontalis, orbicularis oris, and triangularis muscles. This arrangement tests the temporal, zygomatic, and mandibular branches of the facial nerve. If a wire electrode is used, the reference electrode is placed on the contralateral side of the face. In the frontalis muscle, the optimal site is found at a point midway between the hairline and the eyebrow, along a line passing vertically through the pupil. In the orbicularis oris muscle, the recording site is 2 mm above the lip, midway between the midline and the corner of the mouth. In the triangular muscle, the site is at the base of the ramus of the mandible, on a vertical line 15 mm lateral to the corner of the mouth.

STIMULATION: The nerve is stimulated using 25 mm long uninsulated stainless steel needles 0.5 mm in diameter. The active electrode is placed near the facial nerve just distal to its exit from the stylomastoid foramen where the nerve trunk is still undivided. The shortest route to this point of the nerve is obtained by inserting the needle just anteriorly to the tip of the mastoid process at right angles to the skin to a depth of about 20 mm. The reference electrode is placed subcutaneously 25 mm posterior and inferior to the near-nerve electrode.

MEASUREMENT: The latency is measured from the stimulus onset to the initial deflection of the CMAP. Amplitude of the CMAP is measured from the peak to peak. Distance is measured by the conventional method (see Chapter 4).

TEMPERATURE: Skin temperature is 34.3°–34.6°C.

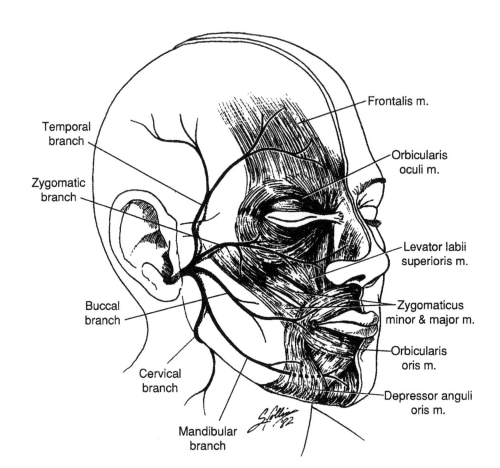

Figure 11.3. Anatomical course and innervation of the facial nerve.

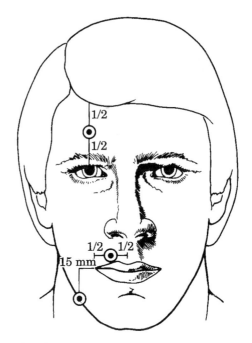

Figure 11.4. Zander Olsen's method of motor nerve conduction of the facial nerve.

NORMAL DATA: See Table 7.39.

INTERPRETATION: Latency should be judged according to the distance from stimulating and recording electrodes.

COMMENT: The latency to the potential recorded with the concentric electrode is 0.1–0.5 msec longer than the latency with a wire electrode.

Oh's Method

This method uses the surface electrode as both stimulating and recording electrodes (Fig. 11.5).

RECORDING: An active surface electrode is placed over the midpoint of the lower portion of the obicularis oculi, and a reference electrode is placed above the eyebrow along the same vertical plane of the active electrode.

STIMULATION: The zygomatic branch of the facial nerve is stimulated anterior and inferior to the tragus of the earlobe.

MEASUREMENT: Latency is measured from the stimulus onset to the initial deflection of the CMAP.

TEMPERATURE: Skin temperature is 31°–33°C.

NORMAL DATA: Number of subjects: 30. Age range: 21–50 yr.

Measurement	Mean ± SD	Normal Limit
Latency (msec)	2.38 ± 0.35	3.08
Amplitude (mV)	3.2 ± 1.1	1.1

COMMENTS: This site of stimulation is easier and less painful than the site inferior and posterior to the external acoustic meatus.

De Meirsman's Method

De Meirsman et al. (3) described a technique for obtaining CMAPs on the posterior auricular muscle (Fig. 11.6).

RECORDING: A coaxial needle electrode is inserted into the posterior auricular muscle located at the midpoint of the posterior aspect of the pinna. By bending the ear for-

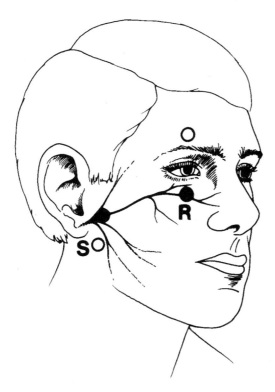

Figure 11.5. Oh's method of motor nerve conduction of the facial nerve.

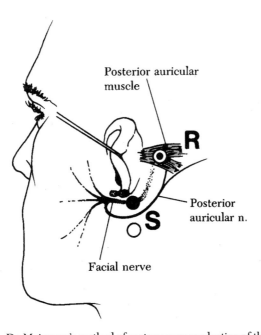

Posterior auricular muscle

R

Posterior auricular n.

S

Facial nerve

Figure 11.6. De Meirsman's method of motor nerve conduction of the facial nerve.

ward, the skin fold that contains the muscle becomes visible. The ground electrode is placed on the contralateral forehead.

STIMULATION: The nerve is stimulated by a surface electrode just below the ear and anterior to the mastoid process.

MEASUREMENT: Latency is measured from the stimulus onset to the first negative deflection of the CMAP.

TEMPERATURE: Skin temperature varies from 34° to 35°C.

NORMAL DATA: Number of subjects: 40. Age range: 15–65 yr.

Measurement	Mean ± SD	Normal Limit
Latency (msec)	1.92 ± 0.35	2.62
Amplitude (mV)	2.5 –10 (Range)	2.5

COMMENTS: De Meirsman et al. (3) stated that this method tests the functional status of the most proximal part of the facial nerve because the posterior auricular muscle is innervated by the first branch of the facial nerve that splits from the whole nerve trunk immediately after passing through the stylomastoid foramen. We are not sure whether this test has any advantage over other methods.

Redhead's Method

Redhead and Mugliston (4) described a technique of the facial nerve conduction with recording electrodes on the risorius muscle (Fig. 11.7).

RECORDING: Bipolar surface electrodes with an interelectrode distance of 2 cm are used. An active surface electrode is placed on the nasolabial fold (the risorius muscle) and a reference electrode close to the corner of mouth.

STIMULATION: The facial nerve is stimulated anterior to the tip of the mastoid process.

MEASUREMENT: Peak-to-peak amplitude is measured. Latency is measured by the conventional method.

TEMPERATURE: Not controlled.

NORMAL DATA: Number of subjects: 50. Age range: 3–56 yr.

	Right	Left	R/L ratio	
Measurement	Mean ± SD	Mean ± SD	Mean ± SD	Normal Limit
CMAP (mV)	3.16 ± 1.08	2.97 ± 1.86	1.12 ± 0.40	
Latency (msec)	3.30 ± 0.48	3.20 ± 0.42	1.01 ± 0.11	4.26

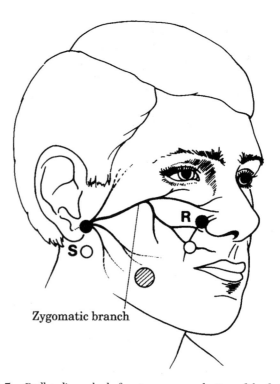

Figure 11.7.   Redhead's method of motor nerve conduction of the facial nerve.

COMMENTS: Many otolaryngologists use this method (5, 6). They are more interested in the amplitude difference between the normal side and the affected side in Bell's palsy. A 25% difference in the amplitude is noted in normal subjects (6). The highest amplitude is obtained with an interelectrode distance of 2 cm for the recording electrodes (5).

Facial Nerve Excitability Test

The facial nerve excitability test does not require any objective recording. The target sign is the minimal twitching of muscle, thus involving a subjective judgment.

STIMULATION: The facial nerve is stimulated by placing an active electrode below the external auditory meatus and behind the angle of the jaw. This stimulates all the facial muscles.

An alternative method of stimulation, which we prefer, is to place an active electrode just anterior and inferior to the tragus of the earlobe. By stimulating this site, each branch of the facial nerve can easily be stimulated with minimal intensity.

Different authors use different durations of stimulus (Table 11.1). The Hilger stimulator (7) (Hilger Facial Nerve Stimulator, Model 2 or 2R. WR Medical Electronics Co., St. Paul, Minnesota) which is specifically designed for this test, uses 0.6 msec duration. As the intensity is gradually increased, there should be minimal twitching of the orbicularis oculi muscle. If this is not visible with sufficient stimulation, the examiner should look for twitching of the orbicularis oris.

MEASUREMENT: When the first minimal twitching of muscle is noted, record the intensity value in milliamperes. The test should be repeated three times and the three values averaged.

TEMPERATURE: Not controlled.

INTERPRETATION: With a 1-msec stimulus duration, Campbell et al. (8) observed that in normal individuals the intensity value is in the range of 3–8 mA. The intensity values of the two sides should be compared to judge if the nerve excitability on one side is diminished. Various investigators have used different stimulus durations and therefore different criteria to judge nerve excitability (Table 11.1). In general, we consider a *4-mA or greater nerve excitability difference significant* for 0.6- to 1-msec stimulus durations. An absence of nerve excitability beyond 20 mA indicates complete nerve degeneration.

COMMENTS: Because of the subjective observation of muscle twitching, it is imperative to distinguish a genuine response from false responses. Three possible errors can be made in this regard. It is best to follow these guidelines:

1. Twitching around the stimulating electrode should not be regarded as a genuine response;

2. When increased intensity is used, care should be taken that contraction of the masseter is not mistaken for a genuine response of the facial muscles; and

3. By virtue of the position of the stimulating electrode, the platysma may respond by direct stimulation when increased intensity is used. It is important to realize that this does not imply the presence of a genuine response.

Table 11.1.
Nerve Excitability Test: Duration of Stimulus and Criteria for Poor Prognosis

Investigators	Duration of Stimulus (msec)	Criteria for Poor Prognosis (mA)
Campbell et al. (8)	1	2
Hilger (7)	0.6	3.5
Laumans (143)	1	3.5
Saade and Karem (144)	1.2	2
Alford et al. (145)	1	3
Adour et al. (146)	0.6	2.5
Devi et al. (147)	0.1	5

Recurrent Laryngeal Nerve

Peytz et al. (9) describe the method for measuring recurrent laryngeal nerve conduction (Fig. 11.8).

RECORDING: The CMAP is obtained by a concentric needle electrode from the vocal muscle (internal and external thyroartenoid muscles). The electrode is introduced either through a laryngoscope (majority of individuals) or directly during total laryngectomy (a few patients). Before laryngoscopy, the pharynx and larynx are sprayed with a mixture of tetracaine (1:200) and adrenaline (1:200,000), and 80–120 mg pethidine are given intravenously. Laryngectomies are performed under general anesthesia (nitrous oxide/nembutal/fluothane/pethidine).

STIMULATION: The recurrent nerve is stimulated near the trachea (Fig. 11.8A) and the vagus nerve just before branching of the recurrent nerve (Fig. 11.8B). An active stimulating needle is inserted paratracheally 2.5 cm below the most prominent point of the cricoid arch. A reference needle electrode is placed in the subcutaneous tissue of the jugular fossa. Another active stimulating needle is inserted at the same level as A at the posterior edge of the sternocleodomastoid muscle. The depth of these electrodes should be adjusted until the lowest threshold of the CMAP is obtained.

MEASUREMENT: The latency is measured from the stimulus onset to the onset of the initial negative or positive deflection of the CMAP. The measurement of amplitude and duration is conventional. The distance between A and B is extrapolated from measurements in cadavers 155–173 cm in height. A cadaver study showed that the distance between A and B increases with height. In subjects 155 to 173 cm in height the distance on the right ranged from 9 to 11.5 cm and on the left from 20 to 25 cm. Nerve conduction velocity (NCV) is calculated from the distance between A and B, which is extrapolated from the cadaver data.

TEMPERATURE: Not controlled.

NORMAL DATA:

Measurement	Mean ± SD	Normal Limit	No. of Subjects
Terminal latency (msec)	2.1 ± 0.05^a	2.2	26
Amplitude (mV)	6.8 ± 0.7		
Duration (msec)	6.6 ± 0.5		20
NCV (m/sec)	60–70 (range)	60	8

[a]Mean distance: 5.9 cm.

COMMENTS: To ascertain that the CMAP is in fact recorded from the vocal muscles without superimposition of potentials from other muscles, the CMAPs are recorded simultaneously on the other channels from the sternocleidomastoid, the platysma, or the infrathyroid muscles. When a potential is recorded from these muscles, it has a longer latency and much lower amplitude than the vocal muscle.

Accessory Nerve

Cherington's Method

Cherington's technique (10) for examining the accessory nerve (Fig. 11.9) uses surface electrodes (Fig. 11.10).

RECORDING: An active surface electrode is placed in the upper trapezius muscle, approximately 5 cm lateral from the C7 spinous process.

STIMULATION: The nerve is stimulated with surface electrodes *slightly above the midpoint between the clavicle and mastoid process along the posterior border of the sternocleidomastoid muscle (Fig. 11.10A).*

MEASUREMENT: Conventional method.

TEMPERATURE: Skin temperature is not controlled.

NORMAL DATA: Number of subjects: 25. Age range: 10–60 yr. The latency is 1.8–3.0 msec for a distance of 5.0–8.2 cm.

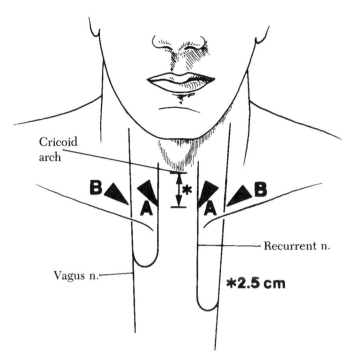

Figure 11.8. Recurrent laryngeal nerve conduction (*A*, *B*). See text.

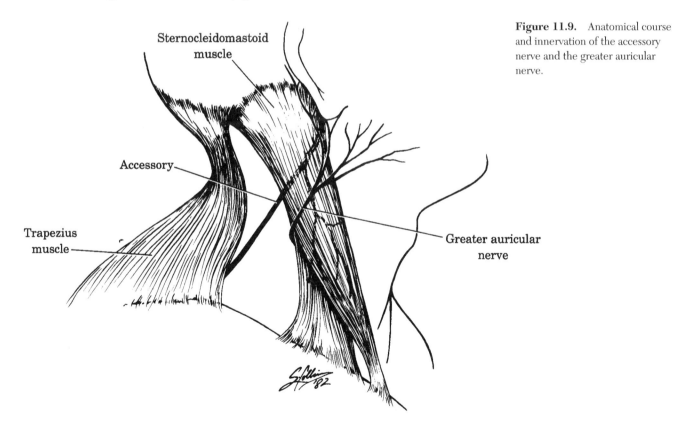

Figure 11.9. Anatomical course and innervation of the accessory nerve and the greater auricular nerve.

INTERPRETATION: If the latency is above the upper normal range, it is considered abnormal.

Fahrer's Method

The technique of Fahrer et al. (11) uses a needle electrode as the recording electrode (Fig. 11.10).

Figure 11.10. Motor nerve conduction of the accessory nerve. **A,** Stimulation with a surface electrode. **B,** Stimulation with a needle electrode (Petrera's method). **C,** Cherington's method. **D,** Fahrer's and Petrera's method.

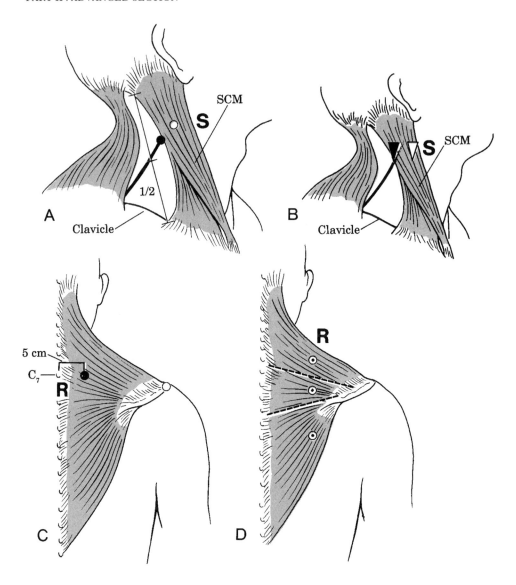

RECORDING: Concentric electrodes are inserted in three parts (ascending, horizontal, and descending) of the trapezius muscle. (No other details were given.)

STIMULATION: The nerve is stimulated with surface electrodes in the posterior triangle of the neck.

MEASUREMENT: Distance measurement is conventional. Latency is measured from the stimulus onset to the onset of the first deflection of the CMAP.

TEMPERATURE: Skin temperature is not controlled.

NORMAL DATA: There is a linear correlation between latency and distance (correlation coefficient r = 0.946).

Latency = 0.689 + 0.158 × distance (cm). SD = 0.47

INTERPRETATION: Latency is judged depending on the distance (Fig. 11.11).

COMMENTS: In five of eight patients with accessory nerve injury, the latency was either prolonged or the CMAP was not obtainable.

Petrera's Method

Petrera and Trojaborg's method (12) is different from Fahrer's method in that a stainless steel needle is used as the stimulating electrode (Fig. 11.10).

RECORDING: Concentric needle electrodes are inserted into the upper, middle and lower part of the trapezius muscle. Bipolar needle electrodes (Dantec 13 K13) are used

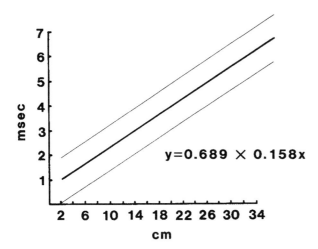

Figure 11.11. Linear relationship between the latency (*y*) and the distance between the stimulating and recording electrodes (*x*). The *thick line* is the regression line of mean latencies. The *thin line* is the regression line of mean latencies ± 2 SD. (From Fahrer H, Ludin HP, Mumenthaler M, Neiger M. The innervation of the trapezius muscle: an electrophysiological study. J Neurol 1974;207:185.)

when the CMAP response is contaminated by volume-conducted activity from nearby muscles.

STIMULATION: A near-nerve needle electrode (Dantec 13L60-13L64) is used as the stimulating electrode just above the midpoint of the posterior border of the sternocleidomastoid muscle and is adjusted close to the nerve, as indicated by the threshold of the CMAP (0.5–1 mA with 0.2 msec stimulus duration) (Fig. 11.10B). The reference needle electrode is placed 1–1.5 cm proximal to the near-nerve needle electrode.

MEASUREMENT: Distance to the upper part is measured with a measuring tape and to the middle and lower parts with an obstetric caliper.

TEMPERATURE: Skin temperature is not controlled. Room temperature is 22°C.

NORMAL DATA: Number of subjects: 22. Age range: 13–66 yr.

Measurement	Mean ± SD	Normal Range	Distance Range
Latency		2.2–6.3 msec	75–305 mm

INTEPRETATION: Latency is correlated with the distance between the stimulating and recording electrodes. Thus, the latency must be judged against the distance-adjusted normal latency (Fig. 11.12). The latency is abnormal when the value is outside the 95% confidence limit.

COMMENTS: In 10 of 16 patients with accessory nerve palsy, the latency to the upper trapezius muscle was prolonged.

Krogness's Method

Krogness's method (13) is different from the above methods in that the proximal portion of the accessory nerve is stimulated, evoking a response from the sternocleidomastoid as well (Fig. 11.13).

RECORDING: A concentric needle electrode is placed in the distal part of the upper third of the trapezius as well as in the sternocleidomastoid muscle at the level of the cricothyroid junction.

STIMULATION: A long-legged active electrode is placed in front of the mastoid process, stimulating the accessory nerve near the jugular foramen.

MEASUREMENT: The latency is measured from the stimulus onset to the first positive deflection. The distances from the midpoint between the active and the reference stimulating electrodes to the recording needle are measured.

TEMPERATURE: Not controlled.

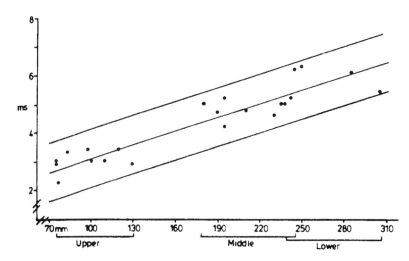

Figure 11.12. Latency to the upper, middle, and lower part of the trapezius muscle as a function of conduction distance. The *center line* represents the regression line (n = 22, r = 0.89), the *outside lines* the 95% confidence limits. (From Petrera JE, Trojaborg W. Conduction studies along the accessory nerve and follow up of patients with trapezius palsy. J Neurol Neurosurg Psychiatry 1984;47:631.)

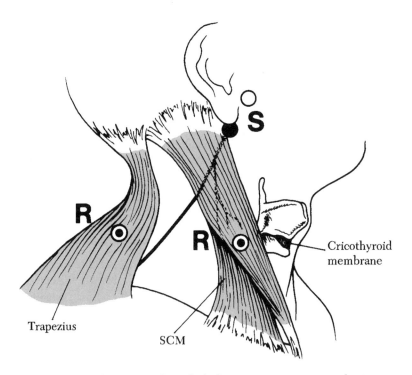

Figure 11.13. Krogness's method of accessory nerve motor conduction.

NORMAL DATA: Number of subjects: 21. Age range: 23–72 yr.

Measurement	Mean ± SD	Normal Limit
Sternocleidomastoid muscle		
Terminal latency (msec)	2.3 ± 0.5[a]	3.3
Amplitude (mV)	8.7 ± 4.6	
Trapezius muscle		
Terminal latency (msec)	3.5 ± 0.5[b]	4.5
Amplitude (mV)	10.7 ± 5.6	

[a]Mean distance: 9.6 cm.
[b]Mean distance: 12.5 cm.

COMMENTS: If the lesion is proximal to the posterior triangle, this is the method of choice.

Hypoglossal Nerve Conduction

Redmond and Di Benedetto (14) described a technique of measuring motor nerve conduction in the hypoglossal nerve.

POSITION OF SUBJECT: The test is performed with the subject seated.

RECORDING: A specially designed orthoplast bite bar is used to secure the recording surface electrodes over the anterior surface of the tongue in the midline (Fig. 11.14). An active recording electrode (distal) and a reference recording electrode (proximal) are impregnated into this bar along the midline 2 cm apart. This bar can be gas-sterilized. The tongue is dried with a gauze sponge and the bar is inserted into the mouth. The mouth is closed so that the bite bar is held securely between the teeth, with enough space for the electrodes wires to pass (Fig. 11.15). The subject is instructed to relax and allow the tongue to rest against the inner aspect of the lower teeth. Once inserted into the mouth, the active recording electrode should be 1 cm posterior to the lower incisors. The side bars facilitate easy insertion and allow the examiner to monitor positioning and movement during the study.

STIMULATION: The hypoglossal nerve is stimulated with the surface electrodes at a point one-third the distance along the inferior surface of the mandible from the angle to the apex and 1 cm medial to the inner aspect of the mandible (Fig. 11.16).

MEASUREMENT: The latency is measured by the conventional method. The CMAP amplitude is measured from baseline to negative peak.

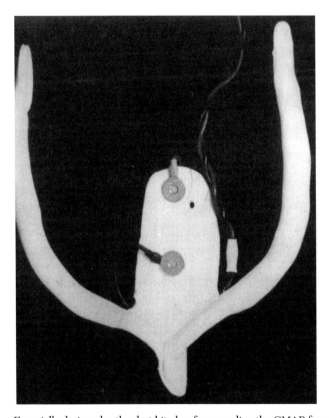

Figure 11.14. Especially designed orthoplast bite bar for recording the CMAP from the hypoglossal muscle. Critical dimensions include a 2-cm separation between the recording and reference electrodes, with the electrodes arranged in the midline. Once inserted into the mouth, the recording electrode should be 1 cm posterior to the lower incisors, with both electrodes upon the anterior surface of the tongue. (From Redmond MD, Di Benedetto M. Hypoglossal nerve conduction in normal subjects. Muscle Nerve 1988;11:448.)

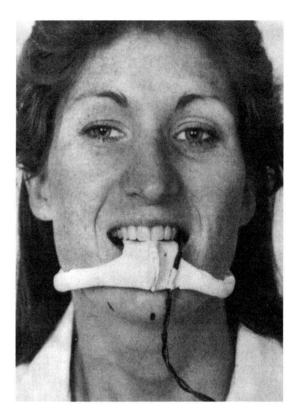

Figure 11.15.   The recording apparatus is inserted into the mouth such that the surface electrodes rest upon the anterior surface of the tongue. The subject bites the middle bar along the electrode wires to exit the mouth without damage. The side bars facilitate easy insertion and allow the examiner to monitor positioning and movement during the study. (From Redmond MD, Di Benedetto M. Hypoglossal nerve conduction in normal subjects. Muscle Nerve 1988;11:449.)

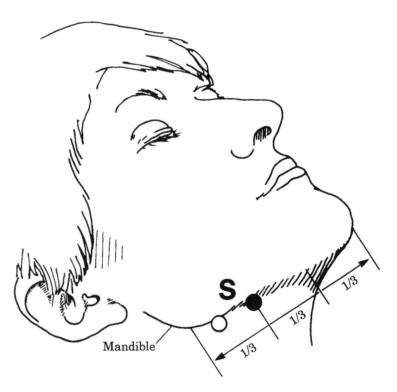

Figure 11.16.   Position of the stimulating electrodes on the hypoglossal nerve.

TEMPERATURE: Skin temperature is not controlled.

NORMAL DATA: Number of subjects: 30. Age range: 19–56 yr.

Measurement	Mean ± SD	Normal Limit
Latency (msec)		
Left	2.1 ± 0.4	2.9
Right	2.2 ± 0.4	3.0
Amplitude (mV)		
Left	3.8 ± 1.6	0.6
Right	3.9 ± 1.6	0.7

COMMENTS: According to authors, the latency was reproducible despite tongue motion, but the amplitude was less reliable because of the variability (18). Tongue movement, however, precludes employing this method for repetitive stimulation studies.

Greater Auricular Nerve

Palliyath's Method

Palliyath (15) described a technique for measuring the sensory nerve conduction of the greater auricular nerve (Fig. 11.9) using a surface electrode (Fig. 11.17A).

RECORDING: An active surface electrode is placed over the back of the earlobe. The reference is placed 2 cm away from the active electrode.

STIMULATION: The nerve is stimulated with a bipolar stimulating electrode held firmly against the lateral border of the sternocleidomastoid muscle at a point 8 cm proximal to the active recording electrode. *The reference electrode is best located at the midpoint between the clavicle and mastoid process along the posterior border of the sternocleidomastoid muscle with an active electrode toward the ear.*

MEASUREMENT: Latency is measured from the stimulus onset to the peak of negative deflection of the CNAP. The amplitude is measured from the take-off to the negative peak.

TEMPERATURE: Skin temperature is between 33–35°. Room temperature is set at 26.6°C (80°F).

NORMAL DATA: Number of subjects: 20. Age range: 21–66 yr.

Measurement	Mean ± SD	Normal Limit
Latency (msec)	1.7 + 0.2	2.1
NCV (m/sec)	46.8 ± 6.6	33.6
Amplitude (μV)	12.7 + 4.1	
Duration (msec)	0.8 + 0.2	1.2

COMMENTS: This technique was able to confirm a greater auricular sensory neuropathy due to an injury of this nerve by a central venous line insertion during surgery in a single case (15).

Kimura's Method

Kimura et al. used a fixed distance between the recording and stimulating electrodes (16). No essential difference is noted between this method and Palliyath's method (15) (Fig. 11.17B).

POSITION OF SUBJECT: Subject lies on his side with the neck relaxed completely.

RECORDING: An active surface electrode is placed on the back of the lower ear lobe. The reference electrode is placed 2 cm away from the active electrode.

STIMULATION: The nerve is stimulated with bipolar stimulating electrodes held firmly against the posterior border of the sternocleidomastoid muscle 8 cm caudally

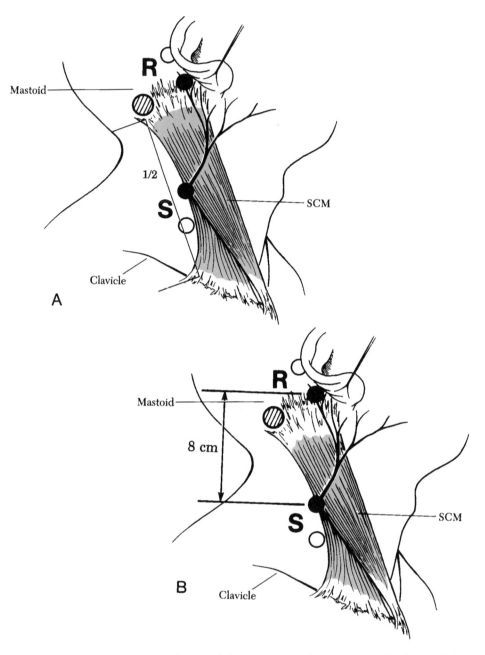

Figure 11.17.   Sensory nerve conduction of the greater auricular nerve. *A*, Palliyath's method. *B*, Kimura's method.

from the recording electrode. If the stimulating electrode is placed too caudally, the accessory nerve is stimulated.

MEASUREMENT: The conventional method of measurement is used.

TEMPERATURE: Skin temperature is not controlled.

NORMAL DATA: Number of subjects: 64. Age range: 14–88 yr.

Measurement	Mean ± SD	Normal limit
Onset latency	1.3 ± 0.2	1.7
Peak latency	1.9 ± 0.2	2.3
Amplitude	22.4 ± 8.9	8.0[a]
Duration	1.1 ± 0.2	1.5

[a]Lower range.

COMMENTS: According to the authors, with this method a well-defined CNAP is obtained in subjects of all ages without using an averager. Amplitude of the CNAP has a tendency to decrease with the patient's age. This nerve conduction can be used for diagnosis of greater auricular neuropathy as well as in differentiation between pre- and postganglionic lesions in the 2nd and/or 3rd cervical segments.

Phrenic Nerve

Newsome Davis's Method

Newsome Davis (17) describes a technique to investigate the phrenic nerve (Fig. 11.18) using surface electrodes (Fig. 11.19A).

RECORDING: The diaphragmatic CMAP is recorded with an active surface electrode placed over the 7th, 8th, or 9th intercostal spaces along the anterior axillary line. A reference electrode is placed 3.5–5 cm posteriorly from the active electrode.

STIMULATION: The nerve is stimulated percutaneously at the posterior border of the sternocleidomastoid muscle at the level of the upper margin of the thyroid cartilage. A brief search is sometimes required before the nerve is located. Because the phrenic nerve at this point lies in close relation to the brachial plexus, stimulation sometimes causes excitation of upper limb muscles. However, with careful placing of the stimulating electrode, selective excitation of the phrenic nerve can usually be achieved.

MEASUREMENT: Conventional method.

TEMPERATURE: Skin temperature is not controlled.

NORMAL DATA: Number of subjects: 18. Age range: 20–61 yr.

Measurement	Mean ± SD	Normal Limit
Latency (msec)	7.7 ± 0.8	9.3
Amplitude (μV)	160–500 (range)	160

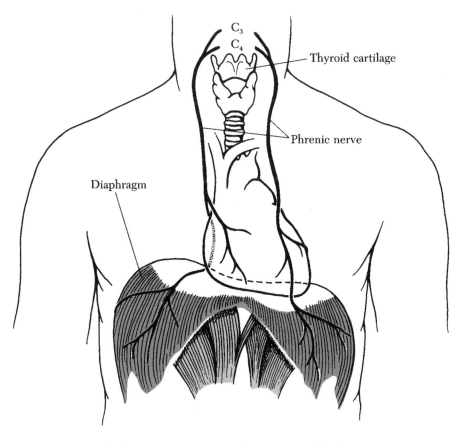

Figure 11.18. Anatomical course and innervation of the phrenic nerve.

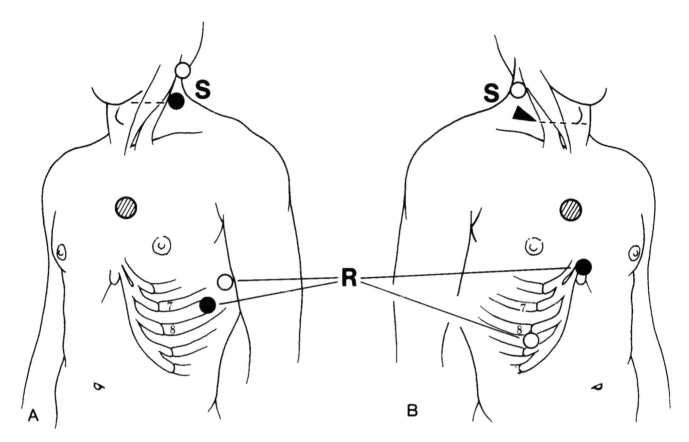

Figure 11.19. Methods of motor nerve conduction of the phrenic nerve. *A*, Newsome-Davis's method. *B*, MacLean's method.

INTERPRETATION: The latency provides a reliable assessment of phrenic nerve function. The amplitude is a less reliable guide.

COMMENTS: There is poor correlation between amplitude and latency. There is no correlation between latency and age.

MacLean's Method

The method of MacLean and Mittioni (18) *uses the needle electrode as a stimulating electrode* (Fig. 11.19B). At the UAB, the phrenic nerve is stimulated with the surface electrode first and, if this does not work, it is stimulated with the needle.

RECORDING: An active electrode is placed over the xiphoid process and a reference electrode over the ipsilateral 8th intercostal space at the costochondral junction.

STIMULATION: A monopolar needle electrode is inserted near the posterior margin of the sternocleidomastoid muscle at the level of the cricoid cartilage (Fig. 11.20). It is angled forward toward the midline so that the tip comes to lie within a few millimeters of the phrenic nerve immediately in front of the anterior scalene muscle. The needle is found to be in proper position when only minimal resistance from loose connective tissue is encountered during insertion to a depth of 15 to 25 mm. During insertion of the stimulating monopolar needle, the needle tracks through the lateral cervical space between fascial planes, thus meeting little resistance from connective tissue and none from muscle. Increased mechanical resistance is encountered only when the needle is angled either too anteriorly into the sternocleidomastoid or too posteriorly into the middle scalene. A reference electrode is placed over the manubrium using a metal plate.

MEASUREMENT: Conventional method.

TEMPERATURE: Skin temperature is not controlled.

NORMAL DATA: Number of subjects: 30. Age range: 18–74 yr.

Measurement	Mean ± SD	Normal Limit
Latency (msec)	7.44 ± 0.59	8.62
Amplitude (μV)	845 ± 405	200
Duration (msec)	48.1 ± 12.1	72.3
Left-right latency difference	0.08 ± 0.42	

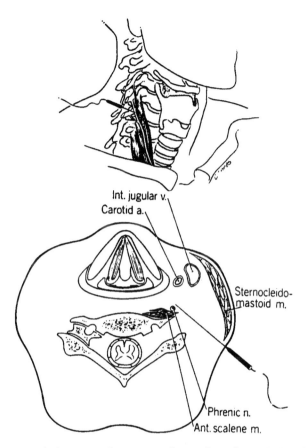

Figure 11.20. Anatomical placement of active stimulating electrode in MacLean's method. (From MacLean IC, Mittoni TA. Phrenic nerve conduction studies: a new technique and its application in quadriplegic patients. Arch Phys Med Rehabil 1981;62:71.)

INTERPRETATION: Any latency of 8.7 msec or more, or any difference in latency of 1.0 msec or more between the normal and abnormal sides, is significant. The measurements of amplitude and duration of CMAPs are highly limited in their usefulness.

COMMENTS: MacLean and Mittioni claimed that this method needs a lower intensity current than percutaneous stimulation, and so the patient tolerates the procedure better. They also claimed that this technique can avoid stimulation of the brachial plexus. They described three potential uses of this technique:

1. Evaluation for electrophrenic respiration. If there is no response, it is unnecessary to proceed with electrophrenic respiration. On the other hand, if there is a near-normal response, implantation of a stimulator will certainly be effective;
2. Localized phrenic nerve lesions; and
3. Any neuromuscular disease that may affect respiration.

Brachial Plexus

Motor Nerve Conduction across the Upper Trunk and the Lateral Cord

Kaplan (19) described a technique for determining the NCV across the upper trunk and the lateral cord of the brachial plexus (Fig. 11.21).

RECORDING: A bipolar surface recording electrode is placed on the brachioradialis

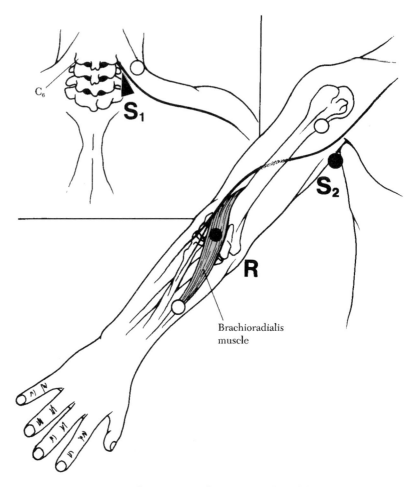

Figure 11.21.   Motor nerve conduction across the upper trunk and the lateral cord of the brachial plexus.

midway between the biceps tendon and the lateral epicondyle along the flexor crease of the antecubital fossa.

STIMULATION: The patient is positioned prone with a pillow under his chest so the cervical spine is moderately flexed while his chin rests on the table. A monopolar stimulating electrode, which is inserted 3 cm lateral to the cephalad margin of the spinous process of the 6th cervical vertebra, stimulates the C6 spinal nerve root. A reference surface electrode is placed 3 cm lateral to an active electrode. As a 2nd site of stimulation, the radial nerve is stimulated in the axilla in the groove between the coracobrachialis and the medial edge of the triceps brachii using a surface electrode.

MEASUREMENT: Latency measurement is conventional. The distance between the point of stimulating the C6 spinal nerve root and that of the radial nerve is measured using sharpened obstetrical calipers, with the patient's arms down by his sides.

TEMPERATURE: Skin temperature is above 34°C.

NORMAL DATA: Number of subjects: 25. Age range: 28–52 yr. The mean NCV is 68 m/sec (SD ± 5.0). The normal limit is 58 m/sec.

COMMENTS: Kaplan stated that nerve root stimulation is easy to perform, accurate, and completely safe. He found slow motor NCVs (40 m/sec) in five patients with neuropathy in the upper trunk.

Motor Nerve Conduction across the Lower Trunk

MacLean and coworkers (20–22) described a technique for determining the NCV by stimulating C8 and T1 roots (Fig. 11.22).

RECORDING: Surface recording electrodes are placed over the hypothenar muscle following the conventional method.

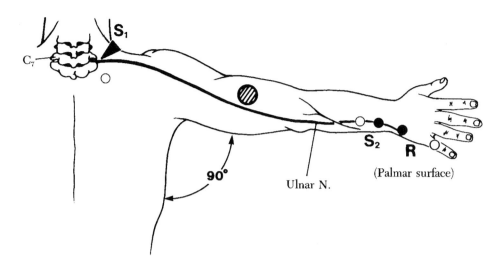

Figure 11.22. Motor nerve conduction of the ulnar nerve with C8 and T1 stimulation.

STIMULATION: A 50-mm monopolar needle is inserted perpendicular to the skin surface in a sagittal plane lateral and slightly caudal to the C7 cervical spine process until the tip rests directly over the C7 transverse process. This needle is used as an active stimulating electrode. A reference stimulating electrode is placed over the bony scapula, close to the stimulating electrode. The distal site of stimulation is at the wrist (8 cm proximal to an active recording electrode).

MEASUREMENT: The conventional method is used for latency measurement. Distance is measured with the arm extended at elbow and the shoulder abducted at 90°.

NORMAL DATA: Number of subjects: not mentioned. Age range: not mentioned. The mean NCV was 54 m/sec (SD ± 2 m/sec). The normal limit is 50 m/sec.

INTERPRETATION: More than 1 msec difference in latency between the sides is abnormal. However, entrapment at the wrist and elbow must be ruled out.

COMMENTS: Theoretically, this test may show slow motor NCV in patients with the thoracic outlet syndrome. This assumes that distal entrapment lesions, e.g., at the elbow, have been ruled out. However, the value of this test in patients with the thoracic outlet syndrome is still questionable.

Motor Nerve Conduction across the Thoracic Outlet

London's Method

London (23) reported a technique of determining the ulnar motor nerve conduction by measuring the distance with a tape.

RECORDING ELECTRODE: Surface electrodes are placed on the abductor digiti quinti (ADQ) muscle by the conventional method.

STIMULATION: The stimulus is applied with surface electrodes 10 cm above the elbow and at Erb's point.

MEASUREMENT: The conventional method is used for the latency measurement. The distance between the point above the elbow and Erb's point is measured by a steel tape and a sharpened obstetrical caliper. The arm position in relation to the trunk is not described. A figure in the article (27) suggests that the arm is kept beside the trunk.

TEMPERATURE: Skin temperature is not controlled.

NORMAL DATA: Number of subjects: 60. Age range: 20–44 yr.

Measurement	Mean ± SD	Normal Limit
Above elbow-Axilla (caliper) (m/sec)	58.9 ± 4.2	50.5
Above elbow-Axilla (tape) (m/sec)	70.2 ± 5.0	60.2

INTERPRETATION: A right-left NCV difference of 9 m/sec or larger is abnormal.

Ginzburg's Method

Ginzburg et al. (24) described a technique for determining median and ulnar motor nerve conduction across the thoracic outlet.

RECORDING: An active surface electrode for median and ulnar nerves follows the conventional method.

STIMULATION: The axilla and Erb's point are stimulated following the conventional method on median and ulnar nerves.

MEASUREMENT: Use the conventional method for the latency measurement. The arm is abducted at the shoulder 60° from the trunk. The distance between the axilla and Erb's point is measured with a caliper.

TEMPERATURE: Skin temperature is not controlled. The room temperature is between 25 and 26.5°C.

NORMAL DATA: Number of controls: 21. Age range: 26–55 yr.

Measurement	Mean ± SD	Normal Limit
Median nerve (m/sec)	65.1 ± 6.1	52.9
Ulnar nerve (m/sec)	63.0 ± 5.5	52.0

INTERPRETATION: The upper limit of normal differences between right and left NCVs is 14 m/sec for the median nerve and 12 m/sec for the ulnar nerve.

COMMENTS: A motor NCV difference of 9–14 m/sec in motor NCV between the right and left arms indicates that motor nerve conduction across the thoracic outlet is *full of technical errors* caused by the changing distance between the electrode and the nerve trunk during stimulation. This difficulty is especially true in obese individuals. In our opinion, *the mixed NCV across the thoracic outlet is a much more reliable measurement.* Thus, we rely more on the mixed NCV than on the motor NCV across the thoracic outlet when determining abnormal nerve conduction.

Krogness's Method

Krogness's technique (25) is different from other techniques in that the ulnar nerve trunk is stimulated near the C8–T1 nerves (Fig. 11.23). Other techniques stimulate Erb's point.

RECORDING: A concentric needle electrode is placed in the ADQ muscle.

STIMULATION: The ulnar nerve is stimulated with an active surface electrode at a point 3–3.5 cm above the ulnar sulcus, in the axilla, and above the clavicle corresponding to the 7th cervical transverse process. At the supraclavicular stimulation point, it is necessary to use a long-legged surface electrode because it must be pressed deeply into the lesser supraclavicular fossa pointing against the 7th cervical transverse process, thus being as close to the C8–T1 nerves as possible.

MEASUREMENT: Latency is measured by the conventional method. Distance is measured by tape from the supraclavicular stimulus point to a point 3–3.5 cm above the elbow (*D1*) and from the axilla to a point 3–3.5 cm above the elbow (*D3*). The arm is abducted 20° from the body, and the elbow is fully extended. The difference between *D1* and *D3* is used as the distance (*D2*) between the supraclavicular stimulating point and the axilla.

TEMPERATURE: Above 33.0°C.

NORMAL DATA: Number of subjects: 27. Age range: 14–49 yr.

Measurement	Mean ± SD	Normal Limit
NCV: above the clavicle-axilla (m/sec)	76.1 ± 5.4	65.3
Latency: above the clavicle (m/sec)	12.5 ± 2.7	17.9

COMMENTS: Krogness (29) claimed that the *D1–D2* difference represents closely the true anatomical length of the nerve and that this method stimulates the ulnar trunk

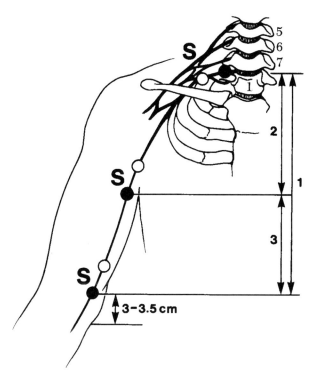

Figure 11.23. Krogness's method of motor nerve conduction of the proximal ulnar nerve.

near its root. He reported slow motor NCV across the thoracic outlet in three of five patients with cervical rib and anticus scalenus syndrome. As discussed in Chapter 5, there are many technical difficulties in obtaining a reliable CMAP response by stimulating the supraclavicular area.

Long Thoracic Nerve Motor Latency

Kaplan's Method

Kaplan (30) described a technique for measuring motor nerve conduction in the long thoracic nerve (Fig. 11.24A).

RECORDING: A monopolar needle electrode is placed as an active electrode into the digitation of the serratus anterior at the T5 rib level at the midaxillary line. The reference surface electrode is placed 2 cm caudally to the active electrode. *Position of the electrode is verified by having the subject's attempt of protraction of the shoulder.*

STIMULATION: The nerve is stimulated at Erb's point by an active surface electrode. The reference electrode is located above and medially.

MEASUREMENT: The latency is measured by the conventional method. Distance is measured with an obstetrical caliper.

TEMPERATURE: Skin temperature is not controlled. Room temperature is 21–23°C.

NORMAL DATA: Number of subjects: 27. Age range: 19–35 yr. The mean latency is 3.9 msec (SD ± 0.6 msec). The normal limit is 5.1 msec.

COMMENTS: Kaplan (26) reported a prolonged mean terminal latency in four athletes with a long thoracic nerve palsy.

Alfonsi's Method

Alfonsi et al. (27) described a technique of motor conduction in the long thoracic nerve with the surface electrode and the concentric needle as the recording electrodes (Fig. 11.24B and C).

RECORDING: If surface electrodes are used, an active electrode is placed on the serratus anterior muscle along the midaxillary line on the 5th rib and a reference electrode

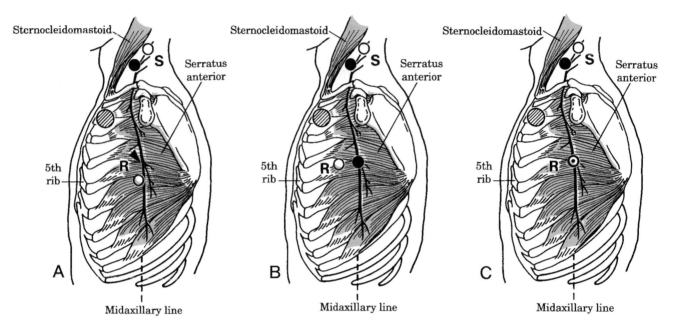

Figure 11.24. Motor nerve conduction of the long thoracic nerve. **A**, Kaplan's method. **B**, Alfonsi's method. **C**, Petrera and Trojaborg's method.

3 cm anterior to the active electrode. If using a needle electrode, a concentric needle is inserted into the serratus anterior muscle along the midaxillary line on the 5th rib.

STIMULATION: The long thoracic nerve is stimulated at Erb's point with bipolar surface electrodes.

MEASUREMENT: Distance between the stimulating and recording electrodes is measured with an obstetric caliper. The latency and the CMAP amplitude are measured using the conventional methods.

TEMPERATURE: Skin temperature is not controlled.

NORMAL DATA: Number of subjects: 44. Age range: 20–65 yr.

	Concentric Needle Electrode			Surface Electrode			
	Latency (msec)[a]		Amp (mV)	Latency (msec)[a]		Amp (mV)	
		Normal			Normal		No. of
Age (yrs)	Mean ± SD	Limit	Mean ± SD	Mean ± SD	Limit	Mean ± SD	Subjects
20–35	3.6 ± 0.3	4.2	7.1 ± 6.0	3.2 ± 0.3	3.8	4.3 ± 3.0	16
36–50	3.8 ± 0.4	4.6	5.7 ± 3.8	3.3 ± 0.3	3.9	3.8 ± 2.4	16
51–65	4.0 ± 0.4	4.8	5.6 + 4.5	3.3 + 0.3	3.9	2.7 ± 1.2	12

[a]Mean distance is 23.6 ± 1 cm (range 22–25 cm).

COMMENTS: Alfonsi et al. stated that the use of a concentric needle as the recording electrode is more accurate and that the CMAP amplitude is unreliable (31).

Petrera's Method

Petrera and Trojaborg (28) described a technique of long thoracic nerve conduction with a concentric needle (Fig. 11.24C).

RECORDING: A concentric electrode is inserted into the serratus anterior muscle over the 5th and/or 6th rib, at a level between the anterior and midaxillary line.

STIMULATION: The nerve is stimulated at the supraclavicular fossa, just above the midpoint of the clavicle, with surface electrodes.

MEASUREMENT: Latency is measured by the conventional method. Distance is measured with an obstetric caliper.

TEMPERATURE: Skin temperature is not controlled. Room temperature is 22°C.
NORMAL DATA: Number of subjects: 21. Age range: 15–70 yr.

Measurement	Mean ± SD	Normal Limit	Normal Range
Latency (msec)	4.5 ± 0.7	5.9	3.6–6.4

INTERPRETATION: The latency increases with the distance between sites of stimulation and recording (Fig. 11.25). The latency is abnormal when the value is outside the 95% confidence limit.

COMMENTS: Among 19 patients with long thoracic nerve palsy, this test showed no response in two, prolonged latency in nine, and normal latency in seven.

Brachial Plexus Motor Latency

Gassel's Method

Gassel (29) described a technique for measuring motor nerve conduction (latency) to the various shoulder girdle muscles using a concentric needle as the recording electrode.

RECORDING: A concentric electrode is placed in the middle of each of the biceps, deltoid, triceps, and supra- and infraspinatus muscles (Fig. 11.26).

STIMULATION: The trunk of the brachial plexus is stimulated with bipolar surface electrodes at Erb's point (a few centimeters above the clavicle in the angle between the posterior border of the sternocleidomastoid muscle and the clavicle at the level of the 6th cervical vertebra). The stimulation is done initially with the cathode as the active electrode and then with the anode as the active electrode. It is important to place the stimulating electrode at Erb's point. Placement of the stimulating electrode a few centimeters away from Erb's point results in an increase in latency.

MEASUREMENT: Latency is measured by the conventional method. The latency values obtained with the stimulating electrode at the opposite polarity of the stimulus pulses are averaged in calculating the final value. The distance is measured with an obstetrical caliper from the center of the bipolar stimulating electrodes to each recording electrode, with the subject's arm at the side of the trunk.

TEMPERATURE: Skin temperature is not controlled.

NORMAL DATA: See Table 7.28.

INTERPRETATION: The latency increases with the distance from the stimulation point. Thus, the distance must be considered when judging the latency to be prolonged.

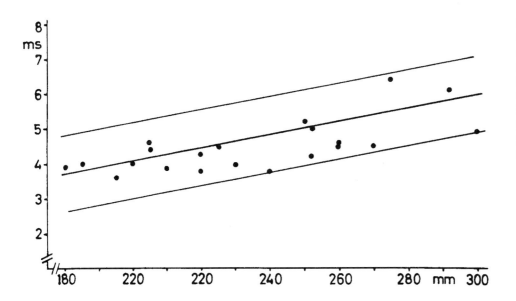

Figure 11.25. Latency to the serratus anterior muscle as a function of conduction distance. The *thick line* represents the regression line (n = 21, r = 0.70); the *thin lines* represent the 95% confidence limits. (From Petrera JE, Trojaborg W. Conduction studies of the long thoracic nerve in serratus anterior palsy of different etiology. Neurology 1984;34:1034.)

Figure 11.26. Brachial plexus motor latency test. Gassell and Kraft's methods are shown here. **A**, Stimulation site. **B**, Concentric needle position in the supra- and infraspinatus and triceps muscles. **C**, Concentric needle and surface recording electrodes in the deltoid and biceps muscles.

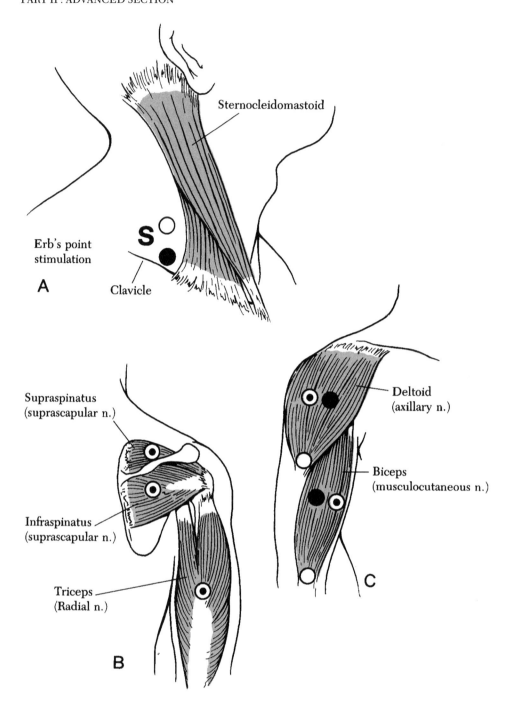

COMMENTS: Submaximal stimulation may produce an H-reflex 10–14 msec after stimulation. The H-reflex may be misinterpreted as a prolongation in latency.

Kraft's Method

Using surface and needle recording electrodes, Kraft (30) obtained the latencies to axillary, musculocutaneous, and suprascapular nerves (Fig. 11.26).

RECORDING: *Axillary nerve:* An active surface electrode is placed over the most prominent portion of the middle deltoid. This area corresponds with the region of greatest muscle mass upon abduction of the shoulder. A reference surface electrode is placed over the junction of the deltoid muscle fibers and its tendon of insertion. The study is performed with the subject lying in a supine position with his arm at his side.

Musculocutaneous nerve: An active surface electrode is placed just distal to the midportion of the biceps brachii muscle at the area of greatest muscle mass. The reference electrode is placed proximal to the antecubital fossa in the region of the junction of the muscle fibers and the biceps tendon.

Suprascapular nerve: A concentric needle electrode is used as the recording electrode in the supra- and infraspinatus muscles. For the supraspinatus muscle, the midpoint of the spine of the scapula is identified by palpation; the needle is inserted medial to this and just above the spine in a downward and foward direction until the scapula is touched. The needle is then withdrawn several millimeters, and the subject is asked to abduct the arm to identify needle placement. Studies of the supra- and infraspinatus muscles are done with the subject sitting with his arm at his side.

Infrascapular muscle: A needle is inserted into the infraspinatus muscle several centimeters below the scapular spine. The needle is gently inserted until the scapular periosteum is touched and then is withdrawn several millimeters. Identification of the muscle is confirmed by having the subject externally rotate his arm at the shoulder.

STIMULATION: The stimulation for all nerves is done at Erb's point. The active electrode is placed slightly above the upper margin of the clavicle lateral to the clavicular head of the sternocleidomastoid muscle, and the reference electrode is oriented superiomedially.

MEASUREMENT: The conventional method for the latency measurement. The distance is measured by conventional means using a modified obstetrical caliper with the arm at the side. The caliper is thought to be the most accurate means of measuring the length of nerve segments across the shoulder.

TEMPERATURE: Skin temperature is not controlled.

NORMAL DATA: Number of controls: 62. Age range: 18–52 yr.

Nerves	Mean ± SD (msec)	Normal Limit (msec)	Distance (cm)
Axillary	3.9 ± 0.5	4.9	14.8–21
Musculocutaneous	4.5 ± 0.6	5.7	23.5–29
Suprascapular nerve			
to supraspinatus	2.7 ± 0.5	3.7	7.4–12
to infraspinatus	3.3 ± 0.5	4.3	10.6–15

Axillary Nerve

The technique for measuring axillary nerve motor conduction was described by Currier (31) (Fig. 11.27).

RECORDING: An active surface electrode is placed over the middle portion of the deltoid muscle 2–9 cm distal to the acromion (corresponding roughly to the belly of the middle portion). A reference electrode position is not clearly mentioned in the text.

STIMULATING ELECTRODE: The nerve is stimulated with an active stimulating surface electrode proximally at Erb's point and distally at the posterior wall of the axilla.

MEASUREMENT: The arm is placed on a padded arm board and held stationary by a strap over the proximal forearm in the 90° abducted position. Distance is measured with an obstetrical caliper. Latency and amplitude measurement is conventional.

TEMPERATURE: Skin temperature is not controlled. Room temperature ranges from 26.7° to 28.3°C.

NORMAL DATA: Number of controls: 40. Age range: 20–35 yr.

Measurement	Mean ± SD	Normal Limit
Latency (msec)		
Erb's point—muscle	4.2 ± 0.4	5.0[a]
Axilla—muscle	2.5 ± 0.4	3.3[b]
NCV (m/sec)	62.2 ± 6.8	48.6
Amplitude (mV)	10.8 - 14.8 (range)	10.8

[a]Mean distance: 11.8 cm.
[b]Mean distance: 9.5 cm.

Figure 11.27.   Motor nerve conduction of the axillary nerve.

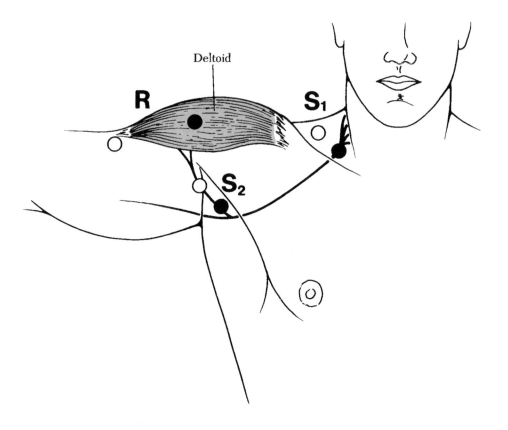

Musculocutaneous Nerve

Trojaborg (32) described a method of determining motor and sensory NCV in the musculocutaneous nerve (Fig. 11.28).

Motor Conduction

RECORDING: The CMAP is recorded with a concentric-needle electrode placed in the end-plate zone and adjusted to the region of maximal response in the brachial biceps muscle (Fig. 11.29).

STIMULATION: The musculocutaneous nerve is stimulated at two sites: (*a*) at the anterior cervical triangle just behind the sternocleidomastoid muscle and approximately 6 cm above the clavicle (Erb's point); and (*b*) at the axilla between the axillary artery and the median nerve medially, and the coracobrachialis muscles laterally, just above the level of the tendon of the latissimus dorsi muscle. The electrical stimulation is applied through an insulated stainless needle electrode which is adjusted close to the nerve as indicated by a threshold of the muscle potential with 0.5–1 mA. A remote needle electrode is placed at the same level as the near-nerve electrode at a transverse distance of 3 cm.

MEASUREMENT: Amplitude measurement is conventional. The distance between the near-nerve stimulating electrodes is measured with an obstetrical caliper. Latency is measured from the stimulus onset to the initial deflection from the baseline of the CMAP. (This is a conventional method for the needle technique.)

TEMPERATURE: Skin temperature is controlled at 36–38°C.

NORMAL DATA: See Tables 7.25, and 7.26, and Fig. 7.7.

Sensory Conduction

RECORDING: Electrodes at the axilla and anterior cervical triangle, positioned by means of the motor threshold, are used for recording sensory CNAPs (Fig. 11.30).

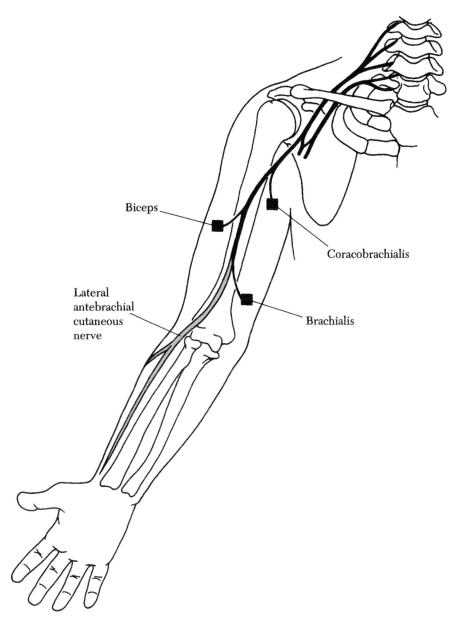

Figure 11.28. Anatomical course and innervation of the musculocutaneous nerve. The lateral ante-brachial cutaneous (lateral cutaneous nerve of the forearm; sensory branch of the musculocutaneous nerve) is also seen.

STIMULATION: The sensory fibers of the musculocutaneous nerve are stimulated with needle electrodes placed along the nerve where it emerges as the lateral cutaneous nerve of the forearm at the level of the elbow crease. Here it can be palpated just lateral to the tendon of the biceps brachii and medial to the brachioradialis muscle. The near-nerve electrode is adjusted, with the amplitude of the sensory potential recorded at the axilla as indicator.

MEASUREMENT: The maximum sensory NCV is determined from the latency to the initial positive peak of the CNAP. When calculating the sensory NCV over the most distal segment, the distance is divided by the latency. When calculating the sensory NCV over the proximal segment, the distance is divided by the latency difference between the distal and proximal latencies. This is a conventional method for the near-nerve needle technique.

TEMPERATURE: Skin temperature is controlled at 36–38°C.

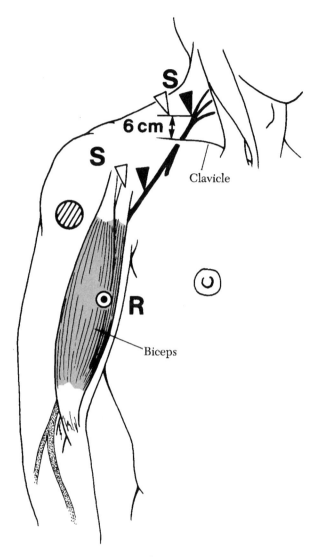

Figure 11.29.   Motor nerve conduction of the musculocutaneous nerve.

NORMAL DATA: See Table 7.27.

INTERPRETATION: When the NCV is below the lower 95% limit, it is considered abnormal in motor and sensory nerve conduction.

Lateral Cutaneous Nerve of the Forearm (Sensory Branch of the Musculocutaneous Nerve)

The antidromic technique for measuring sensory nerve conduction in the lateral cutaneous nerve of the forearm (Fig. 11.28) was described by Spindler and Felsenthal (33) (Fig. 11.31).

RECORDING: An active surface electrode is placed over the anterior branch of the nerve 12 cm distal to the active stimulating electrode along a straight line connecting the active stimulating electrode to the radial artery at the wrist. If the radial artery is difficult to locate, a point midway between the flexor carpi radialis tendon and the radial styloid is used.

STIMULATION: The lateral cutaneous nerve of the forearm is stimulated with a surface electrode at the level of the elbow crease *just lateral to the biceps tendon.* Occasionally, a motor artifact temporarily interferes with the recording when the stimulating

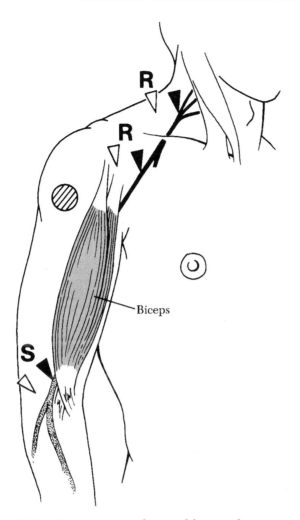

Figure 11.30.   Sensory nerve conduction of the musculocutaneous nerve.

electrode inadvertently slips radially, thus causing contraction of the supinator or bra-chioradialis. However, when the stimulator is kept against the biceps tendon, no motor artifact is seen.

MEASUREMENT: Latency is measured from the stimulus onset to the onset and peak of the negative deflection. The amplitude is measured by the conventional method. Distance is set at 12 cm.

TEMPERATURE: Skin temperature is not controlled. Room temperature is kept at 23.9°C.

NORMAL DATA: Number of subjects: 30. Age range: 20–84 yr.

Measurement	Mean ± SD	Normal Limit
Onset latency (msec)	1.8 ± 0.1	2.0
Maximum NCV (m/sec)	65.0 ± 3.6	57.8
Peak latency (msec)	2.3 ± 0.1	2.5
Amplitude (μV)	24 ± 7.2	12

Right to left latency difference to the onset of the CNAP: 0.30 msec.
Right to left latency difference to the peak of the CNAP: 0.30 msec.
COMMENTS: This test is relatively easy to perform.

Figure 11.31. Sensory nerve conduction of the lateral cutaneous nerve of the forearm.

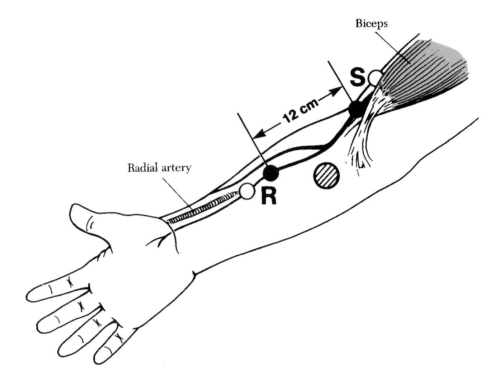

Medial Antebrachial Cutaneous Nerve

Pribyl's Method

The antidromic technique for measuring sensory nerve conduction in the medial antebrachial cutaneous nerve (Fig. 11.32) was described by Pribyl et al. (34) (Fig. 11.33A).

RECORDING: An active surface electrode is placed on the anteromedial surface of the forearm 9–12 cm from the active stimulating electrode, *along the line from the stimulating site to the ulnar styloid.*

STIMULATION: The nerve is stimulated antidromically to *2–4 cm lateral to the medial epicondyle* of the humerus with the active surface electrode located distally. This stimulation site is medial to the location of the median nerve.

MEASUREMENT: Latency is measured from the stimulus onset to the negative peak. Amplitude is measured by the conventional method. Distance is measured from the active stimulating electrode to the active recording electrode.

TEMPERATURE: Skin temperature of the forearm is 31–33°C.

NORMAL DATA: Number of subjects: 40. Age range: 20–67 yr.

Measurement	Mean ± SD	Normal Limit
Latency to the negative peak	2.1	
NCV (m/sec)	49.3 ± 3.8	41.7
Amplitude (µV)	10–30 (range)	10

COMMENTS: With the orthodromic method, the CNAP is smaller and more difficult to obtain. The latency and NCV are approximately the same. This technique was able to confirm the medial antebrachial cutaneous neuropathy in two cases (35).

Reddy's Method

An antidromic technique of sensory nerve conduction on the median antebrachial cutaneous nerve was described by Reddy (Fig. 11.33B) (36).

RECORDING: An active surface recording electrode is placed 18 cm distal to the stim-

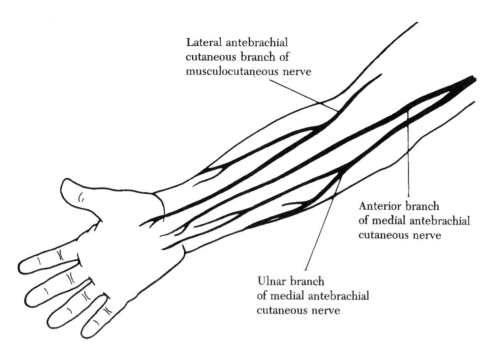

Lateral antebrachial
cutaneous branch of
musculocutaneous nerve

Anterior branch
of medial antebrachial
cutaneous nerve

Ulnar branch
of medial antebrachial
cutaneous nerve

Figure 11.32. Anatomical course of the medial antebrachial cutaneous nerve (the medial cutaneous nerve of the forearm).

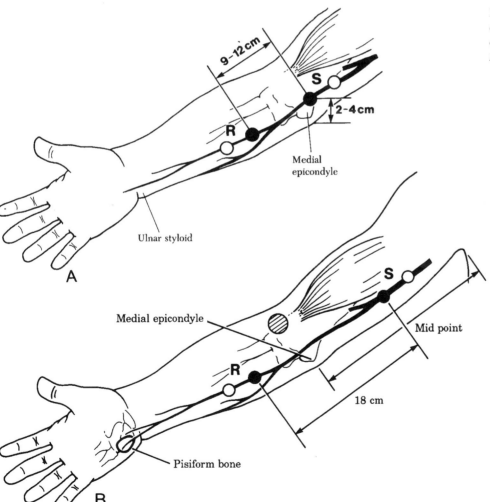

9–12 cm

S

2–4 cm

R

Medial
epicondyle

Ulnar styloid

A

Medial epicondyle

S

Mid point

R

18 cm

Pisiform bone

B

Figure 11.33. Sensory nerve conduction of the medial antebrachial cutaneous nerve. **A**, Pribyl's method. **B**, Reddy's method.

ulating electrode along a straight line connecting a point midway between the bicipital tendon and the medial epicondyle to the anterior aspect of the pisiform bone.

STIMULATION: An active surface stimulating electrode is placed on the nerve over the medial side at about the middle of the arm in the medial bicipital furrow.

MEASUREMENT: Latency is measured to the onset and negative peak of the CNAP. Amplitude is measured from peak to peak. NCV is calculated by dividing 18 cm by the latency to the onset of the CNAP.

TEMPERATURE: Skin temperature is not controlled. Room temperature is controlled at 21–23°C.

NORMAL DATA: Number of nerves: 60. Number of subjects: 30. Age range: 23–63 yr.

Measurement	Mean ± SD	Normal Limit
Onset latency (msec)	2.7 ± 0.2	3.1
Maximum NCV (m/sec)	65.9 ± 4.3	57.3
Peak latency (msec)	3.3 ± 0.2	3.7
Amplitude (μV)	15.4 ± 4.1	8.0

Posterior Antebrachial Cutaneous Nerve

Ma et al. (37) described an antidromic technique of sensory nerve conduction of the posterior antebrachial cutaneous nerve (Fig. 11.34).

RECORDING: An active surface electrode is placed approximately 12 cm distal to the

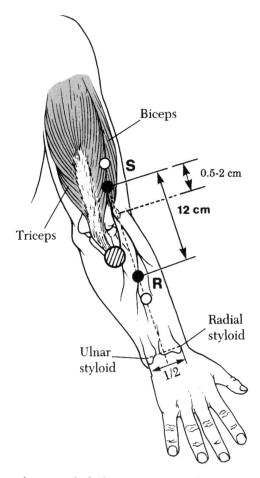

Figure 11.34. Ma's antidromic method of sensory nerve conduction of the posterior antebrachial cutaneous nerve.

active stimulating electrode along a line extending from the stimulation point (see below) to the middorsum of the wrist (midway between the ulnar and radial styloid processes).

STIMULATION: The nerve is stimulated at the elbow, ½–2 cm above the lateral epicondyle, between the biceps and triceps muscles. The stimulation site is closer to the latter, at the medial border of the lateral head of the triceps muscle.

MEASUREMENT: Latency is measured to the onset of negative deflection. Amplitude measurement.

TEMPERATURE: Skin temperature is not controlled. Room temperature is between 23°–26°C.

NORMAL DATA: Number of subjects: 40. Age range: 19–48 yr.

Measurement	Mean ± SD	Normal Limit
Latency (msec)	1.9 ± 0.3	2.5
NCV (m/sec)	64.0 ± 7.4	49.2
Amplitude (μV)	5.0–20 (range)	5.0

COMMENTS: According to Ma et al. (37), the test is best performed with the forearm pronated and it may be necessary to use low intensity or short duration of stimulus to avoid the stimulation artifact or the motor response caused by direct stimulation of the brachioradialis muscle. This technique was able to confirm this neuropathy in three cases (38, 39).

Median Nerve

Anterior Interosseous Nerve Motor Conduction

Nakano et al. (40) described a motor conduction technique for the anterior interosseous nerve (Fig. 11.35).

RECORDING: A concentric needle electrode is inserted into the pronator quadratus muscle.

STIMULATION: Stimulation is delivered percutaneously with a surface electrode above the elbow on the ventromedial aspect of the arm in the region of the biceps brachii muscle and 10 cm below the level of the lateral epicondyle over the flexor superficialis muscle. The patient's arm is stabilized on an arm board.

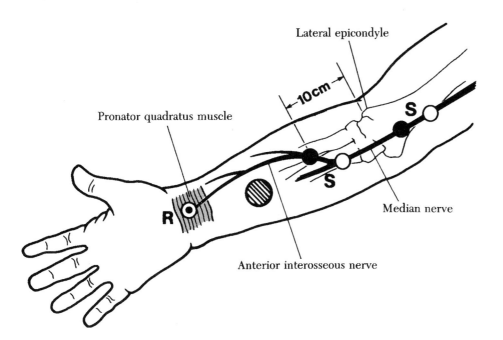

Figure 11.35. Motor nerve conduction of the anterior interosseous nerve.

MEASUREMENT: Latency and distance measurements are conventional. The duration of the CMAP is measured from the initial negative deflection to the isoelectric point of the negative spike.

TEMPERATURE: Skin temperature is not controlled.

NORMAL DATA: Number of subjects: 84. Age range: 9–67 yr.

Measurement	Mean ± SD	Normal Limit
Latency from the elbow (msec)	5.1	6.0
Latency from the below elbow site (msec)	3.6	4.4
Duration of CMAP, negative deflection only (msec)	3.6 ± 1.1	5.8

INTERPRETATION: A 95% lower confidence limit is the lower normal limit.

COMMENTS: Nakano et al. (40) found a prolonged duration of the CMAP (greater than 2 SD) in all of the seven cases of anterior interosseous nerve syndrome studied, prolonged latency from the elbow in five, and considerable attenuation of the amplitude in four. Thus, this test revealed an abnormality in all seven cases.

Median Nerve Motor and Sensory Nerve Conduction with Needle Electrodes

Buchthal et al. (41) described a technique for measuring motor and sensory nerve conduction in the median nerve using needle electrodes.

Motor Conduction

RECORDING: A concentric needle electrode is placed in the end-plate zone, or an 80-μm stainless steel wire is placed transversely near the center of the belly of the abductor pollicis brevis muscle (Fig. 11.36).

STIMULATION: The same needle electrodes that are used for recording the sensory potentials are used for stimulation of the median nerve at the wrist and elbow.

MEASUREMENT: Measurement of latency and amplitude of the CMAP is conventional. The response recorded with a wire electrode is, on the average, half that recorded with a concentric electrode. Terminal latency is corrected to a standard distance of 6.5 cm for the median nerve following the calculation formula (see Chapter 7).

TEMPERATURE: Skin temperature is controlled within 36–38°C.

Figure 11.36. Motor nerve conduction of the median nerve.

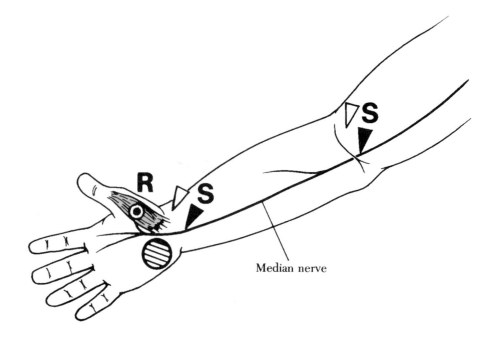

Median nerve

NORMAL DATA: See Table 7.13 and Fig. 7.6.

INTERPRETATION: An upper or lower 95% confidence limit is required to accept a finding as abnormal.

COMMENTS: It is important to remember that the terminal latency increases with the distance between the stimulating cathode at the wrist and the recording electrode in the muscle. Thus, this should be considered in judging an abnormal latency.

Sensory Nerve Conduction

RECORDING: Following the near-nerve technique (see Chapters 7 and 15), an active recording needle electrode is placed at the wrist and elbow along the median nerve (Fig. 11.37). Signal averaging is used for recording CNAPs less than 4 μV in amplitude. Details of this averaging are described in Chapter 5.

STIMULATION: Digit 1 (thumb) and digit 3 (middle finger) are stimulated with an active Velcro stimulating strap. A reference Velcro strap is placed 2–3 cm distal to the active electrode.

MEASUREMENT: Latency is measured from the stimulus onset to the initial positive peak of the CNAP. Amplitude is measured peak to peak. Distance measurement is conventional. When calculating the sensory NCV over the digit-wrist segment, distance (millimeters) is divided by the latency (milliseconds). When calculating the sensory NCV over the wrist-elbow segment, the distance is divided by the latency difference between the elbow and the wrist.

TEMPERATURE: Skin temperature is controlled within 36–38°C.

NORMAL DATA: See Tables 7.14 and 7.15.

INTERPRETATION: Deviations outside the 95% confidence limit are considered abnormal in various parameters of sensory nerve conduction.

COMMENTS: The electrode placed near the median nerve invariably picks up a potential from the radial nerve when digit 1 is stimulated. Ordinarily, the response from the radial nerve does not obscure the onset of the potential from the median nerve.

Segmental Stimulation (Inching) Technique of Sensory Nerve Conduction across the Carpal Tunnel

Kimura (42) described an inching technique of the antidromic sensory nerve conduction across the carpal tunnel (Fig. 11.38).

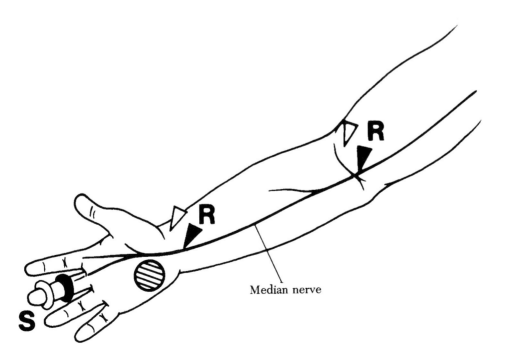

Figure 11.37. Sensory nerve conduction of the median nerve.

Median nerve

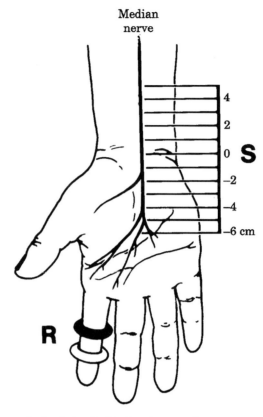

Figure 11.38. Segmental stimulation (inching) technique of sensory nerve conduction across the carpal tunnel.

RECORDING: The sensory CNAP is recorded with ring electrodes placed around the proximal (active) and distal (reference) interphalangeal joints of the 2nd digit.

STIMULATION: The median nerve is stimulated percutaneously at 12 points between the midpalm and the distal forearm in 1-cm increments. The zero level represents the proximal edge of the transverse carpal tunnel ligament.

MEASUREMENT: Latency is measured to the onset of the initial negative response. Amplitude is measured from the baseline to the negative peak.

TEMPERATURE: Skin temperature is 34°C or greater.

NORMAL DATA: Number of subjects: 122 nerves in 61 subjects. Age range: 15–50 yr.

Segment (cm)	Mean ± SD (msec)	Normal Limit (msec)
-5 to -4	0.17 ± 0.08	0.33
-4 to -3	0.22 ± 0.10	0.42
-3 to -2	0.20 ± 0.09	0.38
-2 to -1	0.19 ± 0.08	0.35
-1 to 0	0.16 ± 0.08	0.32

INTERPRETATION: Conduction time exceeding 0.5 msec/cm or more than twice that of the other 1-cm segment is considered abnormal.

COMMENTS: Serial stimulation in 1-cm increments increased the sensory latency almost linearly as the stimulus site was moved proximally. However, the latency increase was slightly but significantly greater in the middle three segments from −4 to −1 compared with the adjacent distal or proximal segments. In 52% of patients with CTS, there was a sharply localized abnormality over a 1-cm segment, which was usually associated with a distinct change in wave-form. With this technique it is possible to find a localized area where most of the slowing is concentrated.

Median Motor Nerve Conduction to the 1st Lumbrical Muscle

Fitz et al. (43) described a technique of motor nerve conduction with the recording electrodes in the 1st lumbrical (L1) muscle (Fig. 11.39A).

RECORDING: An active surface electrode is placed on the L1 muscle 1 cm proximal to the midpalmar crease and to the radial side of the long flexor tendon. Localization of the L1 muscle is done by palpating the long flexor tendon as the subject flexes his index finger. A ring electrode is placed over the base of the index finger as a reference electrode for the L1 muscle and around the base of the thumb for the abductor pollicis brevis (APB) muscle. The APB CMAP is simultaneously recorded in another channel.

STIMULATION: The median nerve is stimulated 12 cm proximal to the recording electrode from the L1 muscle and 8 cm from the APB muscle.

MEASUREMENT: Latency is measured following the conventional method. Amplitude of the CMAP is measured from the isoelectrical line to the peak of the negative deflection.

TEMPERATURE: Skin temperature in the web between the thumb and index finger is above 31°C.

NORMAL DATA: Number of subjects: 80. Age range: 22–66 yr.

Measurement	L1 Muscle		APB Muscle	
	Mean ± SD	Normal Limit	Mean ± SD	Normal Limit
Latency (msec)	3.5 ± 0.34	4.18	3.6 ± 0.31	4.22
CMAP amplitude (μV) at wrist	2241 ± 1150	600	9512 ± 2943	4000
CMAP amplitude decrease across the CT (%)	22 ± 41.5	105	8 ± 25	25

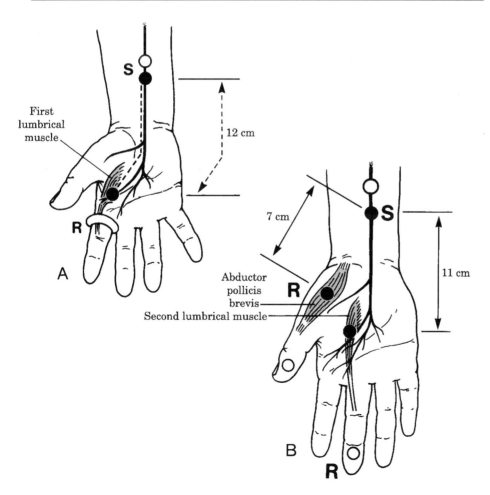

Figure 11.39. Median motor nerve conduction to the first lumbrical muscle (**A**) and to the second lumbrical muscle (**B**).

COMMENTS: Among 36 cases of CTS, the terminal latency was prolonged in the APB in 72% and in the L1 muscle in 66%. In three of 36 cases of CTS, the latency to the L1 muscle was prolonged, whereas the latency to the APB muscle was normal. However, in these patients, the sensory nerve conduction was abnormal. *There is no additional benefit of this method in the diagnosis of CTS.* Greater involvement of the nerve fiber to the APB was found in 58% of these patients compared with 17% for the lumbrical nerve fibers. Thus, this study also showed "lumbrical sparing" in CTS.

Median Motor Nerve Conduction to the 2nd Lumbrical Muscle

Logigian et al. (44) described a technique of motor nerve conduction with the recording electrode in the 2nd lumbrical (L2) muscle (Fig. 11.39B).

RECORDING: An active surface electrode is placed on the motor point over the L2 muscle just radial to the midpoint of the 3rd metacarpal bone. The reference electrode is placed on the distal phalanx of the 3rd digit. The APB CMAP is simultaneously recorded in another channel.

STIMULATION: The median nerve is stimulated 11 cm proximal (straight-line measurement) to the recording electrode in the L2 and 7 cm proximal to the recording electrode in the APB muscle.

MEASUREMENT: Latency is measured following the conventional method. Amplitude of the CMAP is most likely measured from the baseline to the peak of the negative deflection.

TEMPERATURE: Skin temperature in the palm is above 31°C.

NORMAL DATA: Number of subjects: 16. Age range: Not given.

Measurement	Mean ± SD	Normal Limit
Latency (msec)		
L2 muscle	3.3 ± 0.3	3.9
APB muscle	3.3 ± 0.4	3.9
APB-L2 difference	0.0 ± 0.1	0.4
CMAP amplitude (mV)		
APB	8.5 ± 3.2	
L2 muscle	1.6 ± 0.6	
L2/APB	0.21 ± 0.1	

INTERPRETATION: When the latency difference between the APB and L2 muscles is equal or greater than 0.4 msec, the lumbrical muscle is considered "spared."

COMMENTS: In 48 of 66 cases of carpal tunnel syndrome (CTS), the lumbrical muscle is spared. Lumbrical sparing was present in 14 of 17 cases with normal latency to the APB and in five cases with normal palm-to-wrist sensory NCV. Thus, authors claimed that "lumbrical sparing" is a fairly sensitive electrodiagnostic test for CTS. "Lumbrical sparing" is caused by the funicular organization of nerve fibers. The funiculus of the lumbrical muscles is more centrally located than the funiculus to the APB at the level of the radial styloid (45). Thus, in CTS, the nerve funiculus to the lumbrical muscle is spared. Lumbrical sparing in CTS was also observed by Yates et al. (46).

Median Sensory Nerve Conduction (Antidromic Method)

The antidromic method of median sensory nerve conduction is used routinely in a few laboratories. The following method is described in Hamner (Fig. 11.40) (47).

RECORDING: An active clip (or ring) electrode is placed on the midportion of the proximal phalanx of both index and middle fingers and a reference clip (or ring) electrode on the midportion of the middle phalanx of the same fingers, 2.5 or 3 cm from the active electrode.

STIMULATION: The median nerve is stimulated with an active surface electrode at the wrist (13 cm from the active recording electrode or 3–5 cm proximal to the distal wrist

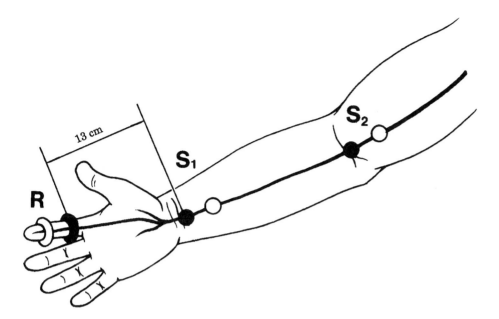

Figure 11.40. Median sensory nerve conduction (antidromic method).

Table 11.2.
Median Sensory Nerve Conduction (antidromic)

Age (yr)	Distal latency (msec)		Amplitude (µV)		NCV (m/sec)	
	Range	Normal Limit	Range	Normal Limit	Range	Normal Limit
0–9	2.0–2.9	2.9	20–70	20	55–73	55
10–19	2.3–3.2	3.2	20–85	20	55–73	55
20–29	2.4–3.3	3.3	20–75	20	55–73	55
30–39	2.3–3.4	3.4	15–80	15	55–73	55
40–49	2.4–3.5	3.5	15–65	15	55–73	55
50–59	2.6–3.6	3.6	15–70	15	55–73	55
60–69	2.8–3.7	3.7	10–50	10	52–68	52
70–	2.8–3.8	3.8	10–45	10	52–68	52

crease), and at the elbow (3–5 cm proximal to the elbow crease). These stimulating points are identical to those for motor nerve conduction of the median nerve.

MEASUREMENT: Distal latency is measured from the stimulus onset to the peak of the negative deflection of CNAP. For NCV calculation in the proximal segment, latency is measured to the takeoff of the CNAP for the distal and proximal stimulation. Conduction time is calculated by subtracting the distal latency (wrist) from the proximal latency (elbow). For the NCV, the distance between proximal and distal stimulations is divided by the conduction time following the conventional method. Amplitude is measured from the baseline to the peak of negative deflection.

TEMPERATURE: Skin temperature is adjusted to 35–37°C.

NORMAL DATA: Number of subjects: Not mentioned.

See Table 11.2.

INTERPRETATION: For the distal latency, 0.2 msec is added or subtracted for each cm difference if a distance other than 13 cm is used.

COMMENTS: Median sensory NCVs should be the same as or faster than the median motor NCVs.

Sensory Nerve Conduction of the Median Nerve over the Palm-Wrist Segment

Buchthal's Method

Using the method of Buchthal and Rosenfalck (48) to measure orthodromic sensory nerve conduction in the median nerve from digit to palm and from palm to wrist, the

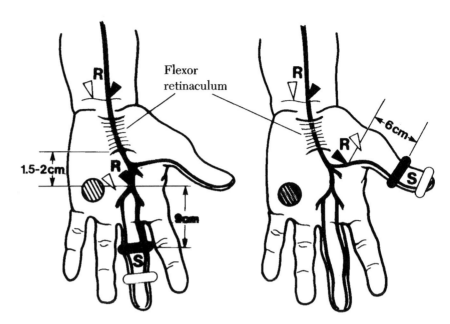

Figure 11.41. Buchthal's orthodromic method of sensory nerve conduction in the median nerve over the palm-wrist segment.

3rd finger is stimulated and the sensory nerve potential recorded by the near-nerve needle technique (Fig. 11.41).

RECORDING: The near-nerve technique is used for recording the sensory CNAP. At the wrist, the electrodes are placed near the nerve by adjusting their position following the conventional method. In the palm, the near-nerve electrode is inserted well outside the zone of compression in the carpal tunnel, 15–20 mm distal to the distal edge of the flexor retinaculum. In the case of digit 3, the electrode is placed 90 mm from the stimulating cathode along a line pointing to the midline of digit 3. To record from the palmar nerve of digit 1, the electrode is placed 60 mm from the cathode at the medial border of the thenar eminence. The palm is cooled by ether before insertion to diminish discomfort.

STIMULATION: An active stimulating ring electrode (or, to diminish the artifact, an uninsulated sensory needle) is placed medially and laterally at the proximal end of the distal phalanx of digit 1 and at the middle phalanx of digit 3. The reference ring electrode is placed 20 mm distally from the active electrode.

MEASUREMENT: The shortest latency is determined from the stimulus onset to the initial positive peak and the longest latency from the stimulus onset to the last separate component of the averaged CNAP. The NCV over the digit-palm segment is calculated by the conventional method. In calculating NCV over the palm-wrist segment, the distance is divided by the latency difference between the wrist and the palm. Distance is measured by the conventional method.

TEMPERATURE: Skin temperature is controlled at 37–38°C.

NORMAL DATA: See Table 7.14.

INTERPRETATION: Sensory NCVs less than 53 m/sec from digit 3 to palm and to wrist, and of less than 52 m/sec across the flexor retinaculum ($p < 0.05$) are considered abnormal.

COMMENTS: The amplitude of the sensory CNAP at the palm evoked by a maximal stimulation to digit III averages 25 µV, about 10 µV higher than at the wrist. Buchthal and Rosenfalck (41) showed a significantly slow sensory carpal NCV across the palm-wrist segment in six of eight patients with carpal tunnel syndrome in whom motor latency was normal and sensory conduction to the wrist was near normal.

Kimura's Method

An antidromic technique of measuring wrist-palm sensory nerve conduction of the median nerve is described by Kimura (49) (Fig. 11.42).

RECORDING: Velcro-strap surface electrodes are placed over the index fingers.

STIMULATION: The nerve is stimulated with surface electrodes at the wrist 3 cm proximal to the distal crease of the forearm and at the palm 5 cm distal to the distal crease of the forearm.

MEASUREMENT: Latency is measured from the stimulus onset to the onset of the initial negative peak. Distance is measured by the conventional method.

TEMPERATURE: Skin temperature is controlled at 34°C or greater.

NORMAL DATA: Number of subjects: 122. Age range: 15–50 yr.

Measurement	Mean ± SD	Normal Limit
Palm-wrist		
Latency (msec)	1.4 ± 0.20	1.8
Sensory NCV (m/sec)	57.3 ± 6.9	43.5
Amplitude (μV)	41.3 ± 19.3	
Digit-palm		
Latency (msec)	1.41 ± 0.22	1.85
Sensory NCV (m/sec)	58.1 ± 7.7	42.7
Amplitude (μV)	44.8 ± 22.0	

Sensory Nerve Conduction over the Finger-Wrist Segment

Oh described a technique of measuring sensory nerve conduction from digits 1, 2, and 3 to the wrist using a surface electrode (50).

RECORDING: An active electrode is placed over the median nerve at the wrist using the conventional method.

STIMULATION: Ring electrodes are placed over digits, 1, 2, and 3. Each digit is stimulated separately.

MEASUREMENT: Latency is measured from the stimulus onset to the onset of the neg-

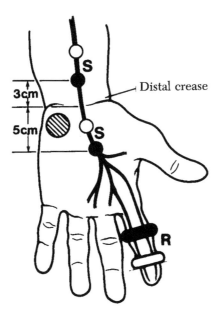

Figure 11.42. Kimura's antidromic method of sensory nerve conduction in the median nerve over the palm-wrist segment.

ative deflection and to the peak of the negative deflection. Distance, amplitude, and duration measurements are conventional.

TEMPERATURE: Skin temperature is kept above 31°.

NORMAL DATA: Number of subjects: 40. Age range: 20–60 yr.

Parameter	NCV (m/sec)		Duration (msec)	Amplitude (μV)
	Onset	Peak		
Digit 1				
Mean ± SD	56.7 ± 5.0	44.0 ± 3.9	1.5 ± 0.4	34.3 ± 14.2
Normal limit	46.7	36.2	2.4	10
Digit 2				
Mean ± SD	60.9 ± 5.1	49.5 ± 4.1	1.6 ± 0.4	30.9 ± 12.1
Normal limit	50.7	41.3	2.4	10
Digit 3				
Mean ± SD	60.2 ± 5.1	48.7 ± 4.1	1.6 ± 0.4	35.1 ± 13.4
Normal limit	50.0	40.5	2.4	10

COMMENTS: In patients with suspected carpal tunnel syndrome, in whom conventional sensory nerve conduction is normal, it is imperative to perform the sensory nerve conduction test from each finger. In some patients, an abnormal value from the sensory branch from one finger is the sole abnormality.

Sensory Nerve Conduction of the Palmar Cutaneous Branch of the Median Nerve

Chang and Lien (51) described a technique of sensory nerve conduction of the palmar cutaneous branch of the median nerve (Fig. 11.43).

RECORDING: The active recording electrode is placed on the median nerve 10 cm from the stimulating electrode.

STIMULATION: The palmar cutaneous nerve is stimulated at the midportion of the hyperthenar muscle with surface electrodes.

MEASUREMENT: Latency is measured to the negative peak, and NCV is calculated following the conventional method.

Figure 11.43. Sensory nerve conduction of the palmar cutaneous branch of the median nerve.

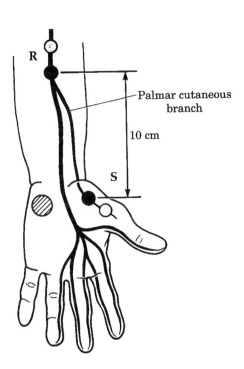

TEMPERATURE: Not controlled.
NORMAL DATA: Number of subjects: 40. Age range: 20–60 yr.

Measurement	Mean ± SD	Normal Limit[a]
Latency (msec)	2.24 ± 0.18	2.69
NCV (m/sec)	43.34 ± 3.52	34.54

[a]Mean ± 2.5 SD.

COMMENTS: According to authors, the nerve conduction study of this nerve should be done with caution and requires more averaging. The stimulation intensity should be increased slowly but not to a supramaximal stimulation in order to prevent the stimulation of the main sensory branch of the median nerve. Comparing the difference in the latency and sensory NCV between the palmar cutaneous branch and first digital branch of the median nerve, Chang and Lien were able to make the diagnosis of CTS in 84% of 50 cases (51). In contrast, the conventional sensory nerve conduction study in the digit-wrist segment successfully diagnosed CTS in 75% of cases.

Ulnar Nerve

Ulnar Motor and Sensory Nerve Conduction with Needle Electrodes

Payan (52) published a method of testing motor and sensory nerve conduction in the ulnar nerve using a needle electrode.

Motor Nerve Conduction

RECORDING: The CMAPs are recorded by concentric needle electrodes in the hypothenar and the 1st dorsal interosseous muscles (Fig. 11.44). When stimulating in the above-sulcus position, the recording concentric needle electrode is also placed in the flexor carpi ulnaris muscle.

STIMULATION: The near-nerve needle electrodes used for recording sensory potentials are used to evoke a CMAP. Thus, the ulnar nerve is stimulated at the wrist, below the sulcus, above the sulcus, and at the axilla.

MEASUREMENT: The latency and amplitude measurements are conventional for the needle method. The distance is measured with the arm extended at the elbow. The distance across the sulcus is set at 10 cm.

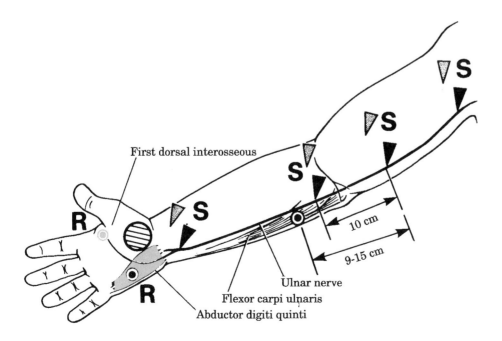

Figure 11.44. Motor nerve conduction of the ulnar nerve.

TEMPERATURE: Skin temperature is controlled at 34–36°C.

NORMAL DATA: See Tables 7.16 and 7.17.

COMMENTS: Terminal latency to the flexor carpi ulnaris is available using this method. The conduction velocity across the sulcus is slower than in the forearm. The terminal latency to the first dorsal interosseous is up to 1.6 msec longer than to the hypothenar muscles.

Sensory Nerve Conduction

We use this method to identify mild ulnar neuropathy when the routine motor, sensory, and mixed nerve conduction tests are normal.

RECORDING: Active recording needle electrodes are placed at the wrist, about 5 cm distal to the medial epicondyle (below-sulcus), about 5 cm proximal to the medial epicondyle (above-sulcus), and about 15 cm proximal to the medial epicondyle (axilla) (Fig. 11.45). The reference needle electrodes are placed subcutaneously radially at a transverse distance of at least 4 cm from the active electrode.

STIMULATION: The digital nerve is stimulated at the little finger (digit 5) with Velcro-strap electrodes.

MEASUREMENT: The latency is measured from the onset of the stimulus to the peak of the first positive deflection. The amplitude, duration, and distance measurements are conventional. The NCV is calculated following the conventional methods for the near-nerve needle technique.

TEMPERATURE: Skin temperature is controlled at 34–36°C.

NORMAL DATA: See Tables 7.19 and 7.20.

COMMENTS: An electronic averager is used except when recording normal CNAPs at the wrist. The conduction velocity across the sulcus is slower than in the forearm. Sensory conduction is faster than motor conduction in the transsulcus segment.

Ulnar Motor Conduction Velocity with the Elbow Flexed

Checkles et al. (53) described ulnar motor nerve conduction with the elbow in the 70° flexed position. They claimed that the true length of the ulnar nerve across the elbow segment is more accurately measured with the elbow flexed (Fig. 11.46).

RECORDING: An active surface electrode is placed on the hypothenar eminence on a point midway between the distal wrist crease and the crease at the base of digit 5, and at the junction of the dorsal and palmar skin.

Figure 11.45. Sensory nerve conduction of the ulnar nerve.

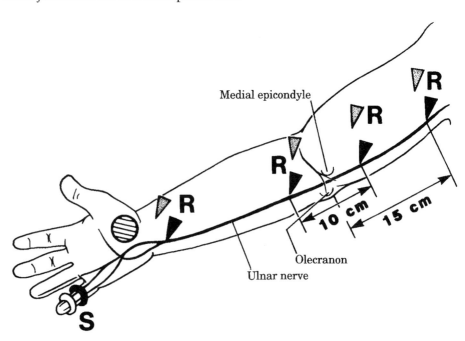

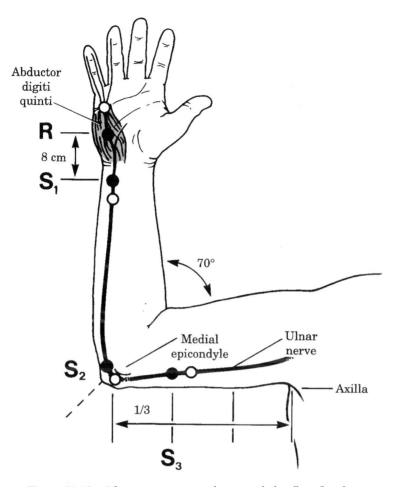

Figure 11.46. Ulnar motor nerve conduction with the elbow flexed.

STIMULATION: The nerve is stimulated with the surface electrode at three points along the course of the ulnar nerve. The distal point of stimulation is 8 cm proximal to the active recording electrode. The midpoint stimulus is delivered just distal to the ulnar groove, and the proximal stimulus at the junction of the middle and distal thirds of the arm.

MEASUREMENT: Latency is measured by conventional means. Distance across the elbow is measured by tape with the elbow flexed at 70°. The average distance is 11.5 cm, in contrast to 8.1 cm with the elbow extended to 180°.

TEMPERATURE: Skin temperature is not controlled.

NORMAL DATA: Number of subjects: 31. Age range: 20–58 yr.

Measurement	Mean ± SD	Normal Limit
NCV (m/sec)		
Forearm segment	61.8 ± 5.0	51.8
Across elbow	62.7 ± 5.5	51.7
Amplitude of negative deflection (mV)	6.14 ± 1.90	2.3

COMMENTS: Though Checkles et al. (53) claimed that this technique measures the NCV more accurately, a majority of investigators, including us, measure the NCV across the elbow in the extended position for convenience. It is important to remember that the NCV across the elbow is equal to or faster than the forearm velocity when the elbow is flexed and slower than the forearm velocity when the elbow is extended.

Short Segmental Incremental Stimulation (SSIS) Method across the Elbow

Campbell et al.'s Method

Campbell et al. (54) described a technique for the short segmental incremental study of motor nerve conduction of the ulnar nerve across the elbow (Fig. 11.47A).

POSITION OF PATIENT: Arm is flexed at a 70–90° angle at the elbow.

RECORDING: The CMAP is recorded with surface recording electrodes from ADQ muscle following the conventional method.

STIMULATION: The ulnar nerve is stimulated successively at 1-cm increments from 5 cm above to 5 cm below the medial epicondyle.

MEASUREMENT: Latency measurement is conventional. Amplitude is measured from the baseline to the negative peak.

TEMPERATURE: Skin temperature is not controlled.

NORMAL DATA: Latency changes over successive 1-cm segments range from 0.05 to 0.25 msec.

INTERPRETATION: By estimating the latency and amplitude changes over each segment, the most impaired segment is identified by a marked increase in latency and by a marked decrease in amplitude (conduction block).

COMMENTS: By this method, tardy ulnar nerve palsy (retrocondylar compression) and cubital tunnel syndrome can be differentiated. Authors were able to localize the lesion at the cubital tunnel in six of 19 cases and to the retrocondylar sulcus in eight cases. In one case, the cubital tunnel and retrocondylar sulcus were equally involved. In four cases, the test was nonlocalizing. By using the SSIS method during surgery, cubital tunnel syndrome was identified in six cases and retrocondylar compression in eight cases. In two patients, both sites were involved equally.

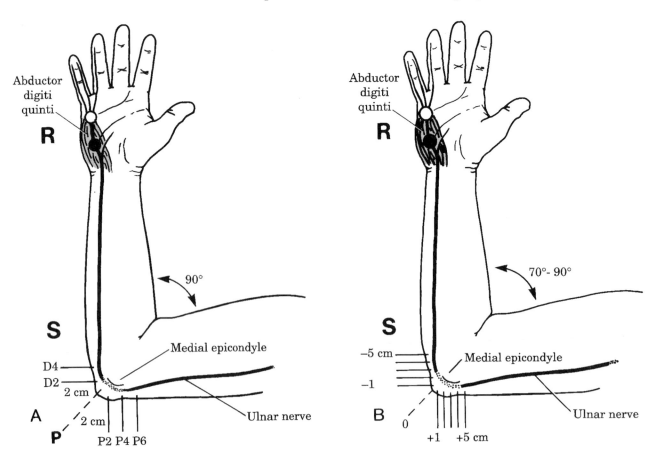

Figure 11.47. Short segmental incremental stimulation method (inching technique) across the elbow. **A**, Campbell's method. **B**, Kanakamedala's method.

Kanakamedala's Method

Kanakamedala et al. (55) described a short-segment stimulation (SSS) method of the motor nerve conduction of the ulnar nerve across the elbow (Fig. 11.47B). *We prefer an inching technique at 2-cm segments with the elbow extended.*

POSITION OF SUBJECT: Arm is flexed at the elbow to 90° with a polypropylene splint.

RECORDING: The CMAP is recorded with surface recording electrodes from the ADQ muscle following the conventional method.

STIMULATION: The ulnar nerve is stimulated successively at 2-cm segments from 6 cm above to 4 cm below the medial epicondyle. The distal points (D2 and D4) are 2 and 4 cm distal to point P (medial epicondyle). The proximal points (P2, P4, and P6) are 2, 4, and 6 cm proximal to point P.

MEASUREMENT: Latency measurement is conventional. Amplitude is measured from the baseline to the negative peak.

TEMPERATURE: Skin temperature is not controlled. Room temperature is kept at 27°C.

NORMAL DATA: Number of subjects: 25 nerves in 14 subjects. Age range: 27–58 yr.

Measurement	Mean ± SD	Normal Limit
Conduction time over 2 cm segment (msec)	0.43 ± 0.20	0.83
Amplitude reduction over 2 cm segment[a] (%)		6%

[a]Distal-to-proximal change.

INTERPRETATION: The most impaired segment is identified by a marked increase in latency and by a marked decrease in amplitude (conduction block). The maximum conduction time is reported to be 0.63 msec. Whether 0.83 or 0.63 msec is used for the normal limit is not clear.

COMMENTS: Among 13 cases of ulnar compression neuropathy at the elbow, the SSS method localized the lesion to the cubital tunnel (D4–D2) to three cases and to the medial epicondyle in nine. Conduction time alone was abnormal in one case, both conduction time and amplitude in nine cases, amplitude only in one case, and conduction time together with a mild reduction in amplitude in two cases. At the EMG laboratory of the University of Alabama at Birmingham, we use a 2-cm SSS method with the arm extended at the elbow.

Latency of the Deep Branch of the Ulnar Nerve in the Hand

Ebeling et al. (56) and Bhala and Goodgold (57) described a method for studying latency in the deep branch of the ulnar nerve in the hand. This test is essential to the diagnosis of a lesion involving the deep branch of the ulnar nerve to the first dorsal interosseous or adductor pollicis brevis muscles.

Ebeling's Method

Ebeling et al. (56) used a concentric needle as the recording electrode (Fig. 11.48).

RECORDING: A concentric needle electrode is inserted into the ADQ and first dorsal interosseous muscles.

STIMULATION: The nerve is stimulated with a surface electrode, which is placed over the nerve approximately 2 cm above the distal wrist crease.

MEASUREMENT: Latency measurement follows the conventional method for the needle technique. The distance between the stimulating electrode and the recording electrode in the ADQ varies from 5.5 to 8.5 cm in different subjects. Latency is not corrected to a fixed distance. The authors stated that it is not possible to estimate accurately the length of the deep branch of the ulnar nerve to the first dorsal interosseous muscle by surface measurement.

TEMPERATURE: Skin temperature is not controlled.

NORMAL DATA: Number of subjects: 50. Age range: not mentioned.

Site of Latency Measurement	Mean ± SD (msec)	Normal Limit (msec)
Abductor digiti quinti	2.9 ± 0.39	3.7
First dorsal interosseous	3.8 ± 0.53	4.9

Figure 11.48. Ebeling's method for motor nerve conduction of the deep branch of the ulnar nerve.

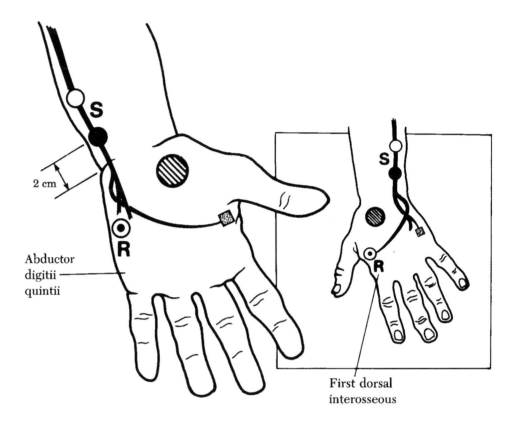

COMMENTS: Because it is impossible to measure accurately the length of the deep branch of the ulnar nerve to the 1st interosseous muscle with surface electrodes, we recommend *caliper measurement*. It is always prudent to compare the latency obtained in the involved hand with that in the opposite hand (using the same distance).

Bhala's Method

Bhala and Goodgold (57) used a surface electrode as the recording electrode (Fig. 11.49).

RECORDING: Surface electrodes are placed along the ulnar border of the hand over the belly of the ADQ and also on the dorsum of the hand between the 1st and 2nd metacarpals over the fleshy belly of the first dorsal interosseous muscle.

STIMULATION: The ulnar nerve is stimulated percutaneously at the wrist using surface electrodes.

MEASUREMENT: Latency measurement is conventional. The distance is not fixed. The latency is not corrected to a fixed distance.

TEMPERATURE: Skin temperature is not controlled.

NORMAL DATA: Number of subjects: 58. Age range: 26–65 yr.

Site of Latency Measurement	Mean ± SD (msec)	Normal Limit (msec)
First dorsal interosseous (msec)	4.0 ± 0.65	5.3
Abductor digiti quinti (msec)	2.7 ± 0.49	3.7

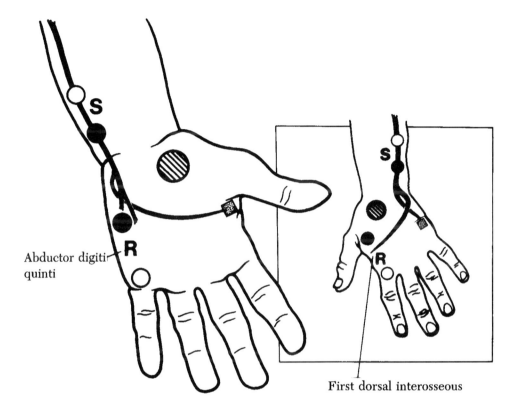

Figure 11.49. Bhala's method for motor nerve conduction of the deep branch of the ulnar nerve.

Abductor digiti quinti

First dorsal interosseous

Ulnar Sensory Nerve Conduction (Antidromic Method)

The antidromic method of ulnar sensory nerve conduction is used routinely in a few laboratories (58, 59). The following method is described by Felsenthal et al. (Fig. 11.50) (60).

POSITION OF SUBJECT: The arm is abducted and the forearm supinated. The elbow is flexed to 90°.

RECORDING: An active ring electrode is placed on the proximal interphalangeal joint of the fifth finger and a reference ring electrode on the distal interphalangeal joint. Below-elbow and above-elbow responses are averaged.

STIMULATION: The ulnar nerve is stimulated with an active surface electrode at the wrist (14 cm from the active recording electrode), below the elbow (immediately distal to the ulnar groove), and above the elbow (10 cm proximal to the below-elbow stimulation site). These stimulating points are idential to those for motor nerve conduction of the ulnar nerve.

MEASUREMENT: Latency is measured to the onset and peak of the negative deflection of the CNAP. If the CNAP is triphasic, onset is measured from the peak of the initial positive deflection from the baseline. For calculation of the NCV in the proximal seg-

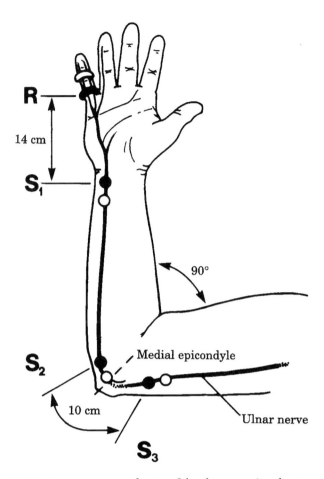

Figure 11.50. Sensory nerve conduction of the ulnar nerve (antidromic method).

ment, the latency is measured to the takeoff of the CNAP for distal and proximal stimulations. Conduction time is calculated by subtracting the distal latency from the proximal latency. For the NCV, the distance between the proximal and distal stimulation points is divided by the conduction time following the conventional method. Amplitude is measured from peak to the peak of the CNAP.

TEMPERATURE: Skin temperature ranged from 30.0 to 33.8°C.

NORMAL DATA: Number of subjects: 20. Number of cases: 40. Age range: 18–46 yr.

Measurement	Onset		Peak	
	Mean ± SD	Normal Limit	Mean ± SD	Normal Limit
Distal latency (msec)	2.6 ± 0.2	3.0	3.2 ± 0.3	3.8
Side-to-side latency difference across-elbow	0.2 ± 0.2	0.6	0.1 ± 0.1	0.3
Forearm NCV (m/sec)	67.5 ± 4.5	58.5	63.6 ± 4.0	55.6
Across-elbow NCV (m/sec)	70.9 ± 10.4	50.1	64.9 ± 6.8	51.3
Amplitude				
At the wrist (μV)			65.1 ± 32.9	20[a]
Below the elbow (μV)			31.1 ± 11.7	6[a]
Above the elbow (μV)			25.4 ± 10.1	6[a]
Forearm decrement (%)			51.4 ± 11.1	74
Across-elbow decrement (%)			18.6 ± 11.2	41

[a]The low normal range.

COMMENTS: Authors reported motor and sensory nerve conductions across the elbow in three patients with ulnar compression neuropathy at the elbow. In all three cases, *the most striking change was the decrement in amplitude of the sensory CNAP across the elbow.* In two patients (one with sensory symptoms and the other with sensory and motor symptoms), the motor nerve conduction showed a prolonged latency across the elbow, confirming the diagnosis. In one patient with sensory symptoms, a decrement in the sensory CNAP amplitude across the elbow was the only abnormality confirming the diagnosis.

Dorsal Cutaneous Ulnar Nerve Sensory Conduction

Kim et al. (61) and Jabre (62) described antidromic techniques for measuring sensory nerve conduction in the dorsal cutaneous ulnar nerve. Their techniques are similar.

Kim's Method

At the UAB EMG Laboratory, we prefer this method with some modification.

RECORDING: An active surface electrode is placed along the 5th metacarpal bone, with the reference electrode over the level of the 5th metacarpophalangeal joint (Fig. 11.51A) (65).

STIMULATION: The nerve is stimulated approximately 8–10 cm above the ulnar styloid, with the stimulating electrodes pressed firmly between the flexor carpi ulnaris tendon and the ulnar bone. If difficulty is encountered in obtaining a response, the following maneuvers are used: (*a*) the stimulating electrodes are moved slowly 2–3 cm above and below the stimulation point; and (*b*) an orthodromic technique is used rather than an antidromic technique. *The best place for the stimulating electrode is 3 cm proximal to the lower border of the ulnar styloid (Fig. 11.51B). Low-stimulus intensity such as less than 20 mA with the stimulus duration of 0.1 msec, is needed to prevent any muscle artifact.*

MEASUREMENT: Latency is measured to the peak of negative deflection. The amplitude measurement is conventional.

TEMPERATURE: Skin temperature is not controlled. Room temperature is 22.8°C.

NORMAL DATA: Number of subjects: 66. Age range: 21–71 yr.

Measurement	Mean ± SD	Normal Limit
Latency (msec)	2.1 ± 0.3	2.7
NCV (m/sec)	47.8 ± 3.8	40.2
Amplitude (μV)	24.2 ± 10.8	

COMMENTS: Sensory CNAP in this nerve is easily obtainable. These authors believe that this technique is useful in documenting a dorsal cutaneous ulnar sensory neuropathy, and localizing a lesion proximal or distal to the branching of the sensory dorsal branch of the ulnar nerve.

Jabre's Method

RECORDING: The active recording electrode is placed over the bottom of the "V" between the 4th and 5th metacarpals, and the reference electrode is placed at the base of the 5th digit (Fig. 11.51B) (62).

STIMULATION: The nerve is stimulated 8 cm from the active electrode, the stimulator probes being either tucked into the space between the ulna and the flexor carpi ulnaris tendon or placed astraddle the bony ulnar, whichever position gives a better baseline.

MEASUREMENT: Jabre's paper did not describe the method of measurement. However, his later paper (63) noted that the amplitude of the response is measured from the takeoff to the peak of the negative phase, and the latency from the stimulus onset to the negative peak. In calculating NCV, the distance is divided by the latency to the takeoff of the CNAP.

Figure 11.51. Sensory nerve conduction of the dorsal cutaneous ulnar nerve. *A*, Kim's method. *B*, Jabre's method.

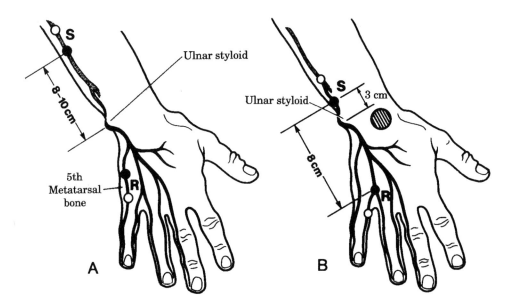

TEMPERATURE: Skin temperature is not controlled.
NORMAL DATA: Number of subjects: 50. Age range: 10–66 yr.

Measurement	Mean ± SD	Normal Limit
Latency (msec)	2.0 ± 0.3	2.6
NCV (m/sec)	60 ± 4.0	52
Amplitude (μV)	20 ± 6	

COMMENTS: About 11% of the subjects had asymmetrical dorsal sensory CNAPs, with a difference of 50% or more in amplitude between the two arms. Jabre believed that this technique is a simple means for: (*a*) localizing a lesion proximal or distal to the takeoff of the sensory dorsal branch of the ulnar nerve; and (*b*) studying the ulnar nerve segment proximal to a wrist lesion when the routine sensory and motor amplitudes are depressed or absent.

Radial Nerve

Motor Conduction

Gassel and Diamantopoulos (64), Jebsen (65), and Trojaborg and Sindrup (66) described a method for determining motor conduction in the radial nerve (Fig. 11.52). Each of these authors used a coaxial needle as the recording electrode. There is no method using surface electrode to measure motor nerve conduction in the radial nerve.

Gassel's Method

The method of Gassel and Diamantopoulos (64) describes motor nerve conduction in the proximal segment of the radial nerve (Fig. 11.53).

RECORDING: The CMAPs are recorded from the brachioradialis, extensor digitorum communis, and anconeus muscles using a concentric needle.

STIMULATION: The radial nerve is stimulated at three sites with surface electrodes:

1. The trunk of the brachial plexus is stimulated a few centimeters above the clavicle in the posterior triangle of the neck in the angle between the posterior border of the sternomastoid muscle and the clavicle (Erb's point);

2. The midposition of stimulation of the nerve is either in the spiral groove, approximately 4 cm posterior to the insertion of the deltoid muscles, or at the lateral part of the humerus where the nerve becomes superficial after having pierced the intermuscular septum; this point is at the

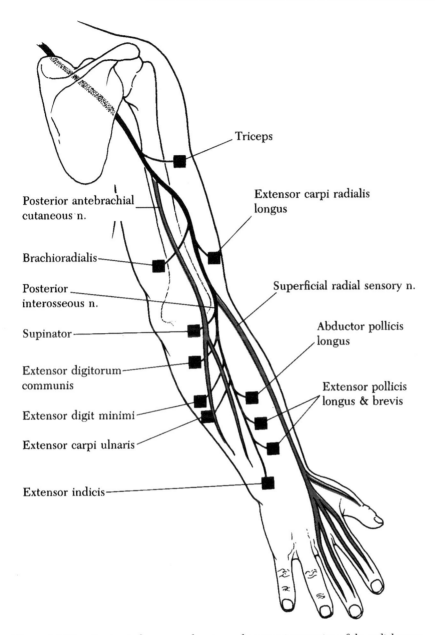

Triceps

Posterior antebrachial cutaneous n.

Extensor carpi radialis longus

Brachioradialis

Posterior interosseous n.

Superficial radial sensory n.

Supinator

Abductor pollicis longus

Extensor digitorum communis

Extensor digit minimi

Extensor pollicis longus & brevis

Extensor carpi ulnaris

Extensor indicis

Figure 11.52. Anatomical course and motor and sensory innervation of the radial nerve.

junction of the upper and middle third of a line drawn between the insertion of the deltoid and the lateral epicondyle of the humerus; and

3. The lower point of stimulation of the radial nerve is about 5 cm above and slightly posterior to the lateral epicondyle of the humerus. The distance between the supraclavicular and midarm point of stimulation varies from 19 to 28 cm, and that between the supraclavicular and lower point of stimulation from 23 to 38 cm.

MEASUREMENT: The latency and amplitude measurements are conventional. The values obtained with the bipolar stimulating electrode at opposite polarity of stimulus are averaged when calculating the final value. The distance from the center of the bipolar stimulating electrodes at each level of stimulation is measured with an obstetrical caliper with the subject's arm at the side.

TEMPERATURE: Skin temperature is not controlled. The temperature of the room is controlled at 21–23°C.

NORMAL DATA: See Table 11.3.

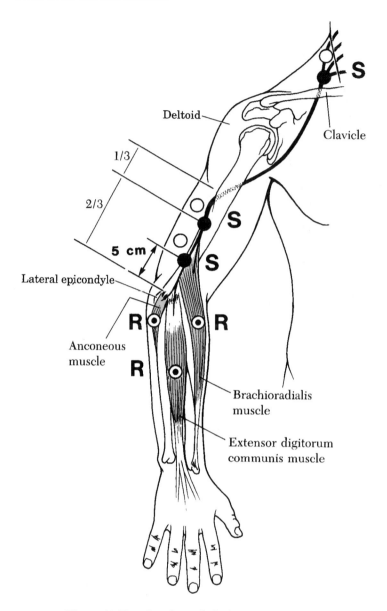

Figure 11.53.   Gassel's method of motor nerve conduction of the radial nerve.

Table 11.3.
Normal Data in 24 Subjects for the Radial Nerve—Gassel's Method (Age: 19–73)

Site	Latency (msec)		NCV (m/sec)	
	Mean ± SD	Normal Limit	Mean ± SD	Normal Limit
Brachioradialis	3.4 ± 0.7	4.8	74 ± 6.7	60.6
Extensor digitorum communis	3.7 ± 0.4	4.5	72 ± 6.1	59.8
Anconeus	3.8 ± 0.5	4.8	66 ± 9.2	47.6

Jebsen's Method

Jebsen (65) described a technique for determining motor NCV in the radial nerve by stimulating three sites and using surface stimulating electrodes (Fig. 11.54).

RECORDING: A concentric needle electrode is inserted into the extensor indicis muscle, lateral to the extensor carpi ulnaris tendon and 4 cm proximal to the styloid process of the ulna. Accurate placement of the coaxial needle electrode may be verified by recording the CMAP picked up by the needle.

STIMULATION: Surface-stimulating electrodes are used for stimulating the nerve at three sites: (*a*) the branch of the radial nerve to the extensor indicis, 3–4 cm proximal to the site of needle insertion; (*b*) the radial nerve 5–6 cm proximal to the lateral epicondyle where it lies in the groove between the brachialis and brachioradialis muscles; and (*c*) the trunk of the brachial plexus at Erb's point.

MEASUREMENT: A tape is used to measure the distance from the distal point of stimulation to the middle point of stimulation (above the elbow). An obstetrical caliper, flattened to an edge, is used to measure the straight-line distance between the site of

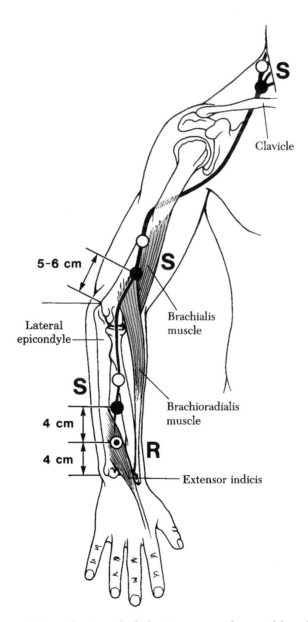

Figure 11.54. Jebsen's method of motor nerve conduction of the radial nerve.

stimulation at Erb's point and the site above the elbow. A latency measurement is done following the conventional method. The arm is abducted approximately 10°, the elbow flexed 10–15°, and the forearm pronated.

TEMPERATURE: Skin temperature is not controlled.

NORMAL DATA: Number of subjects: 98. Age range: not mentioned.

Segment	Mean ± SD (m/sec)	Normal Limit (m/sec)[a]
Proximal	72.0 ± 6.3	59.4
Distal	61.6 ± 5.9	49.8

[a]Latency was not reported.

COMMENTS: In normal individuals, stimulation at Erb's point produces CMAP in the extensor indicis. However, with radial nerve palsy in which compression is at the spiral groove, the stimulation of Erb's point produces a CMAP in the extensor indicis through volume conduction via the median or ulnar nerves. Thus, *it is imperative to stimulate the radial nerve at the spiral groove rather than at Erb's point.*

Motor and Sensory Conduction with Needle Electrodes

Trojaborg and Sindrup (66) described a method of determining motor and sensory conduction in the radial nerve using needle electrodes.

Motor Conduction

RECORDING: The CMAPs are recorded with concentric needle electrodes adjusted to the region of maximal response in the triceps, brachioradialis, extensor digitorum communis, extensor pollicis longus, and extensor indicis muscles (Fig. 11.55).

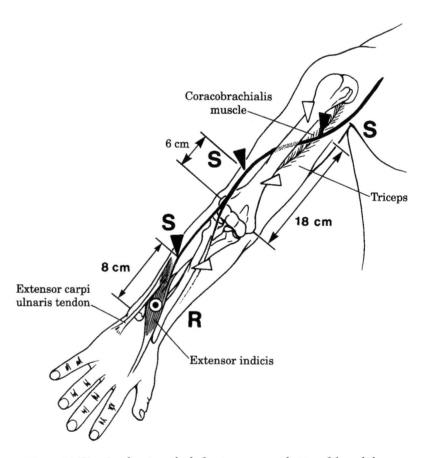

Figure 11.55. Trojaborg's method of motor nerve conduction of the radial nerve.

STIMULATION: The radial nerve is stimulated at three sites with the needle: (*a*) in the forearm, 8 cm proximal to the styloid process of the ulnar bone where the nerve can be palpated just lateral to the extensor carpi ulnaris muscle; (*b*) at the elbow, in the groove between the brachioradialis and the biceps tendon, 6 cm proximal to the lateral epicondyle of the humerus; and (*c*) at the axilla, in the groove between the coracobrachialis and the medial edge of the brachial triceps, 18 cm proximal to the medial epicondyle of the humerus. The stimulus is applied through needle electrodes insulated except for a 3-mm bared tip. An active electrode is adjusted close to the nerve, as indicated by the lowest threshold of the muscle potential.

MEASUREMENT: The conventional method is used for measuring amplitude. The distance between the cathode at the axilla and at the elbow is measured with obstetrical calipers. The latency is measured from the stimulus onset to the initial deflection from the baseline of the CMAP.

TEMPERATURE: Skin temperature averaged 32°C at the thumb, 34°C at the wrist, 35°C at the elbow, and 36°C at the axilla.

NORMAL DATA: See Tables 7.21 and 7.22

Sensory Conduction

RECORDING: Near-nerve needle electrodes are positioned at the axilla and elbow by means of the motor threshold (Fig. 11.56). A near-nerve electrode is placed at the wrist with the amplitude of the sensory CNAP as indicator: (*a*) at the elbow evoked by stimulating the radial nerve at the wrist; (*b*) at the wrist evoked by stimulating the thumb; and (*c*) at the wrist evoked by stimulating the mixed nerve at the elbow. A remote electrode is placed transversely to the near-nerve electrode as far as possible from the median nerve.

STIMULATION: The sensory fibers of the radial nerve are stimulated: (*a*) with a sur-

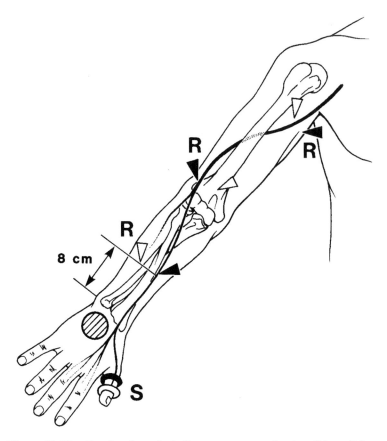

Figure 11.56. Trojaborg's method of sensory nerve conduction of the radial nerve.

face electrode (Velcro-strap or ring), the active electrode placed at the proximal phalanx of the thumb and the reference 20 mm distal to it; (*b*) with needle electrodes, the active one placed over the nerve at the wrist along the lateral border of the radial bone.

MEASUREMENT: The latency is measured between the onset of the stimulus and the initial positive peak of the sensory potential. The amplitude is measured peak to peak.

NORMAL DATA: See Tables 7.21 and 7.22.

COMMENTS: When stimulating the thumb, contamination of the potential recorded above the radial nerve by potential spread from the median nerve is inevitable and makes it impossible to determine if there is a complete block of the radial nerve distal to the wrist. Stimulating the radial nerve at the wrist instead of at the thumb has the double advantage that spread from the median nerve is avoided and the CNAP at the elbow and the axilla is about six times greater because of the larger number of fibers at the wrist and because of the shorter distance of conduction.

When stimulating the thumb, 25% of the sensory potential over the radial nerve at the wrist and elbow and 50% at the axilla are due to spread from median nerve fibers. When the stimulus is applied through needle electrodes to the radial nerve, contamination from the median nerve fibers can be avoided as long as the stimulating current is less than 15 mA.

Motor and Mixed Conduction of the Posterior Interosseous Nerve

Falck and Hurme (67) described a motor and mixed nerve conduction technique for the posterior interosseous nerve of the radial nerve. *We prefer this method with additional stimulation at the spiral groove at midhumerus.*

Motor Conduction

RECORDING: The CMAP is obtained with bipolar surface electrodes on the extensor indicis proprius muscle. The recording electrodes are adjusted to give a slight negative deflection initially (Fig. 11.57A).

STIMULATION: The radial nerve is stimulated at two sites, either with surface electrodes or with needle electrodes (e.g., DISA 13K64): (*a*) in the forearm, 8–10 cm distal to the lateral epicondyle between the bellies of the extensor digitorum communis and extensor carpi ulnaris muscles; and (*b*) at the elbow, 2–3 cm above the lateral epicondyle of the humerus between the brachioradialis and brachial biceps tendons. With needle electrodes, an active electrode is positioned as close to the nerve as possible by using a decreasing stimulus intensity until a stimulus current of 1.0 mA is reached. The reference electrode is placed 10 mm proximal to the active electrode under the skin.

MEASUREMENT: The latency is measured from the stimulus onset to the initial deflection of the CMAP. Distance is measured with sliding calipers.

TEMPERATURE: Skin temperature on the forearm is controlled at 32–34°C.

NORMAL DATA: Number of subjects: 17. Number of nerves: 34. Age range: 31–45 yr.

Measurement	Mean ± SD	Normal Limit
With surface stimulating electrodes		
NCV (m/sec)	68.0 ± 5.4	57.2
Right-left difference (m/sec)	-2.6 ± 7.2	11.8
With needle stimulating electrodes		
NCV (m/sec)	71.4 ± 2.9	65.6
Right-left difference (m/sec)	-1.8 ± 4.7	7.6

COMMENTS: To obtain reliable measurements of the NCV of the posterior interosseous nerve across the arcade of Frohse, authors recommended needle electrodes as the stimulating electrodes (67) because the range of normal values is wider with surface than with needle electrodes. Authors also stated that the opposite side should be examined for comparison.

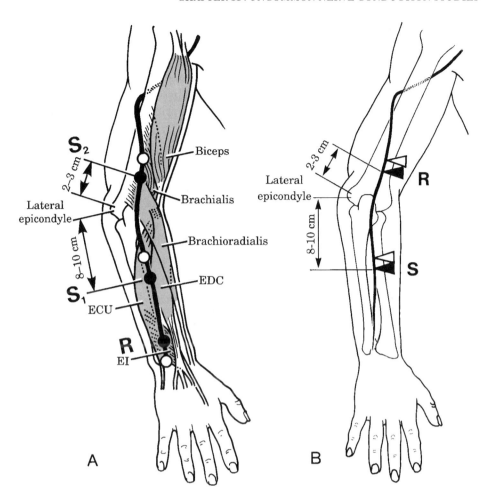

Figure 11.57. Motor (**A**) and mixed conduction (**B**) of the posterior interosseous nerve.

Mixed Conduction

RECORDING: An active near-nerve needle electrode is placed at the elbow 2–3 cm above the lateral epicondyle of the humerus, between the brachioradialis and biceps tendons by means of the minimal motor threshold of 1.0 mA. A reference needle electrode is 10 mm proximal to the active needle electrode (Fig. 11.57B).

STIMULATION: An active near-nerve needle electrode is placed in the forearm, 8–10 cm distal to the lateral epicondyle between the bellies of the extensor digitorum communis and extensor carpi ulnaris muscles by means of the minimal motor threshold of 1.0 mA. A reference needle electrode is placed 10 mm distal to the active needle.

MEASUREMENT: The latency is measured from the stimulus onset to the positive deflection of the CNAP. Distance is measured with sliding calipers.

TEMPERATURE: Skin temperature on the forearm is controlled at 32–44°C.

NORMAL DATA: Number of subjects: 17. Number of nerves: 34. Age range: 31–45 yr.

Measurement	Mean ± SD	Normal Limit
NCV (m/sec)	71.5 ± 3.3	64.9
Right-left difference (m/sec)	-0.7 ± 4.4	8.1

COMMENTS: Authors recommended comparison of the NCV with the normal side (67). In two cases of posterior interosseous syndrome, the NCV across the arcade of Frohse was slow but normalized after surgery (67).

Superficial Radial Sensory Nerve Conduction over the Forearm

Chang's Method

Chang and Oh (68) described a technique of obtaining sensory nerve conduction in the superficial radial nerve over the forearm segment (Fig. 11.58A).

RECORDING: An active recording surface electrode is placed 4–6 cm proximal to the dorsal styloid process of the distal radius.

STIMULATION: The superficial radial nerve is antidromically stimulated with a surface electrode at a point 3 cm proximal to the cubital crease and near the lateral border of the biceps brachii tendon.

MEASUREMENT: The latency is measured to the negative peak of the CNAP and the amplitude from peak to peak.

TEMPERATURE: Skin temperature at the midforearm is controlled above 32°C.

NORMAL DATA: Number of nerves: 76. Number of subjects: 50. Age range: 16–70 yr.

Measurement	Mean ± SD	Normal Limit
NCV (m/sec)	53.3 ± 3.6	46.1
Amplitude (μV)	15.2 ± 9.8	5.0

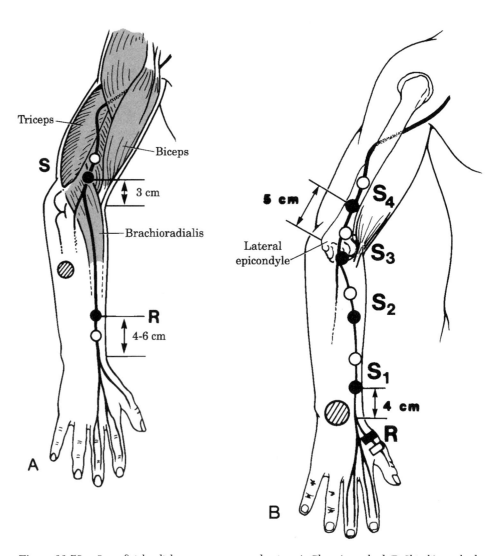

Figure 11.58. Superficial radial sensory nerve conduction. *A*, Chang's method. *B*, Shirali's method.

COMMENTS: On the dorsoradial aspect of the hand, there was overlapping innervation by the lateral antebrachial cutaneous nerve and the distal superficial radial nerve (69). With this method, authors were able to stimulate the superficial radial nerve independently.

Shirali's Method

Shirali and Sandler (70) described an antidromic technique for recording radial sensory CNAPs below the elbow (Fig. 11.58B).

RECORDING: The recording electrodes consist of a pair of 16-gauge fine silver rectangular plates, $8 \times 22 \times 2$ mm, mounted on clear plastic and spaced 13 mm apart. The recording electrodes are placed in the area on the dorsum of the hand proximal to the web between the thumb and the index finger.

STIMULATION: Four proximal sites are stimulated with surface electrodes: (a) the entire radial nerve is stimulated in the groove 5–6 cm proximal to the lateral epicondyle; (b) the superficial sensory branch is stimulated at the elbow lateral to the biceps tendon; (c) in the midforearm where it lies lateral to the radial artery, and (d) at a point about 4 cm proximal to the wrist, where it is superficial and easily palpable on the lateral border of the forearm.

MEASUREMENT: The latency is measured from the stimulus onset to the first upward deflection of the CNAP. Distance is measured by the conventional method. In calculating NCV, the distance is divided by the latency difference between the proximal and distal latencies.

TEMPERATURE: Skin temperature is not controlled.

NORMAL DATA: Number of controls: 32. Age range: 21–65 yr.

Measurement	Mean ± SD	Normal Limit
NCV (m/sec)		
Spiral groove-elbow	77.0 ± 8.8	59.4
Elbow-wrist	62.0 ± 4.2	53.6
Latency (msec)	1.33 ± 0.23	1.79
Amplitude (µV)	54.3 ± 25.9	20

COMMENTS: Shirali and Sandler (70) stated that satisfactory sensory CNAPs were obtained in all subjects except for a few obese individuals in whom there was difficulty stimulating at the musculospiral groove. We have experienced difficulty in locating the radial nerve at the midforearm because the radial artery cannot be located. It is technically easy to obtain sensory CNAPs by stimulating above the wrist and at the elbow.

Intercostal Nerve

Caldwell's Method

Caldwell et al. (71) described a technique for measuring intercostal motor conduction (Fig. 11.59).

POSITION OF SUBJECT: The patient is placed under light general anesthesia and then is positioned to lie on the uninvolved side.

RECORDING: A coaxial needle electrode is placed in the intercostal muscle in the desired interspace in the midaxillary line.

STIMULATION: Stimulating 37-mm monopolar needles are inserted into the corresponding interspace as near the spinal column as technically possible. The electrode tips are placed adjacent to the intercostal nerve with the active stimulating electrode being located distal to the spinal cord. As the stimulus voltage is increased, the recording and stimulating electrodes are adjusted to give the maximal response.

MEASUREMENT: Conventional method.

TEMPERATURE: Skin temperature is not controlled.

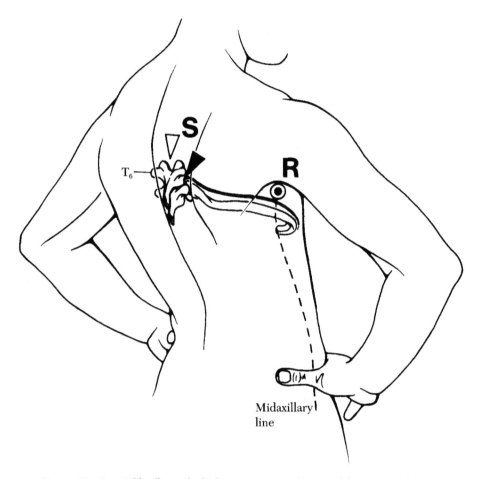

Figure 11.59.   Caldwell's method of motor nerve conduction of the intercostal nerve.

NORMAL DATA: Number of subjects: 134. Age range: 20–75 yr. The mean latency is 3.5 msec (SD ± 0.9), with a normal limit of 5.3 msec.

INTERPRETATION: The criteria for abnormality are as follows (72): (*a*) a delay greater than 5.0 msec with dispersion of evoked response; (*b*) a delay greater than 6.0 msec; and (*c*) a delay 2.0 msec greater than the mean delay for that patient.

COMMENTS: There are two major disadvantages in this technique: The patient should be placed under light general anesthesia, and pneumothorax may be a side effect. Johnson et al. (72) reported an 8.8% rate of posttest pneumothorax and recommended pre- and poststudy chest x-rays as a routine procedure. According to their report, this test must be performed on a few intercostal nerves above and below the suspected nerve to pinpoint the involved nerve. Johnson et al. (72) made an accurate diagnosis of thoracic radiculopathy in 161 patients. Eighty of their patients had subsequent posterior rhizotomy, and pain was relieved in 81% of those undergoing surgery. We prefer a thoracic paraspinal needle EMG study in patients suspected of having a thoracic radiculopathy.

Pradhan's Method

Pradhan and Taly (73) described a method of intercostal nerve (ICN) conduction study using surface electrodes without putting the subject under light general anesthesia (Fig. 11.60).

POSITION OF SUBJECT: The patient lies on the side opposite that being examined with the arms extended over the head. Intercostal spaces are made wide and prominent by putting a pillow under the chest. The arms are placed high in front of the face, as this

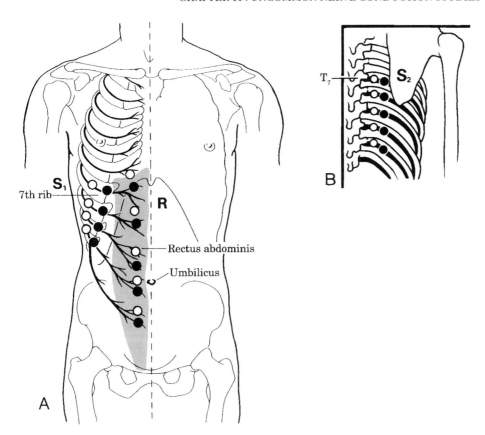

Figure 11.60.   Pradhan's method of motor nerve conduction of the intercostal nerve.

position moves the scapula and the attached muscles forward and upward, allowing easy access to the 7th and 8th ICNs.

RECORDING: An active recording surface electrode is placed at the middle of the width of the rectus abdominalis at the following sites:

Intercostal Nerve	Recording Site
7th	0–1 cm above the level of the xiphoid process
8th	1–3 cm below the level of the xiphoid process
9th	2–5 cm above the level of the umbilicus
10th	1 cm above to 4 cm below the level of the umbilicus
11th	midway between the umbilicus and pubic symphysis

The reference electrode is placed 5 cm above the active electrode.

STIMULATION: The ICN is stimulated with 0.5 msec duration. The distal points of stimulation are about 6 cm behind the costal margin (S_1), and the proximal sites are just lateral to the paraspinal muscles in the same space (S_2). The stimulating electrodes are gently pressed deep and rostral.

MEASUREMENT: Latency is measured by the conventional method. Distance between the two points of stimulation is measured with an obstetric caliper.

TEMPERATURE: Skin temperature is not controlled.

NORMAL: Number of subjects: 30 (Number of tests: 60). Age range: 14–52 yr. See Table 11.4

COMMENTS: Pradhan and Taly stated that this technique can be applied to measure the NCVs of the lower five ICNs with fairly reliable results (73). Among five cases of the Guillain Barré syndrome, they found abnormal NCVs in three. A stimulus duration of 0.5 msec was found to be better than the usual 0.2 msec. Highly obese or muscular patients sometimes required even higher stimulus duration to obtain a proper CMAP.

Table 11.4.
Intercostal Nerve Conduction

Measurement	Latency (msec)		NCV (m/sec)		Amplitude (mV)	Duration (msec)
	Mean ± SD	Normal Limit	Mean ± SD	Normal Limit	Mean ± SD	Mean ± SD
7th ICN	3.5 ± 0.7	4.9	75.1 ± 6.3	62.5	5.6 ± 2.4	14.5 ± 2.7
8th ICN	3.7 ± 0.5	4.7	74.9 ± 6.0	86.9	4.6 ± 2.2	16.4 ± 3.5
9th ICN	4.0 ± 0.3	4.6	75.5 ± 6.4	62.7	2.8 ± 1.5	18.4 ± 3.6
10th ICN	4.6 ± 0.7	6.0	74.8 ± 6.1	62.6	2.4 ± 1.5	19.8 ± 3.6
11th ICN	5.0 ± 0.6	6.2	71.7 ± 7.4	56.9	2.6 ± 1.4	21.5 ± 4.2

Sometimes, owing to a small 12th rib, not enough distance could be obtained to measure the velocity of the 11th ICN. In these cases, distal stimulation was carried out by putting the stimulating electrode over the abdominal wall just in front of the 11th intercostal space.

Lumbar Plexus

Motor Nerve Conduction across the Lumbosacral Plexus

Kaplan (78) described a method of motor nerve conduction across the lumbosacral plexus (Fig. 11.61).

RECORDING: A surface bipolar electrode is placed on the short head of the biceps femoris, 7 cm cephalad to the popliteal crease.

STIMULATION: The L5 root is stimulated with an active monopolar needle that is inserted 3 cm lateral to the caudal margin of the 5th lumbar vertebra. The reference surface electrode is placed 3 cm lateral to the active monopolar needle electrode. For distal stimulation, the sciatic nerve is stimulated with an active monopolar needle that is inserted midway between the greater tuberosity and ischial tuberosity at the gluteal fold. The reference surface electrode is placed on the gluteal fold near the active monopolar needle.

MEASUREMENT: The latency is measured following the conventional method. The distance between the proximal and distal stimulation sites is measured with a sharp obstetric caliper.

TEMPERATURE: Skin temperature is not controlled.

NORMAL DATA: Number of subjects: 25. Age range: 28–52 yr.

Measurement	Mean ± SD	Normal Limit
NCV (m/sec)	70.0 ± 5.0	60

COMMENTS: Author reported that in 10 cases of sciatic neuropathy, the NCV in the lumbosacral plexus was slow (42 ± 8 m/sec) and stated that this finding can distinguish between a lumbosacral neuropathy and a radiculopathy. However, nerve conduction values in the radiculopathy group were not presented. Theoretically, this claim is correct but unproved as yet.

Ilioinguinal Motor Nerve Conduction

Ellis et al. (75) described a technique of motor conduction of the ilioinguinal nerve (Fig. 11.62).

RECORDING: The CMAP is recorded with a monopolar needle inserted 1 cm lateral to the midline and 1–2 cm above the pubic symphysis over the lower abdomen.

STIMULATION: The ilioinguinal nerve is stimulated with a needle electrode medial to the anterior superior iliac spine.

MEASUREMENT: Latency and amplitude of the CMAP are measured by the conventional methods.

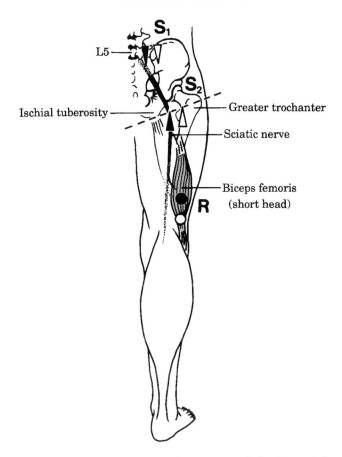

Figure 11.61.   Motor nerve conduction across the lumbosacral plexus.

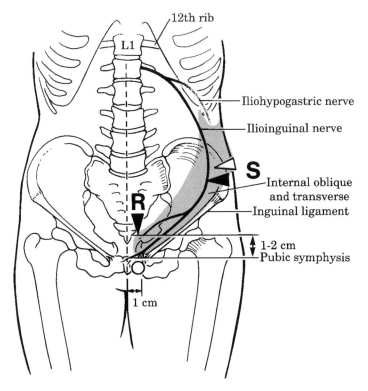

Figure 11.62.   Motor nerve conduction of the ilioinguinal nerve.

TEMPERATURE: Skin temperature is not controlled.

NORMAL DATA: Number of subjects: 10. Number of tests: 20. Age range: 19–50.

Measurement	Mean ± SD	Normal Range	Normal Limit
Terminal latency (msec)	4.2 ± 0.6	3.5–6.0	5.4
Amplitude (mV)	2.0	0.5–10.0	0.5

INTERPRETATIONS: A difference of 50% or more of the CMAP amplitude between the normal and affected side likely indicates abnormality in the affected side.

COMMENTS: Latency comparison between the left and right sides in individual subjects showed excellent agreement (R = 0.94).

Lateral Femoral Cutaneous Nerve

Sensory nerve conduction tests of the lateral femoral cutaneous nerve are described by Butler et al. (76), Sarala et al. (77), and Lysens et al. (78).

Butler's Method

Butler et al. (76) described an antidromic technique for measuring sensory nerve conduction of this nerve using surface electrodes (Fig. 11.63).

RECORDING: Recording electrodes are two strips of lead (1.2 × 1.9 cm), placed 12 cm directly inferior to the anterior superior iliac spine on the anterior aspect of the thigh.

STIMULATION: The nerve is stimulated 1 cm medial to the anterior superior iliac spine with a Teflon-coated monopolar needle electrode (0.04 cm diameter). A surface electrode is used as a reference electrode. Stimulation with an active surface electrode is adequate in thin individuals.

MEASUREMENT: Latency is measured to the peak of the negative deflection of the CNAP. Amplitude and distance measurements are conventional.

TEMPERATURE: Skin temperature is not controlled.

NORMAL DATA: Number of subjects: 24. Age range: 19–81 yr.

Measurement	Mean ± SD	Normal Limit
Latency (msec)	2.6 ± 0.2	3.0
Amplitude (µV)	10–25 (range)	10

COMMENTS: A double-peak response is obtained in many persons. This is eliminated by making the surface electrode smaller so that the nerve potential from only the larger anterior branch is recorded. A motor artifact is often present, identifiable because the negative deflection is 3–4 msec in duration.

Sarala's Method

Sarala et al. (77) described an orthodromic technique for measuring sensory nerve conduction in this nerve using surface electrodes (Fig. 11.64). If this method is unsuccessful, we use the needle as the recording electrode (Lysen's method), and finally the antidromic method.

RECORDING: An active surface recording electrode is placed 1 cm medial to the anterior-superior iliac spine above the inguinal ligament. The CNAPs are averaged with a signal averager. Thirty-four to 64 averagings are performed.

STIMULATION: The nerve is stimulated with a surface electrode 11–16 cm directly inferior to the anterior iliac spine on the anterior aspect of the thigh. The site of stimulation is selected when paresthesia is induced over the lateral aspect of the thigh by stimulation.

MEASUREMENT: Latency is measured from the onset of the stimulus to the negative peak of the CNAP. The amplitude and distance measurements are conventional.

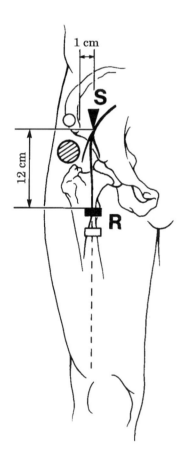

Figure 11.63. Butler's antidromic method of sensory nerve conduction of the lateral femoral cutaneous nerve.

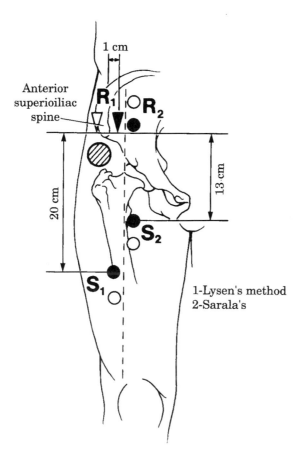

Figure 11.64. Orthodromic method of sensory nerve conduction of the lateral femoral cutaneous nerve. (R_1, S_1) Lysens' method. (R_2, S_2) Sarala's method.

TEMPERATURE: Skin temperature is controlled at 31.0–34.7°C.

NORMAL DATA: Number of subjects: 20. Age range: 20–55 yr.

Measurement	Mean ± SD	Normal Limit
NCV (m/sec)	57.51 ± 8.61	40.3
Amplitude (µV)	2–10 (range)	2

COMMENTS: It is important to localize correctly the site of stimulation by observing paresthesia over the nerve territory. It is not easy to obtain a reliable recording without using the signal averager because of the small amplitude of the CNAP. The orthodromic technique eliminates muscle artifact. It is not easy to obtain the CNAP in overweight individuals. Therefore, it is important to assure technique by comparison with the sensory nerve conduction on the normal side.

Lysens's Method

The method of Lysens's et al. (78) is similar to that of Sarala et al. (81) except that a monopolar needle is used as the recording electrode (Fig. 11.64).

RECORDING: The CNAP is recorded with monopolar needle electrodes (DISA 13L64). The near-nerve electrode is placed above the inguinal ligament 1 cm medial to the anterior superior iliac spine. The potentials, usually 256 responses, are averaged.

STIMULATION: The surface-stimulating electrode is placed 20 cm inferior to the recording point on the course of the nerve, which is determined by locating the areas of lowest threshold for evoking a sensation radiating to the lateral side of the thigh using stimuli of 0.1 msec at 10/sec.

Table 11.5.
Normal Data for the Lateral Femoral Cutaneous Nerve—Lysens's Technique[a]

Age Group (yr)	NCV (m/sec)		Amplitude (μV) (Mean ± SD)	No. of Subjects
	Mean ± SD	Normal Limit		
17–30	60.1 ± 1.5	57.1	4.2 ± 1.5	11
31–40	57.0 ± 3.1	50.8	3.3 ± 1.9	13
41–50	55.4 ± 4.8	45.8	3.8 ± 1.6	18
51–60	54.6 ± 6.2	42.2	2.7 ± 2.3	15

[a]See Lysens et al. (86).

MEASUREMENT: The latency is measured between the stimulus onset and the peak of the first negative deflection. The amplitude and distance measurements are conventional.

TEMPERATURE: The skin temperature is measured at the recording site. Whenever skin temperature is below 32°C, the NCV is corrected using the following equation: NCV corrected = 1.7(32−skin temperature) + observed NCV (m/sec). The skin temperature is kept higher than 32°C.

NORMAL DATA: See Table 11.5.

COMMENTS: By using a needle electrode, Lysens overcomes the technical difficulty in obtaining reliable CNAPs with surface electrodes in obese and pregnant individuals.

Posterior Femoral Cutaneous Nerve

Dumitru and Nelson (79) described a technique of sensory nerve conduction of the posterior femoral cutaneous nerve (Fig. 11.65).

POSITION OF SUBJECT: The subject is in the prone position with the lower extremities completely relaxed.

RECORDING: An active surface electrode is placed in the midline of the posterior thigh 6 cm proximal to the midpopliteal region. The reference electrode is placed 3 cm distally from the active electrode.

STIMULATION: The surface electrode is placed 12 cm proximal to the recording electrode on a line connecting the active recording electrode with the ischial tuberosity in the groove between the medial and lateral hamstring muscles. This intermuscular groove is confirmed by palpating the posterior thigh while asking the patient to flex the knee slightly.

MEASUREMENT: The amplitude of the CNAP is measured from peak-to-peak and the latency to the negative peak.

TEMPERATURE: Skin temperature is controlled between 32 and 33°C.

NORMAL DATA: Number of subjects: 40. Number of nerves: 80. Age range: 20–78 yr.

Measurement	Mean ± SD	Normal Limit
Latency (msec)	2.8 ± 0.2	3.2
Amplitude (μV)	6.5 ± 1.5	4.4

COMMENTS: Complete relaxation of the thigh is mandatory to obtain a reliable response. Latency increases with age.

Femoral Nerve

Gassel (80) and Chopra and Hurwitz (81) calculated the femoral "motor NCV" by stimulating the nerve below the inguinal ligament and recording the CMAPs at two or three locations of the rectus femoris muscle. Because their "NCVs" are not motor NCVs in the truest sense, their methods are not described here.

Johnson et al. (82) stimulated the femoral nerve at three points—superior to the

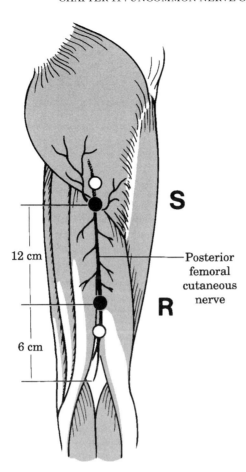

Figure 11.65. Sensory nerve conduction of the posterior femoral cutaneous nerve.

inguinal ligament, inferior to the inguinal ligament, and at Hunter's canal—and recorded the CMAP over the vastus medialis. According to our experience, the stimulation at Hunter's canal is unreliable, and the latency measurement between points "superior" and "inferior" to the inguinal ligament is full of errors because of the short distance between the two sites. Thus, there is no reliable method of measuring the motor NCV in the femoral nerve.

Rigshospitalet's Method

Rigshospitalet's technique uses needles as both stimulating and recording electrodes (83) (Fig. 11.66A).

RECORDING: Recording is from the rectus femoris with concentric electrodes. The distance is not fixed; the median distance is 20 cm.

STIMULATION: The nerve is stimulated just below the inguinal ligament with needle electrodes. The pulsation of the femoral artery is used as a landmark, and the stimulating electrodes are placed vertically immediately lateral to the artery.

MEASUREMENT: Conventional methods for the needle technique.

TEMPERATURE: Skin temperature is kept within 36–38°C.

NORMAL DATA: See Table 7.38 and Fig. 7.8.

INTEPRETATION: Latency should be judged according to the distance from the stimulating and the recording electrodes.

Stohr's Method

The technique of Stohr et al. (84) uses surface electrodes as both stimulating and recording electrodes (Fig. 11.66B).

Figure 11.66. *A*, Rigshospitalet's method of motor nerve conduction of the femoral nerve. *B*, Stohr's method of motor nerve conduction of the femoral nerve.

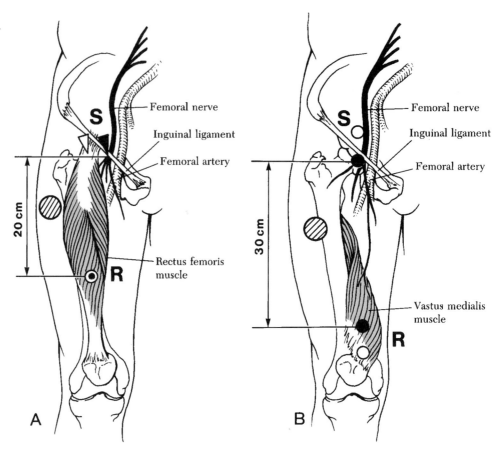

Table 11.6.
Normal Data for the Femoral Nerve—Stohr's Method[a]

Age (yr)	Latency (msec)		Amplitude (mV)		Duration (msec)		No. of Subjects
	Mean ± SD	Normal Limit	Mean ± SD	Normal Limit	Mean ± SD	Normal Limit	
<40	5.2 ± 0.5	6.2	12.1 ± 5.1	3.7	20.9 ± 5.6	32.1	28
>40	5.5 ± 0.5	6.5	9.3 ± 5.2	0.8	10.0 ± 5.9	31.8	40

[a]See Stohr et al. (84).

RECORDING: The response in the vastus medialis is recorded with surface electrodes using the belly-tendon methods. The distance between the stimulating and recording electrodes is best fixed at 30 cm.

STIMULATION: The nerve is stimulated with the surface electrode at the level of the inguinal ligament.

MEASUREMENT: The conventional method is used. The latencies measured are corrected to a standard distance of 30 cm, implying that the distance is not set at 30 cm. However, Stohr et al. did not describe the method of correction.

TEMPERATURE: The mean skin temperature at the inguinal ligament is 36°C with 1.2 SD.

NORMAL DATA: See Table 11.6.

Saphenous Nerve

Wainapel et al.'s Method

Wainapel et al. (85) described an easily performed and reproducible method for the antidromic determination of NCV in the saphenous nerve (Fig. 11.67).

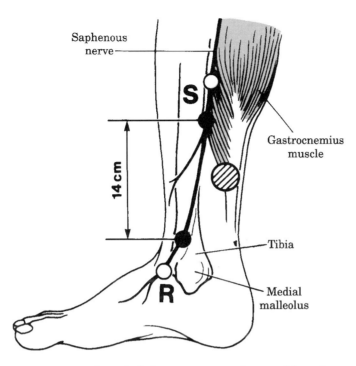

Figure 11.67. Wainapel's method of sensory nerve conduction of the saphenous nerve.

RECORDING: A plastic-mounted bipolar surface electrode with the surface discs 3 cm apart is used for the recording electrode. The reference electrode is placed just anterior to the highest prominence of the medial malleolus in the space between the malleolus and the medial border of the tibialis anterior tendon. The active electrode is located 3 cm above the other and just medial to the aforementioned tendon, whose direction is paralleled by a line drawn between the recording electrodes. *We found the placement of active recording electrode just anterior to the highest prominence of the medial malleolus is more reliable.*

STIMULATION: The site of stimulation is located approximately 14 cm above the active recording electrode, deep to the medial border of the tibia. *Firm pressure should be exerted on the stimulating electrodes, pushing them between the medial gastrocnemius and the tibia.* To facilitate this, the gastrocnemius should be relaxed by positioning the ankle in slight plantar flexion.

MEASUREMENT: Latency is measured from the stimulus onset to the peak of the first negative deflection of the response. The amplitude measurement is conventional.

TEMPERATURE: Room temperature is thermostatically maintained at 22.8°C. Skin temperature is not controlled.

NORMAL DATA: Number of subjects: 40. Age range: 20–79 yr.

Measurement	Mean ± SD	Normal Limit
Latency (msec)	3.6 ± 0.4	4.4
NCV (m/sec)	41.7 ± 3.4	38.3
Amplitude (μV)	9.0 ± 3.4	

COMMENTS: The main problems encountered in saphenous nerve conduction measurements are: (*a*) a low-voltage response of 5 μV or less, which sometimes requires superimposition of tracings or electronic averaging; and (*b*) difficulty obtaining clear responses in subjects with edematous or obese ankles.

This technique offers the following advantages: (*a*) it is less painful, eliminating the need for needle electrode or prior localization of the femoral nerve by electrical stimulation through the needle; (*b*) the mean amplitude of the CNAP is 2–2.5 times greater than Ertekin's method (90); and (*c*) it is technically simpler to perform. Conversely, Ertekin's method does offer greater precision in localization along the course of the saphenous nerve.

Ertekin's Method

Ertekin's method (86) describes the orthodromic technique of obtaining the CNAP over the knee- and ankle-inguinal ligament segments (Fig. 11.68).

RECORDING: The needle electrode is inserted using the near-nerve technique at the inguinal ligament about 0.5–1.5 cm lateral to the maximum pulsation of the femoral artery, and the reference electrode is inserted 3.0 cm laterally. Twenty superimposed sweeps, as well as single sweeps, are photographed.

STIMULATION: With a surface electrode, the nerve is stimulated at the knee below the lower edge of the patella on the medial surface of the leg. Electrodes are held

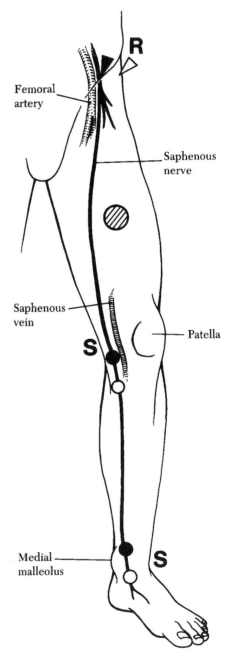

Figure 11.68. Ertekin's and Stohr's methods of sensory nerve conduction of the saphenous nerve.

firmly in place by surgical tape. Before application of the electrodes, the skin is cleaned with ether and gently rubbed with sandpaper. At the ankle, the nerve is stimulated above the medial malleolus. A 0.2-msec duration and stimulus intensity of 40–60 mA stimulus intensity are needed for an adequate sensory response.

MEASUREMENT: The latency is measured from the beginning of the stimulus to the peak of the first positive deflection. The amplitude measurement is conventional.

TEMPERATURE: The skin temperature is kept between 36–37°C.

NORMAL DATA: See Table 11.7.

COMMENTS: Electrical stimulation at this site has the advantage of not activating muscle tissue around the electrodes, and hence artifacts from muscles are avoided. The sensory CNAP was recorded in all individuals up to 63 years and in some patients over 65 years as well. The method does not require an averaging computer.

Stohr's Method

The method of Stohr et al. (84) is identical to Ertekin's method except for using the signal averaging in all individuals (Fig. 11.68).

RECORDING: Teflon-coated needles (DISA 13L64) are used for recording the sensory CNAP. The active electrode is placed near the femoral nerve at the inguinal ligament and the reference electrode 3 cm more laterally. The electronic averaging of 32–512 tracings is used to record the sensory CNAP.

STIMULATION: The saphenous nerve is first stimulated on the medial aspect of the knee with a surface electrode (DISA 13K62), and then in exactly the same manner just above the medial malleolus.

MEASUREMENT: The latency is measured from the stimulus onset to the first positive peak of the CNAP. The amplitude measurement is conventional.

TEMPERATURE: Mean skin temperatures at the inguinal ligament, knee, and medial malleolus are 33.6°, 32.3°, and 31.6°C, respectively.

NORMAL DATA: See Table 11.8.

Table 11.7.
Normal Data for the Saphenous Nerve—Ertrekin's Method[a]

Age (yr)	NCV (m/sec)		Amplitude (µV) (mean ± SD)	No. of Subjects
	Mean ± SD	Normal Limit		
Knee-inguinal ligament				
17–38	59.6 ± 2.3	55.0	4.2 ± 1.8	33
41–63	57.1 ± 2.3	52.5	3.6 ± 2.4	20
Ankle-knee				
17–36	52.3 ± 2.3	47.7		10
Ankle-inguinal ligament				
17–36	56.6 ± 2.0	52.6		10

[a]See Ertrekin (87).

Table 11.8.
Normal Data for the Saphenous Nerve—Stohr's Method[a]

Age (yr)	NCV (m/sec)		Amplitude (µV)		Duration (msec)		No. of Subjects
	Mean ± SD	Normal Limit	Mean ± SD	Normal Limit	Mean ± SD	Normal Limit	
Knee-inguinal ligament segment							
<40	58.9 ± 3.2	52.5	5.5 ± 2.6	1.2	4.9 ± 1.8	8.5	28
>40	57.9 ± 4.0	49.9	5.1 ± 2.7	0.7	5.1 ± 2.0	9.1	41
Ankle-knee segment							
<40	51.2 ± 4.7	41.8	2.1 ± 1.1		8.2 ± 3.3	14.8	22
>40	50.2 ± 5.0	40.2	1.7 ± 0.8		9.1 ± 3.2	15.5	32

[a]See Stohr et al. (88).

Senden's Method

Senden et al. (91) described an orthodromic sensory nerve conduction technique for the distal segment of the saphenous nerve (Fig. 11.69).

RECORDING: An active needle electrode (DISA 13L64) is inserted at the knee below the lower edge of the patella on the medial surface of the leg. The reference needle electrode is inserted more than 3 cm lateral to the active needle electrode. Signal averaging is used to record the CNAP. Usually 256 responses are averaged.

STIMULATION: The nerve is stimulated anteriorly to the medial malleolus with a bipolar surface electrode. Two ground electrodes are used, one around the limb near the stimulation point and the other near the recording site.

MEASUREMENT: The latency is measured from the stimulus onset to the peak of the first negative deflection. The amplitude is measured from peak to peak.

TEMPERATURE: The room temperature ranged from 21°C to 25°C. The skin temperature is measured at the medial aspect of the knee. The mean temperature was 32°C. Whenever skin temperature is below 32°C, the sensory NCV is corrected using the following equation:

$$\text{Corrected NCV} = 1.7 \, (32 - \text{skin temperature}) + \text{measured NCV (m/sec)}$$

NORMAL DATA: See Table 11.9.

COMMENTS: No CNAP was obtained in six normal controls (8.5%). The rate of finding no CNAP increases with age: 0% at 18–30 yr, 9% at 31–40 yr, 10% at 41–50 yr, and 50% at 51–56 yr. Thus, the inability to obtain the CNAP is common in individuals older than 50 years. "Dispersion" (polyphasic potential) is observed in 24% of the normals and occurs more frequently in the older age groups. These normal variables must be considered when interpreting the data.

There is no significant difference in sensory NCV between the different age groups. However, there is a significant difference of the amplitudes between the groups.

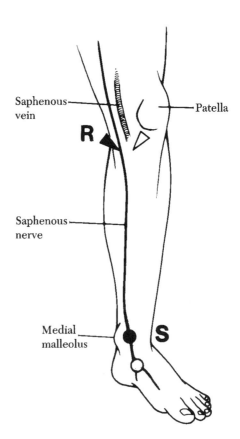

Figure 11.69.   Senden's method of sensory nerve conduction of the saphenous nerve.

Table 11.9.
Normal Data for the Saphenous Nerve—Senden's Method

Age (yr)	NCV (m/sec)		Amplitude (μV) (Mean ± SD)	No. of Subjects
	Mean ± SD	Normal Limit		
18–30	54.9 ± 2.8	49.3	4.4 ± 1.28	34
31–40	53.1 ± 6.6	39.9	3.5 ± 1.50	11
41–50	55.6 ± 3.8	48.0	2.94 ± 0.43	20
51–56	52.1 ± 9.3	33.5	1.6 ± 0.6	6

Sciatic Nerve

Yap's Method

Yap and Hirota (88) described a technique for measuring sciatic nerve motor conduction using a surface electrode (Fig. 11.70).

RECORDING: Two recording sites are selected: the medial gastrocnemius and the ADQ muscles. The conventional method for placing the recording surface electrodes is used for the ADQ muscles. For the medial head of the gastrocnemius muscle, needle and surface electrodes are used for the active recording electrodes, which are placed over the belly of the medial gastrocnemius (13–17 cm from the stimulating point at the sciatic nerve at the popliteal fossa). The reference electrode is placed over the lateral malleolus.

STIMULATION: The proximal sciatic nerve is stimulated at the gluteal fold using a needle electrode as an active electrode and an electrocardiogram rectangular plate (3 × 5 cm), a reference electrode, placed on the flexor surface near the gluteal fold. Distal sciatic nerve stimulation is at the popliteal fossa proximal to the branching of the posterior tibial and common peroneal nerves.

MEASUREMENT: Conventional methods are used.

TEMPERATURE: Skin temperature is not measured.

NORMAL DATA: See Table 11.10.

COMMENTS: Needle electrode stimulation is essential in stimulating the sciatic nerve at the gluteal fold. This produces much less discomfort and no after-effects. There is no problem in locating and applying a supramaximal stimulus on the nerve trunk.

Gassel's Method

The method of Gassel and Trojaborg (93) is essentially the same as Yap and Hirota's method (92) except that needle electrodes are used as the recording electrodes (Fig. 11.70).

RECORDING: CMAPs are recorded intramuscularly using a concentric needle from the anterior tibialis, gastrocnemius, and soleus in the legs, and from the extensor digitorum brevis and abductor hallucis in the feet.

STIMULATION: *Sciatic notch:* The sciatic nerve is stimulated proximally in the buttock or upper thigh either between the greater trochanter of the femur and the tuberosity of the ischium, or directly below the middle of this position on a line drawn downwards to the apex of the popliteal fossa. The stimulation on the nerve at the buttock is done with uninsulated stainless steel needle electrodes 0.4 mm in diameter and 8 cm in length. The needles are placed 2.5 cm apart at a depth of 3–6 cm.

Knee: The lower position of stimulation of the sciatic nerve is in the apex of the popliteal fossa at the level of the upper border of the femoral condyles. Stimulation at the knee is done with a surface electrode.

MEASUREMENT: The conventional motor nerve conduction method for the needle technique.

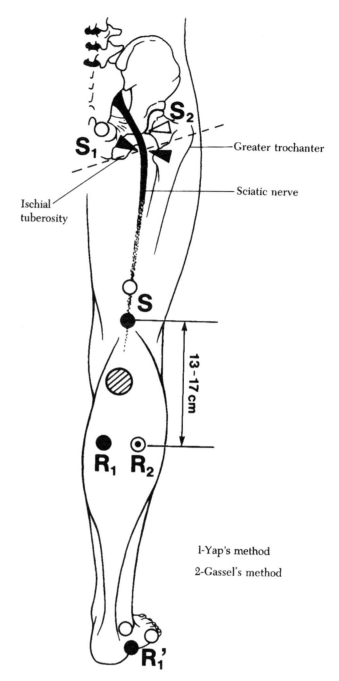

Figure 11.70. Yap's and Gassel's methods of motor nerve conduction of the sciatic nerve. Yap's method is represented by S_1 and R_1; Gassel's method is represented by S_2 and R_2.

Table 11.10.
Normal Data for the Sciatic Nerve in 10 Subjects—Yap's Method (Ages 21–66)

Site	Latency (msec)		NCV (m/sec)	
	Mean ± SD	Normal Limit	Mean ± SD	Normal Limit
Medial gastrocnemius	4.7 ± 0.6^a	4.9	53.8 ± 3.3	47.2
Abductor digiti quinti	15.7 ± 2.2^b	20.1	51.3 ± 4.4	42.5

[a]Mean distance 15 cm.
[b]Mean distance 33 cm.

Table 11.11.
Normal Data for the Sciatic Nerve in 24 Subjects—Gassel's Method (Ages 19–67)

Site	Latency from Popliteal Fossa (msec)		Buttock-Popliteal Fossa NCV (m/sec)		No. of Subjects
	Mean ± SD	Normal Limit	Mean ± SD	Normal Limit	
Abductor hallucis			51.0 ± 5.8	39.4	20
Extensor digitorum brevis			51.0 ± 7.0	37.0	18
Anterior tibialis	5.4 ± 0.7	6.8	55.0 ± 4.5	46.0	15
Soleus	5.4 ± 0.8	7.0	56.0 ± 5.5	45.0	20
Gastrocnemius	5.5 ± 0.7	6.9	56.0 ± 5.6	44.8	19

TEMPERATURE: The intramuscular temperature at 2, 3, and 4 cm depths in the mid-posterior thigh ranges from 34.6° to 36.6°C.

NORMAL DATA: See Table 11.11.

COMMENTS: Unlike Yap's method (92), there is a 20–22% higher conduction velocity in the nerves to the proximal muscles (anterior tibialis, soleus, and gastrocnemius) than to the distal muscles (extensor digitorum brevis and abductor hallucis) of the lower extremity.

Peroneal Nerve

Peroneal Motor Conduction with Needle Electrodes

Singh et al. (90) described a technique for measuring peroneal motor conduction with needle electrodes (Fig. 11.71).

RECORDING: A concentric needle electrode is placed in the end-plate zone of the extensor digitorum brevis, anterior tibial, and peroneus longus muscles.

STIMULATION: Near-nerve electrodes placed in the popliteal fossa and distal to the capitulum fibulae for the sensory nerve conduction are used to stimulate the motor nerve (see Peroneal Sensory Conduction, below). In addition, electrodes are placed near the deep peroneal nerve at the ankle.

MEASUREMENT: Conventional methods are used for latency and amplitude measurements with the needle technique. The latency from the ankle to the extensor digitorum brevis muscle is corrected to a standard distance of 9 cm. (The method is discussed in Chapter 7.) The average distance between "below the fibular head" and the popliteal fossa is 11 cm.

TEMPERATURE: Skin temperature is controlled at 36–37°C.

NORMAL DATA: See Tables 7.29 and 7.30.

Proximal Peroneal Motor NCV

Devi et al. (91) described a method of determining the motor NCV over the fibular head-popliteal fossa by recording the CMAP from the anterior tibialis and peroneus brevis muscles (Fig. 11.72).

RECORDING: For the anterior tibial muscle, the active surface electrode is placed at the junction of the upper third and lower two-thirds of the line between the tibial tuberosity and the tip of the lateral malleolus. The reference electrode is placed over the medial aspect of the tibia at a position 4 cm distal to the active recording electrode. For the peroneus brevis, the active recording electrode is placed at the junction of the upper two-fifths and lower three-fifths of a line between the head of the fibula and the tip of the lateral malleolus. The reference electrode is placed 4 cm distal on the muscle tendon.

STIMULATION: The peroneal nerve is stimulated from above the head of the fibula, just inside the lateral border of the popliteal space at the level of the midpatella. It is

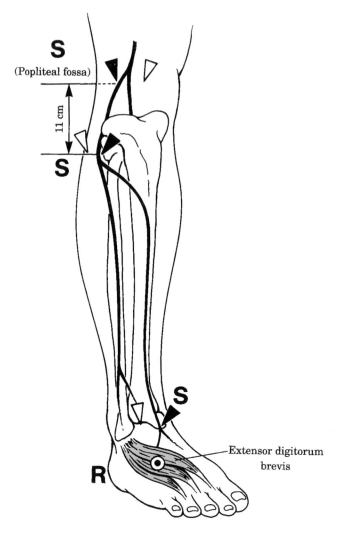

Figure 11.71.   Motor nerve conduction of the peroneal nerve.

also stimulated below the head of the fibula approximately 10 cm distal to the first stimulation point.

MEASUREMENT: Conventional methods are used.

TEMPERATURE: Skin temperature is not controlled.

NORMAL DATA: See Table 11.12.

COMMENTS: This test is indicated in the presence of complete atrophy of the extensor digitorum brevis.

Short-Segment Stimulation of Peroneal Nerve across the Fibular Head

Kanakamedala and Hong (92) described a short-segment stimulation method for the motor nerve conduction of the peroneal nerve across the fibular head (Fig. 11.73).

RECORDING: Surface electrodes are placed on the extensor digitorum brevis by the belly-tendon method.

STIMULATION: The peroneal nerve is stimulated across the fibular head at 2-cm increments, starting 4 cm distal (D4 and D2) and ending 6 cm proximal (P2, P4, and P6) to the fibular head prominence (P).

MEASUREMENT: Latency measurement is conventional. Amplitude is measured from the baseline to the initial negative peak.

TEMPERATURE: Skin temperature is controlled at 32°C.

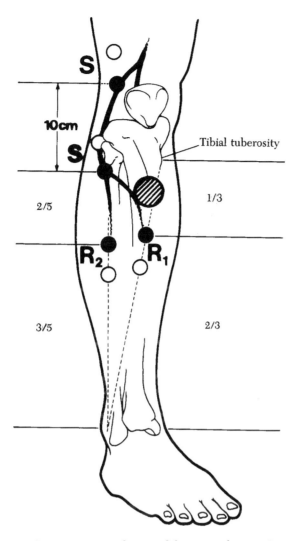

Figure 11.72. Proximal motor nerve conduction of the peroneal nerve. R_1, recording electrode in the anterior tibialis. R_2, recording electrode in the peroneus brevis.

Table 11.12.
Normal Data for the Peroneal Nerve in 34 Subjects—Devi's Method (Ages 17–44)

Site	NCV		Terminal Latency		Amplitude (mV) (Mean ± SD)
	Mean ± SD	Normal Limit	Mean ± SD	Normal Limit	
Anterior tibialis	66.3 ± 12.9	40.5	3.0 ± 0.6	4.2	3.9 ± 1.2
Peroneus muscle	55.3 ± 10.2	34.9	3.0 ± 0.8	4.6	5.9 ± 2.4

NORMAL DATA: Number of subjects: 44 nerves in 28 subjects. Age range: 25–59 yr.

Measurement	Mean ± SD	Normal Limit
Conduction time over 2-cm segments (msec)	0.43 ± 0.17	0.94
Amplitude reduction over 2-cm segments[a] (%)	0.9 ± 3.0	9.9%

[a]Distal-to-proximal change.

INTERPRETATION: More than 3 SD from the mean is used as the criterion for abnormality.

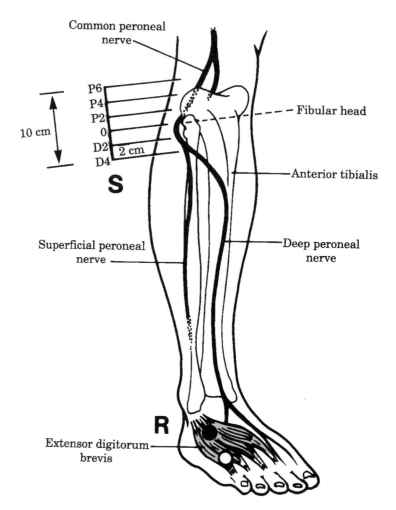

Figure 11.73. Short-segment stimulation (inching) technique of the peroneal nerve across the fibular head.

COMMENTS: Of 18 patients with peroneal nerve palsy, 14 had prolonged conduction time and abnormal amplitude reduction, three had prolongation of conduction time only, and one had abnormal reduction in amplitude only. In this study, a majority of the lesions were located just proximal to the fibular head.

Superficial Peroneal Sensory Nerve Conduction

Jabre's Method

Jabre (63) described an antidromic method for the sensory nerve conduction over the intermediate dorsal cutaneous branch of the superficial peroneal nerve (Fig. 11.74A).

RECORDING: An active surface recording electrode is placed at the ankle level one fingerbreadth medial to the lateral malleolus.

STIMULATION: The nerve is stimulated at a point 12 cm proximal to the active recording electrode, with the stimulator probes firmly held against the anterior edge of the fibula.

MEASUREMENT: The amplitude of the CNAP is measured from the take-off to the peak of the negative phase, and the latency is taken to the negative peak. When NCVs are calculated, the latency is measured to take-off. In calculating NCV, the distance is divided by the latency to the take-off of the potential.

TEMPERATURE: Skin temperature is not controlled. The ambient room temperature is kept at 22°C.

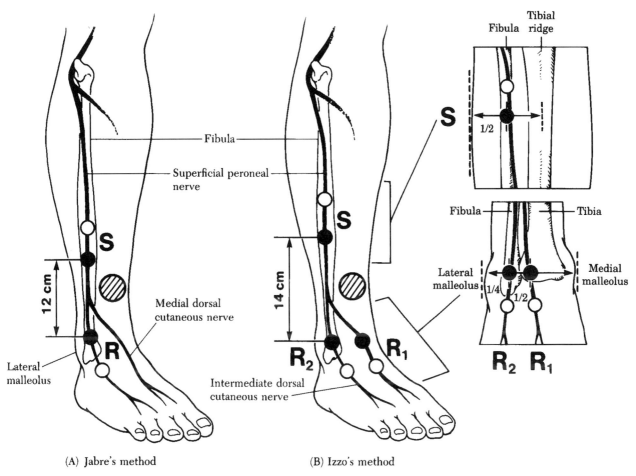

(A) Jabre's method   (B) Izzo's method

Figure 11.74. Sensory nerve conduction of the superficial peroneal nerve. **A**, Jabre's method. **B**, Izzo's method.

NORMAL DATA: Number of subjects: 56. Age range: 3–60 yr.

Measurement	Mean ± SD	Normal Limit
Latency (msec)	2.9 ± 0.3	3.5
NCV (m/sec)	65.7 ± 3.7	58.3
Amplitude (μV)	20.5 ± 6.1	

ADVANTAGES: No averaging is needed, nor is visualization or palpation of the nerve. Because of the recording electrode's position, troublesome motor artifacts from the extensor digitorum brevis are avoided. Jabre was able to record a response in every healthy adult he studied.

Izzo's Method

Izzo et al. (93) described an antidromic method for sensory nerve conduction over the intermediate and medial dorsal cutaneous branches of the superficial peroneal sensory nerve (Fig. 11.74B).

RECORDING: An active surface recording electrode is placed at the ankle level over the medial and intermediate dorsal cutaneous branches, which are located by inspection and palpation during plantar flexion and inversion of the foot. *For best results, a line connecting the medial and lateral malleolus is divided into four equal parts. For the intermediate branch of the nerve, an active recording electrode is placed one-fourth of the distance from the lateral malleolus toward the medial malleolus. For the medial branch, the active recording electrode is placed at the midpoint of this line (Fig. 11.74B, insert).*

STIMULATION: The nerve is stimulated 14 cm from the proximal recording electrodes on the anterior lateral aspect of the leg. *The best stimulating site is at the midpoint between the ridge of the tibia and the lateral border of the calf muscle (Fig. 11.74B, insert).*

MEASUREMENT: The latency is measured from the onset of the stimulus to both the onset of the first negative deflection and to its peak. The conduction velocity is calculated by dividing the distance by the latency to the onset of the first negative deflection. The amplitude is measured by the conventional method.

TEMPERATURE: Skin temperature is higher than 28°C. The room temperature is maintained at 23°C.

NORMAL DATA: Number of subjects: 80. Age range: 20–69 yr.

Measurement	Mean ± SD	Normal Limit
Medial dorsal cutaneous nerve		
NCV (m/sec)	51.2 ± 5.7	39.8
Onset latency (msec)	2.8 ± 0.3	3.4
Peak latency (msec)	3.4 ± 0.4	4.2
Amplitude (μV)	18.3 ± 8.0	5
Intermediate dorsal cutaneous nerve		
NCV (m/sec)	51.3 ± 5.4	40.5
Onset latency (msec)	2.8 ± 0.7	4.2
Peak latency (msec)	3.4 ± 0.4	4.2
Amplitude (μV)	14.1 ± 8.2	4

COMMENTS: No averaging is needed. Nerve potential is obtained from the medial dorsal cutaneous branch in all subjects and from the intermediate branch in 98% of subjects. These are in contrast to the CNAP being found in 100% of sural nerves and 87% of saphenous nerves. When one branch of the superficial peroneal nerve is to be studied, Izzo et al. advocated the use of the medial dorsal cutaneous branch because it is easily located by palpation, often just lateral to the extensor hallucis longus tendon.

Behse's Method

Behse and Buchthal (94) described an orthodromic method for measuring sensory nerve conduction over the medial dorsal cutaneous branch, the fibular head-ankle segment, and the fibular head-popliteal fossa of the superficial peroneal nerve (Fig. 11.75).

RECORDING: With the near-nerve needle technique, the needle is used as an active recording electrode. A reference needle electrode is inserted subcutaneously at least 30 mm transversely from an active electrode.

At the ankle: The needle electrode is placed at the medial branch of the nerve, 2–3 cm proximal to a line connecting the medial and lateral malleoli and 1–2 cm lateral to the tendon of the anterior tibial muscle ("superior extensor retinaculum"). If the nerve cannot be palpated, the site of insertion is found by stimulation with a surface electrode.

At the fibular head: The needle electrode is placed 1 cm below the fibular head near the superficial peroneal nerve by adjusting its position until the threshold of the long peroneal muscle below 1 mA and lower than that of the anterior tibial muscle.

At the popliteal fossa: The needle electrode is placed in the popliteal fossa medial to the tendon of the biceps femoris muscle, 9.5–12.5 cm proximal to the electrode below the fibular head. The reference electrode is placed laterally.

Single-sweep, photographic superimposition of 20 responses or, when the responses are less than 2 μV, averaging of 300–500 responses is used for recording.

STIMULATION: Surface ring electrodes are placed on the big toe. A needle electrode is used as a stimulating electrode at the ankle.

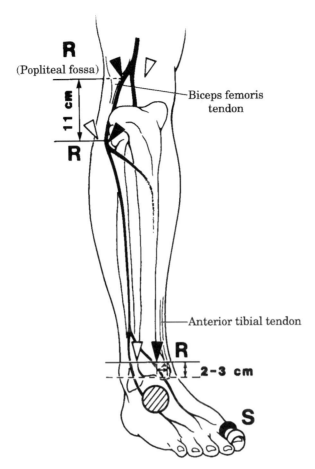

Figure 11.75. Behse's method of sensory nerve conduction of the superficial peroneal sensory nerve.

MEASUREMENT: The shortest latency of the sensory CNAP is measured from the onset of the stimuli to the first positive peak. The NCV is calculated by dividing the distance by the shortest latency or by the conduction time calculated from the difference between latencies, measured at the two recording sites.

TEMPERATURE: Skin temperature on the leg is controlled to 36–37°C.

NORMAL DATA: See Tables 7.31 and 7.32.

COMMENTS: When the superficial peroneal nerve is compressed at the ankle or over the dorsum of the foot, this may be the only test available for confirmation.

Deep Peroneal Sensory Nerve Conduction

Lee et al. (95) described a technique of antidromic sensory nerve conduction for the deep peroneal sensory nerve (Fig. 11.76).

RECORDING: The active surface electrode is placed at the interspace between the 1st and 2nd metatarsal heads. The reference electrode is placed 3 cm distally on the 2nd toe.

STIMULATION: An active surface electrode is placed at the ankle, 12 cm proximal to the active recording electrode and just lateral to the extensor hallucis longus tendon.

MEASUREMENT: The latency is measured from the stimulus onset to the onset of the first negative deflection and the negative peak. The NCV is calculated by dividing the distance by the onset latency.

TEMPERATURE: Skin temperature is kept above 29°C.

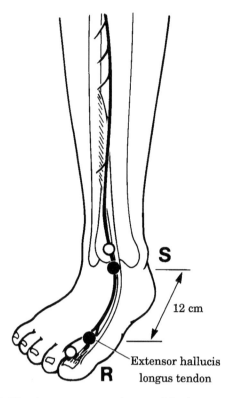

Figure 11.76.   Sensory nerve conduction of the deep peroneal nerve.

NORMAL DATA: Number of subjects: 40. Age range: 21–50.

Measurement	Mean ± SD	Normal Limit
Latency to onset (msec)	2.9 ± 0.4	3.7
Latency to peak (msec)	3.6 ± 0.4	4.6
NCV (m/sec)	42.0 ± 5.0	32.0
Amplitude (μV)	3.4 ± 1.2	1.6

COMMENTS: Authors stated that this technique may be helpful in diagnosing deep peroneal neuropathies in the anterior tarsal tunnel and local deep peroneal nerve injury, and in early detection of peripheral neuropathy. One patient with an entrapment of the sensory branch of the deep peroneal nerve showed a low CNAP amplitude (0.6 μV) and prolonged latency (4.6 msec), confirming this neuropathy (96).

Mixed Nerve Conduction in Peroneal Nerves

The mixed CNAPs in peroneal and posterior tibial nerves are small compared with the CNAPs in median and ulnar nerves. *It is difficult to obtain the CNAP in these nerves without using signal averaging.* However, there are two studies that described the method and reported normal data.

Gilliatt's Method

Gilliatt et al. (97) reported a method of obtaining the mixed CNAP using a needle as the recording electrode (Fig. 11.77A).

RECORDING: Two small stainless steel needles are placed at right angles to the course of the nerve and inserted to a depth of 1.5 cm. No attempt is made to pierce the nerve sheath, the lower needle being immediately behind the neck of the fibula and the upper needle behind the tendon of the biceps femoris at its insertion. With this arrangement each electrode lies just behind the nerve trunk, the interelectrode dis-

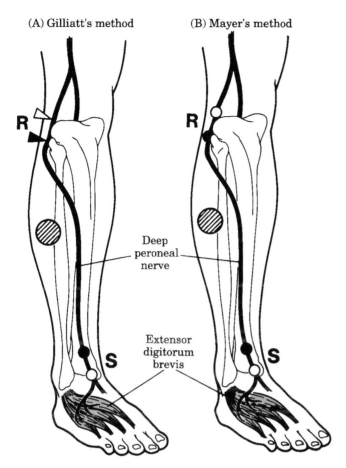

Figure 11.77. Mixed nerve conduction of the peroneal nerve. **A**, Gilliatt's method. **B**, Mayer's method.

tance varying between 3 and 4 cm in different experiments. Photographic recordings of the 100 successive sweeps at low brilliance are superimposed.

STIMULATION: A stimulating surface electrode is placed over the anterior tibial nerve on the dorsum of the ankle, its position being such that stimulation produces brisk contractions of the extensor digitorum brevis and paresthesias radiating into the first interdigital cleft.

MEASUREMENT: Latency to the peak of negative deflection is measured. Amplitude is measured by the conventional method.

TEMPERATURE: Skin temperature is not controlled.

NORMAL DATA:

Measurement	Mean ± SD	Normal Limit	No. of Subjects
NCV (m/sec)			
<50 yr	45.5 ± 3.5	38.0	19
>50 yr	42.6 ± 4.6	33.4	20
Amplitude (μV)	2–15.5 (range)	2	

COMMENTS: The amplitude of the mixed CNAP is lowest in elderly subjects. The conduction velocity is also slightly reduced in older subjects.

Mayer's Method

Mayer's method (98) is different from that of Gilliatt and Goodman (97) in that it uses a surface electrode as the recording electrode (Fig. 11.77B).

RECORDING: Surface electrodes applied to the skin are used for recording. In cases in which the CNAPs are extremely small, needle electrodes are used for recording. These consist of either concentric needles insulated to the tip or solid needles. The needles are inserted through the skin and placed in the vicinity of the nerve to be tested with an interelectrode distance of 3–4 cm. Recording electrodes are placed at the head of the fibula.

STIMULATION: Surface electrodes are placed at the peroneal nerve at the ankle.

MEASUREMENT: The latency is measured from the onset of the stimulus to the junction of the negative deflection potential and the baseline of the potential. Because the amplitude of the potential depends on uncontrollable variables, e.g., skin resistance and distance between nerve and electrodes, it cannot be standardized.

TEMPERATURE: The skin temperature is controlled between 33° and 36°C.

NORMAL DATA:

Age (yr)	NCV (m/sec)	
	Mean ± SD	Normal Limit
10–35	53.0 ± 5.9	41.2
36–50	50.4 ± 1.0	48.0
51–80	46.4 ± 4.0	36.4

Posterior Tibial Nerve

Motor, Sensory, and Mixed Nerve Conduction with Needle Electrodes

Behse and Buchthal (94) described techniques to measure nerve conduction in the posterior tibial nerve with a needle electrode.

Motor Nerve Conduction

RECORDING: A concentric needle electrode is inserted into the abductor hallucis muscle (Fig. 11.78).

STIMULATION: The near-nerve needle electrodes used for recording the CNAP are used to stimulate motor fibers: distally at the ankle above the flexor retinaculum and proximally at the popliteal fossa.

MEASUREMENT: Conventional methods are used to measure latency and amplitude.

TEMPERATURE: Skin temperature is controlled at 36–37°C.

NORMAL DATA: See Table 7.33.

Sensory Nerve Conduction

RECORDING: The near-nerve needle electrode is inserted above the flexor retinaculum behind the medial malleolus and 4–5 cm proximal to the skinfold in the middle of the popliteal fossa (Fig. 11.79).

STIMULATION: The sensory nerve is stimulated by surface ring electrodes on the big toe.

MEASUREMENT: Amplitude is measured by the conventional method. The latency is measured from the onset of the stimulus to the first positive peak. The NCV is calculated by the conventional method for the near-nerve needle technique.

TEMPERATURE: Skin temperature is controlled at 36–37°C.

NORMAL DATA: See Table 7.34.

Mixed Nerve Conduction

RECORDING: The near-nerve needle electrode is inserted at the crease in the popliteal fossa.

STIMULATION: The nerve is stimulated by the near-nerve needle electrode at the ankle.

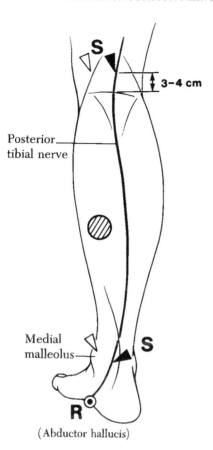

Figure 11.78.   Motor nerve conduction of the posterior tibial nerve.

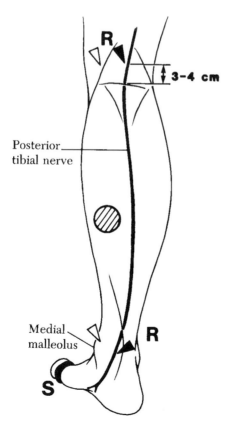

Figure 11.79.   Sensory nerve conduction of the posterior tibial nerve.

MEASUREMENT: Same as for sensory nerve conduction.
TEMPERATURE: Same as for sensory nerve conduction.
NORMAL DATA:

Measurement	Mean ± SD	Normal Limit	No. of Subjects
NCV (m/sec)			
13–30 yr	58.6 ± 3.8	51.0	17
40–52 yr	57.4 ± 4.5	48.4	7
Amplitude (μV)			
15–30 yr	18.0 ± 10.2	5.0	17
40–65 yr	9.9 ± 4.6	1.0	7

Mixed Nerve Conduction with Surface Electrodes

Mayer (98) used a surface electrode to record mixed CNAPs (Fig. 11.80).

RECORDING: Surface electrodes are placed at the popliteal fossa. When the CNAPs are small, concentric needles or solid needles are used for recording.

STIMULATION: The nerve is stimulated at the ankle by a surface electrode.

MEASUREMENT: Latency is measured from onset of the stimulus to the onset of the negative deflection. The amplitude varies, and so it is not measured.

TEMPERATURE: Skin temperature is controlled between 33° and 36°C.

NORMAL DATA:

Age (yr)	Mean ± SD (m/sec)	Normal Limit (m/sec)
10–35	58.6 ± 4.4	48.1
36–50	49.0 ± 3.8	41.4
51–86	48.9 ± 2.6	43.7

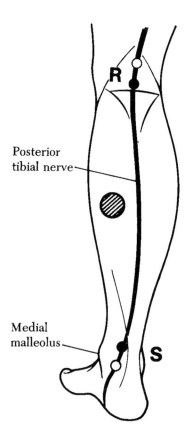

Figure 11.80. Mayer's method of mixed nerve conduction of the posterior tibial nerve.

Plantar Nerve

Motor Nerve Conduction

Oh's Method

Oh et al. (99) described a technique for measuring motor nerve conduction in plantar nerves (Fig. 11.81).

RECORDING: For the medial plantar nerve, an active surface electrode is placed on the belly of the abductor hallucis and the reference electrode on its tendon. The distance between the recording electrode and the stimulating electrode is kept constant at 10 cm. For the lateral plantar nerve, an active surface electrode is placed on the belly of the ADQ muscle. The distance between the stimulating electrode and the recording electrode is kept constant at 12 cm.

STIMULATION: An active stimulating electrode is placed over the posterior tibial nerve above the flexor retinaculum at the ankle.

MEASUREMENT: Latency and amplitude measurements are conventional. The distance for the medial plantar nerve is measured by tape and that for the lateral plantar nerve by caliper.

TEMPERATURE: Skin temperature ranges from 29.5° to 33.5°C.

NORMAL DATA: Number of subjects: 20. Age range: 19–50 yr.

Measurement	Mean ± SD	Normal Limit
Medial plantar nerve		
Latency (msec)	4.10 ± 0.64	5.4
Amplitude (mV)	7.45	3.50
Latency plantar nerve		
Latency (msec)	4.70 ± 0.78	6.3
Amplitude (mV)	7.25	3.00

COMMENTS: To reduce the error associated with the distance, the distance is kept constant between the recording and stimulating electrodes.

Fu's Method

Fu et al. (100) described a method for measuring latencies of the medial and lateral plantar nerves (Fig. 11.82).

RECORDING: *Medial plantar nerve:* The active surface electrode is placed over the abductor hallucis muscle 1 cm behind and 1 cm below the navicular tubercle (medial side of foot).

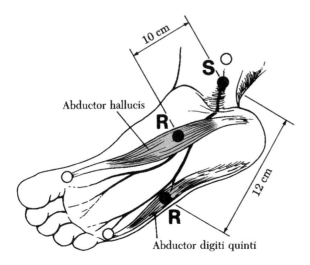

Figure 11.81.   Oh's method of motor nerve conduction of the plantar nerves.

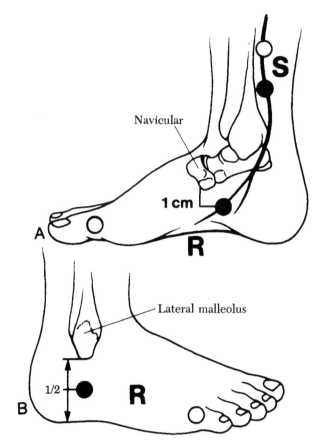

Figure 11.82.   Fu's method of motor nerve conduction of the plantar nerves.

Table 11.13.
Normal Data for the Plantar Nerve in 37 Subjects—Fu's Data (Ages 20–71)

Site	Electrode at 8 cm		Electrode at 10 cm	
	Mean ± SD	Normal Limit	Mean ± SD	Normal Limit
Flexible tape				
Medial plantar nerve	3.4 ± 0.5	4.4	3.8 ± 0.5	4.8
Lateral plantar nerve	3.6 ± 0.5	4.6	3.9 ± 0.5	4.9
Caliper				
Medial plantar nerve	3.6 ± 0.4	4.4	4.0 ± 0.4	4.8
Lateral plantar nerve	3.9 ± 0.6	5.1	4.3 ± 0.6	5.5

Lateral plantar nerve: The active surface electrode is placed over the ADQ muscle at half the distance from the sole of the foot to the tip of the lateral malleolus. The reference electrodes are placed over the big toe for the medial plantar nerve and on the little toe for the lateral plantar nerve.

STIMULATION: The active surface electrode is placed posterior to the medial malleolus and above the flexor retinaculum 8 or 10 cm proximal to the active recording electrode over the abductor hallucis muscle. The same site of stimulation is used for the lateral plantar nerve.

MEASUREMENT: The distance for the medial plantar nerve is measured with both calipers and flexible tape. When using flexible tape, the examiner must follow the anatomical course of the plantar nerve 1 cm posterior to the malleolus. The distance for the lateral plantar nerve is not measured. Latency is measured by the conventional method. Latencies are corrected to 28–32°C.

TEMPERATURE: Mean skin temperature below the median malleolus is 32.1° ± 1.4°C.
NORMAL DATA: See Table 11.13.

COMMENTS: Fu et al. (104) reported latencies corrected to 28–32°C. Unfortunately, the correction method used was not described.

Felsenthal's Method

Felsenthal et al. (101) described a technique of motor nerve conduction of the posterior tibial nerve across tarsal tunnel (Fig. 11.83).

RECORDING: For the lateral plantar nerve, an active surface electrode is placed over the ADQ muscle along the lateral aspect of the foot, midway between the head and the base of the 5th metatarsal bone. A reference electrode is placed distally on the little toe. For the medial plantar nerve, an active electrode is placed over the medial belly of the flexor hallucis brevis (FHB) muscle, which is located proximal and medial to the tendon of the flexor hallucis longus muscle and proximal to the base of the proximal phalanx of the big toe. The reference electrode is placed on the big toe.

STIMULATION: The distal tarsal tunnel stimulation point is localized just proximal to the navicula along the volar margin of the talus. An active electrode is initially placed in this position, and then its placement is adjusted until a supramaximal response is unequivocally obtained. Usually, the stimulation points for the lateral and medial plantar nerves are located within 1 cm of each other. From this distal stimulation point, and with the ankle in a neutral position (90°), a 10-cm straight-line distance is measured across the tarsal tunnel proximal to the medial malleolus and toward the Achilles tendon. At this 10-cm point, the proximal tarsal tunnel stimulation is performed.

MEASUREMENT: A peak-to-peak CMAP amplitude is measured. Latency and NCV are calculated by the conventional method.

TEMPERATURE: Room temperature is kept at about 26.7°C. Skin temperature is kept at 29.0–34.0°C.

NORMAL DATA: Number of subjects: 32. Age range: 20–45 yr.

Measurement	Medial Plantar Nerve		Lateral Plantar Nerve	
	Mean ± SD	Normal Limit	Mean ± SD	Normal Limit
Latency				
Distal (msec)	4.5 ± 0.7	5.9	4.5 ± 0.7	5.9
Proximal (msec)	6.9 ± 0.8	8.5	6.9 ± 0.7	8.3
Across tarsal tunnel (msec)	2.4 ± 0.4	3.2	2.4 ± 0.4	3.2
Side-to-side difference		0.9		0.9
Amplitude				
Distal (mV)	7.7 ± 3.6	1.7	12.0 ± 5.6	3.0
Proximal (mV)	6.9 ± 3.3	2.4	10.8 ± 5.3	3.0
Across tarsal tunnel (%)	10.3 ± 9.5	27.6	10.2 ± 8.5	26.5
NCV (m/sec)	49.4 ± 5.3	38.8	50.9 ± 5.2	40.7

INTERPRETATION: An amplitude decrement of more than 30% across the tarsal tunnel is considered abnormal. A side-to-side variation of more than 50% of the amplitude is unusual.

COMMENTS: Because straight-line measurement was used, the latency difference was recommended rather than the NCV because the "true length" of the nerve segment was not measured. In two cases of tarsal tunnel syndrome, this technique was able to confirm the diagnosis: in one case, by the prolonged latency and 75% decrease in amplitude across the tarsal tunnel in the medial plantar nerve; and in the other, by the prolonged latency in the medial and lateral plantar nerves and 33% decrease in the amplitude across the tarsal tunnel.

Sensory Nerve Conduction of the Medial Calcaneal Nerve

Del Toro et al. (102) described a technique of sensory nerve conduction of the medial calcaneal nerve (Fig. 11.84).

RECORDING: An active surface electrode is placed one-third of the distance from the

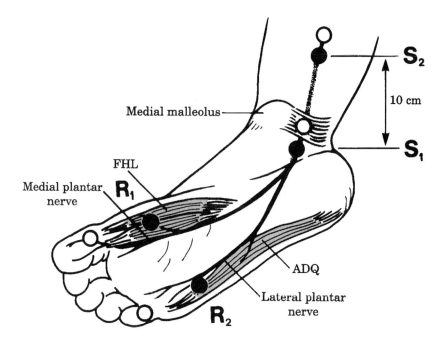

Figure 11.83.   Felsenthal's method of motor nerve conduction of the plantar nerve.

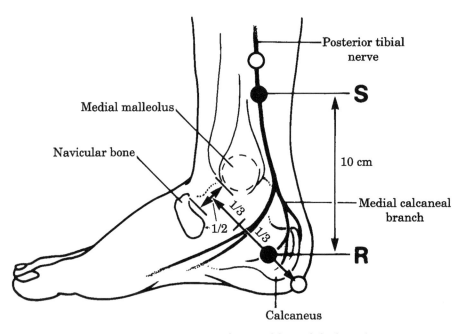

Figure 11.84.   Sensory nerve conduction of the medial calcaneal nerve.

apex of the heel to the midpoint between the navicula and tip of the medial malleolus. A reference surface electrode is placed at the apex of the heel.

STIMULATION: The posterior tibial nerve is stimulated 10 cm proximal to the active electrode.

MEASUREMENT: Latency to the onset and negative peak of the sensory CNAP is measured by the conventional method. Amplitude is measured from baseline to peak.

TEMPERATURE: Skin temperature is not controlled.

NORMAL DATA: Number of subjects: 20. Number of tests: 40. Age Range: Not given.

Measurement	Mean ± SD	Normal Limit
Onset latency (msec)	1.7 ± 0.3	2.3
Side-to-side difference	0.1	
Peak latency (msec)	2.5 ± 0.3	3.1
Side-to-side difference	0.1	
Amplitude (μV)	18 ± 13	8
Side-to-side difference	4	

Sensory Nerve Conduction of Plantar Nerves

Oh's Method

Oh et al. (99) described a technique for measuring sensory nerve conduction of the medial and lateral plantar nerves with surface recording electrode (Fig. 11.85).

RECORDING: An active surface electrode is placed above the flexor retinaculum and medial to the medial malleolus. The site of recording is predetermined during the motor nerve conduction study of the posterior tibial nerve. The 32–256 responses are averaged with a signal averager.

STIMULATION: A ring electrode is used on the great toe to stimulate the medial plantar nerve and on the little toe to stimulate the lateral plantar nerve. The stimulus intensity needed to obtain the maximal amplitude is three times the sensory threshold in the majority of cases.

MEASUREMENT: The distance between the stimulating electrode and the recording electrode is measured by tape for the medial plantar nerve and by caliper for the lateral plantar nerve. Latency is measured from the onset of the stimulus to the negative peak. Amplitude is measured by the conventional method.

TEMPERATURE: Skin temperatures on the plantar surface of the foot range from 29.5° to 33.5°C.

NORMAL DATA: Number of subjects: 20. Age range: 19–50 yr.

Measurement	Mean ± SD	Normal Limit
Medial plantar nerve		
NCV (m/sec)	35.2 ± 3.61	28.0
Amplitude (μV)	3.6	2.0
Lateral plantar nerve		
NCV (m/sec)	31.7 ± 4.9	22.9
Amplitude (μV)	1.9	1.0

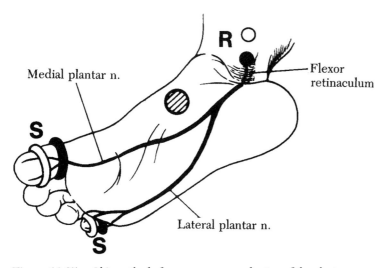

Figure 11.85. Oh's method of sensory nerve conduction of the plantar nerves.

COMMENT: The sensory nerve conduction test of the medial and lateral plantar nerves is essential for confirmation of the tarsal tunnel syndrome. Oh et al. (99) reported abnormal sensory nerve conduction in 90.5% of patients with tarsal tunnel syndrome.

In young normal individuals, the CNAP can be recognized without any averaging in some EMG machines. Because of the small amplitude of potentials, signal averaging is recommended. When no recognizable or constant potential is noted after 256 responses have been averaged, we confirm that there is "no nerve potential." We also always compare the CNAPs between the normal and abnormal sides. This measure ensures the reliability of sensory nerve conduction in plantar nerves.

Guiloff's Method

Guiloff and Sherratt (103) described an orthodromic method for measuring sensory nerve conduction over the medial plantar nerve. This method is similar to that of Oh et al. (Fig. 11.85), with only a few differences.

RECORDING: The recording electrodes are rectangular Ag/AgCl bars covered in saline-soaked gauze mounted 40 mm apart on Perspex. An active recording electrode is placed over a point at which the posterior tibial artery could be palpated, close to the medial malleolus of the ankle. The reference electrode usually rests on the medial edge of the Achilles tendon. Thirty or 32 responses are averaged with a signal averager.

STIMULATION: The medial plantar nerve is stimulated through two ring electrodes of Ag/AgCl covered in saline-soaked gauze, encircling the hallux, which is separated from the other toes by a strip of plastic sheet.

MEASUREMENT: The latency to onset and the negative peak are measured from the stimulus onset. The maximal NCV is calculated by dividing the distance by the latency to the onset of the potential. Amplitude is measured by the conventional method.

TEMPERATURE: Skin temperature on the medial plantar aspect of the foot is 27.0–33°C.

NORMAL DATA: Number of subjects: 69. Age range: 10 to over 70 yr.

Measurement	Mean ± SD	Normal Limit
NCV (m/sec)	35.6 ± 5.6	24.4
Onset latency (msec)	4.8 ± 0.7	6.2
Peak latency (msec)	5.7 ± 1.1	6.8
Amplitude (µV)	2.3 ± 1.4	1.0

COMMENT: The medial plantar sensory CNAP was absent in only three subjects–aged 81, 71, and 60 yr. The disadvantage of this technique is the special electrodes and rings, which should be covered with saline-soaked gauze. This elaborate preparation is unnecessary according to our experience.

Ponsford's Method

Ponsford (104) described an orthodromic method for measuring sensory nerve conduction in the medial and lateral plantar nerves (Fig. 11.86).

RECORDING: An active surface electrode is placed posterior to the medial malleolus, using the posterior tibial artery as a landmark. A reference electrode is placed 2 cm proximal to the active electrode.

STIMULATION: For the medial plantar nerve, an active surface electrode is placed on the sole just lateral to the first metatarsal on the common digital nerve subserving the web surface of toes 1 and 2. A reference electrode is on the metatarsophalangeal joint 2 cm distal to the active electrode. For the lateral plantar nerve, an active surface electrode is placed between the 4th and 5th metatarsals on the common digital nerve subserving the web surface of 4th and 5th toes. A reference electrode is placed on the metatarsophalangeal joint 2 cm distal to the active electrode. Four to 16 responses are averaged.

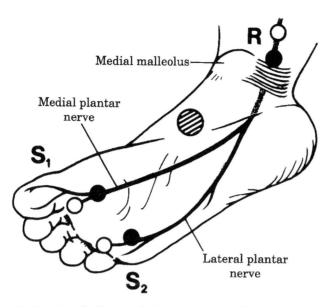

Figure 11.86. Ponsford's method of sensory nerve conduction of the plantar nerves.

Table 11.14.
Medial Plantar Sensory Nerve Conduction

Age (yr)	Onset Latency (msec)		Peak Latency (msec)		Amplitude (µV)		NCV (m/sec)	
	Mean	N Limit[a]	Mean	N Limit	Range	N Limit	Mean	N Limit
10–19 (N = 14)	2.7	3.4	3.3	3.9	10–26	10	49.4	39.9
20–29 (N = 13)	2.5	2.8	3.1	3.6	10–30	10	54.2	45.5
30–39 (N = 16)	2.5	3.0	3.2	3.9	7–20	7	54.1	45.9
40–49 (N = 18)	2.7	3.7	3.4	4.7	5–20	5	52.2	42.0
50–59 (N = 11)	2.9	4.3	3.6	5.4	3–15	3	52.3	45.4
60–69 (N = 11)	2.8	3.5	3.4	4.2	4–8	4	48.7	37.4
70–79 (N = 10)	3.3	5.4	4.2	7.0	2–5	2	49.4	22.3
≥80 (N = 7)	3.7	5.5	4.8	7.0	2–7	2	40.6	29.1
Total (N = 100)	2.9	3.9	3.6	4.9	2–30	2	50.1	38.5

[a]N limit, Normal limit. For the latencies, mean + 2 SD. For the amplitudes, the lower range. For the NCVs, mean - 2 SD.

MEASUREMENT: The latency to onset and the negative peak are measured from the stimulus onset. The maximal NCV is calculated by dividing the distance by the latency to the onset of the potential. Amplitude is measured by the conventional method. The method for distance measurement is not given.

TEMPERATURE: Skin temperature is controlled at 30–32°C at the medial malleolus and sole.

NORMAL DATA: See Tables 11.14 and 11.15.

COMMENTS: Medial plantar CNAPs were readily obtained in all normal subjects, including those aged over 80 yr. Lateral plantar CNAPs were obtained in all normal subjects below the age of 60 but were absent in the majority above this age. Compared with Oh and Guiloff's methods (99, 103), these authors claimed that the amplitude of CNAPs was larger. The amplitude of CNAPs decreased with age. There was no difference between NCVs with increasing age.

Mixed Nerve Conduction

Saeed and Gatens (105) described a technique for recording mixed nerve conduction in the medial and lateral plantar nerves (Fig. 11.87).

RECORDING: An active surface electrode is placed on the posterior tibial nerve just proximal to the flexor retinaculum.

Table 11.15.
Lateral Plantar Sensory Nerve Conduction

Age (yr)	Onset Latency (msec)		Peak Latency (msec)		Amplitude (μV)		NCV (m/sec)	
	Mean	N Limit[a]	Mean	N Limit	Range	N Limit	Mean	N Limit
10–19 (N = 14)	2.8	3.6	3.4	4.2	4–16	4	49.8	37.4
20–29 (N = 13)	2.5	2.7	3.2	3.7	5–12	5	53.9	46.3
30–39 (N = 16)	2.6	3.1	3.3	4.0	2–10	2	54.2	45.8
40–49 (N = 14)	2.7	3.6	3.5	4.6	3–6	3	51.6	39.4
50–59 (N = 10)	3.0	4.6	3.7	5.5	1–6	1	51.3	45.6
60–69 (N = 11)	3.1	4.6	3.7	5.3	0–4	0	47.3	31.7
70–79 (N = 10)	3.9	7.8	4.7	9.0	0–2	0	47.5	20.9
≥80 (N = 7)					0–1	0		
Total (N = 95)	2.9	4.2	3.6	5.2	0–16	0	50.8	38.1

[a]N limit, Normal limit. For the latencies, mean + 2 SD. For the amplitudes, the lower range. For the NCVs, mean - 2 SD.

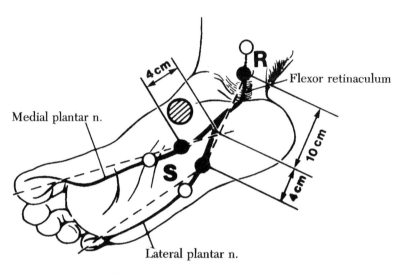

Figure 11.87.   Mixed nerve conduction of the plantar nerves.

STIMULATION: The medial plantar nerve is stimulated with an active electrode at a distance of 14 cm from the recording electrode. The lateral plantar nerve is stimulated with an active electrode 14 cm from the recording electrode.

MEASUREMENT: The latency is measured to the negative peak of the CNAP. The distance is measured with a flexible metal tape as demonstrated in Fig. 11.87.

TEMPERATURE: Skin temperature ranges from 26° to 32°C.

NORMAL DATA: Number of subjects: 4.1. Age range: 20–76 yr.

	Mean ± SD	Normal Limit
Medial plantar nerve		
Latency (msec)	3.16 ± 0.26	3.68
Amplitude (μV)	10–30 (range)	10
Lateral plantar nerve		
Latency (msec)	3.15 ± 0.25	3.65
Amplitude (μV)	8.20 (range)	8

COMMENTS: The most consistent and reproducible response (100% in normal subjects) is obtained at 14 cm. The authors did not use the signal averager and claim that this is an advantage over Oh et al.'s technique. They reported absent CNAPs in median and lateral plantar nerves in both feet in one patient with tarsal tunnel syndrome. According to our experience, the muscle response often obscures the CNAPs, making the recording difficult.

Interdigital Nerves of the Foot

Oh's Method

Oh et al. (99) described a technique for sensory nerve conduction in the interdigital nerves of the foot using the near-nerve needle and signal averaging techniques (Fig. 11.88). We use this technique for the workups of tarsal tunnel syndrome or interdigital neuropathy.

RECORDING: The active needle electrode is inserted close to the posterior tibial nerve in the ankle posterior to the medial malleolus above the flexor retinaculum. This site is chosen with the aid of a surface-stimulating electrode. The active electrode is inserted closer to the medial plantar fascicle in the posterior tibial nerve. The adequacy of the needle position is determined by stimulation of the nerve through the active electrode. When the great toe (1st digit) is contracting minimally with less than 5 mA for a stimulus of 0.05 msec duration, the needle is considered to be accurately positioned. A reference needle electrode is inserted subcutaneously at the same level as the active electrode at a transverse distance of 3–4 cm.

The 64–256 stimuli are averaged with a signal averager in each recording. To ensure reproducibility, three recordings are made for each CNAP. When no recognizable and constant potential is noted after 256 stimuli have been averaged in three recordings, it is determined that there is no nerve potential.

STIMULATION: The 1st and 5th digital nerves are stimulated with ring electrodes. The interdigital nerves are stimulated with interdigital stimulating surface electrodes that are especially designed to stimulate two branches of the interdigital nerve simultaneously (see Fig. 3.6). Each interdigital nerve is stimulated separately by placing the interdigital stimulating electrodes between the toes. The toes are then held tightly together by a rubber band or tape. The supramaximal stimulation intensity is usually at least three times the sensory threshold level and above 60 mA for a stimulus duration of 0.05 msec.

MEASUREMENT: Latency is measured from the stimulus onset to the first positive peak for the maximum NCV, to the highest negative peak for the negative peak NCV, and to the last negative peak of the potential for the minimum NCV. Distance is measured by caliper. The duration is measured from the onset of the first positive peak to the baseline return of the last component of the potential. Amplitude is measured by the conventional method.

TEMPERATURE: Skin temperature is controlled at 32°C.

NORMAL DATA: See Tables 11.16 and 11.17.

COMMENTS: Compared with the 20- to 49-year-old groups, in the 50- to 59-year-old

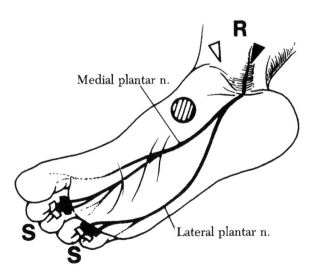

Figure 11.88. Oh's method of interdigital sensory nerve conduction of the foot.

Table 11.16.
Sensory NCVs in the Interdigital Nerves in Normal Subjects—Oh et al.'s Method[a]

	Ages 20–49 (N = 30)		Ages 50–59 (N = 10)		Ages 60–69 (N = 10)		Ages 70–79 (N = 8)	
	Mean	N Limit	Mean	N Limit	Mean	N Limit	Mean	N Limit
Maximum NCV (m/sec)								
I	40.5	35.1	37.8	32.8	36.1	29.7	33.5	24.1
I–II	38.4	32.5	35.7	28.5	33.8	27.6	32.7	22.7
II–III	36.3	30.0	33.3	25.9	31.5	25.5	30.0	22.0
III–IV	35.9	29.6	33.7	25.7	30.4	24.8	28.8	20.8
IV–V	37.2	31.8	34.8	24.1	32.0	25.2	28.7	20.4
V	38.4	30.4	34.8	24.6	31.6	26.4	30.0	23.4
Negative peak NCV (m/sec)								
I	34.8	30.3	32.1	27.0	31.3	25.6	28.7	21.3
I–II	33.0	28.2	30.3	23.5	29.7	22.1	28.3	19.9
II–III	31.1	26.2	28.9	26.1	26.8	22.0	24.7	17.3
III–IV	30.7	25.4	29.7	21.7	26.6	20.0	24.3	15.7
IV–V	32.2	25.7	30.5	22.4	26.8	21.8	25.3	19.1
V	32.3	25.9	29.9	21.6	26.9	19.5	25.5	18.8

[a]N Limit, normal limit (Mean - 2 SD).

Table 11.17.
Amplitude and Duration of Sensory CNAPs in the Interdigital Nerves in Normal Subjects—Oh et al.'s Method[a]

	Ages 20–49 (N = 30)		Ages 50–59 (N = 10)		Ages 60–69 (N = 10)		Ages 70–79 (N = 8)	
	Mean	N Limit	Mean	N Limit	Mean	N Limit	Mean	N Limit
Amplitude (μV)								
I	5.3	2.5	2.6	1.3	1.2	0.5	1.1	0.3
I–II	5.3	1.5	1.4	0.8	1.2	0.5	1.0	0.2
II–III	4.1	1.3	2.2	0.7	1.0	0.5	0.7	0.2
III–IV	3.7	1.3	1.7	0.7	1.1	0.4	0.8	0.3
IV–V	3.0	1.0	1.7	0.7	0.8	0.4	0.8	0.4
V	3.0	1.0	1.7	0.7	0.8	0.4	0.8	0.4
Duration (msec)								
I	3.6	5.2	5.2	9.2	6.7	11.5	5.5	8.3
I–II	4.0	6.2	4.8	7.8	7.2	10.4	6.1	9.5
II–III	4.4	6.8	5.5	9.3	8.0	12.0	5.9	9.3
III–IV	4.0	6.2	5.0	8.6	7.2	9.6	6.4	10.2
IV–V	4.0	6.4	5.4	7.2	5.8	9.2	5.5	8.5
V	3.3	5.5	5.6	10.6	6.9	11.7	6.0	9.0

[a]N Limit: Normal limit for the amplitude, the lowest range. Normal limit for the duration, mean + 2 SD.

group there is a significant decrease in the maximum, negative peak, and minimum NCVs, a significant prolongation in the duration, and a significant decrease in the amplitude of sensory CNAPs. In five cases of interdigital neuropathy, the most prominent abnormality was "dip phenomenon," a selective decrease in the amplitude of the CNAP in the involved interdigital nerve compared with neighboring nerves (106). This technique is able to confirm the diagnosis of tarsal tunnel syndrome in 24 (96%) of 25 cases (107).

Falck's Method

Falck et al. (108) described a technique for sensory nerve conduction in the interdigital plantar nerves of the foot (Fig. 11.89).

RECORDING: The active needle electrode is placed close to the posterior tibial nerve behind and usually somewhat below the medial malleolus. The reference needle electrode is placed subcutaneously 1–2 cm above the recording electrode. The exact location of the recording electrode is found by stimulating the nerve through these electrodes while the CMAP of the ADQ is recorded with a surface electrode. When a

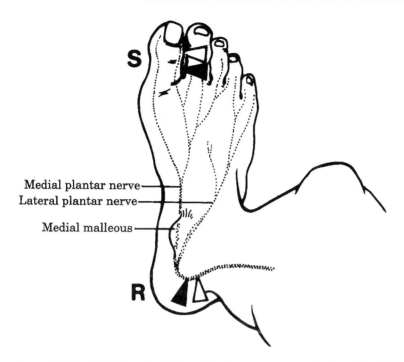

Figure 11.89.   Falck's method of interdigital sensory nerve conduction of the foot.

Table 11.18.
Interdigital Nerve Conduction Study of the Feet

Measurement	Ages (20–34) (N = 12)		Ages (35–49) (N = 8)		Ages (50–65) (N = 8)	
	Mean ± SD	Normal Limit[a]	Mean ± SD	Normal Limit	Mean ± SD	Normal Limit
I–II IDN (m/sec)	40.9 ± 2.8	33.9	38.3 ± 2.8	31.3	33.1 ± 3.0	25.6
II–III IDN (m/sec)	39.9 ± 3.0	32.4	39.7 ± 2.8	32.7	32.8 ± 2.7	26.1
III–IV IDN (m/sec)	41.0 ± 2.7	34.3	38.5 ± 2.0	33.5	32.2 ± 3.5	23.5
IV–V IDN (m/sec)	41.5 ± 3.2	33.5	38.5 ± 2.2	33.0	32.2 ± 3.5	23.5
Difference (m/sec)[b]	2.8 ± 1.2	5.8	2.8 ± 1.4	5.6	3.1 ± 1.2	6.1
Amplitude (μV)[c]	2.9 ± 1.2		2.8 ± 1.4		2.0 ± 0.7	

[a]Normal limit, mean ± 2.5 SD.
[b]Difference between the fastest and slowest NCVs in the interdigital nerves in each subject.
[c]Mean amplitude of CNAPs.

maximal response is recorded from the muscle with a stimulus current of 1.0 mA (duration 0.2 msec) or less, the location of the electrode is accepted.

STIMULATION: An active needle electrode is inserted on the medial side of the proximal phalanx of the toe. The needle electrode is advanced until the tip is felt through the skin on the plantar side. The reference needle electrode is placed about 1 cm distally on the same side of the toe. The stimulus current is 3–4 mA for 0.2 msec duration. When an active electrode is properly placed close to the interdigital nerve, the subject feels a sharp pain radiating toward the tip of the toe with each stimulation. Usually 128 or 256 responses are averaged.

MEASUREMENT: The latency is measured to the onset of the CNAP. There is no specific mention of distance measurement. Amplitude is measured by the conventional method. The difference between the fastest and slowest NCVs in the interdigital nerves of each subject is calculated.

TEMPERATURE: Skin temperature on the sole of the foot is controlled at 28–30°C.

NORMAL DATA: Number of subjects: 28. Age range: 20–64 yr. See Table 11.18.

INTERPRETATION; When the NCV is more than 2.5 SD from the normal mean or 5.4 m/sec slower than the other plantar interdigital nerves in that patient, it is considered abnormal.

COMMENTS: In normal subjects, there was no significant difference between the NCVs in the four different interdigital nerves. In older subjects, the NCVs were significantly slower, and the amplitudes smaller. The CNAP was not always triphasic in shape, but in slightly more than one-third of the nerves, a polyphasic response was seen. In the diagnosis of Morton's neuroma, authors suggested comparing the NCVs of the four interdigital nerves with each other, rather than comparing individual interdigital nerves with the normal mean. In this way the variance caused by age and temperature is minimized. A polyneuropathy might give rise to a slowing of the sensory NCV in all four nerves. In patients with Morton's neuroma, the NCV of the affected nerve was abnormally slow in six cases. This is in contrast to Oh et al. (106), who found that the amplitude is selectively decreased in the affected nerve ("dip phenomenon") in Morton's neuroma. This difference is due to the fact that Oh et al. used an interdigital surface electrode as a stimulating electrode.

Sural Nerve

Sural Sensory Nerve Conduction with Needle Electrodes

Behse and Buchthal (94) described a technique for measuring sural nerve conduction with a needle electrode (Fig. 11.90).

RECORDING: The near-nerve electrode is inserted behind the lateral malleolus, 15 cm proximal to the lateral malleolus and lateral to the Achilles tendon, and 4–5 cm proximal to the skin fold in the middle of the popliteal fossa.

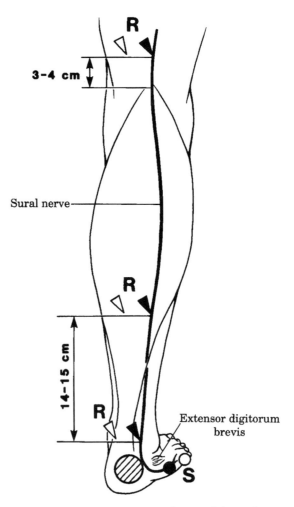

Figure 11.90. Sensory nerve conduction of the sural nerve.

STIMULATION: An active stimulating surface electrode is placed on the dorsal aspect of the foot at least 2 cm distal to the border of the extensor digitorum brevis muscle. The response is maximal with a stimulus of 10–20 mA; a stimulus of more than 20 mA activates the intrinsic muscles of the foot, and their CMAPs interfere with the sensory potential. The nerve can also be stimulated at the lateral malleolus level.

MEASUREMENT: Amplitude is measured by the conventional method. The latency is measured from the stimulus onset to the positive peak of the CNAP. The NCV is calculated by the conventional method for the near-nerve needle technique.

TEMPERATURE: Skin temperature is controlled at 36–37°C.

NORMAL DATA: See Tables 7.35 and 7.36.

INTERPRETATION: Any value outside of the 95% lower limits of the NCV is considered abnormal.

Pudendal Nerve

Internal Pudendal Motor Nerve Conduction

Chantraine's Method

Chantraine et al. (109) described a method of measuring motor nerve conduction in the internal pudendal nerve (Fig. 11.91A and B).

POSITION OF SUBJECT: The subject is placed in a ventral decubitus position.

RECORDING: The concentric needle is inserted into the urethral and anal sphincters.

STIMULATION: Monopolar 70 mm long Teflon-coated needles (except at the tip) are used for stimulation. For the proximal stimulation site (A), a line is drawn joining the posterior superior iliac spine and the upper border of the greater trochanter. A second line, parallel to the first, is drawn 4 cm below it. A point on this second line, 8 cm lateral to the natal cleft, is the surface landmark of the internal pudendal artery and nerve, which is next to it. Two needle electrodes are inserted vertically down to the sciatic

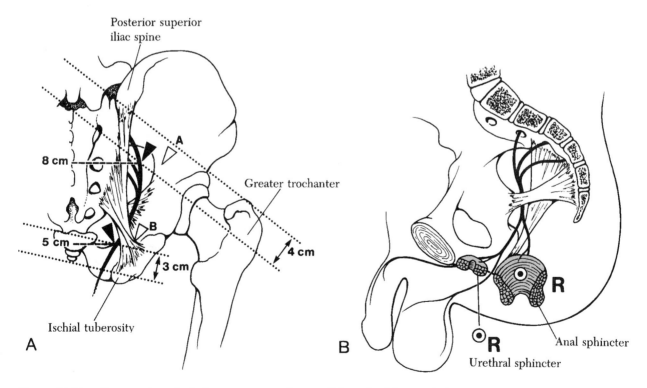

Figure 11.91. Chantraine's method of motor nerve conduction of the pudendal nerve. **A**, Anatomical course of the internal pudendal nerve and landmarks for the stimulating sites. **B**, Recording muscles.

spine, where they lie next to the nerve (A). For the distal stimulation (B) site, a line is drawn from the ischial tuberosity to the point of the coccyx. Then a second line is drawn parallel to but 3 cm above this line. The pudendal nerve in the lesser sciatic notch (B) lies 5 cm from the midline on this second line. The needle electrodes are inserted vertically at this point (B).

MEASUREMENT: Distance and latency are measured by conventional methods. The distance between the two landmarks (A) and (B) ranged from 5.5 to 7.8 cm.

TEMPERATURE: Skin temperature is not controlled.

NORMAL DATA: Number of subjects: 10. Age range: 20–83 yr.

Measurement	Mean ± SD	Normal Limit
Proximal latency (msec)		
Urethral branch	5.1 ± 0.2	5.4
Anal branch	5.5 ± 0.3	6.1
Mean NCV (m/sec)		
Urethral branch	56.8 ± 3.9	49.0
Anal branch	56.3 ± 2.8	50.7

INTERPRETATION: Motor NCV in the pudendal nerve is of the same order of magnitude as the NCV in the limb nerves. The mean values for proximal latencies and NCV are consistently equal for left and right sides. According to Chantraine et al. (109), motor nerve conduction is slowed or sometimes even blocked in patients with a lesion of the nerve trunk; measurement of the pudendal NCV is particularly useful in traumatic disorders of the spinal cord for confirming or denying the presence of a coexistent nerve trunk lesion.

COMMENTS: Chantraine et al. stated that this is a painful test. Nonetheless, they recommend it for all neurological syndromes. Measurement of the latency from the proximal stimulating point has been valuable in itself, whereas the latency from the distal stimulation point is difficult to measure. The correct localization of landmarks for insertion of the stimulating electrodes is important, according to Chantraine et al. (109).

Kiff's Method

Kiff and Swash (110) described a technique of motor conduction in the pudendal nerve (Fig. 11.92).

POSITION OF PATIENT: The patient lies on his left side and a ground electrode is placed on the right upper thigh.

RECORDING AND STIMULATION: An intrarectal digitally-directed technique is used to stimulate the pudendal nerve at the level of the ischial spine, using stimulating and recording electrodes mounted on a glove (St. Mark's pudendal electrodes: Dantec 13L40). The device, mounted on the index finger, is inserted into the rectum and the ischial spine palpated. Stimuli of 0.1 msec duration and 30 V are given at 1-sec intervals. The tip of the device is slowly moved until the sphincter is felt to contract firmly around the base of the finger and the CMAP amplitude is maximally achieved. A supramaximal stimulus, usually 50 V, is then given and two consecutive series of five recordings are made. The procedure is repeated on the opposite side of the pelvis. The CMAP is obtained from the external anal sphincter.

MEASUREMENT: Latency is measured by the conventional method. Latency is calculated from the shortest of five latencies measured on each side. The mean value from each side is used as the final value.

TEMPERATURE: Skin temperature is not controlled.

NORMAL DATA: Number of subjects: 28. Age range: not given.

Measurement	Mean ± SD	Normal Limit	Normal Range
Latency (msec) Right	2.0 ± 0.3	2.6	1.5–2.6
Left	1.9 ± 0.3	2.5	1.5–2.6

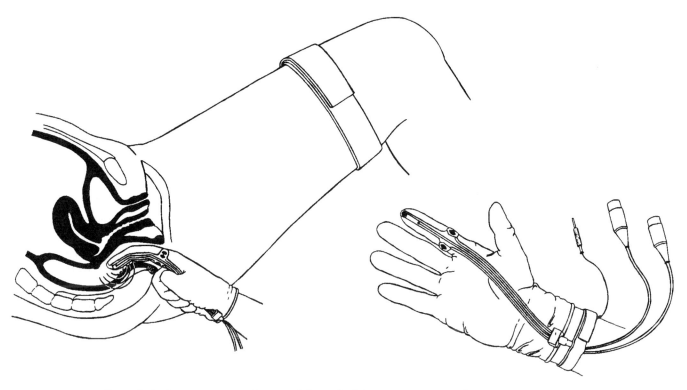

Figure 11.92. Kiff's method of motor nerve conduction of the pudendal nerve using St. Mark's pudendal electrodes. (From: Fowler CJ. Pelvic floor neurophysiology. In: Methods in clinical neurophysiology, No. 1. 1991:19.)

Motor Conduction of the Perineal Nerve

Snooks and Swash (111) described a technique for motor nerve conduction of the perineal nerve.

RECORDING: The CMAP is recorded from the periurethral striated sphincter muscle using an intraurethral electrode (Disa 21L11) mounted on a 14-gauge Foley catheter placed in the urethra by using a sterile, no-touch technique. The intraurethral electrode has two platinum recording surfaces of 5 mm diameter.

STIMULATION: The stimulating technique is the same as for the pudendal nerve (Fig. 11.92).

MEASUREMENT: Same as for the pudendal nerve.

TEMPERATURE: Skin temperature is not controlled.

NORMAL DATA: Number of subjects: 20. Age range: not given.

Measurement	Mean ± SD	Normal Limit
Latency (msec)	2.4 ± 0.2	2.8

Sensory Nerve Conduction of the Dorsal Nerve of the Penis

Bradley's Method

Bradley et al. (112) described the technique of sensory nerve conduction of the dorsal nerve of the penis at rest and with stretching.

POSITION OF SUBJECT: The subject is in a supine position with the penis in an unstretched, flaccid state. The penis is stretched with 1-lb weight applied through a penile clamp to the glans and attached to a traction apparatus.

EMG MACHINE SET-UP: Filter: 1–1.5 KHz. Averaging: 10–50 times.

RECORDING: The recording electrodes are placed on the dorsum of the penile shaft at its base approximately 2 cm apart with an active electrode distally. A wraparound lead plate is placed between the stimulating and recording electrodes in the shaft.

STIMULATION: The stimulating electrodes are placed on the dorsum of the glans penis with an active electrode proximally.

MEASUREMENT: Latency is measured to the peak of the negative deflection, and the amplitude is measured from peak to peak.

TEMPERATURE: Not controlled.

NORMAL DATA: Number of subjects: 27. Age range: 32–63 yr.

Measurement	Mean ± SD	Normal Limit
NCV (m/sec)		
At rest	27.4 ± 3.2	21.0
Stretched	33.0 ± 3.8	25.4
Amplitude (μV)	12.0 ± 6.1	1.9[a]

[a]Low normal range.

COMMENTS: For obvious reasons, the NCV increases with penile elongation. Lin and Bradley's study showed that with a 1-lb weight the dorsal nerve of the penis is stretched optimally and its NCV reaches maximal value. In 20 diabetic patients with erectile impotence, the mean NCV of the dorsal nerve of the penis was significantly slower than the normal mean, whereas the pudendal SEP and bulbocavernosus reflex were normal (113). The NCV was slow in 10 patients, whereas the pudendal SEP was prolonged in eight and the bulbocavernosus reflex in two patients, demonstrating the potential usefulness of this test in the detection of penile neuropathy. Kaneko and Bradley also compared the NCV of this nerve between 28 impotent diabetics and 29 impotent nondiabetics and found that the NCV was significantly slower in the impotent diabetics (114).

Clawson's Method

Clawson and Cardenas (115) described a technique of sensory nerve conduction of the dorsal nerve of the penis (Fig. 11.93). We use this technique with the penis stretched on an intravein injection board.

POSITION OF SUBJECT: The subject's penis is placed in the concavity of a specially designed orthoplast penile traction device (Fig. 11.94), and the penis is stretched to its full length by gripping the tip of the glans. A firm endpoint can be felt when the penis at its full length. The Cunningham incontinence clamp is placed across the glans and a splint to hold the penis at its stretched length. Care is taken to hold the penis at its full length when clamping.

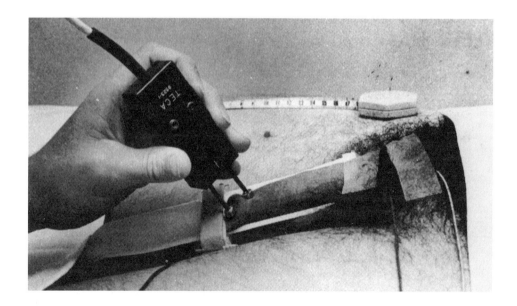

Figure 11.93. Sensory nerve conduction of the dorsal nerve of the penis. Demonstration of electrode placement, stimulation site, and the traction device. (From Clawson DR, Cardenas DD. Dorsal nerve of the penis nerve conduction velocity: a new technique. Muscle Nerve 1991;14:846.)

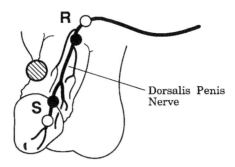

Figure 11.94. Clawson and Cardenas's technique of nerve conduction of the dorsal nerve of the penis.

EMG MACHINE SET-UP: Filter: 30 Hz–2 KHz.

RECORDING: Cupped 1-cm steel electrodes applied with EEG cream are used for the active and reference recording electrodes. An active recording electrode is placed as proximal as possible at the base of the penis, just distal to the symphysis pubis under which the dorsal nerve of the penis runs. A reference electrode is placed 4 cm superior to the active electrode above the symphysis pubis.

STIMULATION: The penis is stimulated orthodromically with an active stimulating electrode just proximal to the dorsal glans, and the reference electrode to the dorsal glans.

MEASUREMENT: Latency is measured to the initial negative peak. The distance is measured following the conventional method.

TEMPERATURE: Skin temperature is above 30°C.

NORMAL DATA: Number of subjects: 20. Age range: 27–58 yr.

Measurement	Mean ± SD	Normal Limit
Latency (msec)	2.3 ± 0.4	3.1
NCV (m/sec)	36.2 ± 3.2	29.8
Amplitude (μV)	2.3 ± 1.1	
Distance (cm)	8.6 ± 1.5[a]	

[a]Normal range: at distance 5.4–11.5 cm.

COMMENTS: No averaging was necessary in the testing of normal subjects. The error in the calculated NCV when the penis was out of traction, versus at its full length, was 44%. Authors stated that this technique is simple and prevents redundancy of the dorsal nerve of the penis. The orthoplast penile traction device can be easily constructed and is inexpensive.

F-Wave

F-Wave Velocity, F-Wave Conduction Time, and F-Wave Ratio

Kimura (116, 117) conducted an F-wave study. The terms he used are defined as follows (Fig. 11.95):

$$\text{F-wave conduction time} = \frac{\text{F-wave latency (msec)} - \text{M-wave latency (msec)} - 1\ \text{msec}}{2}$$

$$\text{F-wave ratio} = \frac{\text{F-wave conduction time (msec)}}{\text{M-wave latency (msec)}}$$

$$\text{F-wave velocity (m/sec)} = \frac{\text{Distance from stimulus point to spinous process (mm)} \times 2}{\text{F wave latency (msec)} - \text{M-wave latency (msec)} - 1\ \text{msec}}$$

RECORDING: An active recording electrode is placed on the conventional sites (see Chapter 5). The collision technique is used at the axilla to obtain the F-wave.

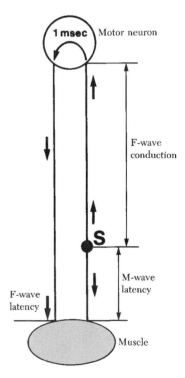

Figure 11.95. Relationship between F-wave latency, M-wave latency, and F-wave conduction time.

STIMULATION: The motor nerve is stimulated at various sites along the nerve, using conventional methods (see Chapter 5).

MEASUREMENT: Latency is measured from the stimulus onset to the initial deflection of the F-wave. The shortest latency among 10 responses is chosen as the latency. The distance is measured as follows:

Upper extremity: The approximate length of the nerve from the stimulus points to the spinal cord is obtained by measuring the distance from the C7 spinous process. Surface tape measurements are taken along the course of the nerve from the wrist to the axilla with the subject in an upright position and the arm abducted to 90°. The hand is supinated for the measurement of the median nerve and pronated for the ulnar nerve. Stimulus points at the axilla are projected posteriorly across the arm in the plane perpendicular to the axis of the arm, and distances between the projected points and the C7 spinous process are determined by tape.

Lower extremity: The approximate length of the nerve from the stimulus point to the spinal cord is obtained by determining the surface distance from the stimulus site to the lower border of the T12 spinous process by way of the greater trochanter of the femur.

TEMPERATURE: Skin temperature is not controlled.

NORMAL DATA: See Table 11.19.

INTERPRETATION: F-wave conduction time is the motor conduction time from the cord to the stimulus site. Thus, the F wave conduction time reflects the motor conduction of the proximal portion of the nerve more accurately than the F-wave latency. The F-wave latency is contaminated by the M-wave latency, the conduction time from the stimulus site to the muscle. Theoretically, the F-wave conduction time is also related to height or leg length. This has not been considered in the interpretation of values. A prolonged F-wave conduction time indicates slower conduction in the segment proximal to the stimulation.

The F-wave ratio is the ratio between the motor conduction time from the cord to the stimulus site (the F-wave conduction time) and that of the remaining nerve segment to the muscle (M-wave latency). Unlike the F-wave conduction velocity, the F-ratio is entirely independent of the total length of the nerve but is based on the assumption that the proportion between the proximal and distal segments is the same among different subjects. If the F-wave ratio is within normal limits, it indicates a more or less equal slowing of nerve conduction between proximal and distal segments. In contrast, if the F-wave ratio is significantly reduced, it indicates that conduction abnormalities are more prominent distally. If conduction abnormalities are more prominent proximally, the F-ratio is increased.

Table 11.19.
Normal Data for the F-wave in 66 Subjects—Kimura's Method[a]

Site	F-wave Latency (msec)		F-ratio (Mean ± SD)	F-wave NCV (m/sec)	
	Mean ± SD	Normal Limit		Mean ± SD	Normal Limit
Median nerve					
Wrist	29.1 ± 2.3	33.4	3.64 ± 0.45	59.2 ± 3.9	67.0
Elbow	24.8 ± 2.0	28.8	1.04 ± 0.09	62.2 ± 5.2	72.6
Axilla	21.7 ± 2.8	27.3	0.40 ± 0.07	64.3 ± 6.4	77.1
Ulnar nerve					
Wrist	30.5 ± 3.0	36.5	4.65 ± 0.75	56.7 ± 2.9	62.5
Below elbow	26.0 ± 2.0	30.0	1.40 ± 0.11	58.2 ± 2.9	64.0
Above elbow	23.5 ± 2.0	27.5	0.72 ± 0.07	61.1 ± 5.4	71.9
Axilla	21.9 ± 1.9	25.7	0.43 ± 0.06	63.0 ± 5.9	64.8
Peroneal nerve					
Ankle	51.3 ± 4.7	60.7	5.17 ± 0.91	53.3 ± 3.7	60.7
Knee	42.7 ± 4.0	50.7	1.11 ± 0.09	56.3 ± 4.9	66.1
Posterior tibial nerve					
Ankle	52.3 ± 4.3	60.9	5.91 ± 0.90	51.3 ± 2.9	67.1
Knee	43.5 ± 3.4	50.3	1.17 ± 0.10	54.4 ± 3.6	68.8

[a]See Kimura (116, 119).

There is a controversy about the F-wave conduction velocity. Young and Shahani (118) claim that there is no need to introduce additional factors for errors in the F-wave conduction, and that the latency reflects a more accurate measurement than the F-wave conduction velocity. They claim that the calculation of F-wave conduction velocity introduces two additional sources of error: (*a*) distance measurement and (*b*) "turn-around time." The error involved with distance measurement is discussed thoroughly in Chapter 12. Kimura (119) and Panaylotopoulos (120) assume that 1 msec is needed for turnaround time in each motor neuron. This assumption is based on animal data indicating that this time is very close to 1.0 msec and the absolute refractory period of the fastest human motor fibers, which is also about 1.0 msec or slightly less. Readers should be aware of this controversy.

F-Wave and Collision Technique

Kimura (116) used the collision technique to obtain the F-wave proximally at the axilla. Normally, with supramaximal stimulation at the wrist and elbow, the F-waves are distinct from the M-wave. However, when the nerve is stimulated at the axilla, the F-wave is not clearly separated from the M-wave because the latency difference between the M-wave and the F-wave is small. To avoid this difficulty, he used the collision technique, delivering a second stimulation at the wrist, which blocks the M-wave elicited by axillary stimulation. With this technique, the orthodromic impulse from the axilla and the antidromic impulse from the wrist can be extinguished by collision, leaving the M-wave from the wrist and the F-wave from the axilla intact. Because these two remaining muscle responses are clearly separate, the F-wave elicited by axillary stimulation can be detected and its latency easily measured.

Details of the Technique

This technique requires two stimulators in the EMG machine (Fig. 11.96). Therefore, many small EMG machines equipped with a single stimulator cannot perform this test.

RECORDING: An active surface electrode is placed on the thenar muscle for the median nerve and on the hypothenar muscle for the ulnar nerve study.

STIMULATION: The first stimulating electrode (S_1) is placed at the wrist and the second stimulating electrode (S_2) at the axilla. Both sites are stimulated simultaneously. At times, detection of the F-wave is easier if the stimulation at the axilla is delivered a few milliseconds after, rather than simultaneously with, the wrist stimulation.

COMMENTS: It is essential to use supramaximal stimulation at the wrist to achieve a complete antidromic block of the M-wave. When wrist stimulation is less than adequate, a small, partially blocked M-wave remains and is confusing because of its great resemblance to an F-wave in shape and latency. Application of the collision technique to the ulnar nerve is simple. The F-wave elicited by axillary stimulation is recorded in all controls. On the other hand, for the median nerve careful placement of the stimulating electrodes and careful adjustment of the stimulus intensity are needed to achieve satisfactory recordings of the F-wave at the axilla because the stimulation tends to activate the adjacent ulnar nerve simultaneously. Kimura was able to record the F-wave in 21 of the 26 subjects (116).

F-Wave on the Soleus Muscle

Fisher et al. (121) described the technique for measuring the F-wave latency on the soleus muscle. The recording and stimulating sites and leg length measurement are identical to those in Branddom and Johnson's method (122) (see Chapter 17).

RECORDING: An active surface electrode is placed on the medial aspect of the soleus muscle at a point one-half the distance between the stimulating site and the most proximal part of the medial malleolus. A reference electrode is placed 5 cm distally from an active electrode on the muscle belly.

STIMULATION: The posterior tibial nerve is stimulated with a surface electrode in the popliteal fossa.

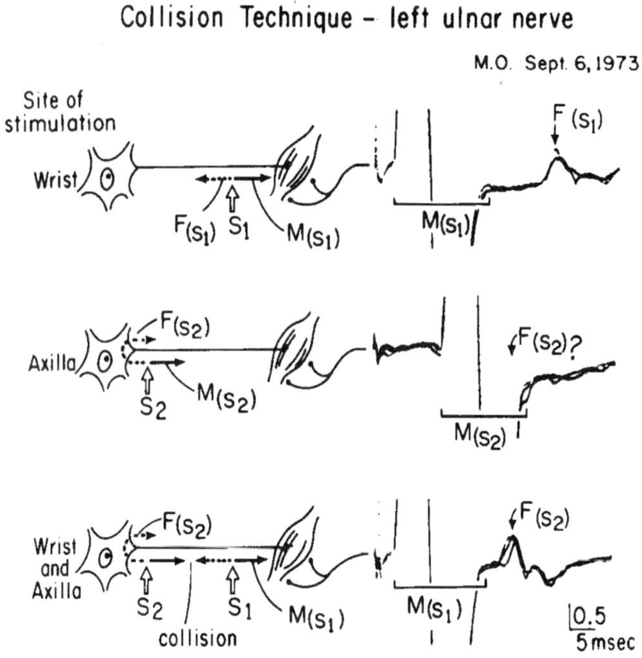

Figure 11.96. Collison technique in the ulnar nerve. A normal M-response *(horizontal brackets)* and F-wave *(small arrows)* are recorded from the abductor digiti quinti through surface electrodes. *Top to bottom:* supramaximal stimulus to the ulnar nerve at the wrist (S_1), at the axilla (S_2), and simultaneous paired stimuli at the wrist and axilla (S_1 and S_2). Three consecutive traces are superimposed for each tracing. The M-wave and F-wave elicited by wrist stimulation were widely separate. With stimulation at the axilla, however, only the M-wave was recorded and the F-wave was apparently absent because the latter occurred before the completion of the former. With paired stimuli, the orthodromic impulse from the axilla and the antidromic impulse from the wrist were extinguished by collision, leaving intact the M-wave ($M_{(S_1)}$) from the wrist and the F-wave ($F_{(S_2)}$) from the axilla. The figures on the left are diagrams showing the orthodromic *(solid arrows)* and antidromic *(dotted arrows)* impulses carrying the M-wave and the F-wave, respectively. In the bottom figure, note the collison between $F_{(S_2)}$ and $M_{(S_2)}$, leaving $M_{(S_1)}$ and $F_{(S_2)}$ intact. (From Kimura J. F-wave velocity in the central segment of the median and ulnar nerves. Neurology 1974;24:541.)

MEASUREMENT: Latency is measured from the onset of the stimulus to the shortest initial deflection of 10 responses. Leg length is measured from the site of stimulation of posterior tibial nerve at the midpopliteal crease to a point over the distal posterior tibial nerve at the most proximal part of the medial malleolus.

TEMPERATURE: Skin temperature is not controlled.

NORMAL DATA: Number of subjects: 19. Age range: 22–58 yr. The linear regression curve and 95% confidence limits comparing F-wave latency and leg length are shown in Fig. 11.97.

INTERPRETATION: The linear regression curve can be used for evaluating absolute prolongation of F-wave latency. An average F-wave latency difference greater than 2 msec between two sides is considered abnormal.

COMMENTS: This technique is unique in that leg length is measured instead of height. Fisher et al. (121) stated that the F-wave from the soleus muscle is helpful in evaluating an S1 injury, and that the F-wave abnormality was the only abnormality in 15% of 41 patients with electrophysiological abnormalities. Using peroneal and posterior tibial F-wave latency in patients with clinically proved lumbosacral radiculopathy, we found that the F-wave latency is not helpful.

F-Wave in the Ulnar Nerve

Weber and Piero (123) developed a formula for calculating F-wave latency in the ulnar nerve (Fig. 11.98).

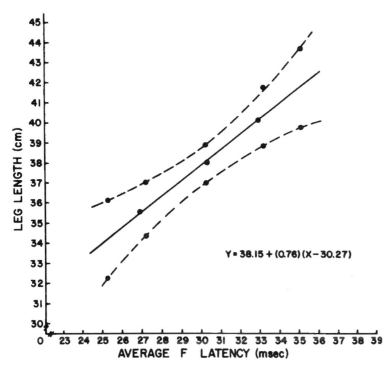

Figure 11.97. Linear regression curve and 95% confidence limits comparing F-wave latency and leg length. (From Fisher MA, Shivde AJ, Terixera C, Grainer LS. The F-response: a clinically useful physiological parameter for the evaluation of radicular injury. EMG Clin Neurophysiol 1979;19:66.)

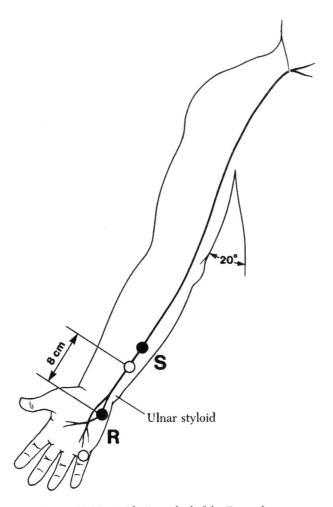

Figure 11.98. Weber's method of the F-wave latency.

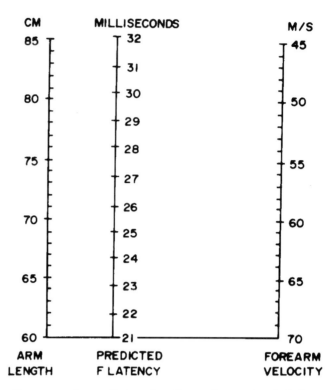

Figure 11.99. Normagram for predicting ulnar F-wave latency. To find the predicted F-wave latency, connect the patient's values for arm length and forearm velocity with a straight line. A value of 2.5 msec (mean + 2 SD) greater than the predicted value is abnormal (m/s = meters/second). (From Weber RJ, Piero DL. F-wave evaluation of thoracic outlet syndrome: a multiple regression derived F-wave latency predicting technique. Arch Phys Med Rehabil 1978;59:467.)

RECORDING AND STIMULATION: The recording and stimulation surface electrodes are positioned just as for the ulnar motor conduction study except that the active stimulation electrode is located proximal to the reference electrode and the reference electrode is 8 cm from the recording electrode.

MEASUREMENT: At least 20 responses are recorded. The shortest latency is measured. "Arm length" is the distance (in centimeters) from the C7 spinous process (vertebra prominens) to the tip of the ulnar styloid process, with the arm abducted at 20° in the coronal plane of the body, the elbow straight, and the palm forward.

TEMPERATURE: Skin temperature is not controlled.

NORMAL DATA: The predicted normal F-wave latency can be calculated in two ways: (*a*) by using the formula:

$$\text{Predicted F-wave latency} = [\text{arm length (cm)} \times 0.30] - [\text{ulnar nerve forearm velocity (m/sec)} \times 0.123] + 11.05$$

and (*b*) by using the normagram in Fig. 11.99.

INTERPRETATION: The mean + 2 SD; the maximum acceptable prolongation above the predicted value is 2.5 msec.

COMMENTS: Weber and Piero (123) stated that with this technique some patients with clinically diagnosed thoracic outlet syndrome had prolonged F-wave latency. However, they did not state how often this abnormality is observed. To make the diagnosis of thoracic outlet syndrome by the F-wave latency, one has to rule out the other common distal ulnar entrapment neuropathy.

F-Wave Latency in the Facial Nerve

Ahiron and Sarova-Pinhas (124) reported the normal value of the F-wave latency and conduction time in the facial nerve.

RECORDING: Active and reference recording surface electrodes are placed on the orbicularis oculi and orbicularis oris muscles following the conventional method.

STIMULATION: The facial nerve is stimulated at the stylomastoid foramen with supramaximal stimulation of 0.2 msec duration following the conventional method. An active electrode is placed proximally.

MEASUREMENT: Latency is measured to the shortest initial deflection of the F-wave following the conventional method. F-wave conduction time is calculated following Kimura's method.

TEMPERATURE: Skin temperature is not controlled.

NORMAL DATA:[a] Number of subjects: 30. Age range: 18–64 yr.

Measurement	Mean ± SD	Normal Limit
F-latency (msec)	9.6 ± 2.4	14.4
F-conduction time (msec)	2.9 ± 1.1	5.1

[a]Since the authors did not mention whether this represents normal data for the orbicularis oculi or oris muscle, these data must be applied to both muscles.

COMMENTS: Among 33 patients with Bell's palsy, 16 patients showed an F-wave latency beyond the 99% confidence line. Six of these 16 patients also had a prolonged M-latency (124).

Minimal Motor Conduction Velocity

Thomas et al. (125) and Hopf (126) described techniques for measuring the NCV of slower motor fibers. Both used the collision technique, which requires an EMG machine with two stimulators. The collision technique is based on two principles: (*a*) when a nerve fiber is stimulated, the nerve excitation travels orthodromically as well as antidromically; and (*b*) when the proximal and distal nerve action potentials meet between two points of stimulation, they cancel each other out.

Thomas's Method

RECORDING: The conventional method is used for the motor nerve conduction (Figs. 11.100 and 11.101) (125).

STIMULATION: The first stimulation electrodes (S_1) are placed at the distal site of stimulation (ankle for the peroneal nerve). The second stimulation electrodes (S_2) are placed at the proximal site (fibular head for the peroneal nerve). To determine the range of motor NCVs, the test is performed as follows:

1. Determine the maximal motor NCV by conventional methods. The conduction time between S_1 and S_2 and the supramaximal intensity of S_2 are then already available;

2. S_2 stimulus is supramaximal during the test;

3. S_1 stimulation precedes S_2 by a few milliseconds (conduction time between two sites is 7 or 8 msec);

4. The intensity of S_1 is gradually increased from zero until the CMAPs from S_2 disappear. When S_1 is zero (Fig. 11.101a), the CMAP is elicited by S_2 stimulation alone. With a gradual increase of S_1 intensity, the response to S_2 is gradually eliminated; with an increasing amplitude of the S_1 response, there is a decreasing amplitude of the S_2 response and a corresponding increase in S_2 latency until in the final tracing the response to S_1 alone remains (Fig. 11.101h).

MEASUREMENT: Latency is measured by the conventional method. Latency for the maximal motor NCV is measured in Fig. 11.101a and for the minimal motor NCV in Fig. 11.101g. The range of motor NCVs can then be calculated.

TEMPERATURE: Skin temperature is not controlled.

NORMAL DATA: The majority of motor fibers in the peroneal nerve conduct at a rate within 15–20% of the maximal NCV, although the lower limit of NCV may be as much as 35–40% below the maximal NCV.

COMMENTS: Thomas et al. (125) claim that, by using this technique, the larger and

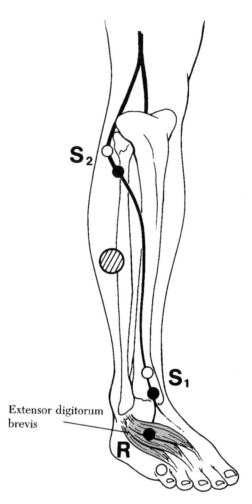

Figure 11.100.   Arrangement of the stimulating electrodes (S₁, S₂) and the recording electrodes to determine the range of NCVs in the motor nerve fibers to the extensor digitorum brevis.

faster motor fibers are selectively blocked by a preceding submaximal distal stimulation, and thus it is possible to study the conduction time of slower fibers in isolation.

Hopf's Method

RECORDING: The conventional method is used for motor nerve conduction (Figs. 11.100 and 11.102) (126).

STIMULATION: The first stimulation surface electrodes (S₁) are placed distally (ankle for peroneal nerve) and the second ones (S₂) proximally (fibular head for peroneal nerve). The technique of stimulation is as follows:

1. The maximal motor NCV is calculated by the conventional method;
2. A nerve is supramaximally stimulated at both sites;
3. The distal stimulation (S₁) is always applied first. This is followed by proximal stimulation (S₂), and the time interval between the two stimuli progressively increased in 0.1-msec (127) or 0.5-msec (128) steps. If S₂ is applied too early after S₁, the only observable response is that of S₁ because the nerve fiber under the S₂ stimulator is either unexcitable, being in refractory period or, if excitable, the S₂ impulse is blocked by the antidromic S₁ impulse (Fig. 11.102A); and

4. With a proper time interval, some of the fibers under stimulus S₂ are again excitable and free to transmit their impulse distally, producing a small wave (Fig. 11.102B). By progressively increasing the time interval between the two stimuli, more and more fibers become available at S₂, until a point is reached when the S₁ response is passed by and the nerve is again capable of transmitting the S₂ impulse fully (Fig. 11.102E). This represents the latency of the slower motor fibers.

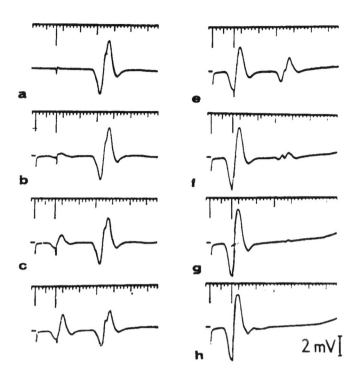

Figure 11.101. Recordings from the extensor digitorum brevis using Thomas' method. *a*, Stimulus onset of S_2 followed by the CMAP. In *b–h*, S_1 precedes S_2 by 6 msec, the stimulus intensity of S_1 being increased progressively from the threshold in *b* to the maximal value in *h*. Time scale: 1 and 5 msec. (From Thomas PK, Seares TA, Gilliatt RW. The range of conduction velocity in normal motor nerve fibers to the small muscles of the hand and foot. J Neurol Neurosurg Psychiatry 1959;22:178.)

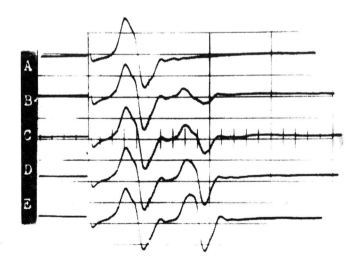

Figure 11.102. Responses from the extensor digitorum brevis using Hopf's method to determine the range of conduction velocity of its motor fibers. The S_1 stimulus is followed by S_2 at progressively increased intervals through 0.1-msec steps. **A**, The interval is too short, and the response to S_2 is completely blocked by the antidromic impulses from S_1. **B–E**, The interval is gradually increased. The first response after the S_2 stimulus in **B** is that conducted through the fastest conducting fibers. The CMAP increases progressively as the time interval increases until it reaches the maximum. Time: 2 msec between two small vertical divisions. (From Miglietta O. Nerve motor fiber characteristics in chronic ischemia. Arch Neurol 1966;14:449.)

Table 11.20.
Range of Normal Minimal Motor Nerve NCVs

Investigation	Tested Nerve	Range of Minimal NCVs (m/sec)	No. of Subjects
Hopf (126)[a]	Ulnar	4–7	20
Miglietta (149)	Peroneal	4–7	50
Miglietta (148)	Ulnar, median	7–12	
Ricker and Hopf (149)	Posterior tibial	10–24	
	Peroneal	8–23	
Blackstock et al. (128)	Ulnar	10–20[a]	8
Betts et al. (129)	Ulnar	6.9–12	25
		15–20[b]	

[a]Allowing a 1-msec refractory period when calculating the NCV.
[b]Allowing a 1.3-msec refractory period when calculating the NCV.

MEASUREMENT: The difference (t) between the moment a minimal S_2 response appears and the moment the S_2 response reaches maximal amplitude is measured. This is the time range needed to calculate the range of NCV, which is calculated by dividing the distance by t.

TEMPERATURE: Skin temperature is not controlled.

NORMAL DATA: Various investigators reported the values noted in Table 11.20.

COMMENTS: Initially, with small intervals, only the impulses in the fastest nerve fibers are not extinguished by the antidromically conducted impulse (Fig. 11.102B). As the interval increases, slower fibers contribute more and more to the S_2 response.

When calculating the NCV range, the absolute refractory periods must be subtracted from t to obtain more accurate results. Hopf's method (126) does not take this into consideration. Betts et al. (129) point out that the determination of the duration of the refractory period is one of the most problematic aspects of this method. Blackstock et al. (128) used 1.0 msec. Applying this value for the refractory period as a correction to the conduction velocity range test gives velocity ranges in the region of 15–20 m/sec. It is evident that, under pathological conditions where the refractory periods are changed, the measurements obtained with this method become somewhat questionable (129).

Refractory Period in Sensory and Mixed Nerve Fibers

The technique of testing the refractory period (RP) in sensory nerve fibers in the median and sural nerves has been described by various authors (130–134). This test is basically the sensory nerve conduction by paired stimulations with varying intervals between the paired stimulations. It is now easily performed with the automated programs on some commercial EMG machine.

RECORDING: A conventional method for the sensory and mixed nerve conduction is used. Some investigators have used the near-nerve needle technique in recording the sensory CNAP (130, 132–134) and others have used surface recording electrodes (131, 135).

STIMULATION: For the median nerve, surface electrodes mounted around the index finger are used (130, 132). For the sural nerve, needle electrodes are placed near the nerve lateral to the lateral malleolus (130). For the mixed ulnar nerve, a surface electrode is used for stimulation at the wrist. Stimulus is supramaximal, of either 0.1 or 0.2 msec duration. The first and second stimuli are equal in intensity and duration. CNAPs are averaged.

For determination of the absolute RP, the stimulus interval (the interval between the first and second stimuli for paired stimulations) is shortened consecutively by 0.1-msec decrements from 2 msec to the interval (absolute refractory period) at which the nerve ceases to conduct the second impulse.

For determination of the relative RP, the stimulus interval is shortened consecutively by 0.25-msec decrements from 5 msec.

MEASUREMENT: Latencies are measured from the stimulus onset to the first positive peak (L) and to the first negative peak (Lp). Amplitude of the CNAP is measured from peak to peak. The absolute RP is the critical stimulus interval at which the nerve ceases to conduct the second impulse. The relative RP is the stimulus interval at which the amplitude of the second response begins to decrease or the latency begins to be prolonged (133). The gradual decrease in the amplitude and gradual prolongation of the latency are plotted against the shortening of the stimulus interval.

TEMPERATURE: Skin temperature is controlled between 33–35°C for Tachmann and Lehmann's method and at 36°C for Buchthal and Rosenfalck's method (130, 132).

NORMAL DATA:

Absolute Refractory Period:

Investigators	Nerve	No. of Subjects	Refractory Period
Gilliatt and Willison (131)	Mixed median nerve	4	0.6–0.7 msec
Buchthal and Rosenfalck (132)	Median sensory	5	0.75 ± 0.04 msec
Lowitzsch and Hopf (133)	Mixed ulnar nerve	28	0.51 ± 0.09 msec
Tackmann and Lehmann (130)	Median sensory		
	20–35 yr	12	0.68 ± 0.06 msec
	40–60 yr	12	0.72 ± 0.05 msec
	Sural sensory		
	20–35 yr	11	0.73 ± 0.08 msec
	40–60 yr	8	0.76 ± 0.07 msec
Ludin and Tackmann (138)	Median sensory nerve	41	0.70 ± 0.08 msec
	Sural nerve	46	0.65 ± 0.12 msec

Relative Refractory Period:

Buchthal and Rosenfalck (132)	Median sensory nerve	5	Three times the absolute refractory period.
Lowitzch et al. (133)	Mixed ulnar nerve	28	
	by latency		3.08 ± 0.25 msec
	by amplitude		2.5 ± 0.47 msec
Hopf et al. (135)	Median sensory nerve		3.21 msec
	Ulnar sensory nerve		3.45 msec

COMMENTS: One study showed that in 22 patients with neuropathy, the relative RP showed more prominent abnormality than the absolute RP or the NCV (133). They were able to show abnormal RP (latency) in 12 patients with neuropathy who had normal NCVs, indicating that the relative RP study is more sensitive in detection of neuropathy than the NCV. Two studies reported abnormalities in the RP in patients with CTS. In 11 nerves in 8 patients with CTS, Tackmann and Lehmann showed that the latency was more prolonged and the amplitude was more depressed in CTS than in normal subjects (136). In 13 nerves of 10 patients with CTS, one study showed that the absolute RP was prolonged and that the relative RP at 50% reduction of amplitude was also prolonged (137).

Refractory Period in Motor Nerve Fibers

Ingram's Method

Ingram et al. (138) described a technique of testing the refractory period in motor nerve fibers. This test can be achieved easily with commercially available automated programs (e.g., Dantec program).

RECORDING: The conventional method of recording for the motor nerve conduction is used.

STIMULATION: Surface electrodes are used for the stimulation. Two active stimulating electrodes (proximal and distal) are placed following the conventional method (Figs. 11.103 and 11.104). For the ulnar nerve, the above-elbow site (4 cm proximal to the cubital tunnel) is used for proximal stimulation and the wrist site for distal stimulation. For the reference electrode, a common saline-soaked strap is placed circumferentially around the limb approximately midway between the proximal and distal active electrodes. Proximal stimuli are set at 120% supramaximal and distal stimuli are set at 150%. The proximal interstimuli interval (ISI) is fixed at 4 msec. Distal ISI increments of 0.1 msec are used.

MEASUREMENT: The test muscle response is first separated from the earlier distally evoked response by a subtraction technique as noted. Averages of test responses (usu-

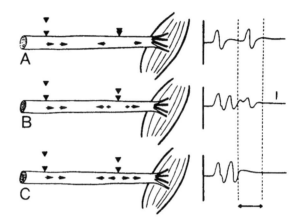

Figure 11.103. Schematic representation of the double collision technique. Paired supramaximal stimuli *(inverted triangles)* are delivered at proximal and distal stimulation sites over a peripheral nerve. The proximal ISI is fixed at a value exceeding the refractory period range, typically at 4 msec. The effect of increasing distal ISI on the late (test) muscle response is shown (**A–C**). Increasing ISI is represented by the increasing spatial separation of stimuli. Maximal nerve volleys are represented by *large arrows,* and submaximal volleys by *small arrows.* The *dashed lines* delineate the analysis window. (From Ingram DA, Davis GR, Swash M. The double collision technique: a new method for measurement of the motor nerve refractory period distribution in man. EEG Clin Neurophysiol 1987;66:227.)

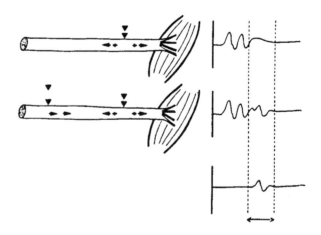

Figure 11.104. Schematic representation of the subtraction technique for step B in Fig. 11.103. The digitized response to the (test) distal stimuli given alone (top trace) is subtracted from the response obtained when the proximal and distal stimuli are delivered simultaneously (middle trace). The resultant late (test) muscle response is shown in the lower trace. (From Ingram DA, Davis GR, Swash M. The double collision technique: a new method for measurement of the motor nerve refractory period distribution in man. EEG Clin Neurophysiol 1987;66:228.)

ally four) for each increment of distal ISI are obtained and these are automatically analyzed to give amplitude and rectified area measurements. Each test response is cross-correlated with the initial maximal response and scaled to give a range of values between 100% and 0%, the latter value being determined by the point at which no further cancellation occurs (refractory period). This is automatically calculated by the automated program.

TEMPERATURE: Skin temperature is controlled at 35°C.

NORMAL DATA: Age range: 22–58 yr.

Measure-ment	Distal ISI required for % cancellation of maximal CMAP (msec)				Range (9–95%)	Ratio (95:5%)	No. of Subjects
	5%	50%	95%	99%			
Median nerve	0.94 ± 0.12	1.03 ± 0.12	1.12 ± 0.14	1.23 ± 0.16	0.18 ± 0.09	1.20 ± 0.09	20
Ulnar nerve	0.85 ± 0.08	0.97 ± 0.10	1.07 ± 0.14	1.28 ± 0.17	0.22 ± 0.08	1.27 ± 0.09	6
Peroneal nerve	1.09 ± 0.15	1.29 ± 0.28	1.59 ± 0.41	1.78 ± 0.45	0.50 ± 0.29	1.47 ± 0.21	8

Kimura's Method

Kimura (139) described a technique for estimating the RP of motor fibers by using a different ISI between the paired stimulations at the proximal stimulation sites (Fig. 11.105).

RECORDING: The conventional method of recording for the motor nerve conduction of the ulnar nerve is used.

STIMULATION: Surface stimulating electrodes are used. Two active stimulating electrodes are placed at the wrist (distal) and at the axilla (proximal) segments of the ulnar nerve, following the conventional method. For proximal stimulation, the stimulus intensity is either maximal or 150% supramaximal and for distal stimulation, 150% supramaximal. Stimulus duration is 0.05 msec. Proximal ISI increments of 0.2 msec are used from 0.5–5.0 msec.

MEASUREMENT: The CMAP, $M(A_2)$, elicited by the second axillary stimulus must be proportional to the number of axons no longer refractory when the second axillary stimulus is applied (Fig. 11.106). The CMAP, $M(A)$, evoked by a single axillary shock alone represents the total number of axons available in the nerve. Hence, the ratio of amplitude, $M(A_2)/M(A)$, gives the excitability of the average motor axon to the second stimulus, i.e., the degree of its recovery from the refractoriness induced by the volley of the first impulse.

TEMPERATURE: Not controlled.

NORMAL DATA: Number of subjects: 24 nerves in 12 subjects. Age range: mean age of 28.

Stimulus Intensity	Absolute RP (msec)[a]	ISI for 100% Recovery (msec)
Maximal	1.00 ± 0.20	2.88 ± 0.57
150% supramaximal	0.77 ± 0.18	2.03 ± 0.57

[a]When M(A2) is first elicited.

Autonomic Function Test

Sympathetic Skin Response

In 1984, Shahani et al. (140) described a technique of obtaining sympathetic skin response with the EMG machine (Fig. 11.107). Uncini et al. (141) employed Shahani et al.'s method with some modifications and reported normal data.

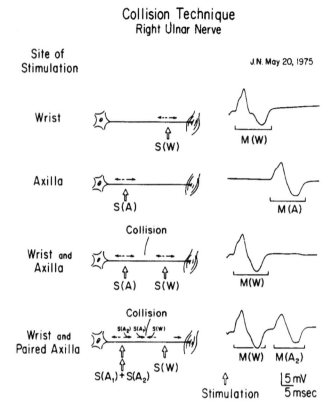

Figure 11.105. Compound muscle action potentials recorded by surface electrodes placed over the abductor digiti quinti after percutaneous stimulation of the ulnar nerve. The figures on the left are schematic diagrams showing orthodromic *(solid arrows)* and antidromic *(dotted arrows)* impulses. Axillary stimulation was given 5.0 msec after the wrist stimulus which triggered sweeps on the oscilloscope. With single stimulation at the wrist and the axilla (the third tracing from the top), the orthodromic impulse from the axilla was extinguished by collision with the antidromic impulse from the wrist. When paired shocks were delivered at the axilla (bottom tracing), $M(A_2)$ appeared because the first axillary stimulus cleared the path for the orthodromic impulse of the second stimulus. The size of $M(A_2)$ is proportional to the number of axons no longer refractory after the passage of a volley of the first axillary stimulus. (From Kimura J. A method for estimating the refractory period of motor fibers in the human peripheral nerve. J Neurol Sci 1976;28:486.)

POSITION OF SUBJECT: The subject is encouraged to relax. The room lights are dimmed.

MACHINE SET-UP: Filter: 0.3–3 KHz. Sweep velocity: 500 msec.

RECORDING: Active and reference surface electrodes are placed on: (*a*) the palm and dorsum of the hand; (*b*) the sole and dorsum of the foot; (*c*) the anterior and posterior surfaces of the upper arm; and (*d*) the patella and popliteal fossa (Fig. 11.108). For each patient, responses are measured in upper and lower extremities. To estimate the conduction velocity, proximal and distal recordings are simultaneously made in the same limb with a distance of approximately 70 cm in the leg and 50 cm in the arm. According to the method of Shahani et al. (140), two surface electrodes are placed 4 cm apart in the 8th intercostal space, with the anterior electrode on the anterior axillary line to record the diaphragmatic EMG during deep inspiration (Fig. 11.108).

STIMULATION: A single stimulus of 0.1-msec duration and 10–30-mA intensity is applied at irregular time intervals to the median nerve at the wrist, to the posterior tibial nerve at the ankle, and to the supraorbital nerve at the forehead. Single auditory clicks (95 dB) are delivered to the ears with a headphone. Electrical and auditory stimuli are administered at irregular intervals greater than 30 sec apart. Shahani et al. (140) also used deep inspiration in place of electrical or auditory stimuli to obtain the response.

MEASUREMENT: Latency is measured from the onset of the stimulus artifact (electrical stimulation) or diaphragmatic EMG activity to the first deflection of the response from the baseline. Amplitude is measured from peak to peak.

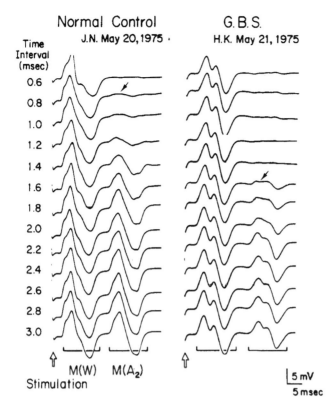

Figure 11.106. Paired axillary shocks of just maximal intensity were combined with a single shock at the wrist (cf. bottom tracing in Fig. 11.105). Interstimulus intervals between two axillary stimuli ranged from 0.6–3.0 msec. The shock intervals were adjusted so that the second axillary shock always occurred 5.0 msec after the wrist stimulus, which triggered sweeps on the oscilloscope. In the normal subject, $M(A_2)$ first appeared *(small arrow)* at the interstimulus interval of 0.8 msec and recovered completely at 3.0 msec. In the patient with Guillain-Barré syndrome, $M(A_2)$ first appeared at the time interval of 1.6 msec and did not recover completely at 3.0 msec. (From Kimura J. A method for estimating the refractory period of motor fibers in the human peripheral nerve. J Neurol Sci 1976;28:487.)

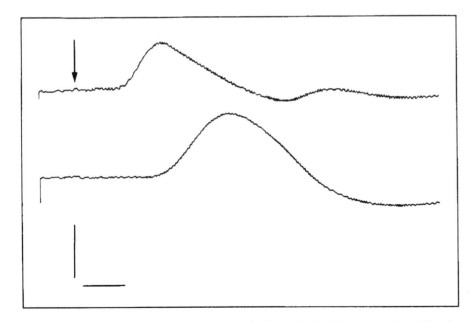

Figure 11.107. Sympathetic skin responses recorded from the hand (upper trace) and foot (lower trace) in response to an electrical stimulus to the contralateral median nerve *(arrow)*. The onset latency of the response is shorter in the hand by 800 msec. A biphasic response of several mV amplitude is recorded at both sites. The tail-end of the foot SSR is truncated because of the long duration of the response. Calibration: 4 and 2 mV for upper and lower traces, respectively; 1 sec. (From Shahani BT, Day TJ, Cros D, Khalil N, Kneebone CS. RR interval variation and the sympathetic skin response in the assessment of autonomic function in peripheral neuropathy. Arch Neurol 1990;47:660.)

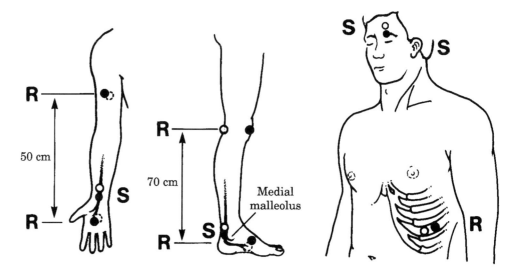

Figure 11.108. Sympathetic response test.

TEMPERATURE: Ambient temperature is controlled at 20–23°C. Skin temperature is controlled at 34–36°C.

NORMAL DATA: Number of subjects: 20. Age range: 27–74 yr.

Measurement	Hand Mean ± SD	Foot Mean ± SD
Latencies (sec):		
Median nerve stimulation	1.5 ± 0.2	2.0 ± 0.3
Posterior tibial nerve stimulation	1.5 ± 0.2	2.1 ± 0.3
Supraorbital nerve stimulation	1.5 ± 0.2	1.9 ± 0.3
Auditory stimulation	1.5 ± 0.2	1.9 ± 0.3
Amplitude (μV):		
Electrical stimulation	985 ± 300	615 ± 236
Inspiration (N = 30)[a]	1193 ± 522	822 ± 421
Unmyelinated axon CV (m/sec) (N = 5)[a]	1.6 ± 0.1	1.0 ± 0.1

[a]Shahani et al.'s values (140). N represents number of subjects.

INTERPRETATION: The sympathetic skin response amplitude varies greatly within and between subjects, including controls, from test to test, making the amplitude an unreliable parameter for the SSR. Thus, only an absent response (no consistent recordings of response) is considered abnormal. Latency or amplitude value is not important.

COMMENTS: The response amplitude varied from test to test, despite efforts to limit habituation (144). The shapes of the response were similar in the arms and legs, but the amplitude was consistently greater in the hand than in the foot and was greater when triggered by deep inspiration than by electrical stimulation. The sympathetic skin response latency correlated well with the subjects' height and was consistently longer in the leg than in the arm.

The RR Interval Variation of the ECG

In 1990, Shahani et al. (142) described a technique of obtaining the RR interval variation (RRIV; the heart rate variability) with the EMG machine.

MACHINE SET-UP: Filters: 16–80 Hz. Sensitivity: 200–500 μV. Sweep velocity: 200 msec. Using the triggering mode and delay line, the oscilloscope display is adjusted by the trigger sensitivity and sweep speed so that two QRS complexes are displayed on the screen.

RECORDING: The surface recording electrodes are placed on the dorsum of each hand. A ground electrode is placed around one wrist.

Since the first QRS complex is the triggering potential, the variation in timing of the

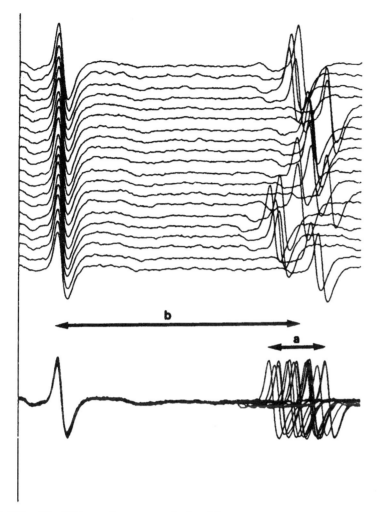

Figure 11.109. The RR interval variation is displayed by superimposing 20 sweeps triggered by the QRS complex of the electrocardiogram. The jitter (***a***) in the second potential is expressed as a percentage of the mean interpotential interval (***b***) as follows: RR interval variation = a/b × 100%. The sweep duration is 1 sec. (From Shahani BT, Day TJ, Cros D, Khalil N, Kneebone CS. RR interval variation and the sympathetic skin response in the assessment of autonomic function in peripheral neuropathy. Arch Neurol 1990;47:660.)

second QRS complex represents the variation in the RR interval (Fig. 11.109). Twenty traces are recorded and superimposed, and a printout is made for subsequent measurement. Five groups of 20 sweeps are recorded at rest, and two during forced deep breathing at 6 breaths/min.

MEASUREMENT: The range in the RR interval (Fig. 11.109a) and the mean RR interval (Fig. 11.109b) are measured. The RRIV is expressed as a percentage of the average RR interval using the following formula: RRIV = a/b × 100. The average of five recordings at rest is termed R%, and that of two recordings during deep breathing, D%. The difference between these two measures (D% − R%) and the ratio of D% to R% (D/R) are also calculated.

TEMPERATURE: Not controlled.

NORMAL DATA: Number of subjects: 53 Age range: 15–73 yr.

Measurement[a]	Mean ± SD
Rest (msec)	18.9 ± 7.2
RRIV HV (msec)	31.0 + 9.3
Difference (msec)	12.1 ± 3.9
Ratio	1.71 + 0.28

[a]Normative Data (Fig. 11.110).

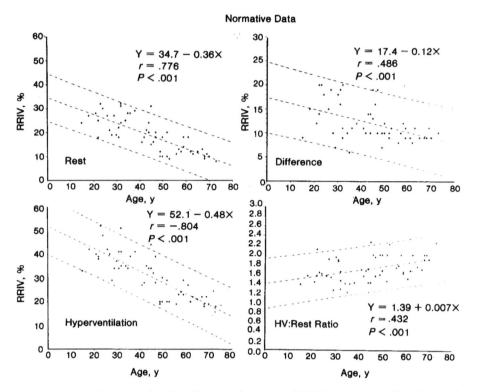

Figure 11.110. Normative data for RR interval variation (RRIV) at rest (to left) and with deep breathing (bottom left) are plotted against age for 53 healthy subjects. Top right, the difference between RRIV at rest and with deep breathing is plotted against age. Bottom right, the ratio between RRIV(HV):RRIV (rest) is plotted against age. The regression line is defined by y = a + bx; the 95% confidence limit interval is shown on both sides of the regression line of best fit; r indicates correlation coefficient for the regression line; and p, probability that the slope is equal to zero. (From Shahani BT, Day TJ, Cros D, Khalil N, Kneebone CS. RR interval variation and the sympathetic skin response in the assessment of autonomic function in peripheral neuropathy. Arch Neurol 1990;47:660.)

INTERPRETATION: When the RRIV% is outside the 95% confidence limit of normal controls, it is abnormal.

COMMENTS: For normal subjects, there was a negative correlation with age for RRIVs for 5%, D%, and D% − R%. For the D/R ratio, there was a weak positive correlation with age. Shahani et al. found that, of 22 patients with peripheral neuropathy and clinical dysautonomia, 15 showed abnormal results on the RRIV and the sympathetic skin response test, and seven had abnormal results on one test only (142). They claimed that these tests are helpful in combination in the assessment of autonomic function in peripheral neuropathies in the EMG laboratory.

REFERENCES

1. Raffaele R, Emery P, Palmeri A, Ricca G, Perciavalle V. Sensory nerve conduction velocity of the trigeminal nerve. EMG Clin Neurophysiol 1987;27:115–117.
2. Zander Olsen P. Prediction of recovery in Bell's palsy. Acta Neurol Scand 1975;52 (Suppl 61):1–121.
3. De Meirsman J, Claes G, Geerdens L. Normal latency value of the facial nerve with detection in the posterior auricular muscle and normal amplitude value of the evoked action potential. EMG Clin Neurophysiol 1980;20:481–485.
4. Redhead J, Mugliston T. Facial electroneuronography: action potential amplitude and latency studies in 50 normal subjects. J Laryngol Otol 1985;99:369–372.
5. Smith IM, Murray JAM, Prescott RJ, Barr-Hamilton R. Facial electroneurography. Arch Otolaryngol Head Neck Surg 1988;114:322–325.
6. Gavilán J, Gavilán D, Sarriá MJ. Facial electroneurography: results on normal humans. J Laryngol Otology 1985;99:1085–1088.
7. Hilger JA. Facial nerve stimulator. Trans Am Acad Ophthalmol Otolaryngol 1964;68:74–77.
8. Campbell EDR, Hickey RP, Nixon KH. Value of nerve excitability measurements in prognosis of facial palsy. Brit Med J 1962;2:7–10.

9. Peytz F, Ramussen H, Buchthal F. Conduction time and velocity in human recurrent laryngeal nerve. Danish Medical Bulletin 1965;12:125–127.

10. Cherington M. Accessory nerve conduction studies. Arch Neurol 1968;18:708–709.

11. Fahrer H, Ludin HP, Mumenthaler M, Neiger M. The innervation of the trapezius muscle: an electro-physiological study. J Neurol 1974;207:183–188.

12. Petrera JE, Trojaborg W. Conduction studies along the accessory nerve and follow up of patients with trapezius palsy. J Neurol Neurosurg Psychiatry 1984;47:630–636.

13. Krogness K. Serial conduction studies of the spinal accessory nerve used as a prognostic tool in a lesion caused by lymph node biopsy. Acta Chir Scand 1974;140:7–11.

14. Redmond MD, Di Benedetto M. Hypoglossal nerve conduction in normal subjects. Muscle Nerve 1988;11:447–452.

15. Palliyath SK. A technique for studying the greater auricular nerve conduction velocity. Muscle Nerve 1984;7:232–234.

16. Kimura I, Seki H, Sasao S, Ayyar DR. The great auricular nerve conduction study: a technique, norma-tive data and clinical usefulness. EMG Clin Neurophysiol 1987;27:39–43.

17. Newsome Davis J. Phrenic nerve conduction in man. J Neurol Neurosurg Psychiatry 1967;30:420–426.

18. MacLean IC, Mittioni TA. Phrenic nerve conduction studies: a new technique and its application in quadriplegic patients. Arch Phys Med Rehabil 1981;62:70–73.

19. Kaplan PE. A motor nerve conduction velocity across the upper trunk the lateral cord of the brachial plexus. EMG Clin Neurophysiol 1982;22:315–320.

20. MacLean IC. Nerve root stimulation to evaluate conduction across the brachial and lumbo-sacral plexus: recent advances in clinical electromyography. AAEE Third Annual Continuing Education Course, 1980:51–55.

21. MacLean IC, Taylor RS. Nerve root stimulation to evaluate brachial plexus conduction. Arch Phys Med Rehabil 1975;56:551.

22. Weber RJ, Piero D. Entrapment syndromes. In: Johnson EW, ed. Practical electromyography. Balti-more: Williams & Wilkins, 1980.

23. London GW. Normal ulnar nerve conduction velocity across the thoracic outlet: comparison of two measuring techniques. J Neurol Neurosurg Psychiatry 1975;38:767–760.

24. Ginzburg M, Lee M, Ginzburg J, Alba A. Median ulnar nerve conduction determinations in the Erb's point-axilla segment in normal subjects. J Neurol Neurosurg Psychiatry 1978;1:444–448.

25. Krogness K. Ulnar trunk conduction studies in the diagnosis of the thoracic outlet syndrome. Acta Chir Scand 1973;129:597–603.

26. Kaplan PE. Electrodiagnostic confirmation of long thoracic nerve palsy. J Neurol Neurosurg Psychiatry 1980;43:50–52.

27. Alfonsi E, Moglia A, Sandrini G, Pisoni MR, Arrigo A. Electrophysiological study of long thoracic nerve conduction in normal subjects. EMG Clin Neurophysiol 1986;26:63–67.

28. Petrera JE, Trojaborg W. Conduction studies of the long thoracic nerve in serratus anterior palsy of dif-ferent etiology. Neurology 1984;34:1033–1037.

29. Gassel MM. A test of nerve conduction to muscles of the shoulder girdle as an aid in the diagnosis of proximal neurogenic muscular disease. J Neurol Neurosurg Psychiatry 1964;27:200–205.

30. Kraft GH. Axillary musculocutaneous and suprascapular nerve latency studies. Arch Phys Med Rehabil 1972;53:382–387.

31. Currier DP. Motor conduction velocity of axillary nerve. Phys Ther 1971;51:503–509.

32. Trojaborg W. Motor and sensory conduction in the musculocutaneous nerve. J Neurol Neurosurg Psy-chiatry 1976;39:890–899.

33. Spindler HA, Felsenthal G. Sensory conduction in the musculocutaneous nerve. Arch Phys Med Reha-bil 1978;59:20–23.

34. Pribyl R, You SB, Jantra P. Sensory nerve conduction velocity of the medial antebrachial cutaneous nerve. EMG Clin Neurophysiol 1979;19:41–46.

35. Chang CW, Oh SJ. Medial antebrachial cutaneous neuropathy: case report. EMG Clin Neurophysiol 1988;28:3–5.

36. Reddy MP: Conduction studies of the medial cutaneous nerve of the forearm. Arch Phys Med Rehabil 1983;64:209–211.

37. Ma DM, Liveson JA. Nerve conduction handbook. Philadelphia: FA Davis, 1983:79–81.

38. Chang CW, Cho HK, Oh SJ. Posterior antebrachial cutaneous neuropathy: case report. EMG Clin Neu-rophysiol 1989;29:109–111.

39. Chang CW, Oh SJ. Posterior antebrachial cutaneous neuropathy. Case report. EMG Clin Neurophysiol 1990;30:3–5.

40. Nakano KK, Lundergan C, Okihiro MM. Anterior interosseous nerve syndromes. Arch Neurol 1977;34:477–480.

41. Buchthal F, Rosenfalck A, Trojaborg W. Electrophysiological findings in entrapment of the median nerve at the wrist and elbow. J Neurol Neurosurg Psychiatry 1974;37:340–360.

42. Kimura J. The carpal tunnel syndrome. Localization of conduction abnormalities within the distal seg-ment of the median nerve. Brain 1979;102:619–635.

43. Fitz WR, Mysiw J, Johnson EW. First lumbrical latency and amplitude. Am J Phys Med Rehabil 1990;69:198–201.

44. Logigian EL, Busis Na, Berger AR, Bryyninckx F, Khalil N, Shahani BT, Young RR. Lumbrical sparing in carpal tunnel syndrome: anatomic, physiological, and diagnostic implications. Neurology 1987;37:1499–1505.

45. Sunderland S. Nerves and nerve injuries. 2nd ed. Edinburgh: Churchill Livingstone, 1978.

46. Yates SK, Yaworski R, Brown WF. Relative preservation of lumbrical versus thenar motor fibers in neurogenic disorders. J Neurol Neurosurg Psychiatry 1981;44:768–774.

47. Hamner K. Nerve conduction studies. Springfield, IL: Charles C Thomas, 1982.

48. Buchthal F, Rosenfalck A. Sensory conduction from digit to palm and from palm to wrist in the carpal tunnel syndrome. J Neurol Neurosurg Psychiatry 1971;34:243–252.

49. Kimura J. The carpal tunnel syndrome: localization of conduction abnormalities within the distal segment of the median nerve. Brain 1979;102:619–635.

50. Oh SJ. Clinical electromyography. Nerve Conduction Studies. Baltimore: University Park Press, 1984:190.

51. Chang CW, Lien IN. Comparison of sensory nerve conduction in the palmar cutaneous branch and first digital branch of the median nerve: a new diagnostic method for carpal tunnel syndrome. Muscle Nerve 1991;14:1173–1176.

52. Payan J. Electrophysiological localization of ulnar nerve lesions. J Neurol Neurosurg Psychiatry 1969;32:208–220.

53. Checkles NS, Russakov AD, Piero DL. Ulnar nerve conduction velocity: effect of elbow position on measurement. Arch Phys Med Rehabil 1971;52:362–365.

54. Campbell WW, Sahni SK, Pridgeon RM, Riaz G, Leshner RT. Intraoperative electroneurography: management of ulnar neuropathy at the elbow. Muscle Nerve 1988;1:75–81.

55. Kanakamedala RV, Simons DG, Porter RW, Zucker RS. Ulnar nerve entrapment at the elbow localized by short segment stimulation. Arch Phys Med Rehabil 1988;69:959–963.

56. Ebeling P, Gilliatt RW, Thomas PK. 1960 A clinical and electrical study of ulnar nerve lesions in the hand. J Neurol Neurosurg Psychiatry 1960;23:1–9.

57. Bhala RP, Goodgold J. Motor conduction in the deep palmar branch of the ulnar nerve. Arch Phys Med Rehabil 1968;49:460–466.

58. Hamner, K. Nerve conduction studies. Springfield, IL: Charles C Thomas, 1982.

59. Kincaid JC, Phillips LH, Daube JR. The evaluation of suspected ulnar neuropathy at the elbow: normal conduction study values. Arch Neurol 1986;43:44–47.

60. Felsenthal G, Freed MJ, Kalafut R, Hilton B. Across-elbow ulnar nerve sensory conduction technique. Arch Phys Med Rehabil 1989;70:668–672.

61. Kim DJ, Kalantri A, Guha S, Wainapel SF. Dorsal cutaneous ulnar nerve conduction: diagnostic aid in ulnar neuropathy. Arch Neurol 1981;38:321–322.

62. Jabre J. Ulnar nerve lesions at the wrist: new technique for recording from the sensory dorsal branch of the ulnar nerve. Neurology 1980;30:873–876.

63. Jabre J. The superficial peroneal sensory nerve revisited. Arch Neurol 1981;38:666–667.

64. Gassel MM, Diamantopoulos E. Pattern of conduction times in the distribution of the radial nerve: a clinical and electrophysiological study. Neurology 1964;14:222–231.

65. Jebsen RH. Motor conduction velocity in proximal distal segments of the radial nerve. Arch Phys Med Rehabil 1966;47:597–602.

66. Trojaborg W, Sindrup EH. Motor and sensory conduction in different segments of the radial nerves in normal subjects. J Neurol Neurosurg Psychiatry 1969;32:354–359.

67. Falck B, Hurme M. Conduction velocity of the posterior interosseous nerve across the Arcade of Frohse. Electromyograph Clin Neurophysiol 1983;23:567–576.

68. Chang CW, Oh SJ. Sensory nerve conduction study in forearm of superficial radial nerve: standardization of technique. EMG Clin Neurophysiol 1990;30:349–351.

69. MacKinnon SE, Dellon AL. The overlap pattern of the lateral antebrachial cutaneous nerve and the superficial branch. J Hand Surg Am 1985;10:522–526.

70. Shirali CS, Sandler B. Radial nerve sensory conduction velocity: measurement by antidromic technique. Arch Phys Med Rehabil 1972;53:457–460.

71. Caldwell JW, Crane CR, Bol GL. Determinations of intercostal motor conduction time in diagnosis of nerve root compression. Arch Phys Med Rehabil 1968;49:515–518.

72. Johnson ER, Powell J, Caldwell J, Crane C. Intercostal nerve conduction and posterior rhizotomy in the diagnosis and treatment of thoracic radiculopathy. J Neurol Neurosurg Psychiatry 1974;37:330–332.

73. Pradhan S, Taly A. Intercostal nerve conduction study in man. J Neurology Neurosurgery Psychiatry 1989;52:763–766.

74. Kaplan PE. A motor nerve conduction velocity across the lumbosacral plexus. EMG Clin Neurophysiol 1982;22:527–530.

75. Ellis RJ, Geisse H, Holub BA, Swenson MR. Ilioinguinal nerve conduction. Muscle Nerve 1992;15:1195.

76. Butler ET, Johnson EW, Kaye AZ. Normal conduction velocity in lateral femoral cutaneous nerve. Arch Phys Med Rehabil 1974;55:31–32.

77. Sarala PK, Nishihira T, Oh SJ. Meralgia paresthesica: electrophysiological study. Arch Phys Med Rehabil 1979;60:30–31.

78. Lysens R, Vandendriessche G, Van Mol Y, Rosselle N. The sensory conduction velocity in the cutaneous femoris lateralis nerve in normal adult subjects and in patients with complaints suggesting meralgia paresthesica. EMG Clin Neurophysiol 1981;21:505–510.

79. Dumitru D, Nelson MR. Posterior femoral cutaneous nerve conduction. Arch Phys Med Rehabil 1990;71:979–982.
80. Gassel M. A study of femoral nerve conduction time. Arch Neurol 1963;9:607–614.
81. Chopra JS, Hurwitz LJ. Femoral nerve conduction in diabetes and chronic occlusive vascular disease. J Neurol Neurosurg Psychiatry 1968;31:28–33.
82. Johnson EW, Wood PK, Powers JJ. Femoral nerve conduction studies. Arch Phys Med Rehabil 1965;49:528–532.
83. Rigshospitalet Laboratory of Clinical Neurophysiology. Electromyography: sensory and motor conduction: findings in normal subjects. Copenhagen, Denmark: RLCN, 1975:43.
84. Stohr M, Shumm F, Ballier R. Normal sensory conduction in the saphenous nerve in man. EEG Clin Neurophysiol 1978;44:172–178.
85. Wainapel SF, Kim DJ, Ebel A. Conduction studies of the saphenous nerve in healthy subjects. Arch Phys Med Rehabil 1978;59:316–319.
86. Ertekin C. Saphenous nerve conduction in man. J Neurol Neurosurg Psychiatry 1969;31:28–33.
87. Senden R, Van Mulders J, Ghys R, Rosselle N. Conduction velocity of the distal segment of the saphenous nerve on normal adult subjects. EMG Clin Neurophysiol 1981;21:3–10.
88. Yap B, Hirota T. Sciatic nerve motor conduction velocity study. J Neurol Neurosurg Psychiatry 1971;30:233–239.
89. Gassel MM, Trojaborg W. Clinical and electrophysiological study of the pattern of conduction times in the distribution of the sciatic nerve. J Neurol Neurosurg Psychiatry 1964;17:351–357.
90. Singh N, Behse F, Buchthal F. Electrophysiological study of peroneal palsy. J Neurol Neurosurg Psychiatry 1974;37:1202–1213.
91. Devi S, Lovelace RE, Duarte N. Proximal peroneal nerve conduction velocity: recording from anterior tibial peroneus brevis muscles. Ann Neurol 1977;2:116–119.
92. Kanakamedala R, Hong CZ. Peroneal nerve entrapment at the knee localized by short segment stimulation. Am J Phys Med Rehabil 1989;68:116–122.
93. Izzo KL, Sridhara CR, Rosenholtz H. Sensory conduction studies of the branches of the superficial peroneal nerve. Arch Phys Med Rehabil 1981;62:24–27.
94. Behse F, Buchthal F. Normal sensory conduction in the nerves of the leg in man. J Neurol Neurosurg Psychiatry 1971;34:404–414.
95. Lee HJ, Bach JR, DeLisa JA. Deep peroneal sensory nerve: standardization in nerve conduction study. Am J Phys Med Rehabil 1990;69:202–204.
96. Posas HN, Rivner MH. Nerve conduction studies of the medial branch of the deep peroneal nerve. Muscle Nerve 1990;13:862.
97. Gilliatt RW, Goodman HV, Willison RG. The recording of lateral popliteal nerve action potentials in man. J Neurol Neurosurg Psychiatry 1961;24:305–318.
98. Mayer RF. Nerve conduction studies in man. Neurology 1963;13:1021–1030.
99. Oh SJ, Sarala PK, Kuba T, Elmore RS. Tarsal tunnel syndrome: electrophysiological study. Ann Neurol 1978;5:327–330.
100. Fu R, De Lisa JA, Kraft GH. Motor nerve latencies through the tarsal tunnel in normal adult subjects: standard determinations corrected for temperature and distance. Arch Phys Med Rehabil 1980;61:243–248.
101. Felsenthal G, Butler DH, Shear MS. Across-tarsal-tunnel motor-nerve conduction technique. Arch Phys Med Rehabil 1992;73:64–69.
102. Del Toro DR, Park TA, Mandel JD, Wertsch JJ. Development of a nerve conduction study technique for the medial calcaneal nerve. Muscle Nerve 1992;15:1194.
103. Guiloff RJ, Sherratt RM. Sensory conduction in medial plantar nerve. J Neurol Neurosurg Psychiatry 1977;40:1168–1181.
104. Ponsford SN: Sensory conduction in medial and lateral plantar nerves. J Neurol Neurosurg Psychiatry 1988;51:188–191.
105. Saeed MA, Gatens PF. Compound nerve action potentials of the medial and lateral plantar nerves through the tarsal tunnel. Arch Phys Med Rehabil 1982;68:304–307.
106. Oh SJ, Kim HS, Ahmad BK. Electrophysiological diagnosis of the interdigital neuropathy of the foot. Muscle Nerve 1984;7:218–225.
107. Oh SJ, Kim HS, Ahmad BK. The near-nerve sensory nerve conduction in tarsal tunnel syndrome. J Neurol Neurosurg Psychiatry 1985;48:999–1003.
108. Falck B, Hurme M, Hakkarainen S, Aarnio P: Sensory conduction velocity of plantar digital nerves in Morton's metatarsalgia. Neurology 1984;34:698–701.
109. Chantraine A, de Leval J, Onkelinx A. Motor conduction velocity in the internal pudendal nerve. In: Desmedt JE, ed. New developments in EMG and clinical neurophysiology, vol. 2. Basel: Karger, 1973:433–438.
110. Kiff ES, Swash M: Slowed conduction in the pudendal nerves in idiopathic faecal incontinence. Br J Surg 1984;71:614–616.
111. Snooks SJ, Swash M: Perineal nerve and transcutaneous spinal stimulation: new methods for investigation of the urethral striated musculature. Br J Urol 1984;56:406–409.
112. Bradley W, Lin J, Johnson B. Measurement of the conduction velocity of the dorsal nerve of the penis. J Urology 1984;131:1127–1129.
113. Lin J, Bradley W. Penile neuropathy in insulin-dependent diabetes mellitus. J Urol 1985;133:213–215.
114. Kaneko S, Bradley WE. Penile electrodiagnosis. Value of bulbocavernosus reflex latency versus nerve

conduction velocity of the dorsal nerve of the penis in diagnosis of diabetic impotence. J Urol 1986;137:933–935.

115. Clawson D, Cardenas D. Dorsal nerve of the penis nerve conduction velocity: a new technique. Muscle Nerve 1991;14:845–849.

116. Kimura J. F-wave velocity in the central segment of the median and ulnar nerves. Neurology 1974;24:539–549.

117. Kimura J. Proximal versus distal slowing of motor nerve conduction velocity in the Guillain-Barré syndrome. Ann Neurol 1978;3:344–354.

118. Young RR, Shahani BT. Clinical value and limitations of F-wave determination. Muscle Nerve 1978;1:248–249.

119. Kimura. Clinical value and limitations of F-wave determination: a comment. Muscle Nerve 1978;1:250–252.

120. Panaylotopoulos CP. Clinical value and limitations of F-wave determinations: a reply. Muscle Nerve 1978;1:252–253.

121. Fisher MA, Shivde AJ, Teixera C, Grainer LS. The F-response: a clinically useful physiological parameter for the evaluation of radicular injury. EMG Clin Neurophysiol 1979;19:65–75.

122. Branddom RL, Johnson EW. Standardization of H-reflex and diagnostic use in S1 radiculopathy. Arch Phys Med Rehabil 1974;55:161–166.

123. Weber RJ, Piero DL. F-wave evaluation of thoracic outlet syndrome: a multiple regression derived F-wave latency predicting technique. Arch Phys Med Rehabil 1978;59:464–469.

124. Ahiron A, Sarova-Pinhas S. The value of F wave in Bell's palsy; a study of F wave response in the facial nerve. EMG Clin Neurophysiol 1984;24:99–106.

125. Thomas PK, Seares TA, Gilliatt RW. The range of conduction velocity in normal motor nerve fibers to the small muscles of the hand and foot. J Neurol Neurosurg Psychiatry 1959;22:175–181.

126. Hopf HC. Electromyographic study on so-called mononeuritis. Arch Neurol 1963;9:307–312.

127. Miglietta O. Motor nerve fibers in amyotrophic lateral sclerosis. Am J Phys Med 1968;47:118–124.

128. Blackstock E, Rushworth G, Gath D. Electrophysiological studies in alcoholism. J Neurol Neurosurg Psychiatry 1972;35:326–334.

129. Betts RP, Johnston DM, Brown BH. Nerve fiber velocity and refractory period distributions in nerve trunks. J Neurol Neurosurg Psychiatry 1976;39:694–700.

130. Tachmann W, Lehmann H. Refractory period in human sensory nerve fibers. Europ Neurol 1974;12:277–292.

131. Gilliatt RW, Willison RG: The refractory and supernormal periods of the human median nerve. J Neurol Neurosurg Psychiatry 1963;26:136–147.

132. Buchthal F, Rosenfalck A. Evoked potentials and conduction velocity in human sensory nerves. Brain Research 1966;3:1-122.

133. Lowitzsch K, Hopf HC, Schlegel HJ. Conduction of two or more impulses in relation to the fiber spectrum in the mixed human peripheral nerve. In: Desmedt JE, ed. New developments in electromyography and clinical neurophysiology, vol. 3. Basel: Karger, 1973:3:272–278.

134. Ludin H, Tackmann W. Sensory neurography. Stuttgart: Georg Thieme Verla, 1981:51.

135. Hopf HC, Le Quesne PM, Willison RG. Refractory periods and lower limiting frequency of sensory fibers of the hand. In: Kunze K, Desmedt JE, eds. Studies on neuromuscular disease. Basel: Karger, 1975:258.

136. Tachmann W, Lehmann HJ: Relative refractory period of median nerve sensory fibers in the carpal tunnel syndrome. Europ Neurol 1974;12:309–316.

137. Holden L, Smith E, Palliyath S. Refractory studies of the median sensory nerve in carpal tunnel syndrome. Muscle Nerve 1987;10:652.

138. Ingram DA, Davis GR, Swash M. The double collision technique: a new method for measurement of the motor nerve refractory period distribution in man. EEG Clin Neurophysiology 1987;66:225–234.

139. Kimura J. A method for estimating the refractory period of motor fibers in the human peripheral nerve. J Neurol Sci 1976;28:485–490.

140. Shahani BT, Halperin JJ, Boulu P, Cohen J. Sympathetic skin response: a method of assessing unmyelinated axon dysfunction in peripheral neuropathies. J Neurol Neurosurg Psychiatry 1984;37:536–542.

141. Uncini A, Pullman SL, Lovelace RE, Gambi D: The sympathetic skin response: normal values, elucidation of afferent components and application limits. J Neurol Sci 1988;87:299–306.

142. Shahani BT, Day TJ, Cros D, Khali N, Kneebone CS. RR interval variation and the sympathetic skin response in the assessment of autonomic function in peripheral neuropathy. Arch Neurol 1990;47:659–664.

143. Laumans EPJ. Nerve excitability in facial paralysis. Arch Otolaryngol 1965;81:478–485.

144. Saade B, Karem F. Simple electrodiagnostic test for Bell's palsy. JAMA 1966;195:824–826.

145. Alford BR, Weber SC, Session RB. Neurodiagnostic studies in facial paralysis. Ann Oto Rhino Laryngol 1970;79:227–234.

146. Adour KK, Winegerd J, Bell DN, Manning J, Hurley JP. Prednisone treatment for idiopathic facial paralysis. New Engl J Med 1972;287:1268–1272.

147. Devi S, Challenor Y, Duarte N, Lovelace RE. Prognostic value of minimal excitability of facial nerve in Bell's palsy. J Neurol Neurosurg Psychiatry 1978;41:646–652.

148. Miglietta O. Nerve motor fiber characteristics in chronic ischemia. Arch Neurol 1966;14:448–453.

149. Ricker V, Hopf HC. Die Leitgeschwindigkeit rasch und langsam leitender Motoneurone der langen Beinnerven beim Menschen. Z EEG EMG 1971;2:125–132.

12

Nonphysiological Factors Affecting Nerve Conduction

There are many factors which introduce variables into nerve conduction. Most of these factors are avoidable; others are not. If they are not understood or avoided, they can easily lead to erroneous results and misdiagnosis. These factors can be grouped into four general categories: technical factors, physiological factors, instrumental factors, and anatomical factors. Anatomical factors are mainly related to anomalous innervations, which are discussed in Chapter 14.

Instrumental Factors

Modern electromyography (EMG) equipment should be properly maintained and calibrated to minimize nerve conduction error caused by equipment malfunction. The most common source of error in the EMG machine is the misreading of the electronic latency indicator, which automatically shows the latency of the potentials when the marker is set at any particular point of the potentials. Clearly, this method has eliminated many sources of errors associated with the old reading method (1, 2). However, to obtain an accurate latency reading, the electronic latency indicator should be checked routinely at regular intervals against the known calibration of the machine. A high index of suspicion should exist if the conduction values contradict what appears to be present clinically.

Technical Factors

The great majority of errors in nerve conduction are due to technical factors (3). In nerve conduction evaluations, we compare the measured nerve conduction values with values obtained from a normal control. For these comparisons to have any meaning, it is imperative that nerve conduction studies be performed according to a standardized technique under the same technical conditions. Any change in technical detail will give different values, as discussed below.

Stimulation

Needle Versus Surface Electrodes

There is no significant difference in motor nerve conduction velocity (NCV) whether stimulation is made with surface or needle electrodes (4). When stimulating with surface electrodes, it is difficult to localize the exact point of stimulation. With needle electrodes this uncertainty is somewhat lessened, and the strength of the stimulus can be reduced about 10 times at the stimulating points. Because of this, the needle electrode has an advantage in that it restricts the spread of the stimulating current to other nerves and eliminates an erroneous estimation of the point of stimulation caused by loose skin. Stimulus interference can be reduced further with the use of bipolar needle electrodes. This technique is especially useful in performing the nerve conduction study over a short segment, e.g., mixed nerve conduction across the elbow (5). The needle electrode is also useful when stimulating a deeply located nerve, e.g., the sciatic nerve in the sciatic notch.

Size of the Surface Electrode

Carpendale (6) found no difference in latency of the compound muscle action potential (CMAP) when stimulating with a circular surface cathode 6 or 20 mm in diameter when the electrodes were centered on the same point on the skin. He concluded that the effective point of stimulation corresponded to the center of the electrode.

Polarity Change of the Electrodes

The change of the stimulus polarity along the nerve results in a change in conduction time of about 0.5 msec in median and ulnar motor nerve conduction (4). With a conduction velocity of 56–68 m/sec, this would correspond to a displacement of the site of stimulation of 28–34 mm, a value that is in reasonable agreement with the 25 mm between the stimulating electrodes. This indicates that although the exact point of stimulation is unknown, the nerve is stimulated within a few millimeters of the cathode. Thus, measurement of the distance from cathode to cathode gives a satisfactory approximation of the conduction distance. It also indicates that *there is no evidence of anodal block when the cathode is placed proximally in motor nerve conduction studies;* the threshold is about the same with both types of stimulation, as are the amplitudes of the CMAP evoked by supramaximal stimuli (4). The same principle applies in the orthodromic sensory nerve conduction study, but we have noticed a difference in the amplitude of the compound nerve action potential (CNAP) when stimulating the digital segments in the median and ulnar nerves (Fig. 12.1). When the cathode is placed distally on the finger, the amplitude is lower, most likely because of stimulation of the thinner sensory fibers.

Monopolar Versus Bipolar Surface Electrodes

If an active electrode is placed over the nerve and a reference electrode at some distance from the stimulated nerve, the conduction velocities differ slightly from those obtained with bipolar stimulation in motor conduction studies. Henriksen (7) found a mean difference of ±0.9 m/sec (range −4.4 to 5.1 m/sec.). On the other hand, Gilliatt et al. (8) found that the CNAP latency was unaffected by changes in the position of the reference electrode with stimulation by surface electrodes. They concluded that *nerve impulses are in fact initiated close to the cathode* and not at some point between the cathode and anode. In practice, bipolar electrodes with an interelectrode distance of 2.5–3.0 cm are recommended for surface stimulating electrodes.

Distance of the Stimulating Electrode from the Nerve

Hodes et al. (9) called attention to the importance of placing the stimulating surface electrodes as near as possible to the nerve to avoid spread to other nerves. Henriksen

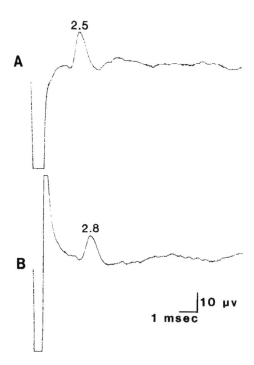

Figure 12.1. Effect of polarity change in sensory nerve conduction. **A**, Proximal electrode is active (cathode). **B**, Distal electrode is active (cathode). Note that there is longer latency (0.3 msec) compared with **A**. If this was not recognized, the NCV would have been slower by 10 m/sec. Numbers represent the negative peak latency in milliseconds.

(7) found a maximum difference of 0.3–0.4 msec in the latency of the motor response when placing the surface electrodes 1–5 cm from the nerve measured perpendicularly. This kind of error can be avoided by placing the active stimulating electrode on the nerve itself.

Stimulus Strength

To obtain meaningful nerve conduction values, supramaximal stimulation is essential. Supramaximal stimulus can be achieved by increasing the intensity by 25–30% above the maximal stimulation. The amplitude and latency of the potentials are affected by the intensity of the stimulus.

With a gradual increase in the stimulus intensity, the amplitude of potentials increases continuously up to the maximum (the maximal stimulation) and then does not increase with further stimulation (supramaximal) (Fig. 12.2). This has been observed in motor as well as sensory nerve conduction with surface and needle recording electrodes (10–13).

On theoretical grounds one would expect the largest fibers to have the lowest threshold and the highest conduction velocity. If this were true, the fastest fibers would be selectively excited with a threshold stimulus, the slower fibers being recruited progressively with the increasing strength of the stimulus. This was found not to be the case (14–16). Dawson (14) observed that *with a gradual increase of stimulus intensity there is a continuous decrease in latency,* which becomes still shorter after the muscle action potential has ceased to increase in amplitude. Preswick (16) compared motor latencies of the median nerve stimulated at the wrist with threshold and supramaximal stimuli in 25 control subjects. With threshold stimuli the mean motor latency was 3.88 ± 0.53 msec, and with supramaximal stimulation the mean latency was 3.33 ± 0.46 msec. The difference between these means was highly significant ($p < 0.001$). This difference is caused by spread of the stimulus from the cathode when strong stimuli are used. Gassel (15) observed that a submaximal motor response might have a considerable delay in latency, and that this occurred with percutaneous as well as needle-stimulating electrodes. In a sensory nerve conduction study with surface recording electrodes, Gilliatt

Figure 12.2. Amplitude change of the sensory CNAP with change of the stimulus intensity. Stimulus duration is 0.05 msec. The stimulus intensity is given at the right of each recording. Note that the amplitude increases with increasing intensity. The shortening of latency is not demonstrated in this figure.

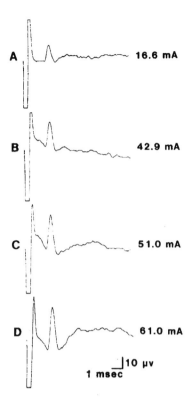

et al. (8) observed similar findings. They found that *the latency of the sensory nerve conduction was shorter with a supramaximal than with a near-threshold stimulus* in six subjects. The difference in latency ranged from 0.05 to 0.15 msec, the mean difference being 0.11 msec. Buchthal and Rosenfalck (11) confirmed this finding in the sensory nerve conduction with the needle recording electrode. With an increase of the stimulus from 10 to 20 mA, the latency at the wrist decreased 1–2%; and with a further increase of the stimulus from 20 to 60 mA, the latency at the wrist decreased an additional 2–5%. They also concluded that this is caused by proximal displacement of the site of stimulation with the supramaximal stimulus intensity.

Stimulus Duration

To reduce the stimulus artifact, the stimulus duration should be as short as possible. The supramaximal stimulus intensity increases with decreasing stimulus duration. *Regardless of the stimulus duration, as long as the supramaximal stimulus is obtained, there is no difference in the latencies.*

"H-Reflex" after Inadequate Stimulation

The H-reflex is consistently obtained without any special facilitation technique from the gastrocnemius-soleus muscle in normal adults. However, the H-reflex can also be obtained in other muscles but usually with some facilitation techniques (See Chapter 17). Because it is elicited by subthreshold stimulation, it may be misinterpreted as being a greatly delayed CMAP if the stimulus is less than threshold level.

Spread of the Stimulus

The spread of the stimulus to a nerve other than that over which the electrode is placed can be an easy source of error in motor nerve conduction studies. It is a rare event under normal stimulation conditions (15), but is not uncommon when a high stimulus intensity is used in patients with nerve lesions (Fig. 12.3). A stimulus may spread to the ulnar nerve after stimulation over the median nerve at the wrist with needle or surface

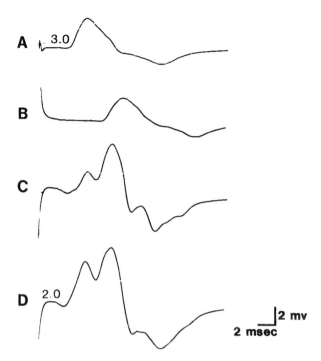

Figure 12.3. "Spread effect" of a strong stimulation intensity on the CMAP. The recording electrode is on abductor pollicis brevis in a case with mild carpal tunnel syndrome. **A**, CMAP with wrist stimulation on the median nerve (0.1 msec stimulus duration). **B**, CMAP with elbow stimulation on median nerve (0.1 msec duration). **C**, CMAP with wrist stimulation on the ulnar nerve (0.1 msec duration), **D**, CMAP with wrist stimulation on the median nerve with a stimulus duration of 0.2 msec. This CMAP is "volume conducted potential" from the ulnar-nerve-innervated thenar muscles activated by the ulnar nerve stimulation via spread of a strong stimulus from the median nerve. Note the initial positive deflection and shortening of terminal latency. The numbers on **A** and **D** represent the terminal latency in milliseconds.

electrodes in patients with carpal tunnel syndrome. Gassel (15) observed a similar spread in a few patients with lesions of the median nerve in the forearm. Stimulus-spread to the median nerve on stimulation over the ulnar nerve at the wrist was found in patients with an ulnar nerve lesion at the elbow. Spread of a stimulus to the ulnar nerve on stimulation of the median nerve at the elbow is common in patients with severe carpal tunnel syndrome in whom a strong stimulus is needed to elicit the response through the compressed carpal tunnel. In this situation, a spurious faster or near-normal motor NCV may be reported if the spread is not recognized.

Another possible error is that this stimulus-spread is interpreted as the Martin-Gruber anastomosis. In case of stimulus-spread, there is no substantial difference in the amplitude of CMAP with wrist and elbow stimulation of the ulnar nerve. On the other hand, in the Martin-Gruber anastomosis the combined amplitudes of proximal median and ulnar stimulation should be approximately equal to the amplitude of the wrist ulnar stimulation (see Chapter 14). Spread of the stimulus on more proximal stimulation in the axilla or supraclavicular region is frequent because of the proximity of the median and ulnar nerves (Fig. 12.4). This is especially crucial in segmental motor and mixed nerve conduction studies across the thoracic outlet in cases of thoracic outlet syndrome in which the ulnar nerve is selectively involved. Careful observation of the contracting muscle in the hand will be of help in deciding whether the ulnar or median nerve is stimulated. This spread of the stimulus is also observed in patients with "Saturday night palsy" when stimulating at the axilla or the Erb's point with the surface electrode. The response on the extensor indicis is due to the spread of stimulus through normal ulnar or median nerves. Thus, if recognized, this spread will also result in faster nerve conduction of the radial nerve. In our experience, it is impossible to obtain any reliable

Figure 12.4. Changing the CMAP by stimulating the wrong nerve. **A**, CMAP from the abductor pollicis brevis with axillary stimulation on the median nerve. **B**, CMAP from the same recording electrode with axillary stimulation on the ulnar nerve. Note the initial positive deflection and two peaks in the negative deflection.

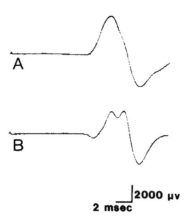

response from the extensor indicis by stimulating at the axilla or Erb's point in patients with Saturday night palsy. Stimulus-spread involving the common peroneal nerve after high-intensity stimulation of the posterior tibial nerve in the popliteal fossa was a frequent occurrence in Gassel's study (15). Spread of the stimulus did not occur upon stimulation at the capitulum fibulae or ankle. Stimulus-spread should be suspected when *there is a sudden change in the shape of the CMAP or the initial positive deflection of the CMAP*. Stimulus-spread should be confirmed by stimulating the neighboring nerve suspected of the spread. This will show a potential identical to that caused by the spread of the stimulus.

Stimulation of a Nerve Other Than the One Intended

This problem occurs in the orthodromic sensory nerve conduction when ring electrodes are used for stimulation on fingers or toes. Ring electrodes on the great toe stimulate the superficial peroneal, deep peroneal, and medial plantar nerves. Ring electrodes on the thumb stimulate the radial and median nerves simultaneously. This is not a source of error as long as the sensory CNAP is recorded at a location far from the other nerve, e.g., at the ankle posterior to the medial malleolus in the median plantar nerve. However, with proximal recording, e.g., at the popliteal fossa or axilla, this creates a problem. Trojaborg and Sindrup (17) estimated that 25% of the sensory potential over the radial nerve at the wrist and elbow and 50% at the axilla were due to spread from median nerve fibers when stimulating the thumb. Thus, it is always prudent to stimulate individual nerves separately if possible.

Recording

Recording methods used in motor nerve conduction studies are vastly different from those used in sensory or mixed nerve conduction studies. This subject is discussed in detail in the following sections.

Motor Nerve Conduction

Needle Versus Surface Electrodes This subject has been well studied by Kaeser (18). With surface electrodes, the amplitude of the CMAP gives a rough estimation of the number of muscle fibers that respond to nerve stimulation (Table 12.1). If the electrodes are arranged in the belly-tendon position with one electrode overlying the endplate region and the other over the tendon, *the CMAP has a simple diphasic shape with an initial negative deflection. Thus, the surface electrode is the only reliable method for documenting the conduction block and the decremental response in the repetitive nerve stimulation, and is an objective measurement of the progressive degeneration of motor nerves. It is also useful for identifying the volume-conducted potential by the initial positive deflection.* Obviously, surface electrodes provide the advantage of nontraumatic recordings and less risk of infection, particularly in patients with hepatitis, Jakob-

Table 12.1.

Comparison of Surface and Needle Recording Electrodes in Motor Nerve Conduction Studies

Measurement	Surface Electrodes	Needle Electrodes
Amplitude	Rough estimation of the total number of muscle fibers responding to stimulation	Estimation of the fractional number of muscle fibers responding to stimulation
Latency	Latency of the fastest motor fibers	The latencies change depending on the site of the needle
Shape	Simple diphasic potentials with the initial negative deflection in the belly-tendon method	Triphasic or tetraphasic potentials with inconsistent initial deflection
Advantages	1. Can detect: (*a*) conduction block; (*b*) decremental response in the repetitive nerve stimulation; (*c*) the volume-conducted potential 2. Best suited for objective-measurement of progressive degeneration of motor fibers 3. Painless 4. No risk of spreading hepatitis, AIDS, or Creutzfeld-Jakob disease	1. CMAP is obtainable from severely atrophied muscle 2. Latency measurement is easier because of steeper onset of the potential 3. Interference from the stimulus artifact is diminished 4. Inteference of the potentials from other muscles is nonexistent
Disadvantages	1. Inability to record CMAP from severely atrophied muscles	1. Painful 2. Risk of spreading hepatitis, Creutzfeld-Jakob disease, or AIDS

Creutzfeldt disease, or AIDS. On the other hand, surface electrodes have a disadvantage in that they may evoke no response from severely atrophied muscles.

With needle electrodes the amplitude of the CMAP does not measure the entire number of muscle fibers responding to nerve stimulation. It records the response from a more limited area of the muscle. This makes the needle electrodes unsuitable for objective measurement of progressive degeneration of motor fibers, localizing a conduction block, and testing neuromuscular transmission. The shape of the CMAP is more complex than that obtained with surface electrodes. *The initial deflection of the potential is not always negative.* The latency varies with the position of the needle electrode. If the needle is not inserted in the end-plate region, a slowing of nerve conduction may be stimulated by the slow conduction in the muscle fibers (4–6 m/sec) (19, 20).

Needle electrodes also have certain advantages. For example, the stimulus artifact that may interfere with the beginning of the CMAP is diminished. Moreover, the steeper onset of the CMAP makes the latency measurements easier than with surface electrodes. Interference from other muscle groups is diminished, which is important when recording from proximal muscles. Even in severely atrophied muscles, it is possible to measure the latency of the muscle response.

In spite of this, it is clear that there are more advantages with surface electrodes than with needle electrodes. Therefore, we prefer the surface electrodes for motor nerve conduction studies.

Size of the Recording Electrodes Henriksen (7) used four sizes of recording surface electrodes: 3, 10, 30, and 40 mm diameter. The conduction time from elbow to hand was not influenced to any significant extent by the size of the electrode, but the amplitude was largest with the smaller electrode. Wee and Ashley found similar results: the latency is unchanged, and the CMAP amplitude decreased with increasing electrode size (21).

Position of the Recording Electrode Standard anatomical locations of recording electrodes provide reproducible potentials that can be compared with normal values. CMAP measurements are most reliable when recordings are made over the end-plate region of the muscle, near the middle of the muscle belly. The recommended positions

Figure 12.5. Changing the CMAP by changing the recording sites. **A**, CMAP from the motor point of the abductor hallucis muscle. **B**, By moving the recording electrode slightly forward away from the motor point, the CMAP shape changes, now with initial positive deflection. The latency and amplitude are not changed.

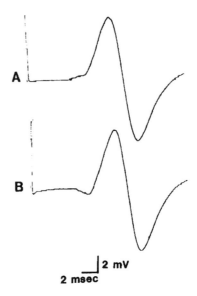

of the recording electrodes are as follows: *the active electrode is placed over the end-plate region and the reference electrode is placed over the tendon (belly-tendon method)*. Henriksen (7) registered the CMAP with surface electrodes in six positions over the hypothenar eminence. When the position of the belly electrodes were changed, the shape and amplitude of the CMAP varied considerably (Fig. 12.5). When the latency was measured to the first positive or negative deflection, the maximum difference was 0.36 msec (range 4.95–5.31 msec). This delay was caused by conduction along muscle fibers. Pinelli (22) showed that the latencies to different motor units in the hypothenar muscle vary from −1.7 to 2.25 msec because of the arrangement of the motor end-plates and the differences in the motor nerve terminals. He found no significant difference in conduction velocities to different motor units, but there were variations of 0.6–2.4 msec in the residual latency.

Sensory Nerve Conduction

Needle Versus Surface Electrodes This subject is discussed in Chapter 15 (Table 15.1).

Orthodromic Versus Antidromic Methods With the orthodromic measurement of sensory NCV, first described by Dawson in 1956 (14), the impulses generated by stimulation travel in the direction in which sensory nerves normally conduct, from the periphery toward the center. Sears (23) was the first to record a diphasic potential from the fingers evoked by stimulation at the wrist. It was identified as an antidromic sensory conduction because the nerve fibers examined conducted in a direction opposite from normal.

Buchthal and Rosenfalck (11) compared the antidromic with the orthodromic sensory nerve potentials. *Recorded with surface electrodes, the antidromic response is larger than the orthodromic* because the digital nerves are nearer the surface than are nerves at the wrist (Fig. 12.6). On the other hand, *the antidromic response is smaller than the orthodromic when recorded with needle electrodes.* Comparing antidromic responses recorded bipolarly with orthodromic responses recorded unipolarly, *antidromic and orthodromic conduction times are identical within the range of error of the method, provided that the stimulating current is just supramaximal for orthodromic stimulation.* When successively stimulating at the wrist, elbow, and axilla, and when the antidromic sensory response can be distinguished from the motor response, the antidromic NCVs are the same as the orthodromic, but the standard deviations are higher.

The major disadvantages of the antidromic method are that the antidromic sensory

CNAPs are often obscured by the muscle potential from a neighboring contracting muscle, and the late phase of the antidromic CNAP may be distorted by a muscle potential, thus making measurement of the peak-to-peak amplitude impossible (Fig. 12.7). For this reason, antidromic CNAPs may be used only when they occur at stimulation intensities that are subthreshold for the motor fibers or when their latencies are clearly shorter than those of the motor potentials.

As a rule, *the diagnostic yield of the antidromic measurement is poorer than that of the orthodromic measurement.* Ludin et al. (24) compared these two methods in (26) patients with carpal tunnel syndrome; antidromic CNAPs were recorded in only 12 patients, whereas definite orthodromic CNAPs were always found. Because of the technical difficulty described above, *the absence of an antidromic potential should not be regarded as a definite pathological finding in the mixed nerve.*

In a study of 30 patients with minimal and early polyneuropathies, Ludin et al. (25) found that the number of components and the duration of the orthodromic CNAPs were the most sensitive indicators of peripheral nerve disease. The maximum conduction velocity and the potential amplitude proved to be relatively unhelpful. The antidromic recording, which can determine only the maximum conduction velocity, is little suited for the diagnosis of a mild neuropathy. Of 30 patients examined, only eight showed a slowing of the antidromic conduction velocity; in 14 patients it was not possible to record measurable potentials. Using the orthodromic method, on the other hand,

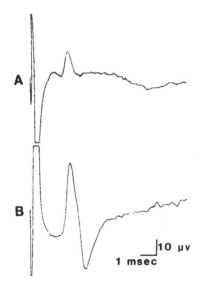

Figure 12.6. **A**, Orthodromic and **B**, antidromic sensory CNAPs. Note the marked difference in the amplitude of CNAP between **A** and **B**. The latency is identical.

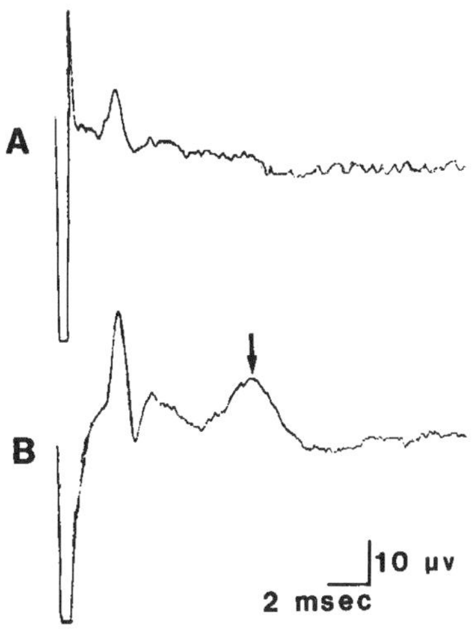

Figure 12.7. Contamination of the CNAP by a muscle artifact. **A**, Orthodromic sural sensory CNAP. **B**, Antidromic sural sensory CNAP followed by a "muscle artifact" *(arrow).* When the CNAP is absent, a muscle artifact" may be mistaken as the CNAP, resulting in the markedly slow sensory NCV.

pathological findings were obtained in 28 of 30 patients. Thus, in patients with early or minimal polyneuropathy, the orthodromic recording is far superior to the antidromic method in confirming the diagnosis. *Therefore, we recommend the orthodromic method for sensory nerve conduction studies whenever possible.*

Distance Between Recording Electrode and Nerve This is a crucial variable because the amplitude of the sensory CNAP decreases progressively as the distance increases. Several studies validate this finding. In one study, with the needle electrode, an increase in depth of 10 mm from the point of maximum amplitude caused the amplitude to fall to one-seventh its former value (11). Thus, the sensory CNAP recorded with a surface electrode was one-third the amplitude recorded with a near-nerve needle electrode in the median nerve at the wrist (26) and one-half the amplitude in the plantar nerve at the ankle (27). Gilliatt et al. (28) also found that with buried needles the amplitude of the mixed CNAP in the peroneal nerve at the fibular head was always greater than that obtained with surface electrodes, the mean increase being 42%. This variable is critical in measuring mixed CNAPs in the axilla or at Erb's point when surface electrodes are used. Because of the loose skin and thick subcutaneous fat in these areas, the distance between the electrode and the nerve becomes variable. Thus, it is important to press the surface electrode tightly to obtain a meaningful amplitude of the CNAP in these areas. When repeated recordings are required on the same individual, surface electrodes give much better reproducibility of the amplitude than needle electrodes because of the considerable changes in amplitude that occur with even small movements of the needle electrode (26).

Distance Between Recording and Stimulating Electrodes Because of different rates of conduction of different-sized myelinated fibers, the CNAP becomes more dispersed as the distance between the recording and the stimulating electrodes is increased. Buchthal and Rosenfalck (11) found that sensory CNAPs recorded with needle electrodes dropped 75% in amplitude in the orthodromic median conduction when the position of the recording electrode was changed from the wrist to the elbow. Using antidromic conduction, Bolton (26) found this drop in amplitude to be approximately 50% when the stimulating electrode was shifted from the wrist to the elbow. Ludin (29) found a longer duration of the sensory CNAP recorded with the needle electrode at the proximal site than at the distal site: The mean duration of the potential at the wrist was 2 msec compared with 4 msec above the elbow in the ulnar nerve.

Bipolar Versus Monopolar Recording In conventional sensory nerve conduction studies, the bipolar recording is used with surface electrodes, whereas monopolar recording is used with the near-nerve needle technique. In a bipolar recording setup, the recording and reference electrodes are placed serially directly over the nerve. In the monopolar recording, instead of placing the reference electrode over the nerve, it is placed away from the nerve at least 30 mm directly lateral to the recording electrode. There is a clear difference in the shape and amplitude of potential between the two recordings (Fig. 12.8). According to Lorente de No (30), the approach of a volley of nerve impulses to an electrode in a volume conductor is signaled by positivity that changes abruptly to negativity as impulses begin to pass under the electrode, and the main negative deflection is followed by a second positive deflection as impulses pass away from the electrode. With needle electrodes, the potential with the monopolar recording is triphasic, with an initial positive deflection in agreement with the volume conduction theory (11, 30). When the two recording electrodes are at the same longitudinal distances from the stimulating cathode, the small potential picked up by the reference electrode does not affect the amplitude or latency of the potential. With bipolar recording, the potential is the algebraic sum of the absolute values of the potential changes occurring at each electrode, depending on the distance between the electrodes and on the conduction velocity. *With a distance of 30–40 mm between electrodes, the bipolarly recorded potential is tetraphasic, the initial positive peak being lower and the amplitude higher than in the monopolar recorded potential. With surface electrodes, similar findings were found* (31).

With surface electrodes, the potentials have been recorded with bipolar placement (8, 14). Gilliatt et al. (8) preferred bipolar recording because it offers much better

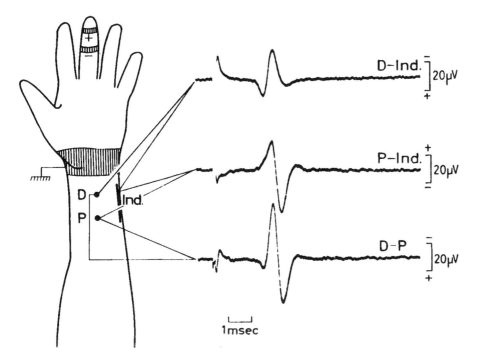

Figure 12.8.   Monopolar and bipolar recorded sensory CNAPs from the median nerve with the near-nerve needle technique. The potentials were successively recorded between an active and a reference electrode (*D-Ind. and P-Ind.,* respectively) and between the two active electrodes (*D-P*). D and P are 30 mm apart at the wrist. The transverse distance to the reference electrode is 35 mm at the wrist and 50 mm at the elbow. Note that the potentials recorded between *P-Ind.* are reproduced with inverted polarity, and that the negative peak in *D-Ind.* is almost simultaneous with the positive peak in *P-Ind.* The stimulus current is 30 mA. The distance from the stimulating cathode at finger III to the leading-off electrode *D* at the wrist is 15 cm. (From Buchthal F, Rosenfalck A. Evoked action potentials and conduction velocity in human sensory nerves. Brain Res 1966;3:24).

rejection of random activity derived from muscle in subjects who do not relax well during the procedure. Under these conditions, the potential often appears with two phases because the small initial and terminal phases cannot be discriminated from noise. The peak of the negative deflection is therefore used as a point of reference to calculate the conduction velocity. This method gives lower values because the bipolar recorded negative peak nearly coincides with the initial positive peak of the potential recorded on the proximal electrode in the monopolar recording.

Distance Between Active and Reference Electrodes   This subject was studied by Gilliatt et al. (8) using surface electrodes. As the interelectrode distance was reduced, they made the following observations: (*a*) the latency to the negative deflection and to the second positive deflection becomes shorter; (*b*) the amplitudes of the initial positive deflection and of the negative deflection decrease; (*c*) the latency to the initial positive peak is independent of the interelectrode distance; and (*d*) with decreased interelectrode distance (less than 3 cm) a diphasic potential is noted. The initial and terminal phases are canceled out. Anderson found similar findings with the orthodromic sensory CNAP (31). He emphasized that there is *no change in sensory NCV* with interelectrode distance. This is because there is no change in the latency to the initial positive peak. Further, he found that the duration of CNAP is longer with greater interelectrode distance but that the rise time is less influenced by different interelectrode distance than the duration. There was no significant difference between 30 mm and 40 mm recording with regard to the peak-to-peak amplitude and rise time. Wee and Ashley found similar results with the antidromic CNAP (32). *In practice, it is important to fix the interelectrode distance in every laboratory and use the fixed distance as the routine. In the UAB EMG laboratory, the 3-cm distance is used.* In that vein, some recommend the use of surface electrodes that are fixed in a saddle that is strapped to or held against the limb instead of electrodes that are individually taped to the skin (33). It is reassuring to know there is no significant difference in the latency, amplitude, or NCV as long as the interelectrode distance is kept between 30 and 40 mm.

Ludin and Tackmann (34) reported similar findings with bipolar needle electrode recordings. Buchthal and Rosenfalck (11) studied the relationship between the CNAPs and the interelectrode distance with needle electrodes. They found that the potentials picked up by the reference electrode placed at transverse distances of 50 and 30 mm from the active electrode were only 10% and 20%, respectively, of the potential on the active electrode near the nerve. This indicates that the small potential picked up by the reference electrode does not appreciably affect the amplitude or the latency of the potential as long as the two recording needles are at the same longitudinal distance from the stimulating cathode. They recommend that *the reference electrode be placed subcutaneously 30–50 mm from the active recording needle.*

Size of the Recording Electrode Conventionally, surface electrodes of 9 mm diameter have been used. Buchthal and Rosenfalck (11) studied the influence of the recording area of the needle electrode. They found that the potentials picked up by the 9-mm long bare tip are 30% lower than by the 1-mm long bare tip. They chose the 3-mm bare tip as an active electrode because there was no difference in amplitude of potential between the 1-mm and 3-mm bare tip, and the difference in distance from the nerve causes less variation in amplitude with the 3 mm bare tip.

Measurement of Latency and NCV

Motor Nerve Conduction

The CMAP evoked by nerve stimulation is often preceded by a small negative wave that may obscure the onset of the CMAP (Fig. 12.9), creating a possible source of error

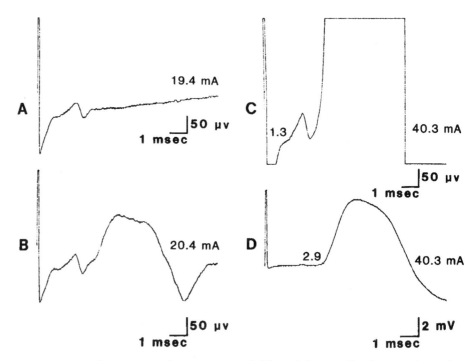

Figure 12.9. Small CNAP preceding CMAP recorded from abductor pollicis brevis with stimulation at the wrist. *A*, CNAP is recordable with a subthreshold (motor) stimulus. *B*, CNAP recorded with a threshold stimulus. *C*, CMAP with supramaximal stimulation. The CNAP is still recordable at the higher sensitivity. *D*, CMAP at low sensitivity. The CNAP is not recognizable at this sensitivity. The numbers at the right of each tracing represent the stimulus intensity in milliamperes. Stimulus duration is 0.05 msec. The number on *C* is the onset latency of the CNAP. The number on *D* is the terminal latency.

when measuring latency (13). This phenomenon was observed in median (12, 35) and ulnar (13) motor nerve conduction. Although Buchthal and Rosenfalck (11), using concentric recording electrodes, suggested that it is derived from motor axons, subsequent studies (13, 35) clearly showed that this small potential represents an antidromically activated sensory CNAP that is picked by the recording electrode. They showed that the threshold of this small potential is constantly below the motor threshold. Fiaschi (35) showed that the sensory CNAP in the median nerve is conducted in volume from the palmar branch of the thumb.

With high sensitivity, Fiaschi (35) was able to recognize this small potential in all of 12 normal individuals in a median motor nerve conduction study, indicating that this is a common occurrence with a high-sensitivity setup. If the sensitivity is changed because the CMAP from one point on the nerve is smaller, this early wave may be taken as the onset of CMAP to one stimulus and not to the other; then, a false NCV may be calculated. Provided it is included in both measurements, no difficulty arises in calculating NCV, as this early wave appears to precede the main deflection by a constant amount (13). It obviously affects the interpretation when only a terminal latency is available, as in the carpal tunnel syndrome (36).

Sensory Nerve Conduction

There are two ways to measure the latency in the sensory nerve conduction studies. As discussed earlier, the approach of a volley of nerve impulses to an electrode in a volume conduction is signaled by positivity, which changes abruptly to negativity as impulses begin to pass under the electrode. If this is the case, it seems reasonable to measure the latency of this point when estimating conduction time for the fastest fibers contributing to the nerve potential, the peak of the initial positive deflection. In fact, Buchthal and Rosenfalck (11) measured the latency to the first positive peak of the unipolarly recorded potential and termed it the maximum NCV. This was possible because the initial positive peak of the potential is prominent when the near-nerve needle technique is used. As discussed previously, this approach is difficult with surface electrodes because of the frequent absence of the initial positive peak.

To circumvent this problem, the onset of the negative deflection or the peak of the negative deflection is used as a point of reference for the latency measurement with surface electrodes. The negative onset used as a point of reference when recording with bipolar surface electrodes is at least 0.4 msec later than the initial positive peak, the delay depending on the distance between the electrode and the nerve and the degree of temporal dispersion. In many laboratories, including our own, the latency is measured to the peak of the negative deflection of the CNAP because it is often difficult to identify the onset of the negative deflection when the potential is small, as noted in most cases where pathology is present. Measurement to the peak of the negative deflection gives more reliable and reproducible results than those obtained by measuring to the onset of the negative deflection according to our data: the standard deviation is wider in the latency to the onset of the negative deflection. There is at least a 0.7 msec difference in latency between the two methods and about a 10 m/sec difference in sensory NCV (27). It should be remembered that the initial positive peak latency represents the conduction velocity of the fastest fibers, and the negative peak latency represents the average conduction of the group Ia fibers. *One advantage of the negative peak latency is that it gives an indication of temporal dispersion because it includes the rise time of the CNAP.*

Using the near-nerve needle technique, it is not uncommon to record a sensory CNAP with many components in patients with peripheral nerve pathology. With such a potential, there could be uncertainty as to whether the maximum NCV should be calculated from the latency of the first positive component even when it is smaller than subsequent ones. Buchthal et al. (36) reported that in cases of carpal tunnel syndrome this uncertainty was observed only when there was marked slowing from digit to wrist, and then both the first and the larger component were so much delayed that the NCV, no matter how calculated, was much slower than normal. This indicates that this situation occurs only in cases of peripheral nerve pathology and, in practice, does not impose any difficulty in the final interpretation of data. Thus, Buchtahl and Rosenfalck (11) recommend that the latency be measured to the first positive peak of the potential, which may or may not be the main component.

This uncertainty could be more disturbing when NCV is calculated from distal to proximal points because components differing in latency may represent different fibers at two points. Buchthal et al. (36) observed that, calculated from the latency of the first component, nine of 144 sensory NCVs from wrist to elbow in cases with carpal tunnel were faster than are found in normal nerve and are hence erroneous.

To avoid this uncertainty, we prefer to measure the latency to the largest positive or negative peak of the CNAP. This is based on our experience in a few cases of tarsal tunnel syndrome in which the NCV calculated from the latency of the first positive component is normal, while the NCV based on the largest positive peak is slower than normal.

Gilliatt et al. (8) compared NCVs obtained by the subtraction method versus the direct latency method. First they stimulated the fingers and recorded the CNAPs at the wrist and elbow in the median nerve. The conduction time between the wrist and elbow was obtained by subtracting the latency to the wrist from the latency to the elbow. This conduction time was compared with the conduction time (latency), which was obtained directly from the potential at the elbow after stimulation of the median nerve at the wrist. There was no consistent difference between the conduction time obtained by subtraction and that measured directly. The mean difference between the two methods was 0.01 msec. Assuming the distance between the wrist and elbow to be 25 cm, the mean NCV difference would be 0.1 m/sec. These results suggest that *no significant error is introduced if the conduction velocity is estimated from a direct latency measurement rather than by subtraction.* We, like Buchthal and Rosenfalck (11), prefer the conduction velocity estimated from the direct latency measurement because we do not have to standardize the distance, and the procedure is much simpler.

Mixed Nerve Conduction

In the past, a number of investigators have used the conduction time of nerve potentials evoked by supramaximal stimulation of mixed nerves as a measure of sensory conduction (37, 38). This method is based on the assumption that the fastest sensory fibers conduct faster and have a lower threshold than the motor fibers. This issue was studied by Gilliatt et al. (8) and by Buchthal and Rosenfalck (11). Gilliatt et al. (8) were unable to stimulate sensory fibers at the wrist without also exciting some motor fibers in the mixed ulnar nerve, where they found a lower threshold in sensory than in motor nerves. Buchthal and Rosenfalck (11) compared the threshold of the antidromic sensory potential with that of the muscle potential in the median nerve at the wrist. Antidromic sensory responses had a lower threshold than motor responses in 56% of 55 digital nerves when the stimulus was applied at the wrist, and in 40% of 37 nerves when the stimulus was applied to the elbow or axilla. These studies show that *the mixed nerve conduction should not be used to measure sensory nerve conduction.* McQuillen and Johns (39) stated that only one-fourth of the mixed CNAP is derived from sensory fibers and that the remaining three-fourths is contributed by motor fibers.

The advantage of the mixed CNAP is obvious because the potential evoked at the elbow when stimulating at the wrist is larger than when stimulating the fingers percutaneouly. We found that mixed nerve conduction is as sensitive an indicator as sensory nerve conduction in the detection of early peripheral lesions, and we have thus continued to use it in routine studies. Because both are CNAPs, anything that affects the CNAPs and conduction also affects the mixed CNAPs and conduction.

Distance

The accurate measurement of distance is one of the two most important factors in the determination of NCV. Conduction distances are measured between the center of the stimulating cathode and the center of the active recording electrode using a flexible measuring tape. However, this straight line is only an approximation of the actual course of the nerve. Thus, we are really only *estimating* the approximate NCV since it is impossible to measure the absolute NCV correctly.

Measured Distance Versus Anatomical Distance

Carpendale (6) demonstrated that in the case of the forearm nerves, the distances measured over the skin are 3–8 mm shorter than those measured on the exposed nerve. Henriksen (7) indicated discrepancies of 1 cm. Behse and Buchthal (40) calculated discrepancies of 1% when measuring the peroneal nerve between the capitulum fibulae and the popliteal fossa in adults. Emery (41) and Wagner and Buchthal (42) made a similar study of children and gave the differences between surface measurement and determination of the actual distance on the exposed nerve as 1.3% and 3.0%, respectively. These differences are negligible as long as the segments examined are long enough and the nerve runs almost straight. The differences become critical, however, when the distance concerned is unusually short (less than 10 cm) and in cases where nerves tend to run spirally, e.g., the radial nerve in the upper arm. According to Maynard and Stolov (2), the error in the motor NCV when conduction distances are 10 cm or less is very high, well over 10 m/sec for all velocities of 40 m/sec or more. This represents a potential error of 25%, which is certainly unacceptable. *This is why 10 cm is the shortest acceptable distance for the segmental conduction velocity.* However, shorter distances have been used by several investigators in studies of the sensory nerve conduction in the palm-wrist segment (see Chapter 11).

When the nerve runs spirally, measurement with obstetrical calipers affords better results than tape measurement in estimating the distance along the nerve. In our laboratory, the obstetrical caliper is routinely used to measure the radial nerve across the spiral groove, the brachial plexus across the shoulder girdle, the ulnar nerve across the thoracic outlet, and the plantar nerves across the plantar surface of the foot. Gassel and Diamantopoulos (43) found a variation of no more than 1 cm between the in situ length of the radial nerve and surface measurement with a caliper determined at three postmortem examinations. When the nerve runs straight, as in the ankle-fibular head segment of the peroneal nerve, there is no significant difference between measuring the distance with a surface tape or with a caliper (44).

Position of the Limbs

It is ideal to position the limb so as to give the best approximation of the anatomic length of the tested nerve. In some situations the distance between two anatomical parts differs, depending upon the position of the limb. The best example of this fact is seen in the effect of the position of the elbow on the measurement of ulnar NCV, as studied by Checkles et al. (45). They found that lower conduction values were obtained when ulnar conduction across the elbow was performed with the elbow extended than with the elbow flexed. This slowing of the NCV across the elbow was caused by shortening of the distance in the extended position. They noted that accurate and reproducible values were obtained when the elbow was maintained at 70° of acute flexion. Cadaver dissections demonstrated that the ulnar nerve was folded upon itself when the elbow was extended, but at 70° of acute flexion, the nerve was straightened but not overstretched along its course. In practice, however, it is difficult to perform the test with the elbow in the flexed position. Thus, many investigators (5, 46–48) estimate the NCV of the ulnar nerve across the elbow in the extended position.

The position of the arm is also a problem in measuring the distance across the thoracic outlet: There is a difference when the arm is abducted to 45° or 90°. *Thus, it is important to perform the nerve conduction test using the recommended position of the limbs each time.*

Examiners' Errors

A more serious problem in obtaining accurate NCV results is the examiners' errors. Simpson (13) stated that examiners may differ by up to 1 cm when measuring the distance between two points on a limb if instructed to lay the tape along the course of a nerve. Buchthal and Rosenfalck (11) reported that the distance between two electrodes was reproducible to within 2 mm. A 2-mm difference gives an uncertainty of about 1.5%. Maynard and Stolov (2) reported the mean and standard deviation for the forearm distance measurement among 15 examiners using the flexible metal Lufkin tape rule to be 222.2 ± 1.8 mm. They concluded that the distance error is primarily the result of skin movement rather than of inaccurate reading of the tape measure. To minimize the distance error factor in serial NCV determinations, Halar and Venkatesh (49) devised a stimulating bar made of two semirigid plastic pieces that can be adjusted to the distance obtained at the time of first testing and used repeatedly for serial NCV determinations on the same nerve. In this way they were able to reduce the distance error factor in serial NCV studies. *In practice, it is best to measure the distance from the center of the cathode to the center of the active recording electrode using the recommended position of the limb being tested.*

Machine Setups

A change in the machine setup is a possible source of error when measuring the latency and amplitude of the potentials. Even though EMG machines are built to reproduce a response accurately with different sweep speeds and sensitivity settings, their measurement of these responses is subject to a certain amount of human error unless performed on a machine that automatically measures both amplitude and latency. Because of this, settings should be constant throughout each individual study whenever possible.

Filter

For the motor nerve conduction study, the recommended filter range is 2–10 kHz, and for the sensory and mixed nerve conduction studies 20–2 kHz. These filter ranges have been selected to ensure exact reproduction of the responses. Obviously, a change in the filter range will affect the amplitude and latency. If the change is excessive, the shape and duration of the potentials are also affected. In general, the narrower the frequency limit the greater is the distortion noted in the potentials (Fig. 12.10). In motor conduction, the lower frequency limit affects the amplitude more than the high frequency limit because of the longer duration of the potentials. Stolov (50) found a 22% decrease in the amplitude, 40% narrowing of the negative spike, an extra phase, and an increased duration of the CMAP when the lower frequency was changed from 8 to 80 Hz. On the other hand, with sensory and mixed nerve conduction, the high frequency is more important because of the shorter duration of the potentials.

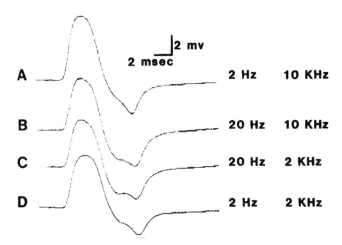

Figure 12.10. Change of the amplitude on the CMAP with a filter change: 19.6% decrease of amplitude between **A** and **D**. Latency is negligible. Hz and kHz represent the filter range.

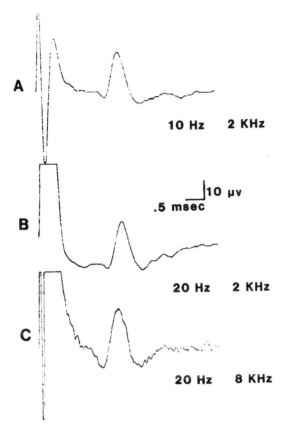

Figure 12.11. Change of the CNAP with the filter change. With the high filter decreased from 8 to 2 kHz, three changes are visible: (*a*) 18% decrease in amplitude; (*b*) 0.075 msec lengthening of latency; and (*c*) elimination of small interferences.

In our experience, reduction of the high-frequency limit decreases the amplitude and increases the latency (Fig. 12.11). When the high-frequency limit was shifted from 8 to 2 kHz, there was about an 18% reduction in amplitude and a 0.08-msec prolongation in latency. Buchthal and Rosenfalck (11) found that in the sensory CNAPs recorded with the near-nerve needle technique, a reduction of the high frequency from 5 to 2 kHz diminished the amplitude recorded at the wrist by only 15%, and the steep positive-negative deflection was prolonged by no more than 0.1 msec; a reduction to 1 kHz reduced the amplitude by 25%. With the near-nerve needle technique, the high-frequency limit might have to be set high to 5–10 kHz to obtain the nerve potentials with many short components. Under pathological conditions, the CNAP may contain components with frequencies of 8–10 kHz. In such instances an excessive lowering of the upper frequency limit causes a reduction in amplitude of these short components. However, it is important to remember that the widening of the frequency range also introduces noise, which may be difficult to eliminate. *In practice, the frequency range should be set as recommended, according to the type of conduction test.*

Change of Sensitivity

With the near-nerve needle technique in sensory nerve conduction, the initial positive peak, used as the reference point for the latency is clearly identifiable. However, with surface recording in motor and sensory conduction, the point of reference for the latency is often curved, making it difficult to decide which point to measure. Recording with high sensitivity minimizes this difficulty but does not remove it. An error can occur when the sensitivity is changed during the performance of a nerve conduction study. Gassel (15) reported a tendency toward a slightly longer latency with low sensitivity than with higher sensitivity (Fig. 12.2). Sensitivity changes can be expected to alter the

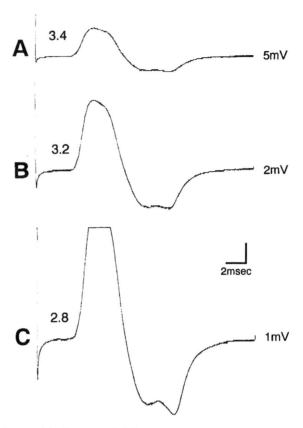

Figure 12.12.   Change of the latency with different sensitivities. Notice that the latency is decreased as the sensitivity increases with 5 mV to 1 mV. This is a CMAP from abductor pollicis brevis with wrist stimulation on median nerve in a normal individual. Numbers above the baseline of each tracing are the terminal latencies.

Figure 12.13.   Change of the latency with different sweep velocities. This is a CMAP from abductor pollicis brevis with wrist stimulation on median nerve in a patient with carpal tunnel syndrome. Numbers above the baseline of each tracing are the terminal latencies.

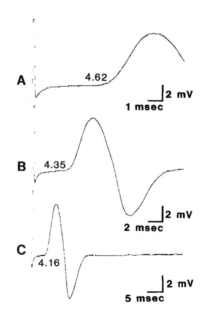

reader's judgment of where a reference point is. *The sensitivity should be consistent for all stimulating sites of a nerve in the same test.*

Change of Sweep Speed

Different sweep speeds can cause differnt latency measurements, which could affect the distal latency and conduction velocity. There is a tendency for a slightly longer latency with higher sweep speed (Fig. 12.13). *The sweep speed should be consistent for all stimulating sites of a nerve in the same test.*

REFERENCES

1. Honet JC, Jebsen RH, Perrin EG. Variability of nerve conduction velocity determinations in normal persons. Arch Phys Med Rehab 1968,49:650–654.
2. Maynard FM, Stolov WC. Experimental error in determination of nerve conduction velocity. Arch Phys Med Rehab 1972;53:362–273.
3. Dumitru D, Walsh NE. Practical instrumentation and common sources of error. Am J Phys Med Rehabil 1988;67:55–65.
4. Trojaberg W. Motor nerve conduction velocities in normal subjects with particular reference to the conduction in proximal and distal segments of median and ulnar nerves. EEG Clin Neuropathol 1964;17:314–324.
5. Nishihira T, Oh SJ. Ulnar neuropathy: an improved method of diagnosis. Arch Phys Med Rehab 1976;57:602.
6. Carpendale MTF. Conduction time in the terminal portion of the motor fibers of the ulnar median peroneal nerves in healthy subjects and in patients with neuropathy. Unpublished Thesis, Mayo Foundation, University of Minnesota, Rochester, 1956.
7. Henriksen JD. Conduction velocity of motor nerves in normal subjects and in patients with neuromuscular disorders. Unpublished Thesis, University of Minnesota, Rochester, 1956.
8. Gilliatt RW, Melville ID, Velate AS, Willison RG. A study of normal nerve action potentials using an average technique (barrier grid storage tube). J Neurol Neurosurg Psychiatry 1965;28:191–200.
9. Hodes R, Larrabee MC, German W. The human electromyogram in response to nerve stimulation and the conduction velocity of motor axons. Arch Neurol Psychiatry 1948;60:340–365.
10. Buchthal F, Rosenfalck A. Action potentials from sensory nerve in man: physiology and clinical application. Acta Neurol Scand 1965;414(Suppl 13):263–266.
11. Buchthal F, Rosenfalck A. Evoked action potentials and conduction velocity in human sensory nerves. Brain Res 1966;3:1–122.
12. Gutmann L. The intramuscular nerve action potential. J Neurol Neurosurg Psychiatry 1969;36:509–513.
13. Simpson JA. Fact and fallacy in measurement of conduction velocity in motor nerves. J Neurol Neurosurg Psychiatry 1964;27:381–385.
14. Dawson GD. The relative excitability of conduction velocity of sensory and motor nerve fibers in man. J Physiol (Lond) 1956;131:436–451.
15. Gassel MM. Source of error in motor nerve conduction studies. Neurology 1964;14:825–835.
16. Preswick G. The effect of stimulus intensity on motor latency in the carpal tunnel syndrome. J Neurol Neurosurg Psychiatry 1963;26:398–401.
17. Trojaborg W, Sindrup EH. Motor and sensory conduction in different segments of the radial nerve in normal subjects. J Neurol Neurosurg Psychiatry 1969;32:354–359.
18. Kaeser HE. Nerve conduction velocity measurements. In: Vinken PJ, Bruyn GW, eds. Handbook of clinical neurology, vol 7. Amsterdam: North Holland Press; 1970:116–196.
19. Buchthal F, Guld K, Rosenfalck P. Innervation zone in propagation velocity in human muscles. Acta Physiol Scand 1955;35:174–190.
20. Buchthal F, Guld K, Rosenfalck P. Propagation velocity in electrically activated muscle fibers in man. Acta Physiol Scand 1955;34:75–82.
21. Wee AS, Ashley RA. Relationship between the size of the recording electrodes and morphology of the compound muscle action potentials. EMG Clin Neurophysiol 1990;30:165–168.
22. Pinelli P. Physical, anatomical, and physiological factors in the latency measurement of the M response. EEG Clin Neurophysiol 1962;17:86.
23. Sears TA. Action potentials evoked in digital nerves by stimulation of mechanoreceptors in the human finger. J Physiol (London) 1959;148:30–31.
24. Ludin HP, Lutschg J, Valsangiacomo F. Vergleichende Untersuchung orthodromer und antidromer sensibler Nervenleitgeschwindigkeiten. 1. Befunde bei Normalen und beim Karpaltunnelsyndrom. Z EEG EMG 1977;8:173–179.
25. Ludin HP, Lutschg J, Valsangiacomo F. Vergleichende Untersuchung orthodromer und antidromer sensibler Nervenleitgeschwindigkeiten. 2. Befunde bei Polyneuropathien und bei status nach Polyradikulitis. Z EEG EMG 1977;8:180–186.
26. Bolton CF. Factors affecting the amplitude of human sensory compound action potentials. AAEE Minimonograph #17, 1981.

27. Oh SJ, Kim HS, Ahmad BK. Electrophysiological diagnosis of the interdigital neuropathy of the foot. Muscle Nerve 1984;7:218–225.
28. Gilliatt RW, Goodman HV, Williamson RG. The recording of lateral popliteal nerve action potentials in man. J Neurol Neurosurg Psychiatry 1961;24:305–318.
29. Ludin HP. Electromyography in practice. Stuttgart: Thieme, 1980.
30. Lorente de No R. Studies from the Rockefeller Institute for Medical Research. New York: Rockefeller Institute, 1947;132:384–477.
31. Anderson K. Surface recording of orthodromic sensory nerve action potentials in median and ulnar nerves in normal subjects. Muscle Nerve 1985:8:402–408.
32. Wee AS, Ashley RA. Effect of interelectrode recording distance on morphology of the antidromic sensory nerve action potentials at the finger. Electromyograph Clin Neurophysiol 1990;30:93–96.
33. Eduardo E, Burke D. The optimal recording electrode configuration for compound sensory action potentials. J Neurol Neurosurg Psychiatry 1988;51:684–687.
34. Ludin HP, Tackmann W. Sensory neurography. New York: Thieme-Stratton Inc., 1981.
35. Fiaschi A. Observations on the sensory nature of the intramuscular nerve action potential. J Neurol Neurosurg Psychiatry 1973;36:509–513.
36. Buchthal F, Rosenfalck A, Trojaborg W. Electrophysiological findings in entrapment of the median nerve at wrist and elbow. J Neurol Neurosurg Psychiatry 1974;7:340–360.
37. Downie AW, Newell DJ. Sensory nerve conduction in patients with diabetes mellitus and controls. Neurology 1961;11:876–882.
38. Mayer RF. Nerve conduction studies in man. Neurology 1963;13:1021–1030.
39. McQuillen MP, Johns RJ. The nature of the defect in the Eaton-Lambert syndrome. Neurology 1967;17:527–536.
40. Behse F, Buchthal F. Normal sensory conduction in the nerves of the leg in man. J Neurol Neurosurg Psychiatry 1971;34:404–414.
41. Emery AW. Conduction velocity in the median nerve of infants and young children, 1963. Unpublished Thesis, British Columbia. Cited in Ludin and Tackmann (34).
42. Wagner AL, Buchthal F. Motor and sensory conduction in infancy and childhood: reappraisal. Develop Med Child Neurol 1972;14:189–216.
43. Gassel MM, Diamantopoulos E. Pattern of conduction times of the radial nerves: a clinical and electrophysiology study. Neurology 1964;14:222–231.
44. Checkles NS, Bailey JA, Johnson EW. Tape and caliper surface measurements in determination of peroneal nerve conduction velocity. Arch Phys Med Rehabil 1969;50:214–218.
45. Checkles NS, Russakov AD, Piero DL. Ulnar nerve conduction velocity—effects of elbow position on measurement. Arch Phys Med Rehab 1971;52:362–365.
46. Eisen A. Early diagnosis of ulnar nerve palsy. Neurology 1974;24:256–262.
47. Miller RG, Hummel EG. The cubital tunnel syndrome: treatment with simple compression. Ann Neurol 1980;7:567–569.
48. Payan J. Electrophysiological localization of ulnar nerve lesions. J Neurol Neurosurg Psychiatry 1969;32:208–220.
49. Halar EM, Venkatesh B. Nerve conduction velocity measurements: improved accuracy using superimposed response waves. Arch Phys Med Rehab 1976;57:451–457.
50. Stolov WC. Instrumentation and measurement in electrodiagnosis. AAEE Minimonograph # 16. Rochester, Minnesota, 1981.

13

Physiological Factors Affecting Nerve Conduction

This chapter discusses the physiological factors that affect the nerve conduction.

Temperature

Among the various physiological factors that affect nerve conduction velocity (NCV), temperature is the most important. Ludin and Tackmann (1) regarded the influence of temperature as the most important source of error.

Nerve Conduction Velocity

The fact that the NCV decreases at lower temperatures was already recognized by Von Helmholtz in 1867 (2). As early as 1925, Rosenberg and Sugimoto (3), working with the sciatic nerve in the frog, observed that conduction velocity decreased from 33 to 5 m/sec as temperatures decreased from 26° to 3.5°C. Tasaki and Fujita (4) and Klensch (5) found that in frog nerve the conduction time as related to temperature followed nearly a straight line between 20° and 5°C. It is known from animal experiments that conduction is eventually completely blocked at low temperatures, the myelinated A fibers being the first affected and the thin fibers of group C the last.

In human nerve conduction, various investigators have reported different values for the rate of increase of NCV per degree (Table 13.1). These studies showed that the NCV increases linearly with the temperature within the physiological range. In motor nerve conduction, the rate of increase ranges from 1.1 to 2.4 m/sec. In sensory nerve conduction with surface electrodes, this rate ranges from 1.2 to 2.3 m/sec. In sensory nerve conduction with needle electrodes, the rate varies from 0.76 to 2.1 m/sec. On the other hand, Todnem et al. found a nonlinear relationship between NCV and temperature: the most pronounced increase of NCV per degree in the nonphysiological 19–25°C range and a less pronounced increase of NCV in the physiological 30–37°C range (6). DeJesus et al. (7) studied the effect of temperature on minimum motor and

Table 13.1.
Relationship Between NCV and Temperature

Investigator	Nerve Tested	Range of Temperature Investigated (°C)	Increase Per Degree (m/sec)
Motor NCV			
Henriksen (70)		29–38	2.4
DeJong et al. (11)	Peroneal	23.5–35	1.8
DeJesus et al. (7)	Median	18–36	2.1
Bolton and Carter (22)	Median	21–31	1.47
Todnem et al. (6)[a]	Median	19–38	0.9–1.4 (20–25°C)
			-0.3–0.4 (30–37°C)
Geerlings (71)	Median	20–34	2.2
Harlar et al. (15)	Posterior tibial	26–32	1.1
Sensory NCV			
With surface electrodes			
Bolton and Carter (22)	Median (orthodromic)	21–31	2.18
	Median (antidromic)	21–31	2.31
Todnem et al. (6)[a]	Median	17–37	1.2–1.9 (20–25°C)
			-0.2–0.6 (30–37°C)
With needle electrodes			
DeJesus et al. (7)	Median	18–36	2.1
Buchthal and Rosenfalck (41)	Median	20–36	2.0
Ludin and Beyler (23)	Median	22–36	1.51
Lowitzsch et al. (72)	Ulnar	20–35	1.3
Alfonsi et al. (26)	Median	20–42	0.76

[a]This study found a nonlinear relationship between the NCV and skin temperature.

sensory NCVs. For the minimum motor NCV, they used a modification of Hopf's method (8, 9). For minimum sensory NCV, the latency was measured to the baseline return of the last component, according to Buchthal and Rosenfalck (10). Although again a linear relationship was observed, the slope of the linear regression line of the fast fibers was steeper than that of the slower fibers (Fig. 13.1). In an attempt to consolidate the findings on fast and slow conduction velocities, these authors found that *the slopes of the regression lines coincided when the semilogarithm of the NCV was plotted against temperature.* This relationship was identical for all motor and sensory fibers. This semilogarithmic relationship between any NCV and temperature formed the basis for a correction formula that could be applied to convert the NCV obtained at one temperature to that at another temperature.

$$Y_2 = Y_1 (Q_{10}) \frac{\Delta T}{10}$$

Q_{10} = ratio of highest to lowest velocity over a 10°C range
Y_2 = corrected velocity as a standard temperature (°C)
Y_1 = observed velocity
ΔT = difference (°C) between standard and observed temperatures

Two variant formulas are as follows. The first, suited to any slide rule possessing an L-scale, is:

$$Y_2 = Y_1 10^{(M_1 \Delta T)}$$

where all symbols have the meanings given above and $M_1 = 0.018$.

The second equation is suitable for calculators having an e^x key:

$$Y_2 = Y_1 e^{(M_2 \Delta T)}$$

where e is the base of the natural log system and $M_2 = 0.0419$.

The averaged Q_{10} for all normalized conduction velocities was 1.51 ± 0.03 over the temperature ranges studied. The Q_{10} in the study of DeJong et al. was 1.6 (11).

These formulas were tested in eight patients who had the NCV determined before

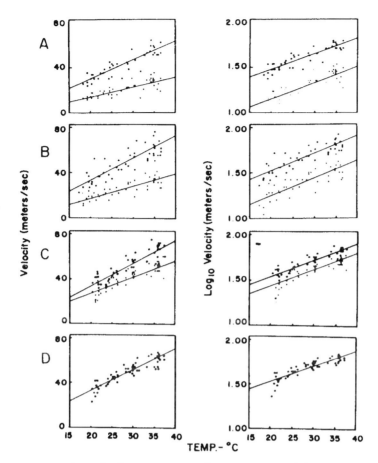

Figure 13.1.   Linear relationship between motor and sensory NCVs and skin temperature. Left column, Arithmetic scale. Right column, semilogarithmic scale. *A*, Thumb to wrist. *B*, Middle finger to wrist. *C*, Wrist to elbow (sensory). *D*, Elbow to wrist (motor). (o)V_{max}, (o)V_{min}. (From DeJesus PV, Hausmanowa-Petrusewicz I, Barchi RL. The effect of cold on nerve conduction of human slow and fast nerve fibers. Neurology 1973;23:1184.)

and after warming of the limbs (7). The NCVs prior to heating were corrected using the formulas above and were found to be close estimates of the postwarming NCVs, indicating the practical usefulness of the formulas. If the temperature had not been determined or the limbs not heated, the slow NCVs in three cases could have been misinterpreted as being caused by pathological conditions. Thus DeJesus's formulas offer a simple method of eliminating diagnostic errors caused by temperature variation of the limbs and require only that the surface temperature be monitored (7).

Skorpil (12) correlated the motor NCV with rectal temperature in three individuals subjected to hypothermia. In the ulnar nerve, the NCV was slowed by an average of 4.6–4.9 m/sec for each degree of decrease in rectal temperature.

Thus, it is clear that temperature variation influences the NCV substantially and that *the NCV increases linearly with the temperature.*

Distal Motor Latency

The distal motor latency is similarly influenced by changes in temperature. Carpendale (13) found that *the distal motor latency increased by 0.2 msec per degree centigrade drop in temperature* between 25° and 35°C in the median and peroneal nerves. DeJesus et al. (7) found that the distal motor latency varied inversely with temperature when the latency was standardized to a mean distance of 6.6 cm. Todnem et al. found a nonlinear increase of the distal latency with a decline in temperature (6). Although the influence of temperature on conduction in the distal segment paralleled that in the main segment of the nerve, the Q_{10} values were slightly higher (1.65 for the distal motor latency versus 1.51 for the maximum motor NCV) when the latency was expressed as "velocity" for the purpose of analysis. The higher Q_{10} for "distal conduction" may have reflected the contribution of events at the neuromuscular junction.

Late Responses

There are only a few studies addressing the effects of temperature on the late responses. A linear increase in the F-wave latency of the median nerve was found with a temperature decline between 17–30°C in 20 subjects (6). There was no significant change in the H-reflex amplitudes measured during the baseline and cooling periods (with an average of 18.4°C decrease in the skin temperature) in 16 subjects (14). Neither was there any significant change in the H-reflex latency from the gastrocnemius muscle between 26–30°C in 25 subjects (15).

Amplitude and Duration of the CMAP

Ricker et al. (16) studied this issue in 25 normal subjects in the temperature range 18–36.6°C and found that *the amplitude of the compound muscle action potential (CMAP) increased* in 24 cases while the isometric twitch force decreased *with lower temperatures*. They concluded that the increase of the CMAP could be caused by the effect of cooling directly at the muscle cell membrane, and the increased twitch by the effect on the contractile apparatus. Similar observations were made by Borenstein and Desmedt (17) in myasthenia gravis patients.

These findings in human subjects are consistent with those in crustacean muscles: Fatt and Katz (18) found that the amplitude of the CMAP clearly increased in crustacean muscle after cooling. Denys (19) showed that *the duration of the CMAP was also increased with lowered temperatures*. DeJesus et al. (7) found that the average duration of the CMAP increased directly with a decrease in temperature.

The explanation proposed for the normal increase in amplitude or surface area of the compound action potential is that cooling has less effect on the initial increase in Na permeability than on subsequent inactivation of Na permeability and increase in K permeability (recovery process). When the recovery process of the action potential is slowed, the amplitude increases (20, 21). An increase in the duration of the compound action potential at the lower temperature is due to the identical Q_{10} figures for the large- and small-diameter fibers (7). Because the entire population of nerve fibers slows proportionally in response to cooling, one would not expect a change in the shape of the evoked response. However, the duration of the evoked response is prolonged. The Q_{10} between 37° and 27°C equals 1.6 for the myelinated fibers of several species (21). Fibers conducting at a speed of 75 m/sec at 37°C therefore conduct at a speed of 72.2 m/sec at 36°C. Over a 50-cm segment, the delay will be increased by 0.25 msec. Also, fibers conducting at 25 m/sec at 37°C will therefore conduct at a speed of 24 m/sec at 36°C. Over the same 50 cm nerve segment the resulting delay will be 0.8 msec. The difference becomes even more significant with slower conducting fibers and lower temperatures.

Latency, Duration, and Amplitude of Sensory CNAPs

With surface electrodes, Bolton et al. (22) found that over physiological temperature ranges (21–31°C), *the sensory compound nerve action potential (CNAP) shows a progressive linear increase in latency, amplitude, duration, and area with decreasing temperature*. The amplitude changes are marked for antidromic CNAPs recorded from the median digital nerves, but for some reason are minor for orthodromic CNAPs recorded from the median nerve at the wrist (Figs. 13.2 and 13.3). The radial CNAP at the wrist recorded antidromically is also sensitive to temperature change. Thus, temperature may be an important variable in amplitude measurement, depending upon the nerve and the type of conduction (22).

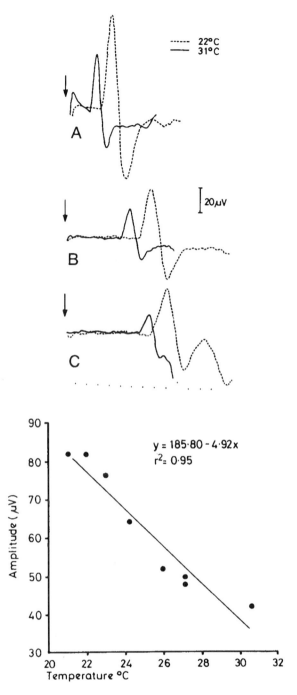

Figure 13.2. Antidromic sensory CNAP (recorded with a surface electrode) of median digital nerves from stimulation at the wrist (*A*), elbow (*B*) and upper arm (*C*) at cool and warm finger temperatures. Note the decrease in the amplitude, duration, and area of the CNAP on more proximal stimulation independent of temperature, but the further decrease in these features at higher temperature. *Dots* in the lower scale are at 1-msec intervals. (From Bolton CF, Carter KM. Temperature effects on the size of human sensory compound action potentials. J Neurol Neurosurg Psychiatry 1981;44:410.)

Figure 13.3. Relationship between the amplitude of the antidromic sensory CNAP (recorded with the surface electrodes) of the median digital nerves of the index finger and rising temperature of the cutaneous surface of that digit in a healthy subject. (From Bolton CF, Carter KM. Temperature effects on the size of human sensory compound action potentials. J Neurol Neurosurg Psychiatry 1981;44:409.)

With needle electrodes, Ludin and Beyler (23) studied these parameters of the sensory CNAPs. The latency, duration (the largest positive-negative deflection), and the potential areas increased linearly between 22° and 36°C as the temperature decreased. Interesting temperature effects on the amplitude were observed. Between 26° and 36°C, the amplitude increased with lowering temperature as noted with surface electrodes. However, between 22° and 26°C, the amplitude decreased with lowering temperature (Fig. 13.4). The decrease of the potential duration is attributed by Ludin and

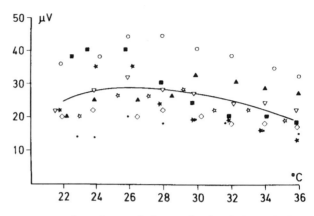

Figure 13.4. Temperature dependence of the amplitude of the orthodromic sensory CNAP (recorded with the near-nerve needle) in the median nerve at the wrist on stimulation at the index finger in eight test cases. (From Ludin HP, Beyler F. Temperature dependence of normal sensory nerve action potentials. J Neurol 1977;216:177.)

Beyler to two different mechanisms. With rising temperature: (*a*) temporal dispersion of the potentials for different fibers becomes smaller; and (*b*) a shortening of the individual spikes occurs. Because dispersion diminishes with increasing temperature, the compound potential amplitude increases. The amplitude increase for temperatures below 25°C is, they explained, caused by decreasing dispersion rather than a real increase in spike height. The negative linear relationship between temperature and duration of sensory CNAP was also observed by DeJesus et al. (7). They did not notice any change in the mean sensory threshold of the thumb or middle finger between 28° and 36°C. The number of potential components was shown to depend relatively little on temperature (1).

Effects of Temperature in Diseased Nerves

Most studies of the relationship between skin temperature and nerve conduction were performed in normal nerves. If the correction formula for temperature is to be used routinely for all cases in the EMG labortory, we have to assume that the effects of temperature in diseased nerves are similar to those in normal nerves. However, diseased nerves may not react in the same way as do normal nerves. Bolton compared the effect of temperature between 23–33°C on the median motor and sensory nerve conduction in 16 normal individuals and in the same number of patients with carpal tunnel syndrome and with uremic neuropathy, respectively (24). In comparison with normal nerves, *there was a tendency for the rate of change with increasing temperature to be less for the sensory CNAP amplitude in patients* with carpal tunnel syndrome and uremic neuropathy and to be greater for the motor distal latency in patients with carpal tunnel syndrome. In uremic neuropathy, the F-wave latency decreased at 3 times the rate in normal individuals or in patients with carpal tunnel syndrome.

Our study in 20 patients with carpal tunnel syndrome yielded the same findings in the CNAP amplitude but not in the distal latency (25). Alfonsi et al. studied this issue in the median sensory nerves in four cases of chronic demyelinating neuropathy associated with paraproteinemia (26) and found the same linear trend of increasing NCV with a temperature rise up to 36°C in both normal and diseased nerves. However, there was a distinct difference between normal and diseased nerves above 36°C: instead of a gradual increase of NCV as noted in normal nerves, there was a decrease of NCV in diseased nerves. At 42°C there was a complete block of nerve conduction in two cases. Unlike normal nerves, there was no increase of CNAP amplitude with a decline of temperature from 36–25°C.

In summary, these studies showed that there are some quantitative differences between normal and diseased nerves in their response to temperature change. This difference is most obvious in the sensory CNAP amplitude. With regard to the NCVs, there is no essential difference. From this we can conclude that *the same NCV correction formula for temperature can be applied to normal as well as to diseased nerves as long as the temperature is within the physiological range up to 36°C.*

Clearly, the skin temperature should be routinely monitored and controlled during nerve conduction tests and taken into account when interpreting the findings. Various methods have been proposed to minimize the temperature variation in nerve conduction:

1. The test should be performed at a standard temperature. This is an ideal method of controlling the temperature effect. The standard temperature in many laboratories is 36–38°C (27–29). It is rare to measure a skin temperature of 36–38° in an individual; it is easy to warm the exposed limb to 36–38°C using a temperature control unit. Although this is the ideal temperature, the method is time-consuming. In our laboratory, skin temperature is controlled at 32°C for the plantar nerve test because the skin temperature of the foot varies enormously from 25° to 32° among individuals.

2. The skin temperature is measured routinely. If it is lower than the controlled temperature, the limb should be warmed to the controlled temperature. In our laboratory, the controlled temperature is 31°C. Normal nerve conduction data were gathered with skin temperatures at 31–34°C. When the skin temperature is lower than 31°C, we warm the area to be tested to 31°C.

3. If the skin temperature is lower than the controlled temperature, the measured NCV may be converted to the correct NCV for the controlled temperature using DeJesus et al.'s correction formula (7). As discussed previously, this formula is applied to the normal as well as diseased nerves as long as the temperature is within the physiological range, up to 36°C. At this time, this is the best alternative if warming is not possible.

4. Before each examination, patients are allowed to adapt to an ambient room temperature, which may vary from 21°C (30) to 30°C (31). Kato (31) suggested that the temperature gradients are greatly reduced when the room temperature is 30°C. Ulnar nerve conduction was 5.3 m/sec faster than at a room temperature of 20°C. DeJesus et al. (7) studied this issue in 44 consecutive patients. Before each examination patients were allowed to adapt to an ambient temperature of 26°C for 30 min. Of 44 patients, 26 (59%) had mean skin temperatures of 25.5–32°C. This study indicates that such a measure alone is not sufficient to control the skin temperature.

In practical terms, we recommend the following:

1. The ambient room temperature should be set at 26°C (78°F). In this way, a majority of patients' skin temperatures are above 31°C.

2. In all nerve conduction studies, the skin temperature should be monitored in the examined areas of the limbs.

3. For routine studies, if the skin temperature is lower than the controlled temperature (above 31°C in our labortory), the area should be warmed to the controlled temperature.

4. If warming is not possible, the measured NCV should be converted to the correct NCV for the standard temperature using DeJesus et al.'s correction formulas (see Chapter 4).

5. For special studies, the skin temperature should be controlled to the standard temperature; e.g., 32°C in plantar nerves in our laboratory; and 35–36° in other EMG laboratories (1, 29).

Age

Age is an important variable in the study of nerve conduction. The changes in the nerve conduction are most impressive in the first few years of life and less marked in later years.

Children Up to 16 Years of Age

Nerve conduction changes in children up to 16 years of age are described in detail in Chapter 8. In short, *the NCVs in motor, sensory, and mixed fibers are about 50% of the normal adult values in the full-term newborn baby, reaching about 75% of the adult value at 1 year of age, and about 100% at 4 years of age.* The motor, sensory, and mixed

NCVs increase in a logarithmic function. By the time a child is 4–6 years old, the NCV has reached values found in young adults. No further increase in the NCV is noted between 4–6 and 16 years of age. The increased NCV during infancy and early childhood is most likely due to two factors: (a) the increase in the number of large fibers between birth and 8 years of age, when the number is the same as in adult nerves (32, 33), and (b) the complete myelination of nerve fibers by 5 years of age (32).

Other than the NCV, the most striking difference in nerve conduction of children and adults is the presence of *"double peaks" in the sensory CNAP in infants and small children,* indicating the presence of two groups of fibers with different degrees of maturation. The double peaks are common in children 3 months to 6 years of age (34). Wagner and Buchthal (33) found that fibers contributing to the second component conducted 20–30% more slowly than the fibers of the first component, and that the amplitude of the second component was 20–30% lower than that of the first component.

Adults

The NCV of motor, sensory, or mixed nerve conduction decreases with age beginning in the twenties (Table 13.2). For motor nerve conduction the rates of decrease in the NCV per decade (Fig. 13.5) range from 0.4 m/sec in the peroneal nerve (29) to 2.3 m/sec in the median nerve (28). For sensory nerve conduction with surface electrodes, the rates range from 2.0 m/sec in the median nerve (35) to 4.0 in the ulnar nerve (36). In sensory nerve conduction with the near nerve needle technique, the rates range from 0.1 m/sec in the ulnar nerve to 1.85 m/sec in the median nerve (28) (Fig. 13.6). In the ulnar nerve the decrease was 1.2 m/sec per decade from 20 to 54 years of age and 3.3 m/sec per decade after age 55 (27). For mixed nerve conduction, the rates were 3.5 m/sec in the ulnar and 4.0 m/sec in the median nerve. In the interdigital plantar nerves of the foot, dramatic slowing of NCV was observed in individuals over 50 years old (37). This may have been caused by subclinical neuropathy of the interdigital nerves in the foot in the older group. From Table 13.2, it is clear that the decreasing rate of the NCV is of the same magnitude in the motor and the sensory NCVs with the near-nerve needle technique. On the other hand, a steeper decrease in NCV is noted in sensory and mixed NCVs with surface electrodes. This relationship between the NCV decline and age is uniformly seen in the proximal as well as in the distal segments of the nerves (1, 28, 29).

Contrary to the predominant view concerning the relationship between age and

Table 13.2.
NCV with Age: Decrease per Decade after Twenties

Nerve	NCV Range (msec)	References
Motor Nerve Conduction		
Median	0.6–2.3	(28, 29, 35)
Ulnar	0.6	(28, 73)
Peroneal	0.4–0.8	(28, 29, 57)
Posterior tibial	1.7	(28)
Sensory Nerve Conduction		
With surface electrodes		
Median, orthodromic	3.0	(36)
Median, antidromic	2.0	(28, 35)
Ulnar, orthodromic	4.0	(36)
With near-nerve technique		
Median	1.8	(27, 28)
Ulnar, up to 54 years	1.2	(27)
Ulnar, over 55 years	3.3	(27)
Ulnar	0.1	(28)
Sural, calf, orthodromic	0.5–1.1	(27, 28)
Mixed Nerve Conduction		
Median	4.0	(36)
Ulnar	3.5	(36)

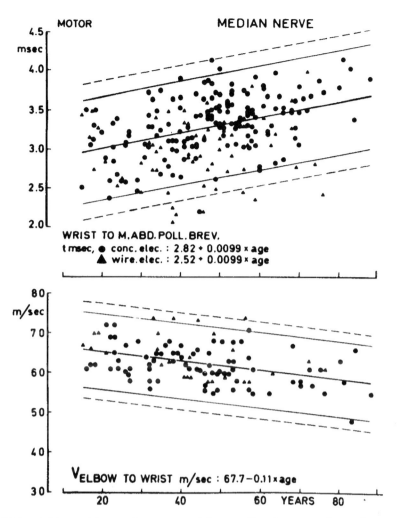

Figure 13.5. **A,** Terminal latency from wrist to abductor pollicis brevis muscle as a function of age. The latencies were corrected to a distance of 6.5 cm. Needle stimulation was applied at the wrist. **B,** Motor NCV from elbow to wrist as a function of age. Needle stimulation at wrist and elbow. The *thick line* is the regression line for values recorded with concentric electrodes. The *solid lines* represent 95% confidence limits, and the *dotted lines* 99% confidence limits. (From Rigshospitalet Laboratory of Clinical Neurophysiology. EMG-Sensory and motor conduction. Findings in normal subjects. Copenhagen, Denmark: RLCN, 1975:29).

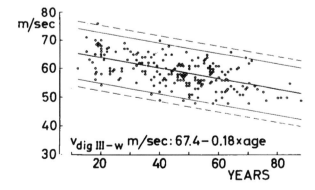

Figure 13.6. Sensory NCV from digit III to wrist with stimulation to digit III. For other explanation, see Fig. 13.5. (From Rigshospitalet Laboratory of Clinical Neurophysiology. EMG-Sensory and motor conduction. Findings in normal subjects. Copenhagen, Denmark: RLCN, 1975:27.)

NCVs, two studies have showed nonlinear effects of age on NCV (38, 39). Wagman and Lesse (38) showed no change in the mean NCV throughout the second to fifth decades with significantly lower values in the sixth to eighth decades. Taylor found that the maximum motor and sensory NCV values are not achieved until the fourth decade, when a progressive decline begins. He stated that the effect of age on the motor and sensory NCVs is represented better by the parabola than the straight line (39).

The distal latency in motor conduction is mildly prolonged with age (Fig. 13.5). In the median nerve, the distal latency was prolonged by 20% in subjects 75–89 years of age compared with those aged 15–24. Taylor did not find any effect of age on terminal latency (39).

The amplitude of the CMAP is also affected by age, showing a gradual decline (Fig. 13.7). This change does not seem to be important in practice because of the wider range of CMAP amplitudes in normal individuals. *The amplitude of the sensory CNAP also decreases with age* (Fig. 13.8). LaFratta (40) reported that the amplitude of sensory CNAPs with surface electrodes decreases as a function of age in man between 23 and 91 years of age. By the age of 60 years, the sensory CNAP amplitude drops by 36%. The amplitude of the sensory CNAP with the near-nerve needle technique decreases linearly in the logarithm with increasing age (1, 27). At 70 years of age, the amplitude was shown to be about half that at 20 years. In the ulnar nerve the decrease in amplitude was greater after 55 years of age than before, probably because of a greater incidence of subclinical damage at the cubital sulcus in older subjects. Similar changes were noted in

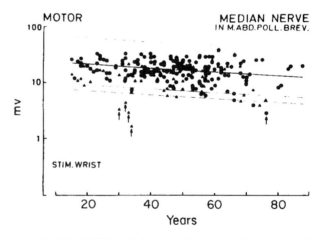

Figure 13.7.   Amplitude of the CMAP in abductor pollicis brevis (log scale) as a function of age. For other explanations, see Fig. 13.5. (From Rigshospitalet Laboratory of Clinical Neurophysiology. EMG-Sensory and motor conduction. Findings in normal subjects. Copenhagen, Denmark: RLCN, 1975:29.)

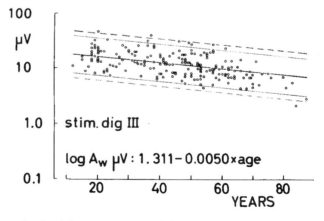

Figure 13.8.   Amplitude of the sensory potential (log. scale) recorded at the wrist as a function of age; the stimulus was at digit III. (From Rigshospitalet Laboratory of Clinical Neurophysiology. EMG-Sensory and motor conduction. Findings in normal subjects. Copenhagen, Denmark: RLCN, 1975:27.)

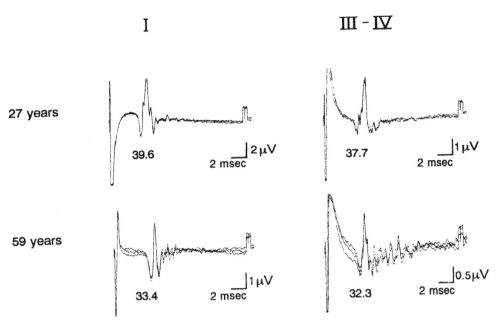

Figure 13.9. The sensory CNAPs of the interdigital nerves recorded with the near-nerve needle technique at the ankle. *I*, The I digital nerve. III-IV, The III-IV interdigital nerves. Note that the CNAPs from the 59-year-old normal control show a prominent abnormal temporal dispersion, a lower amplitude, and a slower NCV. Numbers below the CNAPs represent NCVs in m/sec.

interdigital nerves in the 50- to 59-year-old group: a lower amplitude of potentials and increased temporal dispersion evidenced by the longer duration and the higher number of components (35) (Fig. 13.9). *In older individuals, Buchthal and Rosenfalck (41) also observed a similar increased temporal dispersion.* They reported the duration of the sensory CNAP to be 20–25% longer than in young individuals (41).

In an effort to explain the age-related decrease in the NCV, Lascelles and Thomas (42) and Troghi et al. (43) offered some histological data. They found an increased loss of large fibers, an increased incidence of fibers with segmental demyelination, and a shortening of the internodal segment in the sural nerve of control subjects over 65 years of age. Neary et al. (44) found partial demyelination of the ulnar nerve at the cubital tunnel, which may explain the higher rate of decrease in the ulnar NCV after age 55 years.

From the information given here, it is best to compare all nerve conduction findings in a patient with those from normal nerves matched for age. If such data are not available, the age factors must be considered when interpreting the results. In our laboratory, the normal data have been pooled from normal controls—26–60 years old—with two standard deviations used as the lower or upper limit of the normal nerve conduction values. *When interpreting the results in patients over 60 years of age, 1 m per decade is allowed for the motor NCV and 2 m per decade for the sensory NCV with surface electrodes.*

Proximal and Distal Segments of the Nerve

It has been generally agreed that *the NCV is faster in the proximal segment than in the distal segment of the nerve.* Kaeser (45) compiled data for motor nerve conduction from various sources. According to his data, the NCV in the proximal segment is faster than in the distal segment by 6% in the ulnar nerve and by 12% in the median nerve. A similar difference was observed in the proximal and distal portions of the sciatic nerve (46). For sensory nerve conduction with the near-nerve needle technique, the same proximal-to-distal conduction gradient of NCV was clearly observed in median, ulnar, radial, sural, superficial peroneal, and posterior tibial nerves (1). In the median nerve, the NCV in the forearm is faster by 6% than in the finger-wrist segment (1). No data are available for the sensory nerve conduction with surface electrodes because of the impossibility of recording reliable potentials at the proximal segments of the limbs by stimulating the distal sensory fibers with this technique. However, for mixed nerves the proximal-and-distal gradient of the NCV was documented by Mayer (47), who found the mixed NCV in the upper arm segment to be faster (by 5%) than in the forearm segment in median nerves.

Two factors may explain these findings: (*a*) the temperature gradient along the extremity; and (*b*) a decrease in the average fiber diameter of the fastest conducting fibers because of branching and tapering in the distal parts of the nerve. A temperature difference of approximately 1°C exists between the proximal and distal segments (48, 49), which might explain small differences in velocity. Gasser and Grundfest (50) and Tackmann et al. (51) showed that the conduction velocity is proportional to the diameter of the axon. The distal slowing of conduction velocity might then reflect a decrease in diameter of the nerve fibers from the proximal segment to the distal segment. Indeed, such a change in diameter has been demonstrated histologically in rabbits; motor nerves decrease in diameter distally not only because of branching but also because the individual fibers taper distally (52). The internodal distance also becomes shorter in the distal part of the nerve (53).

Upper and Lower Extremities

The NCV is significantly lower in the lower extremities than in the upper ones. For motor nerve conduction, the NCVs in the peroneal nerve are, on average, 7 m/sec slower than those in the median nerve (45). For sensory nerve conduction with surface electrodes, the velocity in the sural nerve is slower by 5 m/sec than in the median and ulnar nerves according to our data. For sensory nerve conduction with the near-nerve needle, the velocities in the sural nerve are slower by 6–10 m/sec than in the median nerves (1). For mixed nerve conduction, the velocities in the peroneal and posterior tibial nerves are slower by 17 m/sec than in the median and ulnar nerves (47). This difference is explained by two factors: (*a*) the temperature difference between the upper and lower extremities; and (*b*) more prominent axonal tapering in the longer lower extremities. We have observed a temperature difference of approximately 2°C between the hand and foot, which accounts for some of the NCV difference. Soudmand et al. (54) and Campbell et al. (55) proposed that more prominent axonal tapering in the distal portion of the leg is responsible for this difference. No data could be found directly comparing fiber size in the upper and lower extremities. O'Sullivan and Swallow (56), however, studied the fiber size and content of radial and sural nerves to establish normal ranges. They found that the radial nerves had a larger mean fascicular diameter and greater mean fiber density. According to Campbell et al.'s analysis, there is a tendency for the radial nerve to contain slightly larger fibers than the sural (55).

Sex

There is no consensus among investigators of nerve conduction concerning the differences between males and females, although Gregersen (57) and LaFratta and Smith (58) found significantly higher values in women than in men. On the other hand, Lang et al. (59) found lower NCVs in women. Wagman and Lesse (38) and Wyrick and Duncan (60) did not find any significant differences in NCV between the sexes. Campbell et al. (55) found faster NCVs in females, a difference which disappeared when correction was made for their lesser height. Bolton and Carter (22) reported that the amplitude of human antidromic sensory CNAPs recorded from median and ulnar digital nerves is greater in females than in males. Their data suggest that this difference between the sexes can be explained entirely on the basis of the circumference of the digits: on the average males have larger-sized digits and wrists than females. This causes the recording electrode to be a greater distance from the underlying nerve, thereby reducing the CNAP amplitude in antidromic sensory conduction studies. Kembel (61) saw a significantly greater age-related decrease in NCV in men than in women. Thus, it appears that sex alone does not influence the NCV.

Body Length

The results of examinations concerning the influence of body length on NCV are contradictory. Kato (31) and Wagman and Lesse (38) saw no connection. Lang and

Bjorkquist (62) and Lang et al. (59) found a significant negative correlation between body length and motor and sensory NCVs, respectively. Strangely, however, in their examinations of the radial nerve of female test subjects, there was a correlation only on the left side while the same examination showed no such correlation on the right side of the body. Campbell et al. (55) and Soudmand et al. (54) found that peroneal and sural NCVs varied inversely with body height, whereas median motor and sensory NCVs failed to show any significant relationship to height. In an expanded study of 104 normal subjects from the same institution, Rivner et al. concluded that a strong inverse correlation was found between height and sural, peroneal, and posterior tibial NCV (63). They presented a complicated NCV correction formula for height as well as for age and temperature for each nerve and cautioned that diagnostic conclusions made from nerve conduction data without correcting for height may be invalid in patients taller or shorter than normal. These authors proposed that this was caused by the abrupt distal axonal tapering in the lower extremities.

Variations in Nerve Conduction in Serial Tests

The NCVs are not the same when the test is performed serially in the same individual. As noted in Table 13.3, for motor nerve conduction the mean differences in the NCV on serial tests range from 1.6 to 4.4 m/sec, and the coefficients of variation (the standard deviation as a percentage of mean) range from 5.4 to 9%. For antidromic sensory nerve conduction, the coefficients of variation are 4.7–9%. For mixed nerve conduction, the mean difference is 4.4 m/sec and the coefficient of variation is 4.7%.

These variations in the NCVs on serial tests are caused by a combination of various technical and physiological factors—called "experimental errors." There are three important experimental errors in the determination of conduction velocity: (*a*) temperature; (*b*) measurement of distance; and (*c*) measurement of conduction time or latency. Maynard and Stolov (64) concluded that 89% of the overall experimental error is accounted for by inaccuracies in the determination of latency. However, their measurements were done with rulers from the recorded potentials. Obviously the latency marker measurement is more accurate than a ruler measurement, thus reducing the error associated with the latency measurement. Hopf (65) estimated a possible discrepancy of 2.5 m/sec (5%) for a hypothetical conduction distance of 30 cm and a conduction velocity of 50 m/sec. For the sensory nerve conduction, Buchthal and Rosenfalck (41) calculated a total experimental error of 5–6%. If the distance could be determined to an accuracy of 5 mm, the extent of the experimental error for a distance of 20 cm would be 2.5%. They stated that measurement of the latency is less critical in sensory NCV than in motor NCV if the first positive peak of the potential is taken as the point of reference. According to Ludin and Tackmann (1), failure to take into account the influence of temperature represents a far greater source of error.

Chaudhry et al. examined the inter- and intraexaminer reliability of the median motor and sensory, peroneal motor, and sural sensory nerve conduction in normal subjects and found that a high degree of intraexaminer reliability was present, but that there are significant interexaminer differences (66). This suggests that, in the serial nerve conduction studies, more reliable nerve conduction data can be obtained by a single examiner.

Nerve conduction variations on serial tests are critical when judging the improvement or worsening of the NCV in disease processes or when evaluating treatment. Halar and Venkatesh (67) devised a semirigid bar with distal and proximal stimulation electrodes that can be placed at a set distance. They were able to reduce the coefficient of variation from 6.1% with the standard technique to 2.0% with this device, thereby reducing the error associated with the distance measurement. Oh et al. (68) used a different method of reducing experimental errors: we determined the NCV in the same nerve in the same extremity during serial testing. Each determination was repeated 10 times, and the mean values were corrected to a skin temperature of 35°C according to the formula of DeJesus et al. (7). This technique has proved reliable in monitoring serial NCVs in a given individual for treatment evaluation (68, 69).

Table 13.3.
Variability in Nerve Conduction with Serial Testing

Investigator	Nerves Studied	Time Interval	Difference Noted (m/sec)	Coefficient of Variation[a] (%)
Henriksen (70)	Ulnar motor	"Different days"	Maximum: 7.5	
			Mean: 1.9 (3.2%)	
Thomas and Lambert (75) (15 infants)	Ulnar motor	"Different days"	Maximum: 2.0	
			Mean: 1.6 (5.7%)	
Honet et al. (76) (27 normals)	Median motor	Greater than one week	Mean: +0.77 ± 4.45[b]	
	Ulnar motor		+0.87 ± 4.26	
	Peroneal motor		+0.93 ± 3.96	
	Median sensory, antidromic		+0.44 ± 4.04	8–9
	Ulnar sensory, antidromic		+0.35 ± 5.82	
Wyrick and Duncan (60) (32 normals)	Ulnar motor	Morning/afternoon	Mean: Male 2.65 (4.7%) Female 2.23 (3.9%)	
Halar and Venkatech[c] (67)	Ulnar, median peroneal motor	Once a week for 4–6 weeks	1.3	2.0
McQuillen and Gorin (77) (5 normals)	Ulnar motor	Twice a week; 9 tests for 3 months	Mean: 4.4 (7.6%) Maximum: 8.8	5.4
	Ulnar mixed		Mean: 4.4 (8.0%) Maximum: 5.5	4.7
	Terminal latency		Mean: 0.66 msec (25%) Maximum: 1.0	15.4
Carpendale (13) (17 normals)	Terminal latency	Paired measurement	Maximum: 0.4 msec	
Bergman (78) (1 normal)	Median motor	Twice a day, 19–21 tests		4.75–4.22
	Ulnar motor			4.4–5.1
	Median sensory, antidromic			4.22–4.75
Christie and Coomes (79) (1 normal)	Ulnar motor	Four different days	Maximum: 14	
	Terminal latency		1 msec	
	Median motor		20	
	Terminal latency		2 msec	
Bleasel and Tuck (74) (1 normal)	Median, ulnar, peroneal, motor	10 times for 3 months		
	NCV:			2.2–5.6
	Amplitude:			8.5–15.7
	Median, ulnar, NCV:	10 times for 3 months		3.8–6.7
	Amplitude:			26.9–32.1

[a]The standard deviation as a percenage of the mean.
[b]The mean difference before and after the interval ± standard deviation.
[c]Double-stimulus technique.

REFERENCES

1. Ludin HP, Tackmann W. Sensory neurography. New York: Thieme-Stratton, 1980.
2. Von Helmholtz H. Mitteilung betreffend Versuche über die Fortpflanzungsgeschwindigkeit der Reizung in den motorischen Nerven des Menschen, welche Herr N. Baxt aus Petersburg im Physiologischen Laboratorium zu Heidelberg ausgeführt hat. Mber Akad Wiss Berlin 1867. 228–234 (Cited from Kaeser (45)).
3. Rosenberg H, Sugimoto T. Uber die physikochemischen Bedingungen der Erregungsleitung im Nerven. Biochem Z 1925;156:262–268.
4. Tasaki I, Fujita M. Action currents of single nerve fibers as modified by temperature changes. J Neurophysiol 1948;11:311–315.
5. Klensch H. Uber die Einflusse von Temperatur und Narkose auf die Erregbarkeit und Erregungsleitung der Kaltbluternerven. Pflugers Arch Ges Physiol 1949;251:513.
6. Todnem K, Knudsen G, Riise R, Hyland H, Aarli JA. The non-linear relationship between nerve conduction velocity and skin temperature. J Neurol Neurosurg Psychiatry 1989;52:497–501.
7. DeJesus PV, Hausmanowa-Petrusewicz I, Barchi RL. The effect of cold on nerve conduction of human slow and fast nerve fibers. Neurology 1973;23:1182–1189.

8. Hausmanowa-Petrusewicz J, Kopec J. An evaluation of the method of antidromic stimulation in human peripheral nerves. EMG Clinic Neurophys 1968;8:105–113.

9. Hopf HC. Electromyographic study on so-called mononeuritis. Arch Neurol 1963;9:307–312.

10. Buchthal F, Rosenfalck A. Sensory potentials in polyneuropathy. Brain 1971;94:241–262.

11. DeJong RH, Hershey WN, Wagman IH. Nerve conduction velocity during hypothermia in man. Anesthesiology 1966;27:805–810.

12. Skorpil V. 1965. Conduction velocity of human nerve structure. Rozpr Cesk Akad Ved 1965 (Cited in Kaeser (45)).

13. Carpendale MTF. Conduction time in the terminal portion of the motor fibers of the ulnar, median, peroneal nerves in healthy subjects and in patients with neuropathy. [Unpublished master's thesis]. Rochester, Minnesota: Mayo Foundation, University of Minnesota, 1956.

14. Bell KR, Lehmann JF. Effect of cooling on H- and T-reflexes in normal subjects. Arch Phys Med Rehabil 1987;68:490–493.

15. Halar EM, DeLisa JA, Brozovich FV. Nerve conduction velocity: relationship of skin, subcutaneous and intramuscular temperature. Arch Phys Med Rehabil 1980;61:199–203.

16. Ricker K, Hertel G, Stodieck G. Increased voltage of the muscle action potential of normal subjects after local cooling. J Neurol 1977;216:33–38.

17. Borenstein S, Desmedt JE. Local cooling in myasthenia. Arch Neurol 1975;32:152–157.

18. Fatt P, Katz B. The electrical properties of crustacean muscle fibers. J Physiol 1953;120:171–204.

19. Denys EH. The role of temperature in electromyography. AAEE Minimonograph # 14, Rochester, Minnesota, 1980.

20. Dawson, H. A textbook of general physiology. 3rd ed. Boston: Little, Brown;1964:725.

21. Hopkins A. Normal and abnormal physiology. In: Dyck PJ, Thomas PK, Lambert EH, eds. Peripheral neuropathy. Philadelphia: WB Saunders, 1975:378–387.

22. Bolton CF, Carter KM. Temperature effects on the size of human sensory compound action potentials. J Neurol Neurosurg Psychiatry 1981;44:407–413.

23. Ludin HP, Beyler F. Temperature dependence of normal sensory nerve action potentials. J Neurol 1977;216:173–180.

24. Bolton CF, Carter K, Koval JJ. Temperature effects on conduction studies of normal and abnormal nerve. Muscle Nerve 1982;5:145–147.

25. Baysal AI, Chang CW, Oh SJ. Temperature effects on nerve conduction studies in patients with carpal tunnel syndrome (Unpublished data).

26. Alfonsi E, Merlini GP, Giorgetti A, Ceroni M, Piccolo G, Agostinis C, Savoldi F. Temperature-related changes in sensory nerve conduction: studies in normal subjects and in patients with paraproteinemia. EMG Clin Neurophysiol 1987; 27:277–282.

27. Buchthal F, Rosenfalck A, Behse F. Sensory potentials of normal and diseased nerves. In: Dyck PJ, Thomas PK, Lambert EH, eds. Peripheral neuropathy. Philadelphia: WB Saunders, 1975:442–464.

28. Ludin HP. Electromyography in practice. New York: Thieme-Stratton, 1980.

29. Rigshospitalet Laboratory of Clinical Neurophysiology. EMG-Sensory and motor conduction. Findings in normal subjects. Copenhagen, Denmark: RLCN, 1975.

30. Kaplan PE. Electrodiagnostic confirmation of long thoracic nerve palsy. J Neurol Neurosurg Psychiatry 1980;43:50–52.

31. Kato M. The conduction velocity of ulnar nerve and the spinal reflex time measured by means of the H-waves in average adults and athletes. Tohoku J Exp Med 1960;73:74–85.

32. Gutrecht JA, Dyck PJ. Quantitative teased fiber and histological studies of human sural nerve during post-natal development. J Comp Neurol 1970;138:117–130.

33. Wagner AL, Buchthal F. Motor and sensory conduction in infancy and childhood: Reappraisal. Devel Med Child Neurol 1972;14:189–216.

34. Cruz Martinez A, Perez Conde MC, Del Campo F, Barrio M, Gutierrez AM, Lopez E. Sensory and mixed nerve conduction velocity in infancy and childhood. 1. Normal parameters in median, ulnar, and sural nerves. Electromyogr Clin Neurophysiol 1978;18:487–504.

35. LaFratta CW. A comparison of sensory and motor NCV as related with age. Arch Phys Med Rehab 1966;47:286–290.

36. Downie AW, Newell DJ. Sensory nerve conduction in patients with diabetes mellitus and controls. Neurology 1961;11:876–882.

37. Oh SJ, Kim HS, Ahmad BK. Electrophysiological diagnosis of the interdigital neuropathy of the foot. Muscle Nerve 1982;5:566–567.

38. Wagman IH, Lesse H. Maximum conduction velocities of motor fibers of ulnar nerve in human subjects of various ages and sexes. J Neurophysiol 1952;15:235–244.

39. Taylor PK. Non-linear effects of age on nerve conduction in adults. J Neurol Sci 1984;66:223–234.

40. LaFratta CW. Relation of age to amplitude of evoked antidromic sensory nerve potentials. Arch Phys Med Rehab 1972;53:388–389.

41. Buchthal F, Rosenfalck A. Evoked action potentials and conduction velocity in human sensory nerves. Brain Res 1966;3:1–122.

42. Lascelles RG, Thomas PK. Changes due to age in internodal length in the sural nerve in man. J Neurol Neurosurg Psychiatry 1966;29:40–44.

43. Troghi H, Tsukagoshi H, Toyokura Y. Quantitative changes with age in normal sural nerves. Acta Neuropath 1977;38:213–220.

44. Neary D, Ochoa J, Gilliatt RW. Subclinical entrapment neuropathy in man. J Neurol Sci 1975;24:283–298.

45. Kaeser HE. Nerve conduction velocity measurements. In: Vinken PJ, Bruyn GW, eds. Handbook of clinical neurology, vol 7. Amsterdam: North-Holland, 1970:116–196.

46. Gassel MM, Trojaborg W. Clinical and electrophysiological study of the pattern of conduction times in the distribution of the sciatic nerve. J Neurol Neurosurg Psychiatry 1964;27:351–357.

47. Mayer RF. Nerve conduction studies in man. Neurology 1963;13:1021–1030.

48. Arrigo A, Cosi V, Savoldi F. The conduction velocity of the human sciatic nerve. EEG Clinic Neurophysiol 1962;(suppl 22):23–25.

49. Trojaborg W. Motor nerve conduction velocities in normal subjects with particular reference to the conduction in proximal and distal segments of median and ulnar nerves. EEG Clin Neurophysiol 1964;17:314–314.

50. Gasser HS, Grundfest H. Axon diameters in relation to the spike dimensions and the conduction velocity in mammalian A-fibers. Amer J Physiol 1939;127:393–414.

51. Tackmann W, Spalke G, Oginszus HJ. Quantitative histometric studies and relation of number and diameter of myelinated nerve fibers to electrophysiological parameters in normal sensory nerves of man. J Neurol 1976;212:71–84.

52. Fernand VSV, Young JZ. The sizes of the nerve fibers of muscle nerves. Proc R Soc London (Biol) 1951;139:38–58.

53. Lehmann HJ. Uber das strukturelle und quantitative Verhalten der Schmidt-Lantermannschen Einkerbungen und der Segmente. Z Zeilforsch 1950;3:213. (Cited in Kaeser (45)).

54. Soudmand R, Ward C, Swift TR. The effect of height on nerve conduction velocity. Neurology 1982;32:407–410.

55. Campbell WW, Ward C, Swift TR. Nerve conduction velocity varies inversely with height. Muscle Nerve 1981;4:520–523.

56. O'Sullivan DJ, Swallow M. The fiber size and content of the radial and sural nerves. J Neurol Neurosurg Psychiatry 1968;31:464–470.

57. Gregerson G. Diabetic neuropathy: influence of age, sex, metabolic control, and duration of diabetes on motor conduction velocity. Neurology 1967;17:972–980.

58. LaFratta CW, Smith OH. A study of the relationship of motor nerve conduction study in the adult as to age, sex, and handedness. Arch Phys Med Rehab 1964;45:407–412.

59. Lang AH, Forsstrom J, Bjorkquist SE, Kuusela V. Statistical variation of nerve conduction velocity. J Neurol Sci 1977;33:229.

60. Wyrick W, Duncan A. Within-day trends of motor latency and nerve conduction velocity in males and females. Am J Phys Med 1970;49:307–315.

61. Kemble F. Conduction in the normal adult median nerve: the different effect of aging in men and women. EMG 1967;7:275–287.

62. Lang AH, Bjorkquist SE. Die Nervenleitgeschwindigkeit peripherer Nerven beieinflussende Konstitutionelle Factoren beim Menschen. Z EEG-EMG 1971;4:162–170.

63. Rivner MH, Swift TR, Crout BO, Rhodes KP. Toward more rational nerve conduction interpretations: the effect of height. Muscle Nerve 1990;13:232–239.

64. Maynard FM, Stolov WC. Experimental error in determination of nerve conduction velocity. Arch Phys Med Rehab 1972;53:362–372.

65. Hopf HC. Impulstertung im peripheren Nerven. In: Hopf HC, Struppler A, eds. Electromyographie. Stuttgart: Thieme, 1974:110.

66. Chaudhry V, Cornblath DR, Mellits ED, et al. Inter- and intra-examiner reliability of nerve conduction measurements in normal subjects. Ann Neurol 1991;30:841–843.

67. Halar EM, Venkatesh B. Nerve conduction velocity measurements: improved accuracy using superimposed response waves. Arch Phys Med Rehab 1976;57:451–457.

68. Oh SJ, Clements RS, Lee YW, Diethelm AG. Rapid improvement in nerve conduction velocity following renal transplantation. Ann Neurol 1978;4:369–373.

69. Clements RS, Vouganti B, Kuba T, Oh SJ, Darnell B. Dietary myo-inositol intake and peripheral nerve function in diabetic neuropathy. Metabolism 1979;28(suppl 1, no 4):477–483.

70. Henriksen JD. Conduction velocity of motor nerves in normal subjects and in patients with neuromuscular disorders. [Unpublished master's thesis]. Rochester, Minnesota: University of Minnesota, 1956.

71. Geerlings AHC, Mechelse K. Temperature and nerve conduction velocity, some practical problems. EMG Clin Neurohysiol 1985;25:253–260.

72. Lowitzsch K, Hopf HC, Galland J. Changes of sensory conduction velocity and refractory periods with decreasing tissue temperature in man. J Neurol 1977;216:181–188.

73. Norris AH. Age changes in the maximum conduction velocity of motor fibers of human ulnar nerve. J Appl Physiol 1953;5:589–593.

74. Bleasel AF, Tuck RR. Variability of repeated nerve conduction studies. Electroencephalogr Clin Neurophysiol 1991;81:417–420.

75. Thomas JE, Lambert EH. Ulnar nerve conduction velocity and H-reflex in infants and children. J Appl Physiol 1960;15:1–9.

76. Honet JC, Jebsen RH, Perrin EB. Variability of nerve conduction velocity determinations in normal persons. Arch Phys Med Rehab 1968;49:650–654.

77. McQuillen, MP, Gorin FJ. Serial ulnar nerve conduction velocity measurements in normal subjects. J Neurol Neurosurg Psychiatry 1969;32:144–148.
78. Bergman J. On variability of conduction velocity measurements on repeated examination. EMG 1971;11:143–148.
79. Christie BGB, Coomes EN. Normal variation of nerve conduction in three peripheral nerves. Ann Phys Med 1980;5:303–309.

14

Anomalous Innervation of the Nerves

Normal variations in peripheral nerve innervation are not unusual. The clinician must recognize several common variations in the performance of nerve conduction and electromyographic (EMG) studies to prevent faulty interpretation of the electrophysiological data. The most important variations in the peripheral nerves are: (*a*) median-ulnar anastomosis (Martin-Gruber anastomosis); (*b*) ulnar-median anastomosis; and (*c*) an accessory deep peroneal nerve.

Median-Ulnar Anastomosis of the Motor Fibers

The median-ulnar anastomosis is the most common form of anomalous innervation. This anomaly was first described by Martin in 1763 and later by Gruber in 1870 and thus is referred to as the Martin-Gruber anastomosis.

In a study of cadavers, Gruber (quoted by Mannerfelt (1)) found an anastomosis in 38 of 250 arms (15.2%) and Hirasawa (quoted by Mannerfelt (1)) found one in 13 of 124 arms (10.5%). Various nerve conduction studies have found an anastomosis in 15–39% of normal controls (Table 14.1) and in 8–26% of patients with carpal tunnel syndrome. This anastomosis involves axons leaving either the main trunk of the median nerve or the anterior interosseous nerve, crossing through the forearm to join the main trunk of the ulnar nerve, and ultimately innervating the intrinsic hand muscles (Fig. 14.1). Although a significant number of axons may participate in this anomalous route, all the axons of the median nerve are not involved. The axons in this anastomosis may innervate any of the intrinsic hand muscles, most commonly the first dorsal interosseous (Table 14.2). This anomaly seems to be inherited in an autosomal dominant mode. Crutchfield and Gutmann (2) reported that 62% of 29 relatives of five subjects with this variation also had this anomaly.

This anatomical variation can be easily confirmed by placing the recording electrodes on three muscles—the thenar, hypothenar, and first dorsal interosseous—and by stimulating the median and ulnar nerves at the wrist and elbow. With these settings, in normal individuals the compound muscle action potentials (CMAP) from the abductor digiti quinti or the first dorsal interosseous muscle in the ulnar nerve is slightly higher in

Table 14.1.
Frequency of the Median-Ulnar Anastomosis

Investigator	Criteria of Anastomosis	Group Studied	Frequency (%)
Crutchfield and Gutmann (2)	1. CMAP amplitude upon median stimulation: at the elbow > at the wrist[b] 2. CMAP amplitude upon ulnar stimulation: at the wrist > at the elbow[b]	Normal	18 (N = 50)[a]
Iyer and Fenichel (6)	Near-normal latency upon elbow median stimulation and prolonged terminal latency	Carpal tunnel syndrome	7.7 (N = 65)
Gutmann (4)	Initial positive deflection in thenar CMAP upon median elbow stimulation	Carpal tunnel syndrome	25 (N = 63)
Kimura et al. (9)	Collision technique[c]	Unselected subjects	17 (N = 328)
Mannerfelt (1)	Electrical stimulation and sensory nerve block		14.6 (N = 41)
Sun and Streib (26)	1. First DI. CMAP amplitude upon median stimulation: at the elbow > at the wrist[d] 2. Thenar M. CMAP amplitude upon median stimulation: at the elbow > at the wrist[e] 3. Hypothenar M. Any CMAP with negative deflection upon median stimulation at elbow[f]	Hospital volunteers and patients referred to the EMG laboratory, including patients with carpal tunnel syndrome	34 (N = 150): 26% (N = 63) for CTS; 39% (N = 87) for normal

[a]N = number of cases tested.
[b]At least 1.0 mV larger.
[c]See Kimura et al.'s original article for details (10).
[d]At least 25% larger.
[e]Or CMAP decreased by more than 25% with ulnar stimulation above the elbow rather than at the wrist.
[f]Potentials quite different and larger with median stimulation at the elbow rather than at the wrist.

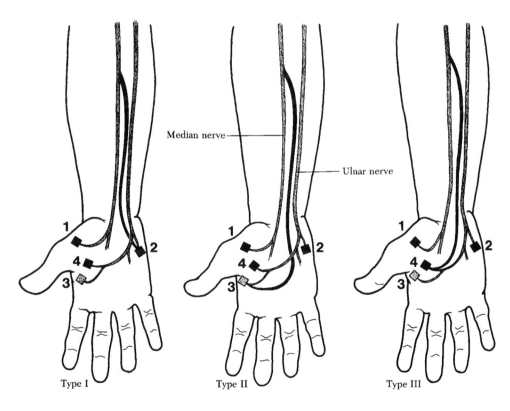

Figure 14.1. Martin-Gruber anastomosis. Type I: The crossover fibers terminate in the hypothenar muscle. Type II: The crossover fibers terminate in the first dorsal interosseous muscle. Type III: The crossover fibers terminate in the thenar muscle. The *solid line* represents the anastomosis. **1**, Abductor pollicis brevis. **2**, Abductor digiti quinti. **3**, First dorsal interosseous. **4**, Adductor pollicis.

amplitude with supramaximal stimulation of the nerve distally as compared with more proximally (3). This is because of increased synchronization at distal stimulation. The amplitude of the CMAP with wrist stimulation is normally 90–120% of the amplitude with elbow stimulation. With median nerve stimulation, the response from the abductor digiti quinti and the first dorsal interosseous muscle is either absent or small in amplitude with the initial positive deflection. The response from the abductor pollicis brevis in ulnar nerve stimulation is similar. The initial positive deflection in these mus-

Table 14.2.
Frequency of Martin-Gruber Anastomosis in Intrinsic Hand Muscles

Investigator	No. of Cases Studied	Frequency in Muscles Innervated by Anomalous Innervations		
		Thenar	First Dorsal Interosseous	Hypothenar
Crutchfield and Gutmann (2)	26	6	26 (20)[a]	4
Kimura et al. (9)[b]	96	64 (1)		76 (13)
Wilbourn and Lambert (27)	22	3	21	9
Mannerfelt (1)	6	4	6	2
Sun and Streib (26)	51	18	51	23

[a]Numbers in parentheses in last three columns represent the number of cases innervating one muscle alone.
[b]The first dorsal interosseous muscle was not studied.

cles is caused by volume conduction spread from the adjacent muscle, which is innervated by the stimulated nerve.

The Martin-Gruber Anastomosis in Normal Individuals

In the presence of a Martin-Gruber anastomosis in normal individuals, *the CMAP from the first dorsal interosseous, hypothenar, and/or thenar muscles is larger (at least 1.0 mv) upon median nerve stimulation at the elbow than at the wrist, and the CMAP from one or more of these muscles is larger (at least 1.0 mV larger) when stimulating the ulnar nerve at the wrist than at the elbow* (2) (Figs. 14.2 and 14.3). This is so because there are more axons available for stimulation in the median nerve at the elbow than at the wrist and in the ulnar nerve at the wrist than at the elbow. During this test, it is important to fulfill a few technical requirements: (*a*) the stimulation at each site should be supramaximal; (*b*) the recording electrodes should be placed on a motor point of the muscles; and (*c*) there should not be any cross-spread of the stimulation at the wrist or elbow between the median and ulnar nerves.

The response of each muscle depends on the type of anastomosis. There are three main types of Martin-Gruber anastomosis, each of which can be found separately or in combination. Each is dealt with as a separate type for the purpose of explanation.

Type I—Hypothenar Innervation

The crossover fiber terminates in the hypothenar muscle in type I anastomosis. Thus, the Martin-Gruber anastomosis manifests during routine ulnar motor studies. This type should be suspected when the amplitude of the CMAP on the hypothenar muscle is disproportionately higher when the ulnar nerve is stimulated at the wrist than when done at the elbow. *The most characteristic finding is a higher amplitude (at least 1.0 mV) of the CMAP of the hypothenar muscle upon wrist stimulation than with elbow stimulation in the ulnar nerve study (Fig. 14.2).* Stimulation of the median nerve at the elbow confirms the anastomosis by showing an unexpected CMAP. Stimulation of the median nerve at the wrist evokes no CMAP or only a shallow response with the initial positive deflection from the hypothenar muscle. Because the nerve conduction pattern in this type of anastomosis simulates a conduction block at the elbow (if stimulation is above the elbow) or at the forearm (if stimulation is below the elbow), it is important to rule out the Martin-Gruber anastomosis by appropriate stimulation of the median nerve at the elbow. This anastomosis can also be confirmed by calculating the crossover contribution of axons. This is done by adding the amplitudes of the CMAPs upon stimulation of the ulnar and median nerves at the elbow and then comparing this to the response obtained with ulnar stimulation at the wrist. The combined amplitude of the proximal median and ulnar stimulation should be approximately equal to the amplitude of the distal ulnar stimulation.

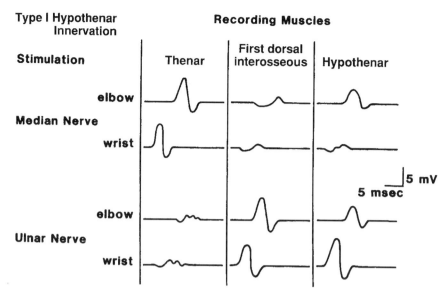

Figure 14.2. CMAPs from the thenar, first dorsal interosseous, and hypothenar muscles in type I Martin-Gruber anastomosis in an otherwise normal individual. Note the CMAP from the hypothenar muscle after median nerve stimulation at the elbow. Wrist stimulation did not elicit any CMAPs with the initial negative deflection.

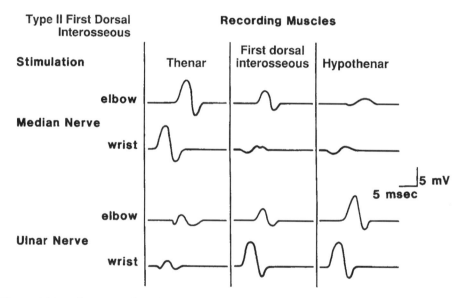

Figure 14.3. The CMAPs from the thenar, first dorsal interosseous, and hypothenar muscles in type II Martin-Gruber anastomosis in an otherwise normal individual. Note the first dorsal interosseous CMAP with initial negative deflection on median nerve stimulation at the elbow. This CMAP is not seen with wrist stimulation.

Type II—First Dorsal Interosseous Innervation

Type II is the most common Martin-Gruber anastomosis. It does not present any difficulty in routine ulnar nerve conduction studies because the recording electrodes are not placed on this muscle. A potential difficulty arises in cases of suspected lesions in the deep palmar branch of the ulnar nerve because the recording electrodes should be placed on the dorsal interosseous muscle. In normal individuals with this type of anastomosis, *the most prominent finding is a larger CMAP from the first dorsal interosseous muscle on wrist stimulation than upon elbow stimulation of the ulnar nerve*

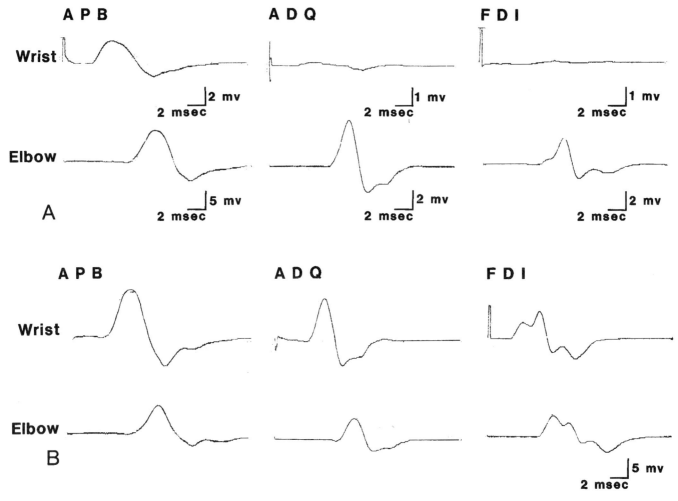

Figure 14.4. The CMAPs from the thenar (APB: abductor pollicis brevis), hypothenar (ADQ: abductor digiti quinti), and first dorsal interosseous (FDI) muscles in a case of left thoracic outlet syndrome and type I and II Martin-Gruber anastomosis in the right forearm. ***A***, Median nerve stimulation. ***B***, Ulnar nerve stimulation.

(Figs. 14.3 and 14.4). Again, this anastomosis can be confirmed by median nerve stimulation at the elbow, resulting in an unexpected CMAP. To calculate the crossover contribution of axons, the median wrist amplitude must be subtracted from the median elbow amplitude; this difference should then be added to the ulnar amplitude at the elbow. The result should approximately equal the ulnar wrist amplitude.

Type III—Thenar Muscle Innervation

Type III, the least common type of anastomosis, manifests in routine median motor conduction studies with the recording electrodes on the abductor pollicis brevis. It is the most difficult type to recognize and document. It should be suspected when the CMAP on the thenar muscle is unusually larger after elbow stimulation than with wrist stimulation of the median nerve. *The most prominent finding in normal individuals is a larger CMAP amplitude (at least 1 mV) from the thenar muscle upon elbow stimulation of the median nerve compared with wrist stimulation (Fig. 14.5)*. Stimulation of the ulnar nerve produces a CMAP with an initial positive deflection that is higher distally at the wrist than proximally at the elbow. This positive deflection is a volume conduction response from the ulnar innervated muscle in the thenar muscle group. It is important to remember that even though the thenar muscle group is routinely used for the median motor nerve conduction study, it also contains the adductor pollicis and the

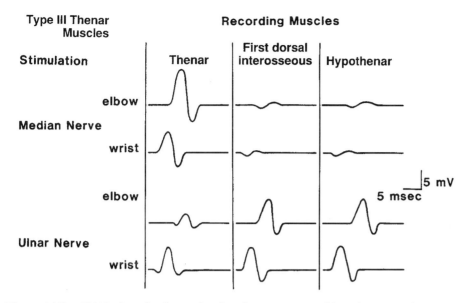

Figure 14.5. CMAPs from the thenar, first dorsal interosseous, and hypothenar muscles in type III Martin-Gruber anastomosis. Note the higher amplitude of the thenar CMAP upon elbow stimulation compared with wrist stimulation in the median nerve.

deep head of the flexor pollicis brevis, which are usually innervated by the ulnar nerve. To calculate the crossover contribution, subtract the elbow ulnar amplitude from the wrist ulnar amplitude and add this difference to the wrist median amplitude. This should approximately equal the median elbow amplitude.

The Martin-Gruber Anastomosis in Carpal Tunnel Syndrome

In carpal syndrome, the Martin-Gruber anastomosis may produce additional electrophysiological changes that make interpretation of the nerve conduction difficult unless the electromyographer is aware of this anomaly. *Three different conduction patterns are noted:*

1. *Median nerve stimulation at the elbow evokes a thenar CMAP with an initial positive deflection not seen on stimulation at the wrist (4) (Fig. 14.6);*
2. *There is an erroneously normal proximal (elbow) motor latency in the median nerve with prolongation of the distal motor latency; and*
3. *A thenar CMAP with two components is seen upon median nerve stimulation at the elbow (Fig. 14.7).*

Gutmann (4) reported a thenar CMAP with the initial positive deflection on median elbow stimulation as the pathognomonic electrophysiological finding indicative of the Martin-Gruber anastomosis in the presence of carpal tunnel syndrome. This initial positive deflection is recorded despite the fact that the recording electrode lies over the motor point; it is not seen upon median nerve stimulation at the wrist. Median and ulnar nerve stimulation studies—with recording the responses from thenar, hypothenar, and first dorsal interosseous muscles—document that this characteristic change in the carpal tunnel syndrome is caused by the Martin-Gruber anastomosis. Gutmann noted this change in 20% of median nerves in 62 consecutive patients with bilateral carpal tunnel syndrome (3). He explained the initial positive deflection of the CMAP on median elbow stimulation but not on wrist stimulation as follows: Conduction in the median nerve axons going through the carpal tunnel and innervating thenar muscles is slower than in those median nerve axons crossing to the ulnar nerve and supplying the first dorsal interosseous, adductor pollicis, abductor digiti quinti, and flexor pollicis brevis (3). The CMAP from the latter muscles, upon median nerve stimulation at the elbow, is generated prior to that from the thenar muscles innervated by median

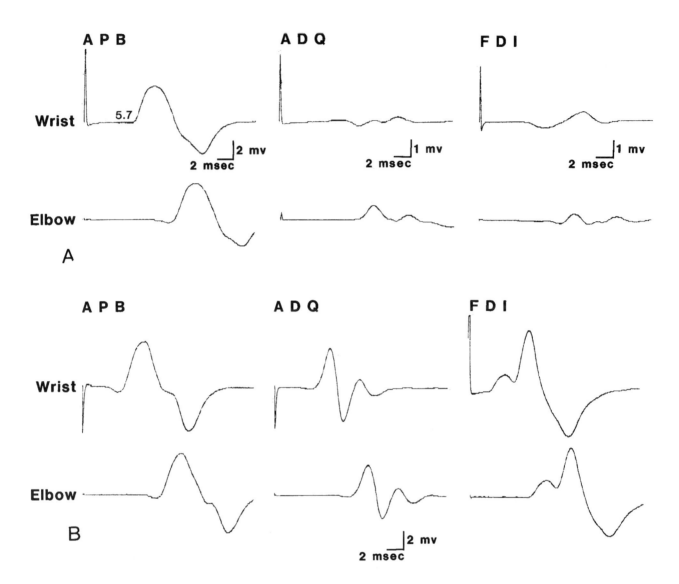

Figure 14.6. The CMAPs from the thenar (APB), hypothenar (ADQ), and first dorsal interosseous (FDI) muscles in a case of carpal tunnel syndrome and type I Martin-Gruber anastomosis. The thenar CMAP on median elbow stimulation is preceded by a positive deflection not seen on wrist stimulation. The initial positive deflection on median elbow stimulation is the cardinal clue. Terminal latency of median nerve is 5.7 msec. *A*, Median nerve stimulation. *B*, Ulnar nerve stimulation.

axons going through the carpal tunnel. The earlier appearing CMAP is incorporated into the overall thenar CMAP, but because it originates at some distance from the recording electrode, it produces an initial positive deflection. This initial positive deflection is caused by the volume conduction effect and is not present when stimulating the median nerve at the wrist, below the level of the anomalous interchange.

Thus, *the thenar CMAP with an initial positive deflection upon elbow stimulation of the median nerve alone, in the presence of a carpal tunnel syndrome, is indicative of the Martin-Gruber anastomosis (3).* In fact, Gutmann suggested this initial positive deflection as an electrophysiological diagnostic index for mild carpal tunnel syndrome (5). He reported six cases of mild carpal tunnel syndrome in which motor and sensory nerve conductions were essentially normal and a positive deflection preceding the thenar CMAP on elbow stimulation, but not on wrist stimulation, was the sole electrophysiological abnormality.

Iyer and Fenichel (6) reported five cases of carpal tunnel syndrome in which near-

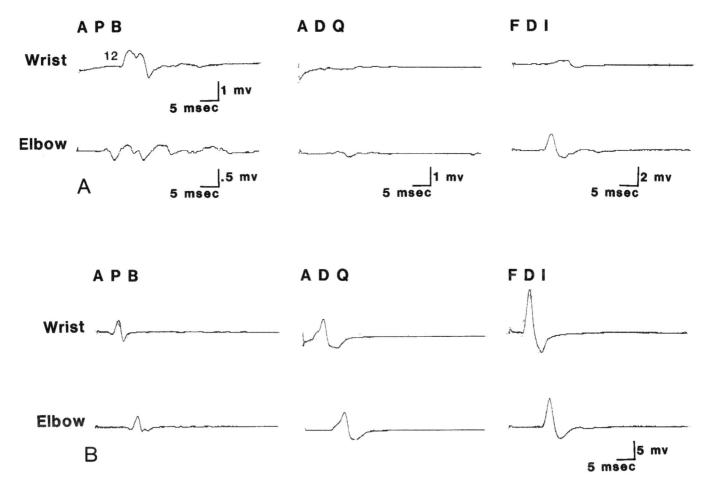

Figure 14.7. The CMAPs from the thenar (APB), hypothenar (ADQ), and first doral interosseous (FDI) muscles in a case of marked carpal tunnel syndrome and type II Martin-Gruber anastomosis. The thenar CMAP with two components and the initial positive deflection on median elbow stimulation is a prominent finding. Terminal latency of median nerve is 12 msec. **A,** Median nerve stimulation. **B,** Ulnar nerve stimulation.

normal latency was found upon proximal stimulation of the median nerve, although the distal motor latency was prolonged. The presence of the Martin-Gruber anastomosis leads to partial or total sparing of the thenar muscles from the effects of compression of their nerve supply in a case of carpal tunnel syndrome. In cases of partial sparing, the distal latency of the median nerve is prolonged, but upon stimulation at the elbow the latency is normal because the stimulus can travel along the noncompressed fibers constituting the anastomosis and bypass the retinaculum via the ulnar nerve. This is the cause of the near-normal proximal latency resulting in the apparent short conduction time in the forearm segment of the median nerve and the spuriously high calculated NCV. It is important to remember that the spread of strong stimulus current from the median nerve to the ulnar nerve at the elbow may produce similar findings. Often in cases of severe carpal tunnel syndrome, a high-intensity stimulus current is needed to evoke the CMAP across the compressed carpal tunnel. The Martin-Gruber anastomosis should be confirmed by the method described above. According to Gutmann (3), this finding is less common in carpal tunnel syndrome in the presence of the anomaly. He observed this finding only once in 63 consecutive patients studied and concluded that it is not a very useful finding.

Additionally, Lambert (7) described a thenar CMAP with two components upon median nerve stimulation at the elbow, again related to the slower conduction in the median nerve at the wrist and the faster conduction in those axons that have crossed to the ulnar nerve. The ulnar nerve component is absent when the median nerve is stimulated at the wrist. According to our experience, this is seen in severe carpal tunnel syndrome (Fig. 14.7). This too seems to be an uncommon finding.

Median-Ulnar Anastomosis of the Sensory Fibers

There has been a report of one case of carpal tunnel syndrome in which the forearm ulnar-median anastomosis of sensory fibers was documented in addition to the Martin-Gruber anastomosis (8). This patient had carpal tunnel syndrome and a Martin-Gruber anastomosis to the abductor digiti quinti muscle. In addition, a small (0.5 μV) sensory CNAP was recorded in the median nerve at the elbow (Figs. 14.8 and 14.9) with stimulation of digit 5, which was not recordable after procaine infiltration of the ulnar nerve at the wrist. Since the CNAP was not recorded at the median nerve at the wrist with stimulation of digit 5, Santoro et al. believed that this case represents the first example of a median-ulnar anastomosis of sensory fibers in the forearm (8).

Ulnar-Median Nerve Anastomosis of the Motor Fibers

In contrast to the frequent occurrence of the median-ulnar nerve anastomosis (Martin-Gruber anastomosis), ulnar-median nerve anastomosis is rare (Fig. 14.10). Kimura et al.

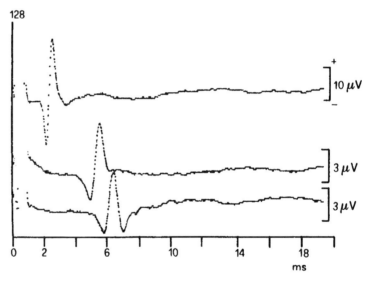

Figure 14.8. Sensory CNAP along the course of the ulnar nerve (above, at the wrist; middle, at the elbow below the sulcus; and below, at the elbow above the sulcus) on supramaximal stimulation of digit V. (From Santoro L, Rosato R, Caruso G. Median-ulnar nerve communications: electrophysiological demonstration of motor and sensory fiber cross-over. J Neurol 1983;229:229.)

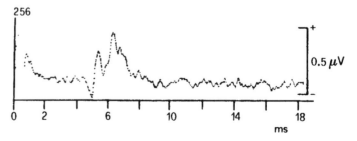

Figure 14.9. Supramaximal stimulation on digit V.; sensory CNAP at the elbow, at the median nerve position. (From Santoro L, Rosato R, Caruso G. Median-ulnar nerve communications: electrophysiological demonstration of motor and sensory fiber cross-over. J Neurol 1983;229:229.)

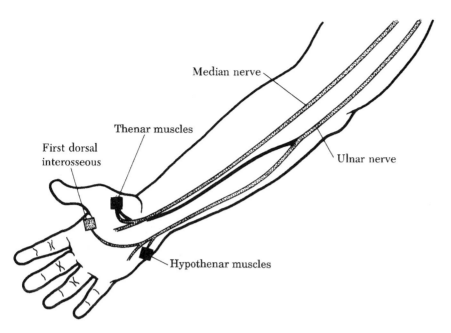

Figure 14.10.   Ulnar-median nerve anastomosis *(solid line)*.

stated specifically that crossover from the ulnar to the median nerve in the forearm was not found electrophysiologically in any of the 656 hands they studied (9). Marinacci found this anomaly in two patients among 298 cases of ulnar nerve lesions (10).

So far, only three cases of ulnar-median nerve anastomosis in the forearm have been reported. Marinacci described one patient who sustained a traumatic severance of the median nerve in the elbow (10) that resulted in EMG signs of partial denervation in the flexors of the forearm. The thenar muscle remained intact clinically and electromyographically. Stimulation of the right median nerve above the elbow produced no muscular contraction in the forearm or hand. In contrast, stimulation of the ulnar nerve at the elbow elicited a muscular contraction in the flexors of the forearm and the hypothenar and thenar groups in the hand.

Kómár et al. reported a patient with a complete transection of the median nerve above the elbow and clinically only partial median nerve palsy (11). EMG examination indicated a forearm anastomosis of motor axons from the ulnar to the median nerve.

Streib reported an incidental finding of an ulnar-median anastomosis in a woman with myopathy (12) (Fig. 14.11). The CMAP of the thenar muscles was more than 50% higher after stimulation of the ulnar nerve at the elbow than at the wrist. Median nerve stimulation gave opposite results: a large amplitude after wrist stimulation and a smaller one after stimulation at the elbow. No CMAP was recorded from the hypothenar muscles upon median nerve stimulation at the wrist or elbow. Motor and sensory NCVs of the median and ulnar nerves were normal. Digital sensory compound nerve action potentials (CNAPs) were of normal amplitude and latency.

To identify this anastomosis, the recording electrode should be placed on the thenar muscle and the stimulation applied at the wrist and elbow along the median and ulnar nerves. This produces characteristic findings:

1. *The CMAP of the thenar muscle is considerably higher (20%) after stimulation of the median nerve at the wrist than at the elbow; and*

2. *The CMAP of the thenar muscle is considerably higher after stimulation of the ulnar nerve at the elbow than at the wrist.*

These electrophysiological findings are associated with brisk contraction of the thenar muscles.

Ulnar-median nerve anastomosis should be suspected when the hand muscles are clinically intact in the presence of a severe median nerve lesion in the forearm, as illus-

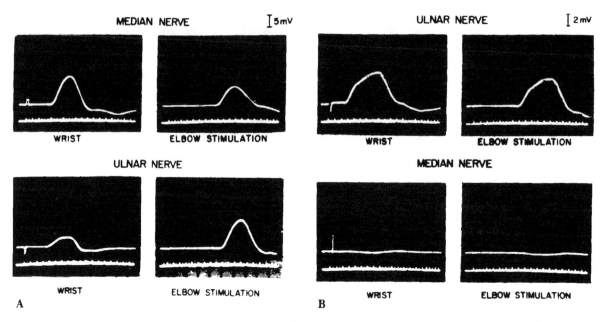

Figure 14.11.   The CMAPs from thenar (**A**) and hypothenar (**B**) muscles in a case of ulnar-median anastomosis. (From Streib EW. Ulnar-to-median nerve anastomosis in the forearm: electromyographic studies. Neurology 1979;29:1536.)

trated in Marinacci and Kómár's cases (10, 11). The presence of this anomaly may cause confusion when evaluating median nerve lesions under the following clinical situations:

1. In the presence of an ulnar-median nerve anastomosis a complete lesion of the median nerve at the forearm might erroneously be interpreted as a partial lesion of the median nerve. The EMG in the thenar muscle shows normal findings, whereas in the forearm flexors it shows full-blown denervation. However, stimulation of the median nerve above the lesion shows a marked abnormality across the lesion, whereas stimulation of the ulnar nerve at the elbow shows a good response.

2. Stimulation of the median nerve at the elbow causes a lower-amplitude CMAP than after stimulation at the wrist, which may be erroneously interpreted as evidence of a conduction block. A high index of suspicion of this anomaly prevents misinterpretation of the findings.

Ulnar-Median Nerve Anastomosis of the Sensory Fibers

Hopf reported a case of forearm ulnar-to-median nerve anastomosis of sensory axons (13). This was discovered as an incidental finding during serial investigations of the sensory distribution of the ulnar nerve of the hand in 30 healthy subjects. There was no ulnar-to-median anastomosis of motor fibers in this individual. With stimulation of the digital nerves of the 4th finger (radial side) and the 3rd finger (ulnar side), at the wrist, CNAPs of 10 and 15 μV were recorded on the median nerve but none on the ulnar nerve; at the elbow, CNAPs of 7 and 10 μV were recorded on the ulnar nerve but none on the median nerve (Fig. 14.12). This is the first reported case of an ulnar-median anastomosis of sensory fibers in the forearm.

Variations in Innervation of Hand Muscles

All of the intrinsic muscles of the hand are innervated by the ulnar and median nerves. Most commonly, the abductor pollicis brevis and opponens pollicis are innervated by the median nerve, and the first dorsal interosseous, adductor pollicis, and abductor digiti quinti by the ulnar nerve. The flexor pollicis brevis often has a dual innervation: the superficial head by the median nerve and the deep head by the ulnar nerve.

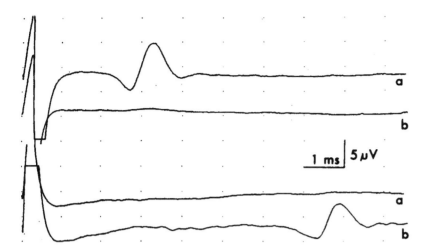

Figure 14.12. Sensory CNAP from ulnar and median nerves to stimulation of the middle finger on the radial side. Recording from median (**A**) and ulnar (**B**) nerves at the wrist (upper two tracings) and elbow (bottom tracings). (From Hopf HC. Forearm ulnar-to-median nerve anastomosis if sensory axons. Muscle Nerve 1990;13:655.)

There are many variations of the innervation in hand intrinsic muscles. This anomalous communication was described by Riches and Cannieu and so is referred to as the Riches-Cannieu anastomosis (3). It is not clear whether these communications are sensory, motor, or mixed. Mannerfelt noted these communications in three of nine hand dissections (1).

Roundtree (14) found significant variations in the standard pattern of innervation in 20% of 226 cases studied and the pattern of innervation described in standard textbooks in only 33% of cases. The most common variation seen in 33% of patients with anomalous innervation was all thenar muscles (flexor pollicis brevis, abductor pollicis brevis, adductor pollicis, and opponens pollicis) to be entirely innervated by the median nerve. The next common variation (32% of patients) was median nerve innervation of the abductor pollicis brevis and opponens pollicis and the entire flexor pollicis brevis by the ulnar nerve. Fifteen percent of patients showed innervation of the abductor pollicis brevis and opponens pollicis by the median nerve and dual innervation of the flexor pollicis brevis. Two percent had all intrinsic hand muscles innervated by the ulnar nerve. In 1%, the entire thenar muscle, adductor pollicis and first dorsal interosseous were innervated by the median nerve. In 2%, the entire thenar muscle and adductor pollicis were innervated by the median nerve, and the first dorsal interosseous and abductor digiti quinti by the ulnar nerve. According to Gutmann (3), the hypothenar muscle at times has innervation from the median nerve.

In the presence of a Riches-Cannieu anastomosis, the clinical findings and the needle EMG findings in the muscles of a patient with a complete nerve lesion may be identical to those seen with a partial injury to the nerve.

It is difficult to recognize this anomaly by the nerve conduction studies alone unless all intrinsic hand muscles are innervated either by ulnar or median nerves. In the "all median hand," the CMAP from the hypothenar muscle shows a decent response with the initial negative deflection upon wrist stimulation of the median nerve (15). In the "all ulnar hand," the CMAP from the thenar muscle shows a decent response with the initial negative deflection upon wrist stimulation of the ulnar nerve. In both situations, the anastomosis on the forearm should be ruled out by stimulation of the median and ulnar nerves in the elbow. There should not be any substantial difference in the CMAP amplitude with wrist and elbow stimulation of the same nerve.

Kimura and Ayyar addressed this issue and suggested an electrophysiological method of identifying the Riches-Cannieu anastomosis (16). By stimulating the median and ulnar nerves at the wrist and recording the CMAP on the abductor pollicis brevis, first dorsal interosseous, and abductor digiti quinti muscles, they calculated the ulnar or median nerve innervation ratio as follows:

Ulnar nerve innervation ratio (%) in the abductor pollicis brevis equals to:

$$\frac{\text{the CMAP amplitude with ulnar stimulation}}{\text{the CMAP amplitude with ulnar stimulation} + \text{the CMAP with median stimulation}} \times 100$$

Median nerve innervation ratio (%) in the first dorsal interosseous or abductor digiti quinti muscle equals to:

$$\frac{\text{the CMAP amplitude with median stimulation}}{\text{the CMAP amplitude with median stimulation} + \text{the CMAP ulnar stimulation}} \times 100$$

It should be noted that they measured the negative peak as the amplitude. They did not specify the criteria of ulnar-to-median or median-to-ulnar-nerve communication. However, any ratio beyond 10% seems to be regarded as an index of such communication. Using this criterion, they found ulnar-to-median communication in 125 (83.3%) of 150 hands and median-to-ulnar communication in 65 (43.3%) of 150 hands from the first dorsal interosseous muscle and in 24 (16.0%) from the abductor digiti quinti muscle.

This method is not valid for identification of the Riches-Cannieu anastomosis because it does not consider the volume-conducted response as a contributing factor in the CMAP amplitude. The only reliable method is to record the CMAP response with subcutaneous needles from the intrinsic hand muscles and to stimulate the ulnar and median nerves at the wrist and elbow with the near-nerve needle in order to reduce the artifact generated by volume conduction-induced stimulation and responses. This has to be further confirmed by the same study after blocking the normally innervating nerve at the wrist. In fact, Dumitru et al. confirmed one case of ulnar-to-median-nerve communication by such a study before and after blocking the median nerve with a local anesthetic (Fig. 14.13) (17).

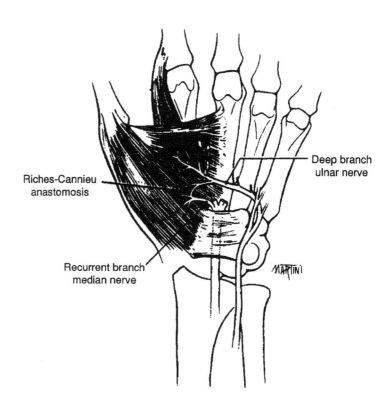

Figure 14.13. The Riches-Cannieu anastomosis between the deep ulnar nerve and the recurrent branch of the median nerve. (From Dumitru D, Walsh NE, Weber CF. Electrophysiologic study of the Riches-Cannieu anomaly. EMG Clin Neurophysiol 1988;28:28.)

Anomalous Innervation of the Musculocutaneous Nerve

The musculocutaneous nerve usually innervates the biceps branchii and coracobrachialis. However, on rare occasions this nerve has been found to innervate the flexors of the median nerve in the forearm and to extend to innervate a part of the thenar muscle group (18) (Fig. 14.14). There was one case reported by Marinacci (19): A 39-year-old laborer fell and injured the right upper extremity. A needle EMG study showed 50% denervation activity in the biceps, about 25% denervation activity in the flexors of the forearm, and about 5% denervation activity in the thenar muscle group. Motor NCV in the median and ulnar nerves was normal. Needle EMG in many muscles innervated by axillary, radial, and ulnar nerves was normal. Marinacci reasoned that the median nerve injury was ruled out because of the fact that the same degree of denervation activity present in the forearm was not present in the thenar muscle group. He concluded that the needle EMG findings in this case were consistent with an isolated anomalous musculocutaneous nerve lesion.

Accessory Deep Peroneal Nerve

The accessory deep peroneal nerve is a common variant of the common peroneal nerve innervating the extensor digitorum brevis (EDB). The EDB is usually innervated exclusively by the deep peroneal nerve, a main branch of the common peroneal nerve. However, in 19–22% of individuals, one or both of the EDBs are innervated partially by the accessory deep peroneal nerve, a branch of the superficial peroneal nerve (20–22) (Table 14.3).

The accessory deep peroneal nerve arises from the superficial peroneal nerve midway on the lateral aspect of the leg; it passes deep and posterior to the peroneus brevis tendon, behind the lateral malleolus, and subsequently innervates the lateral portion of the EDB (Fig. 14.15). This anomaly seems to be inherited in an autosomal dominant mode. Crutchfield and Gutmann (20) showed that 78% of relatives of five subjects also had the anomaly, compared with 22% of unrelated individuals. Awareness of this variation in innervation of the EDB is important for the correct clinical and electromyo-

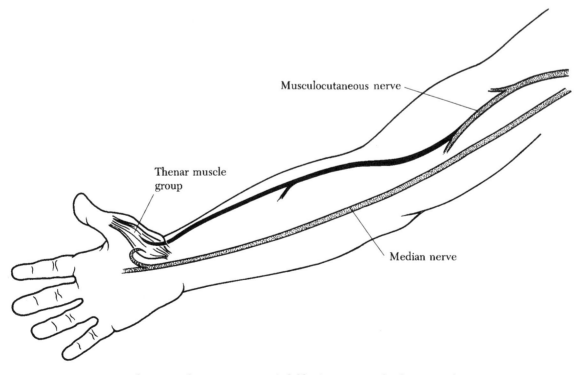

Figure 14.14.   Anomalous musculocutaneous nerve *(solid line)* innervating the thenar muscles.

Table 14.3.
Frequency of the Accessory Deep Peroneal Nerve

Investigator	Group Studied	Frequency (%)
Lambert (22)	50 healthy persons	22
Infante and Kennedy (21)	22 healthy persons	18.7
	82 EMG patients	
Crutchfield and Gutmann (20)	100 healthy persons	22

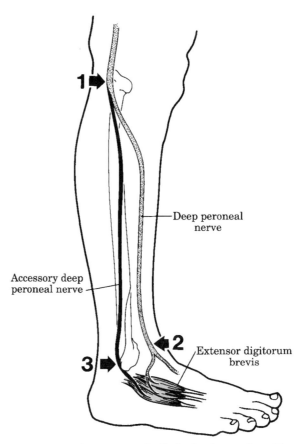

Figure 14.15.   Accessory peroneal nerve. **1**, At the fibular head. **2**, At the ankle. **3**, Behind the lateral malleolus. These are the sites for stimulation to confirm the presence of the accessory peroneal nerve (*solid line*).

graphic evaluation of peroneal nerve lesions.

This anatomical variation can be easily proved by stimulating the peroneal nerve at three locations: the deep peroneal nerve at the ankle, the common peroneal nerve at the fibular head (conventional method), and the accessory deep peroneal nerve posterior to the lateral malleolus.

This anatomical variation should be suspected when the amplitude of the EDB CMAP is considerably smaller when stimulating the deep peroneal nerve at the ankle compared with stimulating the common peroneal nerve at the knee. Normally, the amplitude of the EDB CMAP by stimulating the deep peroneal nerve at the ankle should be 90–120% of the amplitude obtained by stimulating the common peroneal nerve at the knee (3).

In the presence of an accessory deep peroneal nerve, the following typical findings of the nerve conduction are noted (Fig. 14.16):

1. *The amplitude of the EDB CMAP is 0.2 mV or greater upon stimulation of the accessory deep peroneal nerve (2).* This stimulation is associated with a visible EDB twitch. Using the above criteria, Crutchfield and Gutmann (2) found the accessory deep peroneal nerve in 22% of 100 healthy unrelated individuals. In 12 individuals with the accessory deep peroneal nerve, Infante and Kennedy (21) recorded a CMAP amplitude of 0.4–3.0 mV. Stimulation of the accessory deep peroneal nerve posterior to the lateral malleolus produced visible contraction of the lateral part of the EDB. This consisted of contraction of the fourth toe in a majority of cases and, in rare cases, of the third and fifth toes (22). Lambert was able to follow the course of the superficial peroneal nerve from the lateral malleolus to the common peroneal nerve at the knee in steps of 2–5 cm in all cases. The average NCV of the accessory deep peroneal nerve was reported to be 50 m/sec (22).

2. *The EDB CMAP is abnormally smaller (less than 90%) after stimulation of the deep peroneal nerve on the dorsum of the ankle than it is after stimulation of the common peroneal nerve at the knee.* Because Gutmann (3) reported that the amplitude of the EDB CMAP after stimulation at the ankle is 90–120% of that after stimulation at the knee, it is reasonable to judge that less than 90% is abnormal.

3. The amplitude of the EDB CMAP upon stimulation of the accessory deep peroneal nerve at the ankle is approximately equal to the difference between the CMAP of the deep peroneal nerve at the ankle and the common peroneal nerve at the knee. This is evoked by stimulation of the accessory deep peroneal nerve posterior to the lateral malleolus. When the accessory deep peroneal nerve and the deep peroneal nerve are stimulated simultaneously in the same plane at the ankle, the EDB CMAP is essentially the same as that after stimulation of the common peroneal nerve at the knee (22).

4. The EDB CMAP is largest after stimulation of the accessory deep peroneal nerve and the difference between the responses after stimulation of the common and deep peroneal nerves is largest when the recording electrodes are placed over the lateral part of the EDB and smallest when the recording electrodes are placed over the median part of the muscle (22).

Lambert (22) cited one condition in which the response of the EDB to stimulation of the common peroneal nerve may be larger than that evoked by stimulation of the deep peroneal nerve, in the absence of the accessory deep peroneal nerve. He stated that in some patients with a chronic polyneuropathy or with a nerve regenerating after peroneal nerve injury, fibers innervating the EDB may easily be excited at the knee, but

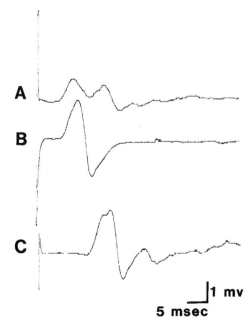

Figure 14.16. Accessory peroneal nerve in a patient with diabetes mellitus without neuropathy. *A,* CMAP upon peroneal ankle stimulation. *B,* CMAP upon accessory peroneal ankle stimulation. *C,* CMAP upon peroneal fibular head stimulation.

they may have a very high threshold to stimulation at the ankle. Fortunately, in these instances a high threshold to stimulation is associated with a low NCV. There is no response after stimulation posterior to the lateral malleolus.

The presence of the accessory deep peroneal nerve may cause confusion in the evaluation of peroneal nerve lesions under the following clinical situations:

1. A lesion affecting the accessory deep peroneal nerve or the superficial peroneal nerve from which it arises might produce fibrillation and positive sharp waves in the EDB. This might erroneously be interpreted as evidence of a lesion in the deep peroneal nerve.

2. In the presence of the accessory deep peroneal nerve, a complete lesion of the deep peroneal nerve might be interpreted erroneously as evidence of a partial lesion of the deep peroneal nerve. The EMG in the lateral belly of the EDB records no fibrillation but a normal number of motor unit potentials (MUPs). Stimulation of the common peroneal nerve at the knee would still produce the response in the EDB. Gutmann reported two such cases (23): Two patients had complete deep peroneal nerve lesions but a good response in the EDB after stimulation of the common peroneal nerve at the knee. The author correctly identified the presence of the accessory deep peroneal nerve by the method described above. He stressed that clinically residual function in the lateral portion of the EDB, in the face of an otherwise complete deep peroneal palsy, should suggest this anatomical variation, and that the needle EMG should substantiate the clinical findings.

3. In a partial lesion involving a physiological block at the knee, the expected smaller CMAP after stimulation above the head of the fibula (compared with at the ankle) may be lost because of the concomitant smaller CMAP upon ankle stimulation of the deep peroneal nerve resulting from this anomaly (3). However, in this circumstance, upon common peroneal nerve stimulation below the head of the fibula, one would expect a larger CMAP than that seen at the other two stimulation sites.

Accessory Superfical Peroneal Sensory Nerve

In normal individuals the superficial peroneal sensory nerve divides into medial and intermediate terminal branches, which run anteriorly over the ankle to supply most of the dorsal foot with sensory innervation. An accessory superficial peroneal sensory nerve has been reported in one case (24). The patient complained of pain over the right lateral malleolus and proximal dorsum of the foot without any weakness or sensory loss. There was a firm, cord-like structure traversing the lateral aspect of the right lateral malleolus in a rostro-caudal direction. There was no Tinel's sign. Antidromic stimulation of the superficial peroneal sensory nerve approximately 12 cm proximal to the ankle at the anterior edge of the fibula elicited a small (2.8 μV) CNAP with slow NCV (33.3 m/sec) over the cord-like structure at the lateral malleolus. Stimulation of the sural nerve in the posterior mid-calf region resulted in no recorded response over this structure. Nerve conduction in the common peroneal, superficial peroneal sensory, and sural nerves was reported to be normal. During surgery a constricting fascial band was found overlying the nerve as it crossed the lateral malleolus. Moving the recording or stimulating electrode even slightly resulted in loss of the CNAP, indicating that the response was from an underlying structure and was not volume-conducted from the distal nerve. Thus, Rubin et al. believed that this nerve is an anomalous sensory branch of the superficial peroneal nerve (24).

Motor Fibers in the Sural Nerve

The sural nerve is generally thought to be composed exclusively of sensory fibers innervating the lateral side of the foot and little toe. Liguori and Trojaborg reported one case in human subjects with an incidental finding of anomalous innervation of the abductor digiti quinti (ADQ) muscle of the foot via the sural nerve (25). In this case a motor branch left the main trunk of the sural nerve 2 cm above the lateral malleolus to innervate the ADQ (Fig. 14.17), and the ADQ muscle was innervated by the sural as well as the posterior tibial nerve. Stimulation of the sural nerve at mid-calf evoked an antidromic sensory CNAP at the lateral malleolus, which was followed by a broad

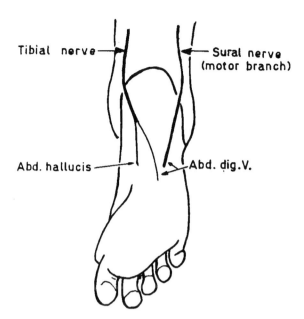

Figure 14.17. Anomalous innervation of the ADQ via sural nerve fibers branching off approximately 2 cm above the lateral malleolus. The lateral plantar branch of the tibial nerve to the ADQ is also indicated. (From Liguori R, Trojaborg W. Are there motor fibers in the sural nerve? Muscle Nerve 1990;13:13.)

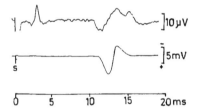

Figure 14.18. *Top,* A sensory CNAP recorded over the sural nerve at the lateral mallelous following stimulation at midleg. The antidromic conducted response was followed by a late response volume-conducted from the abductor digiti quinti (ADQ) muscle. *Bottom,* A CMAP from the ADQ following stimulation of the sural nerve at mid-leg. (From Liguori R, Trojaborg W. Are there motor fibers in the sural nerve? Muscle Nerve 1990;13:13.)

response volume-conducted from the ADQ. By inserting a concentric needle electrode into the ADQ and stimulating the sural nerve at multiple sites proximally along its length, they confirmed that the broad response was generated from the ADQ muscle (Fig. 14.18).

To identify this anomaly, the recording electrode should be placed on the sural nerve at the lateral malleolus and on the ADQ muscle, with stimulation applied at the mid-calf site of the sural nerve. This produces characteristic findings:

1. Sensory CNAP is recorded at the lateral malleolus as usual;
2. Sensory CNAP is followed by a late broad motor response;
3. Motor CMAP is recorded from the ADQ muscle; and
4. Orthodromic sural nerve conduction is normal.

This anomaly could potentially mask a complete lesion of the lateral plantar nerve if erroneously interpreted as a partial lesion. Such a case has not been reported.

REFERENCES

1. Mannerfelt L. Studies on the hand in ulnar nerve paralysis. A clinical experimental investigation in normal and anomalous innervations. Acta Orthop Scand (Suppl) 1966;87:23–142.
2. Crutchfield C, Gutmann L. Hereditary aspects of accessory deep peroneal nerve. J Neurol Neurosurg Psychiatry 1973;36:899–990.
3. Gutmann L. Important anomalous innervations of the extremities. AAEE Minimonograph # 2, Rochester, Minnesota, 1979.
4. Gutmann L. Median-ulnar nerve communications and carpal tunnel syndrome. J Neurol Neurosurg Psychiatry 1977;36:899–990.

5. Gutmann L, Gutierrez A, Riggs JE. The contribution of median-ulnar communications in diagnosis of mild carpal tunnel syndrome. Muscle Nerve 1986;9:319–321.

6. Iyer V, Fenichel GM. Normal median nerve proximal latency in carpal tunnel syndrome: a clue to coexisting Martin-Gruber anastomosis. J Neurol Neurosurg Psychiatry 1976;39:449–452.

7. Lambert EH. Diagnostic value of electrical stimulation of motor nerves. EEG Clin Neurophys (Suppl) 1962;22:9–16.

8. Santoro L, Rosato R, Caruso G. Median-ulnar nerve communications: electrophysiological demonstration of motor and sensory fiber cross-over. J Neurol 1983;229:227–235.

9. Kimura J, Murphy MJ, Varda DJ. Electrophysiological study of anomalous innervation of intrinsic hand muscles. Arch Neurol 1976;33:842–844.

10. Marinacci AA. Anomalous innervation of the small muscles of the hand—"all median" or "all ulnar hand." In: Applied electromyography. Philadelphia: Lea & Febiger, 1968;23–30.

11. Kómár J, Szegvári M, Gloviczky A, et al. Traumatische Durschnitt des N medianus ohne kompletee motoriche Parese: Martin-Grubeische Anastomose. Nervenarzt 1978;49:697–699.

12. Streib EW. Ulnar-to-median nerve anastomosis in the forearm: electromyographic studies. Neurology 1979;29:1534–1537.

13. Hopf HC. Forearm ulnar-to-median nerve anastomosis of sensory axons. Muscle Nerve 1990;13:654–656.

14. Roundtree T. Anomalous innervation of the hand muscles. J Bone Joint Surg 1949;31–B:505–510.

15. Marinacci AA. The problem of unusual anomalous innervation of hand muscles. The value of electrodiagnosis in its evaluation. Bull LA Neurol Soc 1964;29:133–142.

16. Kimura I, Ayyar DR. The hand neural communication between the ulnar and median nerves: electrophysiological detection. Electromyog Clin Neurophysiol 1984;24:409–441.

17. Dumitru D, Walsh NE, Weber CF. Electrophysiologic study of the Riches-Cannieu anomaly. Electromyog Clin Neurophysiol 1988;28:27–31.

18. Haymaker W, Woodhall B. Peripheral nerve injuries. Philadelphia: WB Saunders, 1953.

19. Marinacci AA. Diagnosis of "all median hand." Bull LA Neurol Soc 1964;29:191–197.

20. Crutchfield CA, Gutmann L. Hereditary aspects of median-ulnar nerve communications. J Neurol Neurosurg Psychiatry 1980;43:53–55.

21. Infante E, Kennedy WR. Anomalous branch of the deep nerve detected by electromyography. Arch Neurol 1970;22:162–165.

22. Lambert EH. The accessory deep peroneal nerve: a common variation in innervation of extensor digitorum brevis. Neurology 1969;19:1169–1176.

23. Gutmann L. Important anomalous innervations of the extremities. AAEE Minimonograph # 2, 1979.

24. Rubin M, Menche D, Pitman M. Entrapment of an accessory superficial peroneal sensory nerve. Can J Neurol Sci 1991;18:342–343.

25. Liguori R, Trojaborg W. Are there motor fibers in the sural nerve? Muscle Nerve 1990;13:12–15.

26. Sun SF, Streib EW. Martin-Gruber anastomosis: electromyographic studies. Part 2. Electromyogr Clin Neurophysiol 1983;23:271–285.

27. Wilbourn AJ, Lambert EH. The forearm median-to-ulnar nerve communication; electrodiagnostic aspects. Neurology 1976;26:368.

15

Near-Nerve Needle Technique in Sensory Nerve Conduction

For the recording of sensory compound nerve action potentials (CNAP), early authors (1, 2) suggested the use of a pair of surface electrodes placed 2-3 cm apart along the nerve to be examined. This is still widely accepted as the standard method of testing in the United States and England. In 1966, Buchthal and Rosenfalck introduced the near-nerve needle technique in the nerve conduction study in a classic monograph (3). Since then, this technique has been widely accepted on the European continent. An extensive review of this subject was recently published (4).

There is no question that this technique provides considerable and invaluable information that cannot be obtained with the surface electrode. The surface electrode technique and the near-nerve needle technique are compared in Table 15.1 and Figure 15.1. Even in laboratories where surface electrodes are used routinely in sensory nerve conduction studies, the near-nerve needle technique is definitely indicated: (a) when the surface electrode technique fails to identify the abnormalities in clinically suspected cases of early mild neuropathy. Abnormal temporal dispersion (dispersion phenomenon) or a slowing of the minimal nerve conduction velocity (NCV) can be observed with the needle technique (Fig. 20.10); (b) when the CNAP is unrecordable with the surface electrode. Often the needle technique records a tiny CNAP, thus enabling the NCV to be calculated (Fig. 15.2). This information may be vital in differentiating between axonal degeneration and segmental demyelination.

Technique

Needle Electrode

In order to obtain reproducible potentials, needle electrodes with clearly defined dimensions and characteristics should be used. The most commonly used needle is a Teflon-coated steel needle with an uncoated tip that is made specifically for the sensory CNAP (Dantec 13L60-13L64—Dantec Medical, Inc., Santa Clara, CA). An active elec-

Table 15.1.

Comparison of Recording Techniques with Surface Electrodes and Near-Nerve Needle Electrodes

Parameter	Surface Electrodes	Near-Nerve Needle Technique
Technique		
Pain	Painless	Painful on needling
Time required	Less	Longer
Impedance	High	Low; noise/signal ratio markedly reduced
Small potential (1 µV)	Not recordable	Easily recordable
Proximal nerve conduction	Difficult	Easier
Maximum NCV slower than 20 m/sec	CNAP usually not recordable	Can be calculated
CNAP		
Shape	Usually monophasic or diphasic	Usually triphasic
First positive peak	Difficult to identify	Clearly identifiable
Amplitude	Usually smaller (about 50% of CNAP recorded by the needle; better reproducibility in repeated recordings)	Usually higher
Small components	Not recordable	Easily recordable; minimum NCV can be calculated
Abnormal temporal dispersion	Rarely seen	Easily documented

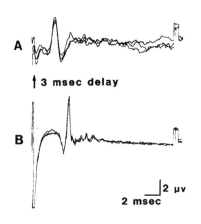

Figure 15.1. Comparison between the sensory CNAP with surface electrodes (**A**) and near-nerve needle electrodes (**B**). The sensory CNAP is from toe I to the medial malleolus. Note the sharp demarcation of the first positive peak, the higher amplitude, and many small components in (**B**) potential. Maximal NCVs [43.5 in (**A**) vs 42.6 m/sec in (**B**)] and negative peak NCVs [36.2 in (**A**) vs 37.3 m/sec in (**B**)] are not different. Minimal NCV (**B**) is calculated to be 19.2 m/sec.

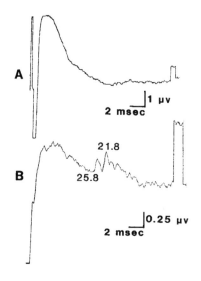

Figure 15.2. Comparison between the sensory CNAP with surface electrodes (**A**) and near-nerve needle electrodes (**B**). No recognizable CNAP is noted with the surface electrodes even after averaging, but a small CNAP is noted in a case of tarsal tunnel syndrome.

trode has an uncoated tip 2 mm in area, and the reference electrode an uncoated tip of 3.5 mm.

To lower the impedance of the needle, regular electrolytic treatments of the electrodes are recommended immediately before use. This is because the impedance of the electrode is greatly increased as a result of repeated use and sterilization. This treatment can be achieved by one of two methods. First, with the current generator (e.g., Dantec 14B48), the impedance of the electrodes is reduced by passing an alternating current of 30 mA for 30 seconds through the active electrode and of 50 mA for 30 seconds through the reference electrode placed in 0.9% NaCl solution at 90°C. Alternatively, with the EMG stimulating unit (e.g., Dantec 15E07/25 stimulator), the electrodes are dipped into a physiological saline solution and a current of up to 50 mA (stimulus duration 1 msec) is allowed to flow for 30 seconds at a stimulation rate of 20/sec. Fortunately, the disposable sensory needles (Dantec 13R22-13R25), which are available now, do not need this electrolytic treatment.

Position of the Needle

The correct position of the active electrode near the nerve is very critical to this technique (Fig. 15.3).

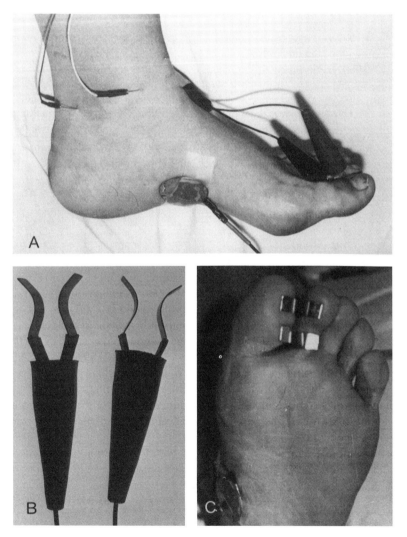

Figure 15.3. Placement of the active recording needle and reference electrodes at the ankle to record the CNAP from the plantar nerves. Note that the reference electrode is placed transversely at least 3 cm away from the active recording needle. (From Oh SJ, Kim HS, Ahmad BK. Electrophysiological diagnosis of the interdigital neuropathy of the foot. Muscle Nerve 1984;7:219.)

1. The correct site for needle placement is chosen first with the aid of the surface-stimulating electrodes. In the ulnar, median, and posterior tibial nerves, a surface-stimulating electrode can pinpoint well the site where the lowest stimulus threshold is required to evoke the motor response. In pure sensory nerves, the stimulating surface electrode can identify the site of the lowest threshold for evoking a sensation radiating into the innervating territory.

2. The active electrode should be inserted at the chosen site to the recommended depth (Table 15.2). If the needle touches the nerve, a radiating electrical sensation is produced along the nerve. This sensation is a sure sign that the needle is near the nerve.

3. To ascertain that the active electrode is as close as possible to the nerve, three procedures are recommended:

  a. The active electrode is used to stimulate motor fibers, and its position is adjusted until the lowest threshold for the compound muscle action potential (CMAP) is reached. The lowest threshold is usually achieved with stimulus intensity between 0.5 mA and 1.0 mA for a 0.2-msec stimulus (3), and between 1 and 5 mA for a 0.05-msec stimulus (5). It is advisable to position the proximal recording electrode first. Otherwise, the distal electrode may be displaced by muscle twitchings caused by proximal stimulation.

  b. The depth and direction of insertion are changed until the maximum amplitude of the sensory CNAP is obtained. Optimal positioning of the active electrode is somewhat difficult in pure sensory nerves. Stimulation is usually carried out distally to evoke the maximum potential in the proximally located active electrode. When recordings are made from more than one point along the nerve, the electrode is used alternately to stimulate the nerve and to record the potential in order to locate the positions with the lowest thresholds of stimulation and the highest potential amplitudes.

  c. The mixed nerve is stimulated distally, and the proximal electrodes are adjusted to obtain maximal amplitude of the CNAP.

According to Buchtahl and Rosenfalck, these three procedures are equally effective in the median, ulnar, and radial nerves; but in the legs a sensory CNAP can be obtained only when the electrodes are brought close to the nerve while stimulating motor fibers or mixed nerves (3). This procedure is naturally difficult and time-consuming in pathological cases where the amplitudes of the sensory CNAP are very small. However, the optimal position-

Table 15.2.
Recording Sites[a]

Nerve	Wrist	Elbow	Axilla
Median	10–20 mm prox. to the border of the flexor retinaculum ulnar to the tendon of m. flexor carpi radialis. Depth: 5 mm	Level of the line between the med. and lat. epicondyli of the humerus, prox. to the bicipital aponeurosis, med. to the brachial artery. Depth: 10–15 mm	Med. bicipital groove, 120–150 mm prox. to the med. epicondylus of the humerus, med. to the brachial artery. Depth: 30 mm
Ulnar	20 mm prox. to the pisiform bone, radial to the tendon of m. flexor carpi ulnaris. Depth: 10 mm	Sulcus on the dorsal aspect of the med. epicondylus of the humerus. Depth: 5–10 mm	Med. groove between the biceps and the coracobrachial and triceps muscles, dorsal to the brachial artery, 120–150 mm prox. to the med. epicondylus. Depth: 30–40 mm
Radial	Lat. border of the radius, 40–50 mm prox. to the styloid process of the radius. Depth: 5 mm	Level of a line between the med. and lat. epicondyli of the humerus in the groove between the brachioradial muscle and the tendon of the brachial biceps muscle. Depth: 20–25 mm	Groove between the coracobrachial muscle and the medial edge of the brachial triceps, 120–150 mm prox. to the med. epicondylus. Depth: 50 mm

Nerve	Ankle	Knee	Buttock
Tibial and sciatic	Equidistant from the med. border of the insertion of the Achilles tendon and the med. malleolus. Depth: 10–15 mm	Popliteal fossa 50 mm prox. to the popliteal plica between semimembranosus and femoral biceps muscles. Depth: ca. 40 mm	Equidistant from the greater trochanter of the femur and the ischial tuberosity at the level of the fold of the buttock. Depth: ca. 70 mm

[a]From Buchthal F, Rosenfalck A. Evoked action potentials and conduction velocity in human sensory nerves. Brain Res 1966;3:110.

ing of the active needle electrode near the nerve is critical because the amplitude is heavily dependent on the nearness of the needle to the nerve.

4. The reference needle electrode should be inserted subcutaneously at the same level as the active electrode at a transverse distance of 3-4 cm. In the case of the median nerve when the thumb is stimulated, the reference electrode is placed "ulnarly" to avoid pick-up from the radial nerve. When a recording potential is evoked by stimulation of the portion of finger 4, which is innervated by the ulnar nerve, the reference electrode should be placed radially (3).

Stimulation and Averaging

The stimulation (0.05-0.2 msec in duration) is given at a rate of 1 sec or less. Supramaximal stimulation must be used to obtain a clinically meaningful CNAP amplitude. In general, to stimulate sensory fibers maximally, the required intensity is at least 40 mA for 0.05 msec stimulus duration (5) and at least 20 mA for 0.1 or 0.2 msec stimulus duration (3). The following guidelines are used to obtain the supramaximal stimulation:

1. When the sensory CNAP is visible on the oscilloscope without averaging, a simple method has proved satisfactory in clinical practice to obtain the supramaximal stimulation. With a gradual increase of stimulation intensity, the point is reached at which the sensory CNAP amplitude is no longer visibly increased (6). If the stimulating intensity is then increased by a further 30-50%, there can be no doubt that supramaximal stimulation has been attained (5, 7).

2. When the sensory CNAP is not easily recognizable without averaging, the sensory threshold is determined by increasing the stimulus intensity slowly until each stimulus is barely felt. The threshold is determined at least three times. Supramaximal stimulation intensity is at least three times the sensory threshold according to our experience (5). Buchthal and Rosenfalck (3) used four to five times the sensory threshold as supramaximal stimulation.

3. In pathological cases where no sensory CNAP is recognizable without averaging and sensory impairment is present, a stimulation intensity of 60-70 mA has to be used. It is true that a greater stimulus intensity is required in patients with neuropathy than in normal subjects.

Sensory potentials of less than 4 μV in amplitude and slow components have been recorded by liberal use of signal averaging. Signal averaging enhances the reliability of the sensory CNAP when it is tiny.

Measurement of Sensory CNAP

The latency is measured from the onset of the stimulus to the initial positive peak of the potential (Fig. 15.4). This latency is used to calculate the maximum sensory NCV. The negative peak latency is measured from the onset of the stimulus to the negative peak

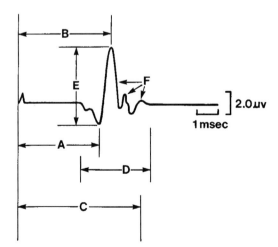

Figure 15.4. Designations of the CNAP. **A**, Latency to the main positive peak for the maximal NCV. **B**, Latency to the negative peak. **C**, Latency to the last negative peak for the minimal NCV. **D**, Duration of the potential. **E**, Peak-to-peak amplitude. **F**, Components.

of the potentials. This negative peak latency is used to calculate the negative peak sensory NCV (5). The amplitude of the potential is marked from peak to peak.

The number of components (peaks) in the potential should also be indicated. According to Ludin et al. (7), only those components that reach at least 10% of the amplitude of the largest components are included. Buchthal et al. (8) identified the small components of the potentials by their shape when they increased in proportion to a calibration signal in subsequent averaging. Shefner et al. required the amplitude of the small components to be at least twice the amplitude of the underlying baseline noise before accepting the small components as a genuine potential (9). We count all superimposable peaks on at least three tracings as the components. The minimum NCV is calculated on the basis of latency to the first positive peak of the last component (8) or to the negative peak of the last component (5).

The duration of the sensory CNAP is measured from the first positive peak to the positive peak of the last component (4) or from the onset of the first positive deflection to the return of the last component to the baseline (3, 5, 6). This measurement is an index of the temporal dispersion.

Artifacts

The most annoying source of artifact is muscle potential generated by the unrelaxed muscle near the needle electrodes. Therefore, it is very important to have the patient as relaxed as possible; to achieve this, an audiomonitor is used. By listening to the baseline noise, the patient can relax better during the study. Muscle potential can also be partially removed by the signal averager, but the "huge muscle potential" (compared with the sensory CNAP) can distort the averaged potential easily. Thus, it is best to eliminate it by complete relaxation of muscles. Some signal averagers are equipped with automatic and manual artifact rejection modes. The use of such a mode greatly reduces the distortion of potential by the muscle potentials.

Another source of artifact is the volume-conducted potentials from other nerves caused by the lack of selective stimulation of the nerve under study. This difficulty

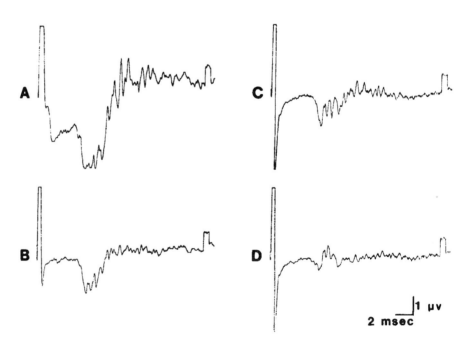

Figure 15.5.   Sensory CNAP contaminated with artifact caused by intraneural insertion of the needle (**A**). Note the extremely high amplitude and the main positive potential. Gradual withdrawal of the needle (**B**, **C**) produces a less distorted CNAP. **D**, Artifact-free CNAP after placement of the needle near the nerve but not in the nerve.

occurs frequently in the fingers, which are innervated by two nerves. In the radial nerve, 25% of the sensory CNAP obtained at the wrist when stimulating the thumb with a ring electrode is due to volume conduction from the median nerve (10). This artifact can easily be eliminated by selective stimulation of the radial nerve at the wrist.

In 1980 Ludin described an artifact that is probably caused by the intraneural position of the needle (7) (Fig. 15.5). This artifact can be recognized by the high amplitude of the first positive peak (two to three times higher than normal) followed by a smaller negative peak. This potential was recorded only when muscle contraction was elicited at a low stimulus intensity during stimulation with the recording electrode in question, and it was always possible to find a normally shaped CNAP when the electrode was slightly withdrawn. As a result, this potential was thought to be due to a reversible conduction block in the nerve fibers caused by pressure from the recording needle. Recognition of this artifact potential is important for avoiding incorrect measurements of latency and amplitude.

Normal Sensory CNAP: Shape and Amplitude

The normal sensory CNAP has a main triphasic potential with a clear initial positive peak followed by a higher-amplitude negative peak. The sensory CNAP recorded at the wrist following stimulation of the finger has an average amplitude of 10-50 μV, with four or five small components of less than 0.5 μV. With a longer conduction distance, the amplitude decreases and temporal dispersion increases. Sensory CNAP at the elbow has an average amplitude of 3-20 μV and seven small components (3, 7). The amplitude of the potential recorded at the ankle and in the popliteal fossa is usually small, about 10% of that recorded at the wrist and at the elbow (8). The potential at the ankle in the posterior tibial nerve evoked by stimuli at the big toe nearly always consists of two to seven components of 0.25-5 μV (5). The sensory CNAP is less dispersed when the sural nerve is stimulated at the dorsum pedis and the potential is recorded at the lateral malleolus (11). The normal values for the sensory nerve conduction are given in Chapters 7 and 11.

REFERENCES

1. Dawson GD. The relative excitability and conduction velocity of sensory and motor nerve fibers. J Physiol (Lond) 1956;131:436-451.
2. Gilliatt RW, Sears TA. Sensory nerve action potentials in patients with peripheral nerve lesions. J Neurol Neurosurg Psychiatry 1958;21:109-118.
3. Buchthal F, Rosenfalck A. Evoked action potentials and conduction velocity in human sensory nerves. Brain Res 1966;3:1-122.
4. Ludin HP, Tackmann W. Sensory neurography. New York: Thieme-Stratton, 1981.
5. Oh SJ, Kim HS, Ahmad BK. Electrophysiological diagnosis of the interdigital neuropathy of the foot. Muscle Nerve 1984;7:218-225.
6. Ludin HP, Lutschs J, Valsansiacomo F. Versleichende Untersuchunsg orthodromer und antidromer sensibler Nervenleitgeschwindigkeiten. 2. Befunde bei polyneuropathien und bei Status nach polyradikulitis. Z EEG-EMG 1977;8:180-186.
7. Ludin HP. Electromyography in practice. New York: Thieme-Stratton, 1980.
8. Buchthal F, Rosenfalck A, Behse F. Sensory potentials of normal and diseased nerves. In: Dyck PJ, Thomas PK, Lambert EH, eds. Peripheral neuropathy. Philadelphia: WB Saunders, 1975:442-464.
9. Shefner JM, Buchthal F, Krarup C. Slowly conducting myelineated fibers in peripheral neuropathy. Muscle Nerve 1991;14:534-542.
10. Trojaborg W, Sindrup EH. 1969. Motor and sensory conduction in different segments of the radial nerve in normal subjects. J Neurol Neurosurg Psychiatry 1969;32:354-359.
11. Behse F, Buchthal F. Normal sensory conduction in the nerves of the leg in man. J Neurol Neurosurg Psychiatry 1971;34:404-414.

16

Intraoperative Nerve Conduction

In every aspect of the management of peripheral nerve injuries, electromyography (EMG) studies are an essential part of the tests, giving the clinician valuable objective information. Serial EMG examinations are critically important in severe nerve injury. Although there are divergent opinions regarding the best timing of surgical exploration and repair of a severe peripheral nerve injury, surgical exploration is recommended if there is no evidence of clinical and electrophysiological improvement within 2–4 months after injury in patients with a complete nerve lesion (absence of any clinical and electrophysiological function of the nerve) (1, 2). In patients with a complete nerve lesion, the clinician is interested in knowing whether there is any discontinuity in the severely injured nerve. Unfortunately, EMG techniques cannot yet provide this information because there are no electrophysiologic parameters that can distinguish between total and partial division of an injured nerve.

About 60–75% of nerve injuries produce a lesion in continuity (1), usually as a result of contusion, severe compression or stretching, fracture, injection injuries, and gunshot wounds. With an injury likely to produce total transection of the nerve, e.g., laceration of the extremity by glass or a knife, relatively earlier surgical exploration is recommended once the complete nerve lesion is documented because the nerve is most likely found to be transected (3).

If a nerve is found to be completely severed during surgical exploration, it does not present any problem in surgical management—it must be sutured. However, with a lesion in continuity, it is difficult to decide whether to resect the lesion. Lesions in continuity may appear as large neuromas but with mature and longitudinally oriented axons centrally, whereas those appearing as small neuromas can have severe intraneural fibrosis and marked axonal disorganization (4). The management of these lesions in continuity has been improved by recording the compound nerve action potential (CNAP) from the surface of the exposed nerve or nerve fascicle in the operating room (3, 5–7).

Technique

Instrumentation and Machine Set-up

Kline's group has used their own assembled equipment since 1968, consisting of the Grass S44 stimulator (Grass Instrument Co., Quincy, MA), which includes a stimulus isolation unit (Grass SIU5), an oscilloscope with differential amplifier (Grass P55), and a Polaroid camera (3, 5, 8). However, there is no longer any need to assemble EMG components for the performance of intraoperative nerve conduction because the modern EMG machine can be used for this purpose without any technical difficulty (9, 10). In fact, modern EMG machines have the added advantage of signal averaging capability.

Many different filter ranges have been used by various investigators: 1 Hz–3 kHz by Kline (8); 20 Hz–20 kHz by Terzis and Publicover (7); 16 Hz–16 kHz by Nelson (10); and 300 Hz–3 kHz by Van Beek et al. (11). We use a standard filter range for the sensory and mixed nerve conduction (20 Hz–2 kHz). Selection of sensitivity depends on the amplitude of the recorded CNAPs. Keep in mind that the amplitude of CNAPs recorded on exposed nerves is higher than routine CNAPs, ranging from 20 μV to 1 mV. In normal exposed nerves, the CNAP amplitude is usually higher than 100 μV. Most investigators did not measure the exact amplitude of the CNAPs in injured exposed nerves because they did not attach too much significance to CNAP amplitude (8, 12, 13). In general, the amplitude of the CNAPs in injured exposed nerves is less than 100 μV. Thus, it is prudent to select *a sensitivity of 50–100 μV at the beginning and adjust the sensitivity according to the amplitude of obtained CNAPs.* Lambert and Dyck stated that, with monopolar in vitro recordings of the sural nerve, the CNAP amplitudes from whole nerves or fascicles are similar and that the amplitude depends on the density of axons (14). This indicates that the amplitude of the CNAP in exposed nerves may directly reflect the number of viable axons in the damaged nerves. Therefore, the amplitude of the CNAP may be more important than previously thought in the intraoperative nerve conduction.

Sweep velocity depends on the distance between the stimulating and recording electrodes. Considering the short interelectrode distance in exposed nerves, 0.5–1 msec is recommended for the sweep velocity set-up. This set-up will usually separate the CNAP from stimulus artifact and reliably measure the latency.

The shortest stimulus duration available on the EMG machine (0.05–1 msec) must be used to reduce stimulus artifact. It is important to remember that a minuscule intensity is needed to evoke a CNAP on the exposed normal nerve compared with that used for surface electrode stimulation in routine nerve conduction studies. *Stimulus intensity for the supramaximal stimulation on the exposed normal nerve is usually 1–10 mA (25–50 V).* If no CNAP is obtained with a stimulus intensity of 20 mA or 125 V, it is unlikely to obtain the CNAP with a higher stimulus intensity. We prefer manual stimulation to adjust the stimulus intensity for the supramaximal stimulation and to allow for adequate analysis of the CNAP. For signal averaging a stimulation of 0.5–1 per sec is recommended.

Stimulating and Recording Electrodes

Stimulating and recording electrodes used for the intraoperative nerve conduction are not commercially available (Fig. 16.1). These electrodes may either be custom-made (see the Appendix) or ordered through special arrangements from Dr. Kline's laboratory (Dr. L. T. Happel, Department of Neurosurgery, Louisiana State University Medical Center, New Orleans, LA). Details of construction were described by Burbank and have been included in the Appendix for the convenience of our readers (15).

Platinum-iridium wire is recommended for the electrodes, although stainless steel wire may be used. The size of the electrodes will vary depending on the nerve tested. For most nerves a 1-mm diameter wire is of sufficient strength and size. For smaller nerves a smaller-diameter steel wire is needed, such as the Grass mounted EEG steel needle electrode (10). For the rootlets or finer nerves a bipolar needle can be used for the stimulating electrode. Whatever size needle is used, these electrodes should meet two important conditions for an adequate intraoperative nerve conduction study: *(a) the end can be hooked so that the nerve can be cradled around the electrode; and (b) the distance between the cathode and the anode can be adjusted.*

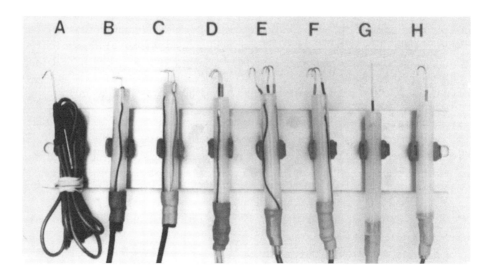

Figure 16.1. Electrodes used for intraoperative nerve conduction. Holder is sterilized with electrodes in place. Towel clips on each end secure holder near the recording site. *A*, Hooked ground, which can be placed directly on the nerve or in adjacent tissues. *B*, Fine recording electrodes for small nerves. *C*, Fine bipolar stimulating electrodes with ground. *D*, Bipolar recording electrodes. *E*, Bipolar stimulating electrodes (bent toward each other) with ground. *F*, Bipolar stimulating electrodes. *G*, Monopolar stimulating probe (active). *H*, Monopolar hook stimulating electrode (reference). (From Nelson KR. Use of peripheral nerve action potentials for intraoperative monitoring. Neurol Clin 1988;6:927.)

The stimulating cathode and anode should be mounted closely together to limit current spread and reduce stimulus artifact. The ground electrode (for which we use an alligator clip) can be placed near or on the nerve between the stimulating and recording electrodes. This is essential to reduce not only muscle potential artifacts but stimulus artifacts as well. Sometimes a hooked ground placed just distal to the stimulating cathode in the same holder helps to reduce stimulus artifact (Fig. 16.1E). Occasionally an active monopolar stimulating electrode is used (Fig. 16.1F), with a reference plate or hook as close as possible to the active electrode to limit current spread and reduce the stimulus artifact (10). Recording electrodes are similar to those used for stimulation. However, a longer distance between the active and reference electrodes is needed to enhance the amplitude of the CNAP. Usually a 1-cm distance is adequate for this purpose.

There must be a definite marker for the active and reference electrodes, usually by color coding of the wires. This facilitates the rapid and proper placement of stimulating and recording electrodes. Active stimulating and recording electrodes should be placed facing each other, following the standard rule for the nerve conduction. The electrode handle must be comfortable enough to facilitate placement and minimize trauma to the nerve, since the electrodes are usually hand-held. *Electrodes with a holder and cable should be gas-sterilized, because autoclaving may damage the cable.*

Preparation

Long before the actual recording, it is important to identify an operating room in which the intraoperative nerve conduction can be satisfactorily performed. From our personal experience, not all operating rooms are equally suited. In certain rooms it is impossible to perform the intraoperative nerve conduction because of electrical interference, usually from 60 Hz artifact. There are many potential sources of 60 Hz artifact in the operating suite. If this occurs, it is best to identify and eliminate the artifact source. The use of shorter recording leads with the preamplifier near the recording electrodes is helpful. We usually attach the preamplifier to the operating table. The connecting cable from the preamplifier to the EMG machine should be electrically shielded (16).

Before each intraoperative nerve conduction test, it is important to check the EMG machine, cables, and electrodes for proper functioning and to prepare enough cables and electrodes for testing. The EMG machine must be placed properly to ensure a clear view of the operating field by the electromyographer, who can confirm the correct placement of the stimulating and recording electrodes by the surgeon and observe the clinical motor response with the stimulation of the nerve.

Three important factors the surgeon must consider for adequate intraoperative nerve conduction testing are: (*a*) the tourniquet; (*b*) neuromuscular blocking agents;

and (c) generous exposure of the nerve. If a tourniquet is used, this should be deflated for a 15– to 20–minute period before beginning intraoperative recordings of the CNAP (17), because ischemia alone can produce a transient absence of CNAP. Neuromuscular blocking agents do not affect the recording of the CNAP. In fact, this is one advantage of intraoperative nerve conduction testing over intraoperative motor nerve stimulation testing. However, surgeons and electromyographers are usually also interested in observing the clinical motor response with stimulation of the nerve. In such cases, neuromuscular blocking agents should not be used during monitoring because this will abolish the motor response. Generous exposure of the nerve is important for a technically satisfactory intraoperative nerve conduction, often requiring a wider exposure than when such testing is not needed. *A minimum of 5–6 cm distance between stimulating and recording electrodes* is needed to record the CNAP adequately with an ordinary EMG machine (9, 10), and sometimes an even greater separation is needed to obtain an adequate CNAP.

Methods of Intraoperative Nerve Conduction

The conventional method of intraoperative nerve conduction has been whole-nerve conduction (Figs. 16.2 and 16.3) (8, 12, 18). Williams and Terzis introduced a single fascicular recording method (7, 13), which differs from whole-nerve conduction in that the study is performed in a single isolated nerve fascicle (Fig. 16.4). They reported that this test can determine precisely the functional integrity of individual fascicles involved in lesions in continuity by comparing the amplitude and shape of the CNAP and the NCV of the involved fascicle with those found in an intact fascicle. Such information on

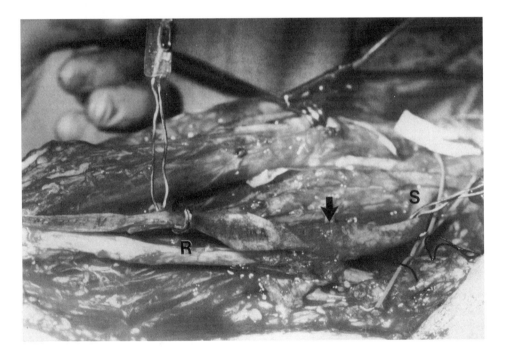

Figure 16.2. Placement of the stimulating and recording electrodes across a neuroma *(arrow)* in the median nerve. **S**, Stimulating electrodes. **R**, Recording electrodes. Courtesy of Dr. Richard Meyer.

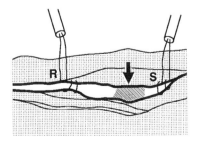

Figure 16.3. Schematic drawing of Figure 16.2.

Figure 16.4. Single fascicular recording technique. (From Williams HB, Terzis JK. Single fascicular recordings: an intraoperative diagnostic tool for the management of peripheral nerve lesions. Plas Reconstr Surg 1976;57:563.)

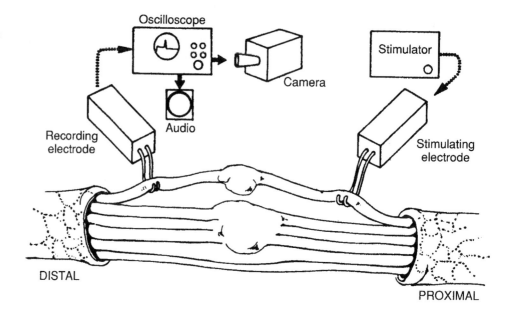

Figure 16.4. Single fascicular recording technique. (From Williams HB, Terzis JK. Single fascicular recordings: an intraoperative diagnostic tool for the management of peripheral nerve lesions. Plas Reconstr Surg 1976;57:563.)

the functional status of each fascicle is needed so that an objective decision can be made to preserve or resect a specific fascicle.

The determination as to which intraoperative nerve conduction method should be used depends on the preoperative clinical and electrophysiological findings. According to Terzis et al. (19), in cases of complete lesion where there are complete motor and sensory deficits distally, only whole-nerve recordings should be used. On the other hand, in cases where there is useful distal function, a combination of whole-nerve and single-fascicular recordings can be utilized (19).

Another method of intraoperative nerve conduction was introduced by Van Beek et al. (11). Their method records percutaneously the somatosensory evoked potentials (SEP) in the cervical spine and the CNAP at the Erb's point after stimulation of the exposed nerve below and above the neuroma. They reported that this technique has an advantage over Kline's method in that general nerve dissection is not needed. We believe that the same information can be obtained before surgery by employing the same technique with an ordinary EMG machine. Thus, this technique does not seem to provide any advantage over a detailed preoperative CNAP study. Further, it should be remembered that the Erb's point recording is not a direct recording from the exposed nerve and may not reflect the actual functional integrity of the tested nerve.

Actual Testing

Once an adequate segment of nerve is exposed, the stimulating and recording electrodes should be placed following the standard method of the nerve conduction. *It is imperative to lift the nerve from the surrounding tissue and fluid with hand-held electrodes.* Blood and spinal fluid (if any) are irrigated away from the electrode. In the case of fascicular nerve conduction, a tested fascicle should be lifted from the other fascicles.

Even with a preoperative equipment check, it is important to check the equipment again after the electrodes are placed on the exposed nerve. Initially, both the stimulating and recording electrodes are placed either proximal to the lesion or on a normal nerve because a CNAP should be recordable at this site if the system is working correctly. Once it is verified that the system is working correctly, the recording electrodes are moved along the injured area and into the distal stump to see if a response can be evoked through the lesion (Fig. 16.2). Stimulation and/or recording at several sites along the nerve will provide the most useful information in attempting to find a conduction block. Stimulation of the nerve is achieved by gradually increasing the stimulus intensity until a maximal CNAP is obtained. Again, it is important to remember that *stimulation on the exposed nerve requires a minimal intensity compared with the routine nerve conduction.* Signal averaging is not used by Kline and DeJonge or Terzis et al. (12, 13, 19), but Van Beek et al. used signal averaging to obtain the CNAP (11).

Measurement of the CNAP

Unlike in routine nerve conduction testing, detailed measurements of the nerve conduction parameters have not been obtained for the intraoperative nerve conduction. *The absence or presence of the CNAP is the most important indicator for or against surgery* (8, 19). Kline's group used a nonaveraged CNAP and felt that an absent response indicates that the nerve lacks the number of axons required for clinically significant recovery (12, 20). With their technique, amplitudes of less than 20 µV are unreliable and yet would indicate neurolysis (20). Terzis et al. measured the amplitudes of the CNAP and NCV and compared those with the data obtained from the intact fascicle (13, 19). A surgical decision was made not on the basis of these data, but on the absence or presence of the CNAP. Thus, except for academic interest there seems to be no need for the calculation of NCV. The temperature in the exposed nerve is considerably less than the patient's core temperature. Also, it is impossible to control nerve temperature in the modern operating suite.

Van Beek et al. used signal averaging to obtain the CNAP and measured the CNAP amplitude in 14 patients with nerve injuries (11). When present, the amplitude of CNAP ranged from 5 to 63 µV. Although absolute neurophysiological data were lacking, they felt that neurolysis was indicated when the amplitude of CNAP exceeded 40 µV and that an NCV below 30 m/sec represented an unfavorable prognosis. The method of NCV calculation and the values were not given. Thus, it seems that there is no need for detailed measurement of the various parameters of nerve conduction in the intraoperative nerve conduction at this time.

Rationale

Experimental studies of crushed or severed and sutured nerves in primates have shown that the presence, and in general the form, of the CNAP along a lesion in continuity are related to the axon population and maturity in regenerating nerves (21). To obtain a CNAP, either moderate (>5 µm diameter) or large (>10 µm diameter) fibers are present at the recording site in the distal stump. With regenerating primate nerves, CNAPs could be recorded 4–6 weeks earlier in severely crushed nerves than in severed and sutured nerves. Potentials were recorded within 6 weeks in crushed nerves and within 10 weeks in sutured nerves. Potentials can also be recorded 2–6 weeks before needle EMG evidence of reinnervation is present. This means that axons of sufficient maturity to conduct a CNAP penetrate well into the distal stump of an injured nerve weeks before sufficient motor end-plate reconstruction occurs to record a CMAP from muscle or for clinical function to be evident. These experiments thus show the clear advantage of CNAP recording over the conventional electrophysiological test for predicting early regeneration.

Such an advantage is also seen in studies of human subjects. Kline's latest analysis of 255 patients with lesions in continuity (1) showed that there is concurrence in the evaluation of complete and incomplete lesions between the clinical and the conventional electrophysiological studies in 80% of cases (Table 16.1). However, intraoperative CNAP monitoring detected evidence of regeneration (by the presence of CNAPs) in 17% of cases in which the clinical and electrophysiological studies showed complete lesions. On the other hand, it also detected evidence of lack of regeneration (by an absence of CNAPs) in 10% of cases in which the clinical examination showed an incomplete lesion. This indicates that intraoperative CNAP monitoring classified 27% of patients into the categories different from those predicted by clinical and EMG/nerve

Table 16.1.
Electrophysiological Studies and Surgical Results of Lesions in Continuity and Brachial Plexus Lesions

	CNAP Present		CNAP Absent	
	No.	Improved No.	No.	Improved No.
Lesions in continuity[a] (N = 255)	145		110	
Neurolysis	142	126 (90%)	14	3 (21%)
Suture	3	1	89	43 (48%)
No repair possible	0	0	7	0
Brachial plexus lesions[b]				
Incomplete lesions (N = 72)				
Neurolysis	69	67 (97%)		
Suture			3	3
Complete lesions (N = 210)				
Neurolysis	63	57 (90%)		
Suture			21	13 (62%)
Graft			89	43 (48%)
Split graft			7	7 (100%)
No repair possible			30	1

[a]Adapted from Kline (1)
[b]Gunshot and stretch injuries. Adapted from Kline and Judice (22).

conduction examinations alone. A similar limitation in the EMG/nerve conduction study is also confirmed by a later study (22).

A histological study of resected nerves showed a difference in axonal organization and maturity between the group with the intraoperative CNAP and the group without it (1). The pathological specimens of the three patients who had undergone resection and suture despite a CNAP showed that axons were relatively mature and well organized, and that had some early myelination, suggesting that recovery might have occurred. In comparison, the 89 specimens resected where a CNAP was absent had a more severe degree of both perineurial and endoneurial scarring as well as a disorganized pattern of axonal regeneration. Axons were poorly organized, fine in caliber, and poorly myelinated. In no resected cases did axonal organization or maturity suggest that functional regeneration would have ever occurred. Based on these data, Kline concluded that the intraoperative CNAP recordings provided reliable information for or against meaningful regeneration when performed 8 weeks or more after the injury (1).

Neurolysis Versus Neurorrhaphy or Nerve Graft

Exploration for a suspected lesion in continuity appears optimal at 2–4 months after injury (1). At this time, with the help of the whole-nerve intraoperative CNAP recordings, a physiological decision can be made about whether to resect the lesion or to leave it alone (Fig. 16.5). In general, if a CNAP can be evoked through the area of injury and recorded distally, careful neurolysis is recommended, leaving the nerve intact. However, if a CNAP cannot be recorded distal to an area of injury, the lesion is resected and neurorrhaphy (suture) or nerve graft is recommended (Fig. 16.6). According to Kline and Nulsen (3), inspection and palpation of many but not all acute lesions in which evoked potentials are absent will confirm the need for resection and suture. If the evoked response can be recorded within a few weeks of an apparently complete nerve injury, it suggests that an element of neuropraxia is present. These lesions usually should not be resected. If 8–10 weeks have passed and a CNAP can be recorded, it means that the lesion was partial to begin with or that effective regeneration has occurred. If, on the other hand, a potential cannot be recorded at this time, satisfactory regeneration is not occurring, and the lesion should be resected.

Following this guideline, Kline has managed lesions in continuity over a period of several years (1). Significant improvement occurred in 89% of those nerves where a

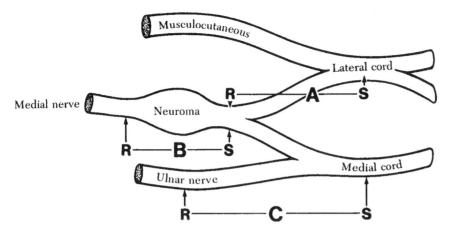

Figure 16.5. A neuroma in median nerve in relation to musculocutaneous and ulnar nerves. **A**, Nerve between the lateral cord and median nerve proximal to neuroma. **B**, Nerve across neuroma in median nerve. **C**, Nerve between medial cord and ulnar nerve. **S**, Stimulating electrodes. **R**, Recording electrodes.

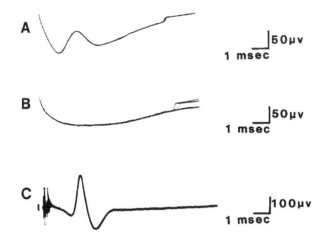

Figure 16.6. CNAP recordings. **A**, **B**, and **C** correspond to A, B, and C segments in Figure 16.5. Note the calibration of the amplitude of CNAP. **A**, Grossly normal CNAP proximal to a neuroma. **B**, No CNAP is recorded across the neuroma. **C**, Completely normal CNAP.

CNAP was recorded and neurolysis performed (Table 16.1). If patients undergoing neurolysis despite the absence of a CNAP are included in the neurolysis group, recovery was seen in 83%. Recovery did not occur in a majority of patients where a CNAP was absent across the lesion 8 weeks or more after an injury and in which neurolysis was done. Exceptions were two patients who had an absent CNAP while surgery was being performed under a tourniquet. A CNAP might have been present in these cases if the recording had been done after the tourniquet had been deflated for a period of time. On the other hand, resection and suture of the nerve produced an improvement in 48% of patients who did not have a CNAP. This is in contrast to an improvement after neurolysis in 21% of patients in the same group (including two cases with tourniquet use).

In 1982, Kline and Judice reported the most complete analysis of intraoperative nerve conduction in 282 gunshot-wounded and stretch-injured brachial plexus lesions in 171 consecutive patients, with at least 1.5 years of follow-up (Table 16.1) (22). Among 282 lesions, 210 were thought to be clinically complete and 72 incomplete. Only 11 (5%) clinically complete lesions showed incomplete lesions in routine EMG and nerve conduction studies, indicating a good correlation between the clinical and routine EMG evaluations in 95% of cases. Depending on the absence or presence of the CNAP in the intraoperative nerve conduction, a surgical decision was made: an absent CNAP indicated a resection of the lesions followed by end-to-end suture or grafting. Recovery was judged satisfactory if a proximal muscle innervated by the injured nerve was 4 and a distal muscle was 3 in strength on the MRC scale. Among 72 incomplete lesions the CNAP was present in the intraoperative nerve conduction in 69, in 67 (97%) of which recovery was satisfactory with neurolysis alone. In two lesions the intraoperative CNAP was absent and an end-to-end suture was performed with good results. Among 210 complete lesions, 63 (30%) showed a CNAP in the intraoperative nerve conduction. Satisfactory recovery occurred in 57 (90%) of 63 cases following neurolysis alone. In 147 cases the CNAP was absent in the intraoperative nerve conduction. Resection followed by end-to-end suture or graft brought a satisfactory outcome in 63 (54%) cases. This study again confirms the sensitivity of intraoperative nerve conduction in detecting axons crossing the injured nerve segment and the reasonableness of Kline and Judice's recommendation that neurorrhaphy or nerve-graft is the treatment of choice in the absence of CNAP by the intraoperative nerve conduction. Similar results were obtained in clinically complete laceration injuries, iatrogenic nerve injuries, and nerve tumors (22). These data further suggest that the surgical decision based on the presence or absence of the intraoperative CNAP, as recommended by Kline and Judice, is reasonable.

Terzis et al. performed the intraoperative nerve conduction of a single fascicle in the damaged nerve segment in seven patients with clinically incomplete lesions but intolerable pain and were able to identify the severely damaged fascicle by the inability to obtain any CNAP across the lesion (13, 19). Resection followed by end-to-end suture or graft relieved the pain and improved sensory function in all seven cases. These authors demonstrated the benefit of the intraoperative nerve conduction of a single fascicle in selective patients with incomplete lesions and painful neuroma.

Thus, the simple intraoperative recording of CNAPs during surgical exploration of the lesions in continuity 8 weeks or more after an injury provides an important practical tip in regard to neurolysis versus neurorrhaphy and makes earlier surgical exploration possible without any potential damage to the surviving or regenerating nerve.

Other Intraoperative Procedures

Compound Muscle Action Potentials (CMAPs)

During peripheral nerve surgery it has been a routine procedure for the surgeon to stimulate the nerve with a hand-held stimulator, looking for the visible motor response of muscles. Instead of depending on a visible motor response, the CMAP can be recorded in the muscle with either disposable surface electrodes, or with intramuscular or subcutaneous needle electrodes. For this purpose a steel needle that can be bent (e.g., a Grass EEG needle) is used in the EMG laboratory at the University of Alabama at Birmingham (UAB). A fine-wire electrode can also be used for this purpose, especially in small muscles.

This procedure tests the integrity of the motor axons of the stimulated nerve in the surgical field and can be easily tested in any hospital where an EMG machine is available. The advantage of this procedure over a visible motor response is obvious: the CMAP can be recorded in muscles where visual observation of a motor response is not possible.

All the technical details of the stimulation are identical with the intraoperative nerve conduction for the CNAP as described above. The only differences are: (*a*) the recording electrodes should be placed in the muscle innervated by the tested nerve; and (*b*) muscle relaxants should not be used. The size of the stimulating electrodes will vary depending on the nerve to be stimulated. For small nerves or roots, the bipolar needle is extremely effective. In the UAB EMG laboratory, a bipolar needle is used routinely to identify the nerve branch in the exposed small meningomyelocele.

This procedure is used for various purposes. During surgery for acoustic neuroma it is important to preserve the integrity of the facial nerve, which is located close by the tumor. To identify the facial nerve, the recording electrodes are placed into the facial muscles, and the CMAP response is monitored during the surgery. With thyroid

surgery it becomes imperative to preserve the superior laryngeal nerve intact. To monitor the superior laryngeal nerve, recording electrodes are placed in the arytenoid muscle in the vocal cord. For meningomyelocele surgery it is often difficult to identify the
sacral nerve roots from the surrounding tissues in the exposed surgical field. For this
purpose we have used a bipolar needle as stimulating electrode and a concentric EMG
needle as a recording electrode in the external anal sphincter muscles.

James et al. used different electrodes: the disposable Nerve-Locator stimulator
(Edward Week & Company, Inc, Long Island City, New York) using 3 volts and 0.5 to 2
mA and an anal plug electrode inserted into the anus or a needle electrode in the anal
sphincter as recording electrodes (23). During the torticollis surgery it is preferable to
cut the nerve innervating the sternocleidomastoid muscle without cutting the nerve
innervating the trapezius muscle. To monitor this procedure, the recording electrodes
are placed in the sternocleidomastoid and trapezius muscles, and stimulation is given
on the accessory nerve rootlets in the exposed surgical field with the bipolar needle. For
the selective posterior rhizotomy for treatment of spasticity, such a technique is also
used to identify the posterior root fascicle, which shows the tonic muscle contraction
(lack of normal inhibition) in the segmental muscles or muscle outside the stimulated
myotome when the root fascicle is stimulated at 10–60/min (24–26). For this procedure
multiple amplifiers (at least eight) are needed to record the motor response from multiple muscles in both legs with the stimulation of a root fascicle. If the tested root fascicle
is known to show "lack of normal inhibition," the tested root fascicle is cut.

Celli and Rovesta performed intraoperative stimulation of the nerve root at its outlet
from the foramen by means of a bipolar stimulating electrode. A bipolar needle recording electrode (or a concentric needle) was introduced about 0.5 cm lateral to the spinous apophysis corresponding to the root to be examined and deep in the paravertebral
muscles (Fig. 16.7) (27). The presence of this response provides proof of the functional
integrity of the posterior dorsal ramus and consequently of the anatomic and functional
continuity of the anterior motor root in the spinal canal. To ensure that the given stimu-

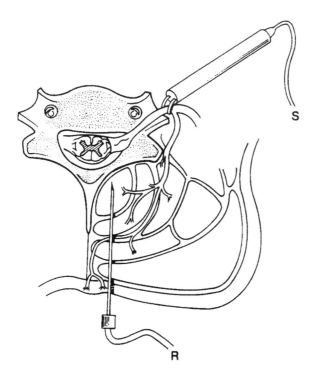

Figure 16.7.   The recording electrode (**R**) is introduced 0.5 cm laterally to the spinous apophysis of
the paravertebral muscles near the lamina, while the stimulating electrodes (**S**) are applied at the root
immediately after its outlet from the foramen. (From Celli L, Rovesta C. Electrophysiologic intraoperative evaluations of the damaged root in tractions of the brachial plexus. Micro-reconstruction of nerve
injuries [Terzis J, ed]. Philadelphia: WB Saunders, 1987:474.)

lus does not spread to the adjacent roots, thus altering the evaluation, they stimulated the roots above and below without moving the recording electrode. The mean values of the CMAP were 2.8 msec in latency, 4.9 mV in amplitude, and 6.9 msec in duration.

A conduction block can be localized to a short segment during surgery for ulnar nerve lesions at the elbow by recording the CMAP from the abductor digiti quinti muscle and stimulating the exposed ulnar nerve serially at 0.5–1 cm segments (Fig. 16.8)

Figure 16.8 Intraoperative direct epineural stimulation, recording from ADQ, easily demonstrated major focal conduction block at the cubital tunnel. Arrow indicates proximal edge of cubital tunnel. (From Campbell WW, Sahni SK, Pridgeon RM, Riaz G, Leschner RT. Intraoperative electroneurography: management of ulnar neuropathy at the elbow. Muscle Nerve 1988;11:78.)

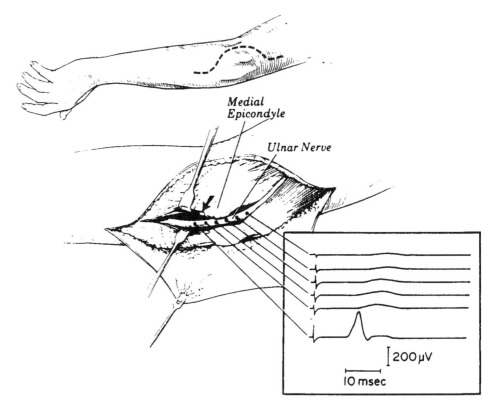

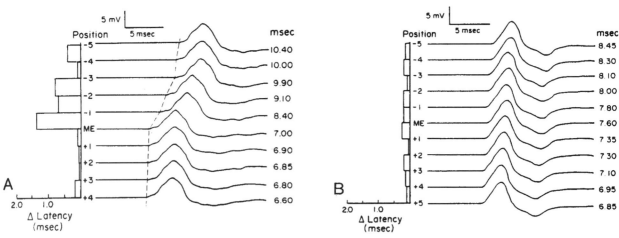

Figure 16.9. **A**, Retrocondylar compression was diagnosed by intraoperative short-segment stimulation. On serial stimulation of 1 cm segments from the most proximal (−) to distal (+) limits of the dissection, recording from ADQ, a marked increase in latency of the CMAP onset occurred just behind and proximal to the medial epicondyle. The patient underwent epineurolysis and microscopically guided limited internal neurolysis followed by anterior subcutaneous transposition. Preoperative study did not show any point of discrete conduction block. **B**, Normal control, percutaneous short segment incremental study over 1-cm segments from proximal (−) to distal (+) to the medial epicondyle (0), recording the CMAP onset latency from the ADQ. Latency change range from 0.05 to 0.25 msec over each segment. (From Campbell WW, Sahni SK, Pridgeon RM, Riaz G, Leschner RT. Intraoperative electroneurography: management of ulnar neuropathy at the elbow. Muscle Nerve 1988;11:79).

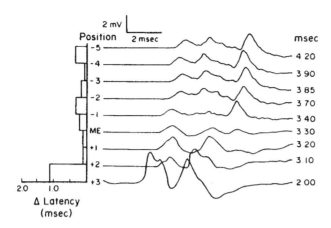

Figure 16.10. The cubital tunnel syndrome was diagnosed by the intraoperative short-segment stimulation with recording from FCU. Preoperative study showed a marked latency change 3 cm distal to the medial epicondyle that was felt to represent the cubital tunnel syndrome. Intraoperative studies confirmed the latency change and demonstrated a major conduction block at the cubital tunnel entrance as well. Surgery was limited to simple decompression of the cubital tunnel (From Campbell WW, Sahni SK, Pridgeon RM, Riaz G, Leschner RT. Intraoperative electroneurography: management of ulnar neuropathy at the elbow. Muscle Nerve 1988;11:79).

(28). Campbell et al. used a stimulus duration of 0.05 msec (rarely 0.1 msec) and a stimulus intensity of 10–30 mA as stimulus parameters (28). With this intraoperative technique, they identified a conduction block at the retrocondylar groove in nine cases, the cubital tunnel in four, at both locations in three, and at the usual distal point in one case (Figs. 16.9 and 16.10). On the basis of these findings the surgical decision was made: anterior subcutaneous transpositions in 12, cubital tunnel releases in four, and distal decompression in one case. In their series, a correct preoperative localization of conduction block was possible in 13 (68%) of 19 cases. Thus, this procedure was critical in six (32%) cases where a preoperative localization of conduction block was not accurately pinpointed, and the surgical decision was made appropriately on the basis of the intraoperative motor conduction study. In one case the intraoperative motor conduction study identified the conduction block at the exit from the flexor carpi ulnaris muscle, and surgical decompression of the fibrous band was performed with good recovery (29).

CNAPs

CNAP recording has been used for purposes other than the intraoperative nerve conduction just described. During meningomyelocele surgery it is important to identify the nerve branch from the surrounding tissue. To identify the sciatic nerve branch, Phillips and Park used a small intraoperative stimulator and recorded the CNAP with a near-nerve sensory needle from the sciatic nerve in the popliteal fossa (30). The somatosensory evoked potential was also monitored caudally from the T11 or T12 levels. Moller et al. recorded the CNAP from the 8th cranial nerve during cerebellopontine angle surgery with the auditory stimulator used for brainstem auditory evoked potentials (31, 32). They reported that the monitoring of the CNAP from the auditory nerve and the BAEP with scalp electrodes decreases the risk of hearing loss in these operations. Richmond and Mahla recorded the CNAP from the exposed facial nerve in the surgical field during surgery for cerebellopontine angle tumor following needle stimulation of the facial nerve at the stylomastoid foramen (33). They noted that the advantage of this technique is that the CNAP can be obtained reliably even in the presence of paralyzing doses of muscle relaxants.

Motor Unit Potentials (MUP)

Needle EMG monitoring records the MUPs generated from muscle. A variety of EMG needles can be used, e.g., a bendable steel EMG needle. Daube stated that the most satisfactory electrodes have proven to be fine wires with 2-mm bare tips (34). Prass and Lüders used an intramuscular bipolar wire electrode (35). To reduce interference from external sources, the electrode connected to the preamplifier must be kept as short as possible. MUP recordings can be made from any somatic muscles, including the facial, extraocular, laryngeal, anal sphincters, intercostal, and any limb muscles. The usual EMG machine setups are 200 μV for the sensitivity and 100 msec for the sweep velocity. The monitoring of multiple muscles is possible and must be performed over a loudspeaker as well as on a monitoring oscilloscope. For facial nerve monitoring, Prass recorded the EMG activity from the frontalis, orbicularis oris, and orbicularis oculi muscles (35). The auditory sound becomes an important monitoring device for the surgeon. *Neuromuscular block must be reduced before EMG monitoring begins, but neurotonic discharges can be recorded with a 50% neuromuscular block* (34). It should be noted that MUP cannot be monitored during cautery.

Neurotonic discharges occur in response to mechanical or metabolic irritation of the nerve innervating the muscle. They are sensitive indicators of nerve irritation and occur more with cranial nerve manipulation than with peripheral nerve manipulation (34). Neurotonic discharges are relatively easily distinguished from 60-Hz artifacts and artifacts produced by nerve stimulators, cavitrons, and respirators. MUP amplitudes ranged from approximately 10 to 200 μV. According to Prass, neurotonic discharges are presented in two distinct patterns: the "burst" pattern and the "train" pattern (35). The burst pattern (Fig. 16.11) is the most frequently observed pattern of EMG activity and is characterized by short, relatively synchronous bursts of MUPs lasting up to a few hundred msec. This pattern is most often associated with direct manipulation of the facial nerve via various dissecting instruments.

The train pattern (Fig. 16.12) is characterized by asynchronous trains of MUPs lasting up to several minutes. MUPs vary in amplitude and frequency, producing "bomber

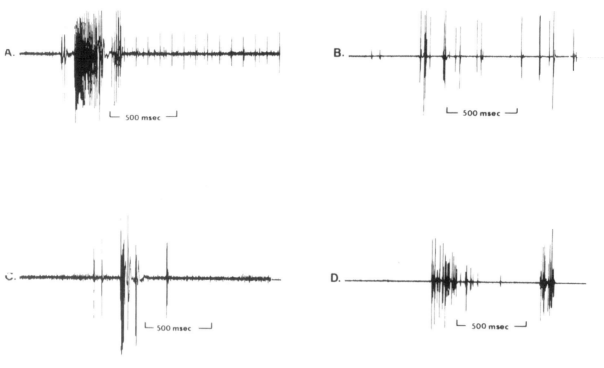

Figure 16.11. Various burst EMG responses. *A*, "limited nerve crush" by an elevating instrument during an attempt to push the facial nerve away from tumor in the cerebellopontine angle. *B*, Blunt facial nerve dissection at the brainstem. *C* and *D*, Two rapid short squirts of Ringer's solution into the surgical field. (From Prass RL, Lüders H. Acoustic (loudspeaker) facial electromyographic monitoring: Part 1. Evoked electromyographic activity during acoustic neuroma resection. Neurosurgery 1986;19:396.).

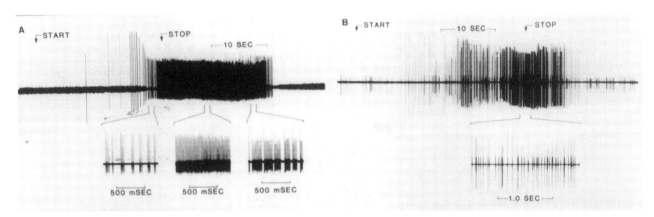

Figure 16.12. Various train EMG responses. Episodes of "bomber" (**A**) and "popcorn" (**B**) train EMG activity associated with lateral-to-medial nerve traction during tumor debulking using a Cavitron ultrasonic aspirator. Arrows indicate approximate times when debulking was started and stopped. The apparent decrease in amplitude observed in the upper trace is an artifact due to the presence of an automatic audio-limiting circuit in the audio section of the particular videotape recorder used. (From Prass RL, Lüders H. Acoustic (loudspeaker) facial electromyographic monitoring: Part 1. Evoked electromyographic activity during acoustic neuroma resection. Neurosurgery 1986;19:397.)

potentials" or "popcorn" sounds. In most instances train activity is associated with the apparent traction of the facial nerve, usually in a lateral-to-medial direction. Because of the typical sounds the surgeon can readily recognize the sounds of neurotonic discharges as soon as he initiates them with surgical manipulation. Using the EMG machine, the monitoring of MUPs can easily be incorporated with the motor nerve conduction monitoring.

APPENDIX: Electrode Construction[a]

Materials:

1. Nylon rod, 0.75 cm (⁵⁄₁₆") diameter (McMaster-Carr Co, Chicago, Illinois; part #8538K 15).

2. Polyolefin shrink tubing of 1.2 cm (½") outside diameter, clear double-wall preferred (Partsmasters, Inc., Dallas, Texas).

3. Platinum-iridium wire, 1 mm (0.04") diameter (18-gauge) (supplied by local jeweler).

4. Belden low-noise instrumentation cable #9452 with graphite-cloth runner (supplied by local electronics distributor).

Methods:

A. A 9 cm (3.5") length of rod is selected. The cable end of the rod is flattened for 1.2 cm (0.5") with a belt sander to one-half the rod's original diameter. Burrs are then removed. A suitable length of cable (e.g., 2 m) is stripped of the outer jacket to expose the inner wires for 10 cm (4"). The inner wires are held along the length of the rod and the unstripped jacket is centered in the flattened area of the rod's cable end. To form a strain relief and anchor, a short ring of polyolefin tubing is shrunk around the cable and rod at the flattened area. The red and black inner wires are stretched along the rod and cut 6 mm (¼") from the rod end. These wires are then soldered to 3.6 cm (1.5") platinum-iridium electrode wire tips. An excellent side-to-side solder joint can be made

[a]This appendix is quoted from Burbank, with author's and publisher's permission (15).

using Superior flux # 30 (water rinse). The wire tips are fixed to the sides of the nylon rod with cyanoacrylate. A 7.2 (3") length of polyolefin is shrunk over the rod and wires. Heat is applied from the electrode to the cable end, moving slowly to avoid bubbles and assure melting of the inner tubing. The electrode wire is then bent to the desired shape with round-nose pliers and polished smooth.

Monopolar electrode holders have a hole centered in the rod's end to hold the electrode wire. This hole is met by a perpendicular side hole 1 mm (⅜") from the electrode end. An endodontic barbed broach (# 45) is used to round the junction of the end and side holes to facilitate insertion of the electrode wire. This wire is cemented in place and the cable connection soldered at the side of the rod. Polyolefin tubing is placed as previously described.

The electrode is gas-sterilized.

REFERENCES

1. Kline DG. Physiological and clinical factors contributing to the timing of nerve repair. Clin Neurosurg 1976;24:425–455.
2. Oh SJ. Electromyographic studies in peripheral nerve injuries. South Med J 1976;69:177–182.
3. Kline DG, Nulsen FE. The neuroma in continuity. Surg Clin North Am 1972;52:1189–1209.
4. Kline DG, Hackett ER. Value of electrophysiologic tests for peripheral nerve neuromas. J Surg Oncol 1970;2:299–310.
5. Kline DG, DeJonge BR. Evoked potentials to evaluate peripheral nerve injuries. Surg Gynecol Obstet 1968;127:1239–1249.
6. Vanderark GD, Meyer GA, Kline DG, et al. Peripheral nerve injuries studied by evoked potential recordings. Milit Med 1970;135:90–94.
7. Terzis J, Publicover N. Clinical application of electrophysiologic recordings. In: Terzis JK, ed. Microreconstruction of nerve injuries. Philadelphia: WB Saunders, 1987.
8. Kline D. Evaluation of the neuroma in continuity. In: Omar G, Spinner M, eds. Management of peripheral nerve problems. Philadelphia: WB Saunders, 1980:450–461.
9. Oh SJ. Intraoperative nerve conduction. In: Clinical electromyography: nerve conduction studies. Baltimore: University Park Press, 1984:319–324.
10. Nelson K. Use of peripheral nerve action potentials for intraoperative monitoring. Neurol Clin 1988;6:917–933.
11. Van Beek A, Hubble B, Kinkead L, Torros S, Suchy H. Clinical use of nerve stimulation and recording techniques. Plast Reconstr Surg 1983;71:225–238.
12. Kline D, DeJonge B. Evoked potentials to evaluate peripheral nerve injuries. Surg Gynecol Obstet, 1968;127:1239–1249.
13. Williams H, Terzis J. Single fascicular recordings: an intraoperative diagnostic tool for the management of peripheral nerve lesions. Plast Reconstr Surg 1976;562–569.
14. Lambert E, Dyck P. Compound action potentials of sural nerve in vitro in peripheral neuropathy. In Dyck PJ, Thomas PK, Lambert EH et al., eds. Peripheral neuropathy, 2nd ed. Philadelphia: WB Saunders, 1984.
15. Burbank P. Electrode construction. Neurol Clin 1988;6:929–930.
16. The International Federation of Societies for EEG and Clinical Neurophysiology. Recommendations for practice of clinical neurophysiology. Amsterdam: Elsevier, 1983.
17. Kline D, Hackett E. Reappraisal of timing for exploration of civilian peripheral nerve injury. Surgery 1975;78:54–65.
18. Kline D, Nulsen F. The neuroma in continuity. Surg Clin North Am, 1972;52:1189–1209.
19. Terzis J, Daniel R, Williams H. Intraoperative assessment of nerve lesions with fascicular dissection and electrophysiological recordings. In Omar G, Spinners M, eds. Management of peripheral nerve problems. Philadelphia: WB Saunders, 1980:462–472.
20. Kline D, Happel L, Hackett E. Clinical use of nerve stimulation. Plast Reconstr Surg 1985;75:764–765.
21. Kline DG, Hackett ER, May PR. Evaluation of nerve injuries by evoked potentials and electromyography. J Neurosurg 1968;31:128–136.
22. Kline DG, Judice DJ. Operative management of selected brachial plexus lesions. J Neurosurg 1983;58:631–649.
23. James H, Mulcahy J, Walsh J, Kaplan G. Use of anal sphincter electromyography during operations on the conus medullaris and sacral nerve roots. Neurosurgery 1979;4:521–523.
24. Fasano VA, Barolat-Romana G, Zeme S, Sguazzi A. Electrophysiological assessment of spinal circuits in spasticity by direct dorsal root stimulation. Neurosurgery 1979;4:146–151.
25. Laitinen LV, Nilsson S, Fugl-Meyer AR. Selective posterior rhizotomy for treatment of spasticity. J Neurosurgery 1983;58:895–899.
26. Phillips LH, Park TS. Electrophysiological studies of selective posterior rhizotomy patients. Neurosurgery: State of the Art Reviews. Philadelphia: Hanley & Velfus Inc, 1989;4:459–469.
27. Celli L, Rovesta C. Electrophysiologic intraoperative evaluations of the damaged root in tractions of the

brachial plexus. In Terzis JK, ed. Microreconstruction of nerve injuries. Philadelphia: WB Saunders, 1987:473–482.

28. Campbell WW, Sahni SK, Pridgeon RM, Riaz G, Leshner RT. Intraoperative electroneurography: management of ulnar nerve at the elbow. Muscle Nerve 1988;11:75–81.

29. Campbell W, Pridgeon R, Sahni K. Entrapment neuropathy of the ulnar nerve at its point of exit from the flexor carpi ulnaris muscle. Muscle Nerve 1988;11:467–470.

30. Phillips L, Park T. Electrophysiological monitoring during lipomyelomeningocele resection. Muscle Nerve 1990;13:127–132.

31. Møller AR, Jannetta PJ. Monitoring auditory functions during cranial nerve microvascular decompression operations by direct recording from the eighth nerve. J Neurosurg 1983;59:493–499.

32. Møller A, Jannetta P. Monitoring auditory nerve potentials during operations in the cerebellopontine angle. Otolaryngol Head Neck Surg 1984;92:434–439.

33. Richmond I, Mahla M. Use of antidromic recording to monitor facial nerve function intraoperatively. Neurosurgery 1985;16:458–462.

34. Daube J. Monitoring neural function during surgery. Advanced Hospital Technology December 1990:33–41.

35. Prass R, Lüders H. Acoustic (Loudspeaker) facial electromyographic monitoring: evoked electromyographic activity during acoustic neuroma resection. Neurosurgery 1986;19:392–400.

17

Reflex Tests

In recent years, reflex tests have become an important element of electrophysiological studies in the proximal segments of peripheral nerves and in the areas where routine nerve conduction tests are not available. In contrast to the nerve conduction test, which measures the nerve conduction of tested nerve segments, the reflex test measures the nerve conduction of the long reflex arc involving the proximal segments of the tested nerve. Additionally, the latency also involves the time required for synaptic relay, whether it is monosynaptic or polysynaptic. Monosynaptic relay is known to be involved in the H- and T-(tendon) reflexes, while oligo- or poly-synaptic relay is a component of other reflexes. Thus, the reflex test is characterized by a longer latency. There are two other distinct characteristics that are not present in the routine nerve conduction study: *(a) habituation phenomenon; and (b) variability of latencies and amplitude.* To avoid the habituation phenomenon, the nerve must be stimulated at 2- or 5-sec intervals, preferably at random. To obtain a more meaningful latency, several recordings should be superimposed and the shortest latency measured. The amplitude is not measured because of its variability. Though the F-wave response is one of the late responses, it is not included in this chapter because it is not relayed through the classic afferent reflex arc, sensory fibers.

H-Reflex

Among the various electrically induced reflexes, the H-reflex is the best known. The H-reflex was named after Hoffmann, who originally described this reflex in the calf muscle (1). The H-reflex is a monosynaptic reflex mediated by the Ia sensory fibers, which synapse with α-motor neurons and its axons (Fig. 17.1). Its neural pathway is similar to that of the T-reflex except that the H-reflex bypasses the muscle spindle of the muscle stretch reflex arc.

The H-reflex of the gastrocnemius-soleus muscle is consistently obtained without any special facilitation technique in adults. However, the H-reflex can also be obtained in other muscles, but usually requires some facilitation techniques (Table 17.1). Among the various muscles, the H-reflex in the vastus lateralis muscle is most easily obtainable: Verhagen et al. obtained the H-reflex in the vastus lateralis muscle in all cases and stated that sometimes it was necessary to use mild voluntary contraction to prime the motor neuron pool sufficiently for reflex activation with minimal contraction (2).

In contrast to adults, the H-reflex in premature and full-term infants is readily

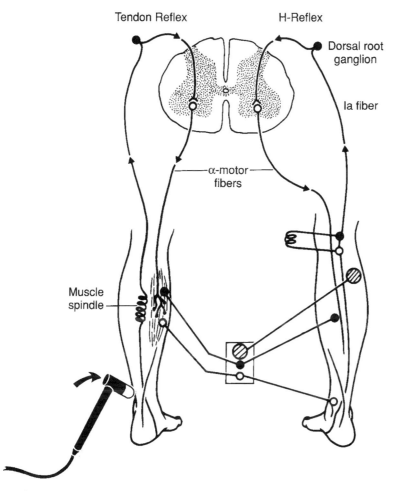

Figure 17.1. Anatomic pathways for the H-reflex and T-reflex: the Ia fibers are the afferent pathways and the α-motor fibers are the efferent pathways with the monosynaptic relay in the anterior horn. For the H-reflex, the stimulation is directly on the Ia fibers themselves. For the T-reflex, the stretch receptors (nuclear bags and chains) in the muscle spindle are activated after stretching the muscle by tapping the muscle tendon with an electronic hammer.

Table 17.1.
The H-Reflex and Facilitation Techniques in Adults

Muscle	Facilitation Technique (FT)
Lower extremity	
Gastrocnemius-soleus	Consistently obtained without FT in all cases
Abd. hallucis or	Obtained in all cases with ankle stimulation
flexor digit. brevis (113)	Not obtained in one of nine normal controls with posterior fossa stimulation
Ext. digit. longus (112)	Obtained with FT (paired stimulation) in all cases
Anterior tibialis (110)	Obtained with FT (paired stimulation) in all cases
Vastus medialis (2)	Obtained in all cases; with FT (mild contraction) in some cases
Upper extremity	
Flexor carpi radialis or	Obtained without FT in 70% of normal controls and with FT (contraction
palmaris longus (109)	of ipsilateral quadriceps) in the remaining 30%
Flexor carpi ulnaris (25)	Obtained with FT (repetitive nerve stimulation at 4/sec rate) in most cases
Ext. digit. communis (110)	Obtained with FT (isometric contraction) in all cases

obtained in many muscles other than the gastrocnemius-soleus muscle (3). The percentage of infants with an H-reflex in the arm decreases progressively during the first year (Table 8.4), until by approximately the age of 1 year it can no longer be found.

Since the H-reflex latency and F-wave latency are similar, it is sometimes difficult to differentiate between these two. Basically, the H-reflex is elicited with subthreshold stimulation, whereas the F-wave is elicited with supramaximal stimulation (Table 4.2). The F-wave latency is a few milliseconds longer than the H-reflex in the same muscle. Differentiation between the H-reflex and F-wave is described in Chapter 4. Guidelines for the identification of the H-reflex are also listed in Chapter 4. The H-reflex is best elicited by a stimulus duration of 0.5–1 msec, which makes it more selective for the afferent Ia fibers (4, 5). Longer duration favors the activation of motor axons. To obtain the H-reflex, the nerve has to be stimulated manually at a rate of once every 2 seconds or longer to avoid the blocking response.

The amplitude of the H-reflex depends on many variables, such as supraspinal influences (6), alertness (7), use of a conditioning stimulus (8), turning of the head (9), eye closure (9), baseline EMG activity (10), and the Jendrassik maneuver (9, 11). Thus, it is not a good criterion of abnormality. *Most authorities use the H-reflex latency as the best index of measurement.* Verhagen et al. compared the H-reflex latency to the HM-interlatency time (the H-reflex latency to the M-response latency) and concluded that the H-reflex latency is superior (2). Factors that increase the amplitude are mild active contraction of the muscle, passive stretch of the muscle, reinforcement maneuvers such as the Jendrassik maneuver, and labyrinthine vestibular stimulation (12). Factors that decrease the amplitude are active contraction of antagonists or strong contraction of the active muscle, passive shortening of the muscle, strong electric stimuli, rapid rate of stimulation (especially more than 1/sec), tapping of the tendon jerk or over the recording muscle, and strong flexion and extension of the neck or other muscles (12). Like any other long reflexes, the H-reflex latency correlates well with height (2, 12–14), leg length (15), or arm length (16). Verhag et al. and Braddom and Johnson found a weak correlation between the H-reflex latency and age (2, 15). Accordingly, *the most important physiological variable in the H-reflex latency is body length* (Fig. 7.5), whether this is measured by the height, leg length, or arm length. The effect of temperature on the H-reflex was studied by two groups (17, 18). They found no significant change in the H-reflex amplitudes measured during the baseline and cooling periods (an average 18.4°C decrease in the skin temperature and 12.1°C decrease in the intramuscular temperature) in 16 subjects (17). There was no significant change in the H-reflex latency from the gastrocnemius muscle between 26°C and 30°C in 25 subjects (18).

Thus, the H-reflex latency in an individual has to be compared at least with the normal value in relation to the body length, usually to the height (Figs. 7.5, 17.14, and 17.18). Since the H-reflex latency varies with body length and less so with age, *a simple and practical way of judging abnormality is to compare the value with the H-reflex latency in the unaffected side* (Table 17.2). It ranges from 1.0 msec in the flexor carpi radialis muscle (19) to 3.6 msec in the vastus medialis muscle (2). This is only applicable when the H-reflex is normal in the unaffected side. The H-reflex latency is quite useful in the detection of a unilateral radiculopathy.

Table 17.2.
Latency Difference of the H-Reflex Between Two Sides

Investigator	Muscle	Latency difference (msec)
Deschuytere et al. (109)	Superficial forearm flexors	1.0
Ongerboer de Visser et al. (26)	Flexor carpi radialis	0.9
Jabre (19)	Flexor carpi radialis	1.0
Verhagen et al. (2)	Vastus medialis	3.6
Deschytere and Rosselle (112)	Extensor digitorum longus	2.0
Braddom and Johnson (15)	Gastrocnemius-soleus muscle	1.5
Lachman et al. (13)	Soleus muscle	2.2

Clinical Applications

The H-reflex test is useful in three clinical situations: radiculopathy and plexopathy, polyneuropathy, and amyotrophic lateral sclerosis.

It has been well established that the H-reflex in the gastrocnemius-soleus (triceps surae) muscle is sensitive in the detection of S1 radiculopathy and helpful in differentiating it from L5 radiculopathy (Table 17.3). The H-reflex in the triceps surae was either absent or prolonged in 50–100% of patients with S1 radiculopathy (15, 20–22). On the other hand, in L5 radiculopathy the H-reflex in the triceps surae was abnormal in 0–26% of cases (23, 24). For the detection of L5 radiculopathy, the H-reflex in the extensor digitorum longus muscle is the test of choice: This test was abnormal in 83% of patients with L5 radiculopathy, whereas it was abnormal in 33% with S1 radiculopathy (25). The H-reflex in the vastus lateralis and medialis muscles successfully confirmed the diagnosis of L4 radiculopathy in all of 54 cases (2, 22). The H-reflex in the flexor carpi radialis is known to be helpful in detection of C6 or C7 radiculopathy, being abnormal in 68–90% of cases (16, 22). The H-reflex in other muscles has not been tested for its diagnostic sensitivity in radiculopathy. These studies proved that *the H-reflex of the appropriate muscle can identify a radiculopathy involving the main root subserving that particular muscle*. In plexopathy, the H-reflex in the flexor carpi radialis was able to identify a brachial plexopathy in all of 25 patients with radiation-induced plexopathy by showing an absent response or delayed latencies (26). This is in contrast to the absent or decreased biceps reflex in 76% of cases.

The H-reflex is either absent or prolonged in latency in the various polyneuropathies (27–30). This is understandable in view of the frequent impairment of muscle stretch reflexes in peripheral neuropathy. The H-reflex from the triceps surae was not obtainable in all patients with absent ankle reflexes (13, 31). There are a few studies comparing the conventional nerve conduction study and the H-reflex test in peripheral neuropathy. In 30 alcoholics, Lefebvre D'Amour et al. showed abnormality in motor nerve conduction in 47% of cases, in late responses (F-wave and H-reflex) in 73% of cases, in sensory nerve conduction in median and ulnar nerves in 73% of cases and in median, ulnar, and sural nerves in 90% of cases (31). This study clearly indicates the greater diagnostic sensitivity of sensory nerve conduction in peripheral neuropathy compared with the late responses when the sural nerve conduction is included.

In 50 patients with various polyneuropathies, Lachman et al. found that the late

Table 17.3.
Diagnostic Sensitivity of the H-Reflex Test in Radiculopathy

Investigator	Test	Diagnostic Sensitivity[a]
Braddom and Johnson (15)	Gastrocnemius-soleus	100% of 25 patients with S1 radiculopathy
Schuchmann (23)	Gastrocnemius-soleus	Mean difference of the H-reflex latency between two sides: 2.9 msec for 13 patients with S1 radiculopathy with absent response in 4 patients; 0.03 msec (normal) for 15 patients with L5 radiculopathy
Rico and Jonkman (24)	Gastrocnemius-soleus	65% of 34 patients with S1 radiculopathy 26% of 27 patients with L5 radiculopathy
Aiello et al. (21)	Gastrocnemius-soleus	100% of 20 patients with S1 radiculopathy[b]
Sabbahi and Kahlil (22)	Gastrocnemius-soleus	100% of 30 patients with S1 radiculopathy
Dhand et al. (20)	Gastrocnemius-soleus	50% of 20 patients with S1 radiculopathy
Deschuytere and Rosselle (112)	Extensor digitorum longus	83% of 35 patients with L5 radiculopathy 33% of 12 patients with S1 radiculopathy
Verhagen et al. (2)	Vastus lateralis	100% of 14 patients with L4 radiculopathy
Sabbahi and Kahlil (22)	Vastus medialis	100% of 40 patients with L4 radiculopathy
Schrimsheimer et al. (16)	Flexor carpi radialis	68% of 25 patients with C6 or C7 radiculopathy 0% of 7 patients with C5 or C8 radiculopathy
Sabbahi and Kahlil (22)	Flexor carpi radialis	90% of 37 patients with C7 radiculopathy

[a]The H-reflex is either absent or prolonged in the latency.

[b]The H-index was used. The H-index = $\dfrac{(\text{Height of subject in cm})^2}{(\text{Time interval H-M in msec})^2} \times 2$

responses (F-wave in the median nerve and H-reflex in the triceps surae) were abnormal in 18% of cases when the routine nerve conduction was normal (13). Based on this finding, they claimed that the late responses (F-wave and H-reflex) are useful in the early detection of peripheral neuropathy. However, their routine nerve conduction studies did not include the sural nerve conduction, which is not acceptable to the present standard of electrophysiological testing for peripheral neuropathy. More convincing evidence in this regard was presented by Schimsheimer et al., who observed the H-reflex in the flexor carpi radialis to be abnormal in 13 (14%) of 93 polyneuropathy patients, whereas the median motor and sensory nerve conductions were normal in these 13 patients (12).

These studies indicate that there are a few cases of peripheral neuropathy in which only the late responses are abnormal while other nerve conduction parameters are normal. This is especially noted in early cases of Guillain-Barré syndrome, which is known to involve predominantly the proximal nerve segments (13). This is one instance in which the H-reflex test is helpful in diagnosis of peripheral neuropathy. Guiheneuc and Bathien studied the H-reflex in alcoholic neuropathy and uremic neuropathy in relation to the maximal amplitude of the H-reflex and M-response versus the NCV (30). Two different patterns of H-reflex abnormalities were found in uremic and alcoholic neuropathies: the early and rapid diminution of the amplitude of the H-reflex in alcoholic neuropathy and the prominent prolongation of the H-reflex latency in the relative absence of change in the amplitude in uremic neuropathy. This difference may represent two different pathogenetic mechanisms: axonal degeneration in alcoholic neuropathy and possibly "demyelination" in uremic neuropathy.

The H-reflex test can be a valuable tool in differentiating between amyotrophic lateral sclerosis (ALS) and primary muscular atrophy or polyneuropathy. In ALS, it is possible to obtain the H-reflex in muscles in which the H-reflex is not normally obtainable without any facilitation technique, because the H-reflex may be released from normal suppression (32). In fact, Norris found the gastrocnemius H-reflex present in almost all cases and in the hand and extensor digitorum muscles in 66–77% of 110 ALS patients (33). In progressive muscular atrophy, he found the H-reflex in the gasctrocnemius in only seven patients and in other muscles in just three of 18 patients. These observations are in sharp contrast to patients with polyneuropathy, in whom the gastrocnemius-soleus H-reflex was absent in almost all cases and in other muscles in all cases.

In Holmes-Adie syndrome (tonic pupils and patchy areflexia), the H-reflex was absent or virtually absent in patients with depressed reflexes whereas the motor and sensory nerve conductions for the peroneal, posterior tibial, and sural nerves were normal (34), indicating that the areflexia in Holmes-Adie syndrome is caused by loss of large spindle afferents or reduced effectiveness of their monosynaptic connections to motor neurons. This observation is partly compatible with the autopsy findings in Holmes-Adie syndrome, which revealed degeneration of dorsal root ganglion cells, fiber loss in the dorsal roots, and nerve fiber degeneration in the lumbosacral portions of the dorsal columns (29, 30).

In tabes dorsalis, the H-reflex and posterior tibial somatosensory evoked potentials were absent, whereas the motor and sensory nerve conductions were normal (37). This observation correlates well with the known pathology of this disease in which the degeneration is confined to the dorsal roots, dorsal funiculi, and posterior columns of the lumbosacral and lower thoracic spinal cord, usually sparing the dorsal root ganglia (38).

T-Reflex

The muscle stretch reflex test, the most important neurological test, is a monosynaptic reflex elicited by a reflex hammer tap to the tendon and is used daily by neurologists as a measure of motor neuron excitability in differentiating between upper and lower motor neuron lesions. The reflex arc consists of Ia fibers as an afferent axon and α-motor fibers as an efferent axon, and is nearly identical to the H-reflex arc. The muscle

Table 17.4.
Physiological Differences Between the H-Reflex and the T-Reflex[a]

Type	H-Reflex	T-Reflex
Stimulation	Direct electrical excitation of the Ia afferent fibers	Muscle stretching and subsequent activation of stretch receptors in the muscle spindle
Afferent pathways	Shorter distance	Longer distance
Sensory volley	No repetitive discharges in the Ia fibers	Repetitive discharges in the Ia fibers
	Afferent volleys are much more synchronous	Afferent volleys are often very asynchronous
Central delay	Shorter because of better synchronization	Could be substantial because of asynchronization

[a]Modified from Brown FW. The physiological and technical basis of electromyography. Boston: Butterworth, 1984;148.

stretch reflex can be objectively documented by the T-reflex, which can be elicited by an electronic hammer tap to the tendon.

Though the H-reflex and T-reflex have the same afferent and efferent pathways, there are, however, important distinctions between the two (Table 17.4; Fig. 17.1). The most obvious difference is the activation site of stimulation: *for the H-reflex, stimulation is directly on the Ia fibers, bypassing the muscle spindle organs, whereas for the T-reflex, the stretch receptors (nuclear bags and chains) in the muscle spindle are activated after stretching the muscle fibers by tapping the tendon with a tendon hammer.* Other differences are listed in Table 17.4. Since the stimulus for the H-reflex bypasses the muscle spindles, Bishop et al. stated that a comparison between the H- and T-reflexes may provide an indirect means of assessing spindle sensitivity controlled by the γ-motor system (33). But this simplistic view has to be interpreted with caution because the H-reflex is also facilitated by the Jendrassik's maneuver (40). The effects of cooling are also different between the H-reflex and T-reflex: there is no change in the H-reflex amplitude, but there is a significant decrease in the T-reflex amplitude during a minimum 14°C cooling period from the normal baseline temperature by the ice water pack over the gastrocnemius-soleus muscle (17).

Technical Aspects

The recording electrodes are not placed following the conventional belly-tendon method used for the nerve conduction study because such placement is associated with a greater movement artifact caused by the tendon tap (41). Certainly, the active recording electrode should be placed on the belly of the muscle. However, the reference electrode is placed either on the muscle tendon opposite the tapped tendon (41, 42) or on a muscle 5–10 cm away from an active recording electrode (24, 43), though a longer interelectrode distance is known to produce a higher T-reflex amplitude (41). As with any other reflex test, the superimposition of more than four or five recordings is essential in the accurate measurement of the shortest latency. Usually, a 5–10 msec sweep velocity and 500–1000 μV sensitivity are the recommended EMG machine setups.

Malcolm studied the various technical aspects of the T-reflex test (44). He found that a delay of up to 4 msec occurred in the reflex latency of the knee jerk to different parts of the quadriceps muscle, emphasizing the importance of the standardization of electrode placement. He suggested that the active recording electrodes should preferably be placed closer to the motor point of the muscles and at symmetrical points on both sides. *The force with which the electronic hammer struck the tendon did not produce any significant difference in latency* as long as the onset of the initial negative deflection was clear. *Reinforcement such as the Jendrassik maneuver increases the amplitude of the tendon response but does not change the latency.* Alterations in the tension of the tendon provoke variations in the amplitude of the tendon response, but the reflex latency remains fairly stable. Thus, Malcolm advised adoption of a standard position of the limbs for T-reflex testing. The amplitude of the T-reflex is generally higher for the brisker reflexes as seen in upper motor neuron lesions, and correspondingly less in diminished reflexes. He concluded that, as a quantitative measure of the reflex response, the eye was approximately as sensitive, for a T-reflex response was not recorded when there was no visible reflex response. *When the examiner places his thumb between the muscle belly and electronic hammer, there is a delay of about 2 msec due to the mechanical delay* introduced by this placement of the thumb (45). Weintraub et al. studied the relationship between the ankle T-reflex and the H-reflex on the gastrocnemius-soleus muscle in 400 limbs and found concordance in 86% (46). When discordant, *the ankle T-reflex was almost always elicitable, whereas the H-reflex was unelicitable, indicating the technical superiority of the T-reflex.* We found the same results in our study of chronic demyelinating neuropathy (38).

There have been only a few studies reporting normal data (41, 44). The ankle T-reflex has been most studied. The amplitude of the T-reflex response varied in normal subjects, but Malcolm reported a negative deflection of approximately 0.3 mV. As expected from any late responses conducting through the long proximal nerve segments, the T-reflex latency is proportional to the height (38, 39, 42, 43), arm length (42), or leg length (43). Thus, *it is important to compare the latency with the height (Figs. 17.23 and 17.26).* The latency difference between two sides is easier to compare (Table 17.5). For the ankle T-reflex, it should not be more than 2 msec according to Rico and Jonkman (24) and 3 msec according to Kuruoglu and Oh (43).

Clinical Applications

The T-reflex test has not been used very often in the clinical setting. This is probably because of the clinician's confidence in his own skill in identifying the segmental lesion in muscle stretch testing with the reflex hammer. The T-reflex test is useful in two clinical settings: (*a*) detection of cervical or lumbosacral radiculopathy (Table 17.6), and (*b*) detection of peripheral neuropathy as a test for the proximal nerve conduction. By using 2 msec asymmetry as a criterion of abnormality between the two sides, Rico and Jonkman found in 61 patients with proven L5 or S1 radiculopathy that the ankle T-reflex test was abnormal in 11% of normal controls, in 21% of patients with L5 radiculopathy, and in 87% of patients with S1 radiculopathy, indicating that this test is particularly useful in detecting S1 radiculopathy (24). They also showed that this test was

Table 17.5.
Latency Difference in the T-Reflex Between Two Sides

Investigators	Tendon Reflex	Latency Difference (msec)
Rico and Jonkman (24)	Achilles	2.0
Kuruoglu and Oh (43)	Achilles	3.0
Stam (48)	Anterior tibialis	4.0
Kuruoglu and Oh (43)	Patellar	2.9
Koenig (45)	Biceps and triceps	2.0

Table 17.6.
Diagnostic Sensitivity of the T-Reflex in Radiculopathy

Investigator	T-Reflex Test	Diagnostic Sensitivity
Malcolm (44)	Ankle	4 (80%) of 5 patients with S1 radiculopathy
	Patellar	1 patient with L4 radiculopathy
Rico and Jonkman (24)	Ankle	Among 61 patients with L5 or S1 radiculopathy:
		21% with L5 radiculopathy
		87% with S1 radiculopathy
Stam (48)	Anterior tibialis	13 (72%) of 18 patients with L5 radiculopathy
De Weerd et al. (49)	Patellar	65% of 20 patients with L3 or L4 radiculopathy
Koenig (45)	Biceps and triceps	11 (73%) of 15 patients with C6 or C7 radiculopathy

more sensitive than the H-reflex test (65%) for the detection of S1 radiculopathy. By demonstrating a prolonged latency of 1–4 msec in the involved side (44), Malcolm found that the ankle T-reflex was able to detect a unilateral lesion, in four (80%) of five patients with S1 radiculopathy, whereas the knee T-reflex was abnormal in one tested patient with L4 radiculopathy. In four patients with bilateral S1 radiculopathy, the ankle T-reflex was able to detect the more involved side in only two cases. Stam found a unilateral absence of anterior tibialis reflex in 13 (72%) of 18 cases of L5 radiculopathy but in only 6% of normal controls (Fig. 17.2) (48). De Weerd and Joost found an abnormal side difference (2.4 msec difference between the patellar T-reflex latency and the M-latency) in 13 (60%) of 20 cases of L3 or L4 radiculopathy (49). Koenig found a pathological biceps and triceps T-reflex in 11 (73%) of 15 patients with unilateral cervical C6 or C7 radiculopathy: prolongation of the latency >2 msec in 10 compared with the normal side and a significant amplitude reduction in one (45). This is in contrast to the EMG abnormality observed in 60% of cases. *All of these studies showed that T-reflex testing is useful in the diagnosis of radiculopathy.*

The usefulness of the T-reflex study in peripheral neuropathy is limited. Eisen et al. studied the T-reflex change in assessing peripheral nerve function following long-term therapy with diphenylhydantoin (50). They found no significant difference in mean T-reflex latency between 45 seizure patients on diphenylhydantoin for more than 10 years and a control group. However, a prolonged T-reflex was found in 65% of cases. This figure is comparable to the sensitivity figures for the H-reflex, sural sensory, and per-

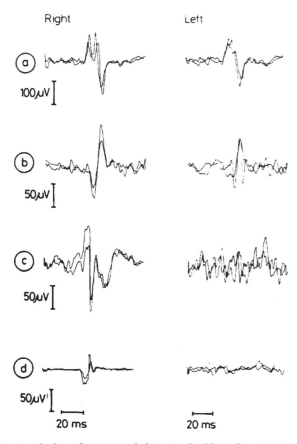

Figure 17.2. Anterior tibialis reflexes recorded in two healthy subjects (***a***) and (***b***) and in two patients with left L5 radiculopathy. Sixteen reflexes were averaged for each recording, and two superimposed recordings are shown for each reflex. In (***a***) and (***b***), reproducible reflexes are recorded on both sides. In (***c***) and (***d***), no response was present on the affected (left) side. Background EMG activity is seen in all recordings, as well as in the muscles without detectable anterior tibialis reflex activity. (From Stam J. The tibialis anterior reflex in healthy subjects and in L5 radicular compression. J Neurol Neurosurg Psychiatry 1988;51:400.)

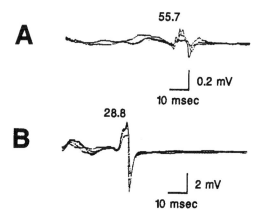

Figure 17.3. Markedly prolonged ankle T-reflex latency (55.7 msec) in a patient with chronic inflammatory demyelinating neuropathy (**A**) in comparison with that (28.8 msec) in a normal control (**B**).

oneal motor nerve conduction tests. We have studied the T-reflex test in 26 patients with chronic inflammatory demyelinating polyneuropathy (CIDP) and found that the T-reflex latency was prolonged in 25 of 26 studied cases; the mean T-reflex latency was more than 150% beyond the normal mean, confirming demyelination as the basic pathologic process (Fig. 17.3) (43). We found this test to be extremely useful in seven patients with CIDP, who had normal or brisk tendon reflexes, by documenting the prolonged T-reflex latency.

As expected, the T-reflex latency is normal in cerebellar, pyramidal, and extrapyramidal diseases (44).

Blink Reflex

The blink reflex is an electrically induced glabellar response that has long been used in clinical neurology. The blink reflex is now known to be a polysynaptic reflex with an afferent arc through sensory fibers of the trigeminal nerve and with an efferent arc through the motor fibers of the facial nerve (51, 52). Kugelberg demonstrated that electrical stimulation of the forehead produces a reflex with two responses: an early response (R1) and a late response (R2) and that, when the supraorbital nerve is stimulated, R1 is present only ipsilaterally, whereas R2 is present bilaterally (52). Clinicopathological studies suggest that R1 is mediated via the main sensory nucleus of cranial nerve V in the pons (53, 54), whereas R2 is mediated via the spinal nucleus and tract of V in the medulla oblongata (Fig. 17.4) (53, 55, 56). From this, Kimura concluded that *a delay of R1 is relatively specific to pontine involvement and R2 is more consistently affected by lateral medullary lesions, though R2 may be affected by pontine lesions* (Fig. 17.5) (57). The R2 of the blink reflex is related to closure of the eyelids. It has a latency similar to that of the corneal reflex (58).

The blink reflex is usually recorded simultaneously from the right and left orbicularis oculi muscles by a stimulation on each supraorbital nerve because of its consistent recording of two responses. The blink reflex from the infraorbital nerve and mental nerves has been described (59). However, because of the lack of a consistent recording, it is not commonly used for clinical purposes. Occasionally, it is difficult to obtain R1, in which case a paired stimulus can be used with an interstimulus interval of 5 msec (60). Three latencies should be measured: (*a*) to the initial deflection of R1 ipsilaterally; (*b*) to the earliest reproducible R2 ipsilaterally; and (*c*) to the earliest reproducible R2 contralaterally. The amplitudes are variable and thus are not important. This technique produces the most information in localizing a lesion to the trigeminal and/or facial nerves.

The latencies of R1 range from 8–14 msec in normal subjects; the difference

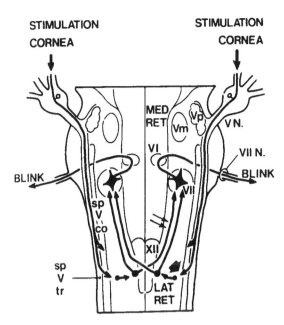

Figure 17.4. Anatomical pathways of the corneal and blink reflexes. In the corneal reflex, there is no early blink reflex equivalent to the early R1 blink response. The R1 response utilizes the more direct central pathway from the trigeminal principal sensory nucleus (V_p) to the facial nucleus (**VII**) (at least one interposed interneuron). The R2 response utilizes the polysynaptic pathway through the spinal trigeminal tract. Inhibition of impulses at the *thick arrow* on the right leads to an afferent block or delay of reflex responses. Inhibition of crossed impulses at the two *small arrows* on the right leads to a blocked or delayed reflex response contralateral to the stimulated cornea on the intact (left) side. VN = trigeminal nerve, Vm = trigeminal motor nucleus, Vp = trigeminal principal sensory nucleus, Sp Vtr = spinal trigeminal tract, Sp Vco = spinal trigeminal complex, VI = abducens nucleus, VII = facial nucleus, VIIN = facial nerve, XII = hypoglossal nucleus, Med Ret = medial reticular formation, Lat Ret = lateral reticular formation. (From Ongerboer de Visser BW. Corneal reflex latency in lesions of the lower postcentral region. Neurology 1981;31:707.)

between the two sides in the same individual is normally less than 1.2 msec. The latencies of R2 range from 23–44 msec; the difference between simultaneously elicited ipsilateral and contralateral responses is less than 5 msec (61). In general, the latency measurement of R2 is not as useful as that of R1 because of the wider range of variability.

Although the abnormality of the blink reflex represents a lesion in the trigeminal and facial nerves and the brainstem, one has to remember that a supratentorial lesion can affect both components of the blink reflex on the opposite side. Fisher observed that the R1 latency of the blink reflex in the involved side was delayed in 38% of 34 patients with stroke and that this usually returns to normal within a few days after the ictus (62). However, the absence of an R2 component, which was observed in 50% of cases, may persist for several weeks after an acute lesion (62). Kimura also observed that, in comatose patients R2 can be suppressed by a lesion at any level of the central nervous system including bilateral supratentorial lesions (57).

Clinical Applications

The blink reflex has been most useful in the evaluation of lesions of the trigeminal nerve and facial nerve, especially in patients with facial dyskinesia or hemifacial spasm.

For the detection of a lesion in the first division of the trigeminal nerve, the blink reflex is the only physiological test available at this time. The classic findings indicative of such a lesion are an *"afferent defect," a prolonged latency of both ipsilateral R1 and R2, and contralateral R2* (Fig. 17.5) (63). Such abnormalities were reported in patients with tumors involving the intracranial portion of the trigeminal nerve, aneurysms, traumatic lesions, and trigeminal sensory neuropathy associated with scleroderma or mixed

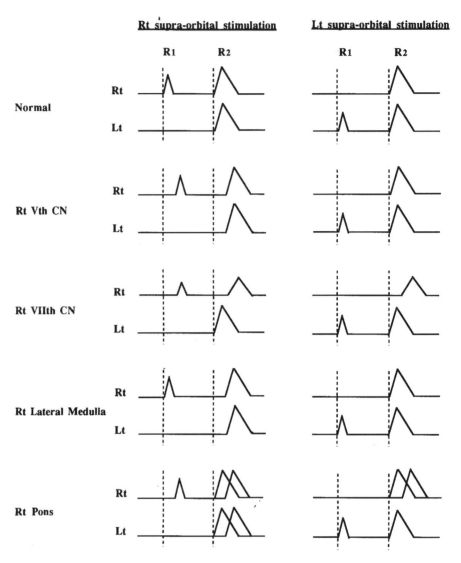

Figure 17.5. Classic abnormalities of the blink reflex in a lesion of the right 5th cranial nerve (afferent type), the right 7th cranial nerve (efferent type), the right lateral medulla, and the right pons. *Dotted lines* represent the normal limit.

connective tissue disease (64–69). On the other hand, the blink reflex is essentially normal in idiopathic trigeminal neuralgia: R1 was abnormal only in 4% of 93 patients (69).

In facial nerve lesions, there is *a delay in the reflex latency only on the affected side, regardless of the side of stimulation ("efferent defect")* (Fig. 17.5). Such abnormalities were found in Bell's palsy or other lesions of the facial nerve (also see Chapter 21) (61, 70). Kimura studied the blink reflex in patients with Bell's palsy in an attempt to predict which patients would subsequently have a poor prognosis (70). The blink reflex was not helpful in the early detection of this group of patients. By simultaneously recording the responses of the orbicularis oculi and orbicularis oris muscles, the phenomenon of facial synkinesis can be assessed. In normal individuals no response is elicited from the orbicularis oris muscle with supraorbital nerve stimulation unless a large stimulus is given (63, 71–73). However, during the aberrant regeneration of the facial nerve after Bell's palsy or other facial nerve injury, a synkinetic response can be recorded in the orbicularis oris as well as other muscles innervated by the facial nerve on the involved side (71).

A similar phenomenon is observed in hemifacial spasm (58, 67–69). *This finding is useful in confirming the presence of hemifacial spasm in doubtful cases and in differentiating hemifacial spasm from other facial movement disorders (Fig. 17.6),* since this

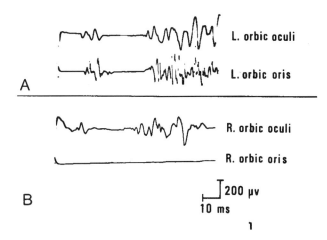

Figure 17.6. Response to supraorbital nerve stimulation in a patient with left hemifacial spasm. Simultaneous recording from orbicularis oculi and orbicularis oris muscles. With left supraorbital nerve stimulation (**A**), the orbicularis oris contracts simultaneously with the orbicularis oculi (that is, synkinesis is present). With supraorbital nerve stimulation (**B**), synkinesis is absent. (From Auger RG. Hemifacial spasm: clinical and electrophysiologic observations. Neurology 1979;29:1284.)

synkinetic response does not occur in the latter. In the past decade, microsurgical decompression of the facial nerve has been performed in the cerebellopontine area in hemifacial spasm (75). Auger et al. (76) and others (77, 78) reported that the synkinetic response accompanying the blink reflex disappeared after surgery, rendering objective confirmation of the effectiveness of such surgery.

In lateral medullary lesions, such as are seen in the Wallenberg syndrome, a distinct pattern of abnormality is seen in the blink reflex (55, 56): both ipsilateral and contralateral R2 are abnormal when the affected side of the face is stimulated, whereas the blink reflex is normal with stimulation on the normal side. Although of interest, these findings have not had much clinical application.

In multiple sclerosis, Kimura found in a study of 260 patients that 78% with clinical pontine signs and 40% with no clinical pontine signs had prolonged R1 (79). The blink reflex may be useful in documenting clinically silent pontine lesions in patients suspected of having multiple sclerosis. Lacquanti et al. demonstrated that abnormalities of the blink reflex closely parallel abnormalities of the brainstem auditory evoked potentials (BAEP), the latter showing abnormalities in 64% of 25 multiple sclerosis patients and blink reflex abnormalities in 60% (80). Others have reported BAEP abnormalities in 50% of MS patients and blink reflex abnormalities in 41% (81). In some cases, they found that the blink reflex was abnormal, while BAEPs were normal, and the converse was also true, so that the techniques occasionally complement each other. However, the blink reflex is no longer used for this purpose.

Blink reflex abnormalities have also been reported in other disorders. In acoustic neuroma, Eisen and Danon observed the abnormality in the efferent component in 11 of 12 patients and in the afferent component in 3 patients (64). More definitive tests have replaced the blink reflex in this disorder. Prolonged R1 and R2 of the blink reflex was reported as additional evidence of a delay in proximal conduction in the Guillain-Barré syndrome and hereditary motor sensory neuropathy (82). No practical additional information is gained from the blink reflex test in patients with peripheral neuropathy.

Masseter (Jaw) Reflex

The masseter reflex is a monosynaptic myotatic reflex, the afferent and efferent pathways of which are the trigeminal nerve via the mesencephalic nucleus of the trigeminal nerve in the midbrain (83). The masseter reflex is elicited less consistently than the electrically elicited blink reflex (69). Using the electronic reflex hammer, which can initiate a sweep on the oscilloscope upon percussion, this reflex can be easily obtained by

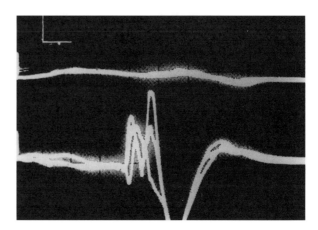

Figure 17.7. Absent jaw reflex on the right and normal latency (7.6 msec) on the left in a patient with a large saccular aneurysm on the syphon of the right internal carotid artery. (From Ongerboer de Visser BW and Goor C. Electromyographic and reflex study in idiopathic and symptomatic trigeminal neuralgias: latency of the jaw and blink reflexes. J Neurol Neurosurg Psychiatry 1974;37:1228.)

the examiner's tapping his finger on the patient's chin and recording the responses from the right and left masseter muscles. This reflex was elicited in normal individuals up to 70 years of age by Ongeboer de Visser and Goor (68). However, Kimura et al. observed no consistent response in three of 23 normal individuals between the ages of 13 and 60 (69). The mean latencies in normal individuals vary from 7.0 to 8.7 msec (68, 84). Since reflex latencies vary with successive trials, comparison between simultaneously recorded right and left responses is more meaningful than absolute values. A difference in latency between the two sides of up to 0.5–0.8 msec is considered to be normal (68, 69, 84). If the masseter reflex is absent bilaterally, no definite clinical significance can be deduced because this may occur in otherwise normal subjects. However, *a persistent unilateral absence of reflexes or significant prolongation of latency is evidence of a lesion involving the motor trigeminal fibers* if the brainstem is normal.

The masseter reflex is clinically useful in two situations: (*a*) localizing lesions in the motor fibers of the trigeminal nerve; and (*b*) documenting the absence of a silent period in patients with tetanus. The masseter reflex was found to be abnormal in trigeminal nerve lesions (68, 69, 85) but was normal in idiopathic trigeminal neuralgia (68, 69). However, in two patients with symptomatic trigeminal neuralgia without any neurological deficit, the masseter reflex was abnormal, detecting a silent trigeminal lesion due to a "mass lesion" (Fig. 17.7) (68). The masseter reflex may be useful in the diagnosis of tetanus. In one patient with chronic tetanus, the silent period of the masseter, elicited mechanically by a jaw tap, was repeatedly absent (86). *An abbreviated or absent silent period of the clinically involved masseter muscle,* which has been attributed to the failure of Renshaw cell inhibition, is *a characteristic feature of tetanus* and is seldom found in other disorders demonstrating motor-unit hyperactivity (87, 88). The masseter reflex may also be useful in the detection of a "silent lesion" in multiple sclerosis (84, 89). Goodwill and O'Tuama detected a "silent lesion" by the masseter reflex, with absent or increased latency on one or both sides in 12 (37.5%) of an unselected series of 32 patients with multiple sclerosis (89). Yates and Brown also found a lack of a reflex response in one or both sides in 12 (30%) of 40 cases of confirmed multiple sclerosis (84). This role of the masseter reflex is now largely replaced by more definitive tests such as the evoked potential and MRI studies.

Sacral Reflexes

The sacral reflex test has become one of three essential tests in the electrophysiological workup of neurological disorders involving the pelvic floor region. The other two tests are the pudendal sensory evoked potential test and the motor evoked potential test in the pelvic floor muscles.

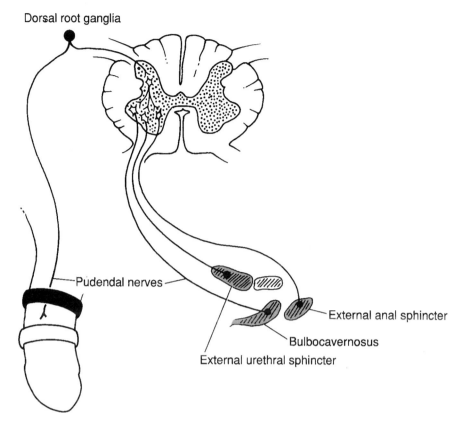

Dorsal root ganglia

Pudendal nerves

External anal sphincter

Bulbocavernosus

External urethral sphincter

Figure 17.8. Anatomical pathways of the bulbocavernosus (BC), pudendoanal, and pudendourethral reflexes. The afferent pathway of the BC reflex arc is the sensory fibers of the pudendal nerve, which is connected to the motor neurons of the pudendal nerve via two or more synaptic relays in the S2–S4 cord. The efferent pathway to the BC, anal, and urethral sphincter muscles is the motor fibers of the pudendal nerve.

The sacral reflexes refer to the reflex responses obtained from the pelvic floor muscles following stimulation of the perineum or genital organs. There are three reflexes: the bulbocavernosus (BC) reflex; the vesicourethral or vesicoanal reflex; and the anal sphincter response. Among these, the BC reflex is the best known and most studied.

The stimulation impulse in the BC reflex arc is transmitted to the S2–S4 spinal segments through the sensory fibers of the pudendal nerves as an afferent pathway, to the motor neurons of the pudendal nerve via two or more synaptic relays in the sacral cord, and to the BC, anal, and urethral sphincter muscles via the motor fibers of the pudendal nerves as the efferent pathway (Fig. 17.8) (90).

Bulbocavernosus Reflex

The bulbocavernosus (BC) reflex is a time-honored reflex test in neurology, testing the neural integrity of sacral spinal segments S2, S3, and S4, and of their afferent and efferent connections in the pelvic floor region through the pudendal nerves. It is clinically elicited by squeezing the glans and digitally palpating the contraction of the BC or external and sphincter (EAS) muscles by means of an index finger inserted into the anal canal. This reflex was used by Bors and Blin as early as 1959 for the examination of neurogenic bladder (91). In 1967, Rushworth described a method of timing the latency of the BC reflex following electrical stimulation of the dorsal nerve of the penis and recording the response from the bulbocavernosus muscle with a needle electrode (92). He found that *the nociceptive reflex recorded from the BC muscle was very stable and did not show habituation* and that its latency was about 35–40 msec in normal male subjects. Krane and Siroky believed the BC reflex to be a specialized flexor reflex similar to the blink reflex (93).

The BC reflex is obtained by stimulating the dorsal nerve of the penis or clitoris and by recording the response from pelvic floor striated muscles, either through needle electrodes or specially designed recording electrodes. Since the terminal branches of the pudendal nerves come into close apposition beneath the symphysis pubis, it is not possible to stimulate the left and the right divisions of this nerve separately. Stimulation to elicit this reflex is easier in men than in women, because the dorsal nerve of the penis is easily stimulated by a ring electrode or bipolar stimulator. In women, the stimulation of the dorsal nerve of the clitoris is delicate. Vodusek recommended using ear-clip electrodes attached to the clitoris and labia (Fig. 17.37 B) (94). Others recommended the use of bipolar stimulators over the clitoris. We prefer a bipolar stimulator because it produces a stimulus strong enough to evoke a more consistent response. Fowler believed that the test was best performed with the subject's cooperation, asking the patient to hold a bipolar stimulator with the active electrode distally over the clitoris (95). He claimed that this minimizes embarrassment and also leaves the subject free to remove the stimulator should the stimulus become uncomfortable.

The intensity of stimulation needed to elicit the BC reflex is variable. *Generally, a 0.2 msec stimulus duration and three to four times the sensory threshold are recommended for an adequate response.* Most studies have used concentric needle electrodes to record the response from the recording muscles but some investigators have used an hourglass plug device to record from the anal sphincter or a catheter-mounted ring electrode to record from the urethral sphincter. When an hourglass plug device, a disposable sphincter electrode, or a catheter-mounted ring electrode is used, averaging is necessary because the response obtained is extremely small. *Compared with the clinical BC reflex, the electrophysiological BC reflex is much more sensitive.* Blaivas et al. recorded the BC reflex electrophysiologically in a small number of urology patients (2% of men and 11% of women) who were presumed to be neurologically normal when it could not detect the BC reflex clinically (96). It is generally agreed that the BC reflex from the BC muscles is obtainable in all males. However, *in females it appears to be impossible to obtain the BC reflex in all individuals.* Vodusek was not able to record the BC reflex from the external urethral sphincter in three of 10 female patients using ear-clip electrodes (94). He admitted that this may have been because of his reluctance to use a higher intensity of stimulation. Citing his personal experience, Fowler also stated that it is often difficult to elicit the reflex in females and that no significance should be given to its absence in a woman (95). This problem is caused by the relatively small response recorded from the external urethral or anal sphincter muscles in female patients. We found that *recording the BC reflex was possible with a concentric needle from the bulbocavernosus muscle even in females and that the amplitude of the BC reflex was higher than when recorded from the EAS.* Even in normal males, the BC reflex was obtained in the EAS in 21% of cases, whereas the BC reflex was obtained in the BC muscle in all normal males (97).

Clinical Applications

Neurogenic Bladder

In patients with neurogenic bladder due to upper motor neuron diseases, the BC reflex is characterized by either normal or shortened latency and an intense after-discharge in some cases. Normal BC latency was reported in 19 patients by Ertekin and Reel (97). However, a significantly shorter mean latency was reported in 44 patients with upper motor neuron lesions by Bilkey et al. (98). Krane and Siroky also observed that the BC latency was on the average lower than normal (93). Krane and Siroky and Ertekin and Reel reported a prominent after-discharge in some cases (93, 97). The former also reported that the reflex threshold was lower than in normal subjects (93).

In patients with neurogenic bladder due to cauda equina and conus medullaris lesions, the BC reflex was either absent or present with a prolonged latency in all of 13 tested cases in Ertekin and Reel's series (97). These patients had neurological deficits including sphincter disturbance and impotence. Mean BC latency was prolonged in cauda equina and conus medullaris lesions (93, 97). The sensory threshold was also much higher in this group of patients compared with normal individuals.

In patients with neurogenic bladder due to polyneuropathy, the BC reflex was either normal or prolonged in Ertekin and Reel's 22 cases (97) and in Krane and Siroky's 17 cases (93), though mean BC latencies were outside the normal limit. The sensory threshold was also abnormal. Most patients with polyneuropathy had diabetes mellitus. Of six males with hereditary motor sensory neuropathy, Vodusek and Zidar found extreme prolongation of the BC reflex in four, none of whom had any sexual dysfunction (99).

Galloway et al. averaged the response from the urethral and anal sphincters following stimulation of the dorsal nerve of penis or clitoris using the surface-mounted electrodes (100). They found an abnormal sacral reflex in 80% of 35 patients with urinary incontinence and a minor defect of the dorsal neural arches of S1 or S2 (101) and in 86% of 14 female patients with acute urinary retention (102).

Impotence

In functional impotence, normal latency was reported in 12 of 13 studied cases in Ertekin and Reel's series (97) and in all of 42 cases in Krane and Siroky's series (93), as

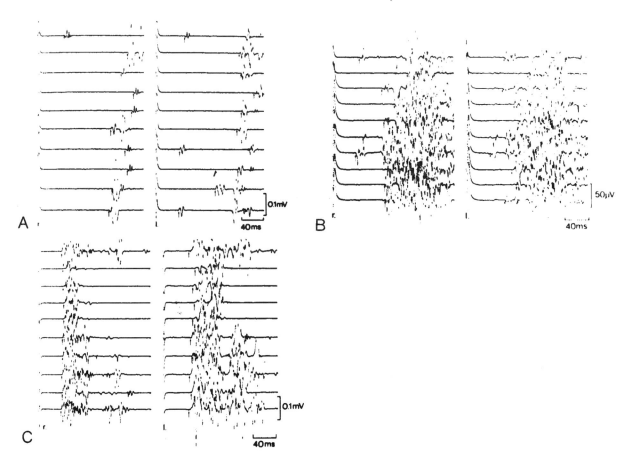

Figure 17.9. Bulbocavernosus (BC) reflex recordings from patients with disturbances of potency due to various etiologies **A**, Increase in minimum and maximum latencies, temporal dispersion on either side, and increase of maximum side differences in a 65-year-old diabetic patient. **B**, Results from a 49-year-old man who had a pelvic fracture 12 years ago. Only the minimum latency on the right side was normal, whereas latencies of the other BC responses were increased. **C**, A 46-year-old man without clinical evidence of a neurological disorder. While the latencies recorded from the right BC muscle are within the normal range, minimum and maximum latencies of the BC reflex recorded from the left side were increased. The latencies of the individual responses in (**B**) are marked by *arrows*. (From Tackmann W, Porst H, Van Ahlen H. Bulbocavernosus reflex latencies and somatosensory evoked potentials after pudendal nerve stimulation in the diagnosis of impotence. J Neurol 1988;235:219–225.)

expected. In 130 male patients with erectile dysfunction in Tackmann et al.'s series, abnormalities of the BC reflex were present in 50% (Fig. 17.9) (103). Among these abnormalities, absence of response and prolonged latency were present in only 24% of cases. In 76% of cases, minor parameters, such as temporal dispersion, were abnormal. From this, they concluded that temporal dispersion should be used as one of several parameters indicating a pathological condition of the pudendal nerve. On the other hand, Lin and Bradley found a prolonged BC reflex in two of 20 diabetic patients with impotence and slow NCV in 10 of 20 patients by the nerve conduction study in the dorsal nerve of the penis (104). Mehta et al. also found that the BC reflex was abnormal in 36% of 111 impotent males (63% of whom were diabetic or alcoholic), whereas the sural nerve conduction was abnormal in 78% and the peroneal motor nerve conduction in 50% (105). These studies emphasize the importance of the routine nerve conduction test as well as the nerve conduction test of the dorsal nerve of the penis in the study of impotence.

Neurogenic Fecal Incontinence

Varma et al. found abnormality in the pudendoanal response in all of 20 patients with neurogenic fecal incontinence: absent response in three, and significant prolongation of latency in 17 (90). Henry and Swash reported an increase in the anal reflex latency in a group of patients with fecal incontinence (106). However, later studies were not able to confirm this finding (107, 108).

Techniques and Normal Values

H-Reflexes

H-Reflex in the Gastrocnemius-Soleus Muscle (Posterior Tibial Nerve)

Braddom and Johnson's Method

Braddom and Johnson described a technique of obtaining the H-reflex in the gastrocnemius muscle and constructed a nomogram for quick prediction of the H-latency in relation to age and leg length (Fig. 5.13) (15).

POSITION OF SUBJECT: Subjects are in the prone position, with knees slightly flexed and a folded pillow under the ankles to keep the ankles in a neutral position.

RECORDING: The active recording electrode is placed halfway along a line connecting the midpopliteal crease (stimulation site) and the most proximal part of the medial malleolus over the medial calf muscle. The reference electrode is placed over the Achilles tendon.

STIMULATION: The posterior tibial nerve is stimulated at the midpopliteal crease with an active stimulating electrode proximally. The stimulus duration used is 0.1 msec and the stimulus frequency is one stimulation every 2 sec.

MEASUREMENT: The leg length is measured as the distance from the site of stimulation of the posterior tibial nerve in the midpopliteal crease to a point over the distal posterior tibial nerve at the most proximal part of the medial malleolus. The H-reflex latency is measured to the first deflection from the baseline from the stimulus onset.

TEMPERATURE: Not controlled.

NORMAL DATA: Number of subjects: 100. Age range: 18–79 yr.

Measurement	Mean ± SD	Normal limit
H-latency (msec)	29.8 ± 2.74	35.3
Difference between two sides (msec)		1.5
H-duration (msec)	16.7 ± 2.86	22.4
H-amplitude (μV)	2635 ± 2249	

Figure 17.10: H-latency compared with leg length in normal subjects of all ages.

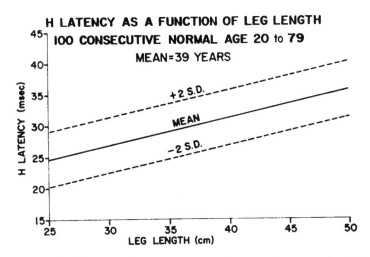

Figure 17.10. H-reflex latency on the gastrocnemius-soleus muscle compared with leg length in normal subjects of all ages (From Braddom RL and Johnson EW. Standardization of H-reflex and diagnostic use in S1 radiculopathy. Arch Phys Med Rehabil 1974;55:163.)

Figure 17.11: Nomogram of the simultaneous regression of H-reflex latency by leg length and age. 5.5 msec is 2 SD.

INTERPRETATION: These authors considered that a 1.5 msec difference between the affected and unaffected sides is significant.

COMMENTS: The H-reflex latency had a fair correlation with leg length ($r = 0.561$) and with age ($r = 0.441$). The H-reflex latency increases approximately 1 msec for each decade of age. Combining the age and height, the following formula is obtained:

H-reflex latency (msec) = 9.14 + 0.46 × leg length (cm) + 0.1 × age (yr).
2 SD = 5.5 msec.

In 25 patients with unilateral S1 radiculopathy, the H-reflex on the affected side was found to be either delayed in latency or absent in each case (15).

H-Reflex in the Flexor Carpi Radialis Muscle (Median Nerve)

Deschuytere et al.'s Method

Deschuytere et al. described a technique of obtaining the H-reflex on the superficial forearm flexor muscle (Fig. 17.12A) (109).

POSITION OF INDIVIDUAL: The subject lies in a supine position on a comfortable couch with the arm slightly abducted and with the elbow joint conveniently positioned at 35° flexion. At times the hand is fixed firmly by tape to ensure isometric contraction.

FACILITATION TECHNIQUE: Contractions of the ipsilateral quadriceps muscle, either isometric or by raising the leg.

RECORDING: The CMAP is recorded with a concentric needle electrode inserted into the flexor carpi radialis and palmaris longus muscles. Ten recordings are superimposed.

STIMULATION: The median nerve is stimulated at the cubital fossa with bipolar surface electrodes with a stimulus duration of 1.0 msec.

MEASUREMENT: The latency is measured by the conventional method.

TEMPERATURE: Skin temperature is not controlled.

NORMAL DATA: Number of subjects: 50. Age range: 18–64 yr.

Measurement	Normal range	Normal limit
The H-reflex latency (msec)	15–17	17
Difference between the sides (msec)	<1	1

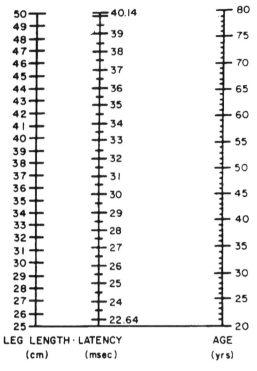

Figure 17.11.   Nomogram of the simultaneous regression of H-reflex latency on the gastrocnemius-soleus muscle on leg length and age. (From Braddom RL and Johnson EW. Standardization of H-reflex and diagnostic use in S1 radiculopathy. Arch Phys Med Rehabil 1974;55:164.)

Figure 17.12.   Methods for the H-reflex on the flexor carpi radialis (FCR) muscle. **A**, With a concentric needle (Deschuytere et al.'s method and Ongerboer De Visser's method). **B**, With a surface electrode on the FCR muscle (Jabre's method).

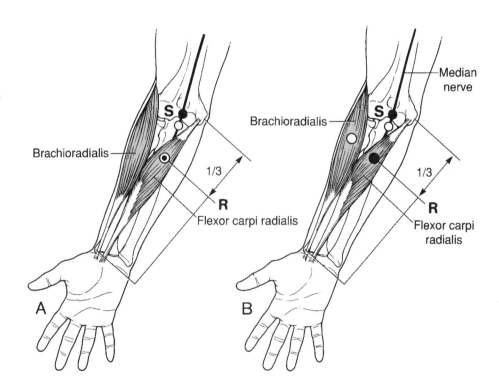

COMMENTS: In every normal individual, the H-reflex was obtained: With the facilitation technique, the CMAP amplitude was increased by 50–100% (104). The H-reflex was obtained without the facilitation technique in 70% of normal controls and with the facilitation (contraction of ipsilateral quadriceps) in the remaining 30%.

Ongerboer de Visser's Method

Ongerboer de Visser's method (20) is essentially the same as Deschuytere et al.'s method. They calculate the interlatency time and the H-reflex conduction velocity (Fig. 17.12A).

POSITION OF SUBJECT: The elbow joint is flexed at 30°.

RECORDING: The CMAP is recorded with a concentric needle electrode inserted into the flexor carpi radialis (FCR) muscle.

STIMULATION: The median nerve is stimulated in the cubital fossa with bipolar surface electrodes. Stimulation is made at a rate of one every 5 sec. Stimulus duration is 0.5 msec. The stimulus sensitivity is gradually increased until a maximal H-reflex is obtained. The active electrode should be placed proximally.

FACILITATION TECHNIQUE: Not mentioned. According to Garcia et al., contraction is performed against resistance, with the hand approximately 30° below the horizontal for the FCR muscle (105).

MEASUREMENT: The H-reflex latency and M-wave latency are measured following the conventional method. The interlatency time (ILT) is determined by subtracting the latency of the maximal M-wave from the maximal H-reflex. The H-reflex conduction velocity (H-RCV) is estimated utilizing the following formula:

$$\text{H-RCV (m/sec)} = \frac{(\text{Distance in mm from stimulus point to C6 spine}) \times 2}{[(\text{H-R latency} - \text{M latency in msec}) - 1]}$$

Monosynaptic delay is 1 msec (106). Distance between the stimulus point to C6 spine is obtained as the sum of the distances from the elbow to the medial end of the deltoid muscle and the latter point to the C6 spine. Arm length is measured from the top of digit 3 to the C6 spine with the arm pronated and abducted to a right angle.

TEMPERATURE: Skin temperature of the upper arm is controlled at 32–34°C.

NORMAL DATA: Number of subjects: 52. Number of tests: 104. Age range: 20–85 yr.

Measurement	Mean ± SD	Normal limit[a]
H-Reflex latency (H-RL)(msec)	16.8 ± 1.1	20.1
Side difference	0.002 ± 0.42	1.26
Interlatency time (IRT)	13.8 ± 1.2	17.4
Side difference	0.11 ± 0.44	1.43
H-RCV (m/sec)	73.7 ± 7.2	52.1
Side difference	0.38 ± 2.4	7.58

[a]Normal limit = mean ± 3 SD.

Figure 17.13: Relationship between arm length and the H-reflex latency and interlatency time (ILT) was studied in 143 controls (16).

Figure 17.14: Relationship between body length (height) and the H-reflex was studied in 80 controls (12).

INTERPRETATION: In both arms the H-reflex was obtained in all controls. Whether this was done without any facilitation technique is not mentioned. There was no relationship between age and H-RL or ILT. In contrast, the H-RCV decreased significantly with increasing age (H-RCV = 88.3 − 0.29 × age).

Jabre's Method

Jabre described a technique of the H-reflex on the flexor carpi radialis muscle using a surface electrode as the recording electrode (Fig. 17.12B) (19).

POSITION OF SUBJECT: The subject is supine and the elbow is slightly flexed.

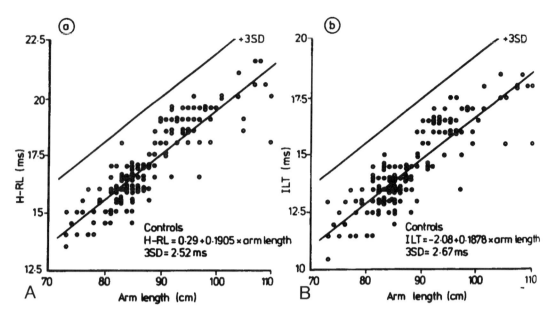

Figure 17.13. Relationship between arm length and (**A**) the H-reflex latency (HRL), and (**B**) the interlatency time (ILT) of the flexor carpi radialis H-reflex. (From Schimsheimer RJ, Ongerboer de Visser BW, Kemp B. The flexor carpi radialis H-reflex in lesions of the sixth and seventh cervical nerve roots. J Neurol Neurosurg Psychiatry 1985;48:446.)

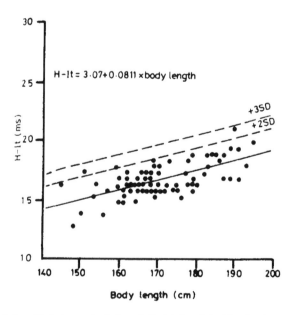

Figure 17.14. Relationship between body length (height) and the H-reflex latency time (H-lt) of the flexor carpi radialis H-reflex. In this study crossing of the upper +3 SD level is considered abnormal. (From Schimscheimer RJ, Ongerboer de Visser BW, Kemp B, Bour LJ. The flexor carpi radialis H-reflex in polyneuropathy: relations to conduction velocities of the median nerve and the soleus H-reflex latency. J Neurol Neurosurg Psychiatry 1987;50:449.)

FACILITATION TECHNIQUE: None mentioned.

RECORDING: An active surface electrode is placed over the belly of the flexor carpi radialis at about one-third of the distance between the medial epicondyle and the radial styloid. The reference electrode is placed over the brachioradialis muscle.

STIMULATION: The median nerve is stimulated at the elbow using bipolar surface electrodes. The stimulus duration is 0.5–1.0 msec. Stimulation rate is once every 2 sec.

MEASUREMENT: Latency is measured using the conventional method. Amplitude is measured from the baseline to the highest negative peak.

TEMPERATURE: Skin temperature is not controlled.

NORMAL DATA: Number of subjects: 39. Age range: 15–59 yr.

Measurement	Mean ± SD	Normal limit
H-reflex		
Latency (msec)	15.9 ± 1.5	18.9
Latency difference between sides	0.4 ± 0.3	1.0 (N = 11)
Amplitude (mV)	1.6 ± 0.4	
M-wave		
Latency (msec)	3.0 ± 0.5	
Amplitude (mV)	7.6 ± 2.5	

COMMENTS: The H-reflex was obtained in 90% of subjects. The responses were always symmetrical. The difference in latency between the two sides (without facilitation) never exceeded 1 msec.

H-Reflex on the Flexor Carpi Ulnaris Muscle (Ulnar Nerve)

Deschuytere et al. described a technique of the H-reflex on the flexor carpi ulnaris (FCU) muscle (Fig. 17.15) (25).

POSITION OF INDIVIDUAL: Same as for the flexor carpi radialis muscle.

FACILITATION TECHNIQUE: Repetitive electrical stimulation at a rate of 4/sec.

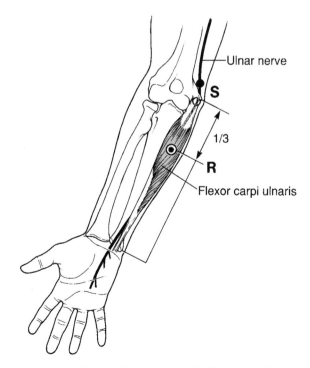

Figure 17.15. Method for the H-reflex on the flexor carpi ulnaris muscle.

RECORDING: The H-reflex response is recorded with a concentric needle electrode in the FCU muscle.

STIMULATION: The ulnar nerve is stimulated with bipolar surface electrodes at the elbow. Stimulus duration is 1.0 or 2.0 msec.

MEASUREMENT: The latency is measured by the conventional method.

TEMPERATURE: Skin temperature is not controlled.

NORMAL DATA: Number of subjects: 50. Age range: 18–62 yr. Normal range: 16–18 msec.

COMMENTS: In all subjects, the H-reflex was obtained from the FCU muscle, either with or without facilitation technique. However, the authors stated that the facilitation technique must be used in most instances to record the H-reflex from this muscle (107).

H-Reflex in the Extensor Digitorum Communis Muscle (Radial Nerve)

Garcia et al. described the technique of obtaining the H-reflex response from this muscle (Fig. 17.16) (110).

FACILITATION TECHNIQUE: Passive movements are performed at the wrist. During voluntary contraction of the forearm muscle, the arm is prone. Voluntary contraction is performed against resistance, with the hand approximately 30° above the horizontal for the extensor digitorum communis (EDC) muscle.

RECORDING: The responses are recorded with concentric needle electrodes from the EDC muscle.

STIMULATION: The radial nerve is stimulated at the lower one-third of the spiral groove with a stimulus duration of 1 msec and a frequency of 0.2 sec (every 5 sec).

MEASUREMENT: Latency is measured by the conventional method.

TEMPERATURE: Skin temperature is not controlled.

NORMAL DATA: Number of subjects: 10. Age range: 25–44 yr. Normal range: 16–20 msec.

COMMENTS: The H-reflex was recorded from this muscle in all subjects during isometric contraction (105).

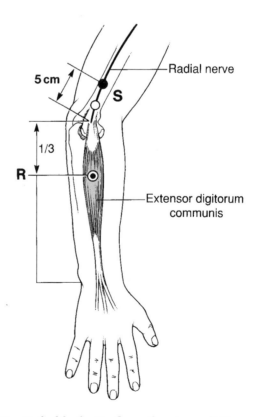

Figure 17.16.   Method for the H-reflex on the extensor digiti communis muscle.

H-Reflex of the Medial Vastus Muscle (Femoral Nerve)

Verhagen et al. described a technique of obtaining the H-reflex of the medial vastus muscle (Fig. 17.17) (2).

FACILITATION TECHNIQUE: Mild voluntary contraction of the vastus medialis muscle.

RECORDING: The H-reflex is recorded with a concentric needle electrode inserted into the muscle at a 4-fingerbreadths distance proximal to the medial upper margin of the patella.

STIMULATION: The femoral nerve is stimulated in the inguinal region with a stimulus of 0.5 msec duration at intervals of at least 5 sec.

MEASUREMENT: The H-reflex latency is measured at the onset of the maximal H-reflex response.

TEMPERATURE: Skin temperature is not controlled.

NORMAL DATA: Number of subjects: 131. Number of nerves: 262. Age range: 20–79 yr.

Measurement	Mean ± SD	Normal limit
H-reflex latency	18.08 ± 1.87	21.82

Figure 17.18: The relationship of height and the H-reflex latency:

The H-reflex latency = 0.0805 × height (cm) + 4.58. 2 SD = 3.4

Figure 17.19: The relationship of age and the H-reflex latency:

The H-reflex latency = 0.025 × age + 16.93. 2 SD = 3.68
The H-reflex latency = 1.44 = 0.047 × age + 0.101 × height (cm). 2 SD = 3.16
Higher H-reflex latency = lower H-reflex latency + 1.77. 2 SD = 1.8

INTERPRETATION: The difference between the right and left sides should be less than 3.6 msec.

COMMENTS: The H-reflex was obtained in all normal subjects, though mild voluntary contraction of the vastus medialis muscle was sometimes necessary to facilitate the recording of the H-reflex (2). In 11 of 14 patients with L4 radiculopathy, the H-reflex

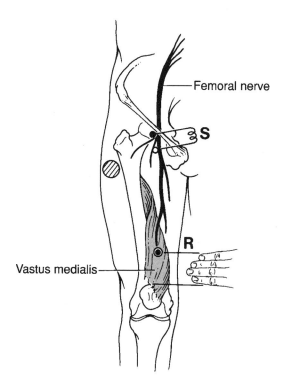

Figure 17.17. Method for the H-reflex on the vastus medialis.

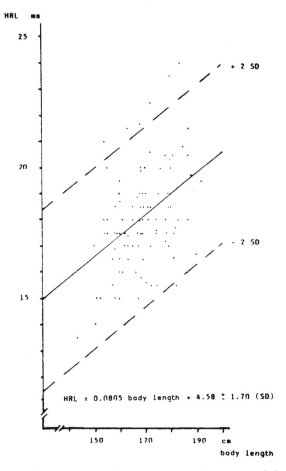

Figure 17.18. Relationship between the H-reflex latency on the vastus medialis muscle and height. (From Verhagen WIM, Schrooten GJM, Schiphof PR, Van Ammers V. The H-reflex of the medial vastus muscle: a study in controls and patients with radiculopathy. EMG Clin Neurophysiol 1988;28:422.)

latencies in the involved side were higher than 3.6 msec compared with those in the noninvolved side.

H-Reflex in the Extensor Digitorum Longus Muscle (Peroneal Nerve)

Deschuytere and Rosselle described a technique of obtaining the H-reflex in the extensor digitorum longus muscle (Fig. 17.20) (112).

FACILITATION TECHNIQUE: The most effective facilitation technique uses paired stimuli at intervals of 170–250 msec. In this way, the second stimulus occurs approximately at the time the muscle relaxes after the contraction elicited by the first stimulus.

RECORDING: The reflex responses are recorded with a concentric needle electrode inserted into the extensor digitorum longus muscle. Most frequently, 10 reflex responses are superimposed.

STIMULATION: The common peroneal nerve is stimulated with surface electrodes in the distal lateral part of the posterior fossa with a stimulus duration of 2 msec.

MEASUREMENT: The latency is measured by the conventional method.

TEMPERATURE: Skin temperature is not controlled.

NORMAL DATA: Number of subjects: 50. Age range: 28–64 yr.

Measurement	Normal range	Normal limit
H-reflex latency (msec)	27–33	33
Difference between sides (msec)	<1	1

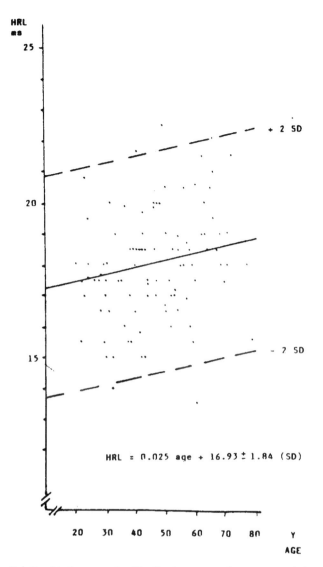

Figure 17.19. Relationship between the H-reflex latency on the vastus medialis muscle and age. (From Verhagen WIM, Schrooten GJM, Schiphof PR, Van Ammers V. The H-reflex of the medial vastus muscle: a study in controls and patients with radiculopathy. EMG Clin Neurophysiol 1988;28:423.)

INTERPRETATION: A 2-msec difference between sides is a definite indication, and a 1-msec difference is a suggestive indication of a root lesion.

COMMENTS: In 47 of the 50 patients with an L5 radiculopathy, the H-reflex was obtained on the extensor digitorum longus muscle, and in 41 cases, the latency difference was more than 2 msec (108). This indicates that this technique is useful in detection of L5 radiculopathy.

H-Reflex on the Anterior Tibialis and Peroneus Muscles (Peroneal Nerve)

Garcia et al. described a technique of obtaining the H-reflex response from the anterior tibialis and peroneus muscles (Fig. 17.20) (110).

FACILITATION TECHNIQUE: Paired stimuli are used to facilitate responses from the anterior tibialis muscle. Passive movements are performed with both ankles. Voluntary contractions of the ankle plantar flexor is made against resistance with the ankle maintained at an angle of 90°.

RECORDING: The responses are recorded with concentric needle electrodes from the muscles as follows: for the anterior tibialis muscle, one-half the distance between the

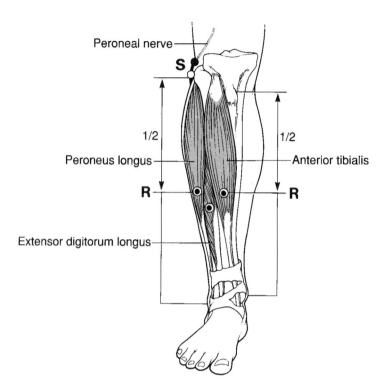

Figure 17.20.   Methods for the H-reflex on the anterior tibialis, extensor digitorum longus, and peroneus muscles.

tibial tubercle and the ankle and for the peroneal muscle, one-half the distance between the fibular head and the ankle.

STIMULATION: The peroneal nerve is stimulated at the fibular head. Stimulation is made with a duration of 1 msec at a frequency of 0.2/sec (every 5 sec).

MEASUREMENT: Latency is measured by the conventional method.

TEMPERATURE: Skin temperature is not controlled.

NORMAL DATA: Number of subjects: 10. Age range: 25–44 yr. Normal range: 28–35 msec.

COMMENTS: The reflexes were recorded from these muscles during isometric contraction.

H-Reflex on the Abductor Hallucis and Flexor Digitorum Brevis Muscles (Posterior Tibial Nerve)

Wager and Buerger described a technique of obtaining the H-reflex with the distal and proximal stimulation of the posterior tibial nerve (Fig. 17.21) (113).

RECORDING: The response is recorded with a surface electrode on the plantar surface of the foot over either the flexor digitorum brevis or abductor hallucis muscle.

STIMULATION: The posterior tibial nerve is stimulated at the ankle and the popliteal fossa with a surface-stimulating electrode with a stimulus duration of 0.2–1.0 msec following the conventional method.

MEASUREMENT: Latency and distance are measured following the conventional method. The latency difference between the ankle and popliteal fossa is divided by the distance to calculate the H-reflex sensory nerve conduction velocity.

TEMPERATURE: Skin temperature is not controlled.

NORMAL DATA: Number of subjects: 8. Age range: Not mentioned.

Measurement	Normal range	Normal limit
H-reflex latency (msec)	43–60	60
H-reflex sensory NCV (m/sec)	39.0–75.0	39

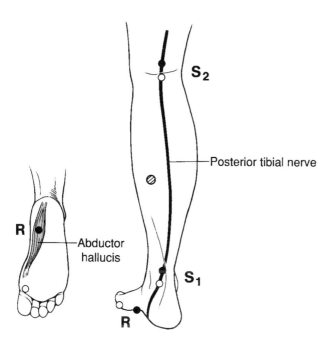

Comments: In nine controls, an H-reflex was obtained in all cases when stimulating at the ankle, but in one of these an H-reflex was not obtained when stimulating at the popliteal fossa (109). There was an inverse linear relationship between the latency and the H-reflex sensory NCVs.

Tendon Reflexes

Ankle T-Reflex (Posterior Tibial Nerve)

Kuruoglu and Oh's Method

Kuruoglu and Oh described the technique of the ankle T-reflex testing (Fig. 17.22A) (43).

Position of Subject: Subject lies on the stomach with a pillow under the ankles to ensure 90° flexion.

EMG Machine Set-Up: Filters: 20–10,000 Hz. Sweep velocity: 10 msec/div. Sensitivity: variable, starting with 1 mV.

Recording: An active surface electrode is placed on the gasrtrocnemius-soleus muscle midway between the popliteal fossa crease and the upper border of the medial malleolus. A reference electrode is placed 5 cm distally from the active surface electrode on the same line.

Stimulation: The Achilles tendon is tapped gently at the ankle with an electronic T-reflex hammer. Four to eight repetitions are made at an interval of 5 sec between each successive stimulation.

Measurement: Latency is measured to the onset of the first deflection from the baseline. Duration is measured from the onset of the baseline deflection to the point where it meets the baseline again. Amplitude is measured from peak to peak. Calf length is measured from the popliteal fossa crease to the upper border of the medial malleolus.

Temperature: Skin temperature in the calf is kept above 31°C.

Normal Data: Number of subjects: 50. Age range: 23–58 yr.

Measurement	Mean ± SD	Normal limit
Latency (msec)	32.1 ± 2.9	37.9
Duration (msec)	14.8 ± 2.5	19.8
Amplitude (μV)	3068	300[a]

[a]Low normal range.

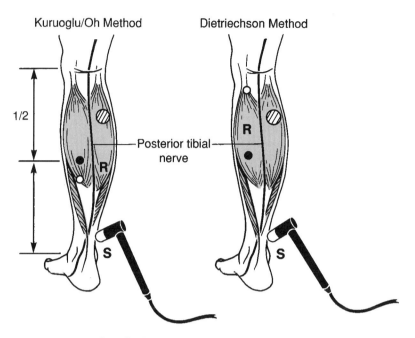

Figure 17.22. **A,** Kuruoglu and Oh's method for the T-reflex on the gastrocnemius-soleus muscle. **B,** Dietrichson and Sorbye's method for the T-reflex on the gastrocnemius-soleus muscle.

Figure 17.23: T-reflex latency with height (cm).

COMMENTS: Latency was well correlated with the height and leg length: Latency = 9.66 + (0.59 × leg length [cm]). 2 SD = 3.9; Latency = −3.74 + (0.21 × height [cm]). 2 SD = 3.9.

Dietrichson and Sorbye's Method

The ankle reflex response was recorded by using the electronic hammer designed by Dietrichson and Sorbye (Fig. 17.22B) (41). This technique was also used by Eisen et al. (50) and Rico and Jonkman (24).

POSITION OF SUBJECT: The subject lies in a prone position with the knees flexed at approximately 120° and the ankles in a resting position of 100° flexion (24).

RECORDING: An active surface electrode is placed on the medial belly of the gastrocnemius muscle and a reference electrode near the popliteal fossa.

STIMULATION: The Achilles tendon is tapped with an electronic T-reflex hammer.

MEASUREMENT: Latency is measured from the stimulus artifact to the onset of the reflex responses.

TEMPERATURE: Skin temperature is not controlled.

NORMAL DATA: This normal values are from Eisen et al. (50). Number of subjects: 50. Age range: mean age: 43 yr.

Measurement	Mean ± SD	Normal limit
Latency	32.4 ± 4.4	41.2

INTERPRETATION: Rico and Jonkman considered that, compared with the normal side, a prolongation of latency of 2 msec or more was abnormal (37).

COMMENTS: By using 2 msec asymmetry as an abnormal finding, Rico and Jonkman found that this test was abnormal in 11% of normal controls, in 21% of patients with L5 radiculopathy, and in 87% of patients with S1 radiculopathy, indicating that this test is useful in detecting S1 radiculopathy (24). They also showed that this test was more sensitive than the H-reflex test (65%) for the detection of S1 radiculopathy.

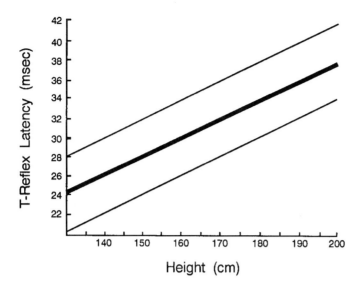

Figure 17.23. Relationship between the T-reflex latency on the gastrocnemius-soleus muscle and height.

Anterior Tibialis T-Reflex (Peroneal Nerve)

Stam described the technique of anterior tibialis T-reflex testing (Fig. 17.24) (48).

POSITION OF SUBJECT: The subjects are in a supine position.

EMG MACHINE SET-UP: Sensitivity is 50–100 μV.

RECORDING: Bipolar surface electrodes (Ag–AgCl, 0.6 cm²; 5 cm apart) are placed on the center of the anterior tibialis muscle 2 cm laterally from the anterior margin of the tibia.

STIMULATION: A wooden spatula is pressed against the first metatarsal and serves to receive the tap. The tap is made with an electronic T-reflex hammer on the dorsal and distal part of the first metatarsal bone.

FACILITATION TECHNIQUE: When no response is recorded from the relaxed muscle, subjects are instructed to maintain slight isometric dorsiflexion of the foot by lightly pressing against the spatula. In these cases, the responses are averaged. In most subjects a reproducible response is present after averaging 16 times. When no reproducible response is visible after averaging 32 times, the reflex is judged to be absent.

MEASUREMENT: Latency is measured to the first deflection of the response from the baseline. Amplitude is the peak-to-peak amplitude.

TEMPERATURE: Not controlled.

NORMAL DATA: Number of subjects: 70. Age range: 19–36 yr.

Measurement	Mean ± SD	Normal limit
Latency: side difference (msec)	1.3 ± 1.1	>4[a]
Amplitude (μV)	150 ± 0.11	<30
Side difference (μV)	50 ± 50	>300

[a]Upper normal range.

COMMENTS: In 83% of normal controls, bilateral reflexes were present. In 11%, reflexes were absent on both sides, and in 6% the reflex was absent unilaterally. There was a good correlation between the latency and height (R = 0.70–0.73). The latency in the anterior tibialis muscle was on average 3.5 msec longer than the soleus reflex. In 13 (72%) of 18 patients with L5 radiculopathy, the T-reflex was absent on the symptomatic side.

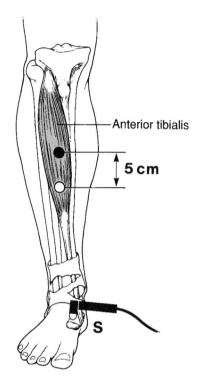

Figure 17.24.   Method for the T-reflex on the anterior tibialis muscle.

Patellar T-Reflex (Femoral Nerve)

Kuruoglu and Oh described the technique of patellar T-reflex testing (Fig. 17.25) (43).

POSITION OF SUBJECT: Subject lies on the back, with a pillow under the knees for a 135° knee flexion.

EMG MACHINE SET-UP: Filter: 20–10,000 Hz. Sweep velocity: 10 msec/div. Sensitivity: variable, starting with 1 mV.

RECORDING: An active surface electrode is placed on the rectus femoris muscle midway between the anterior superior iliac spine and the superior border of the patella. A reference electrode is put 5 cm distally on the same line.

STIMULATION: The quadriceps tendon is tapped gently right below the patella with an electronic T-reflex hammer.

MEASUREMENT: Latency is measured to the onset of the first deflection from the baseline. Duration is measured from the onset of the baseline deflection to the point where it meets the baseline again. Amplitude is measured from peak to peak. Thigh length is measured from the anterior superior iliac spine to the superior border of the patella.

TEMPERATURE: Skin temperature in the thigh is kept above 31°C.

NORMAL DATA: Number of subjects: 50. Age range: 23–58 yr.

Measurement	Mean ± SD	Normal limit
Latency (msec)	17.2 ± 2.0	21.2
Duration (msec)	27.1 ± 5.1	37.2
Amplitude (µV)	1308 ± 872	100[a]

[a]Low normal range.

Figure 17.26. The T-reflex latency (femoral nerve) on the rectus femoris and height (cm).

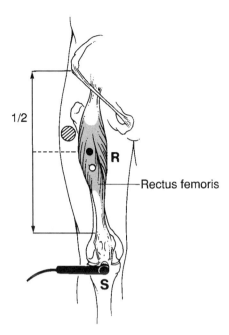

Figure 17.25.   Method for the T-reflex on the rectus femoris muscle.

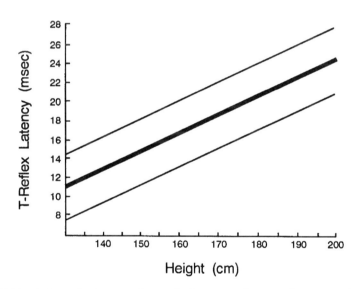

Figure 17.26.   Relationship between the T-reflex latency on the rectus femoris muscle and height.

COMMENTS: Latency was well correlated with the height and thigh length: Latency = −2.55 + (0.12 × height [cm]). 2 SD = 3.12. Latency = 4.19 + (0.28 × thigh length [cm]). 2 SD = 3.52.

Biceps (Musculocutaneous Nerve) and Triceps (Radial) T-Reflexes

Koenig described a technique for obtaining the T-reflex response from the biceps and triceps muscles (Figs. 17.27 and 17.28) (45).

POSITION OF SUBJECT: The subject sits relaxed on a chair with the hands resting on each thigh. Elbows are flexed at an ankle of about 130°. Muscle relaxation is controlled electroacoustically via surface electrodes.

RECORDING: Active surface recording electrodes are placed on the belly of the biceps and the belly of the lateral head of the triceps muscles, respectively. A reference electrode is placed on the acromion.

Figure 17.27. Method for the T-reflex on the biceps muscle.

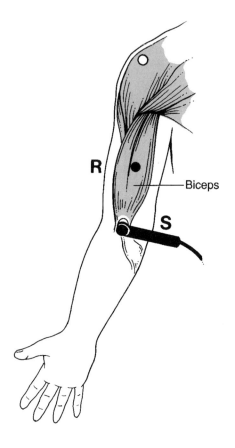

Figure 17.28. Method for the T-reflex on the triceps muscle.

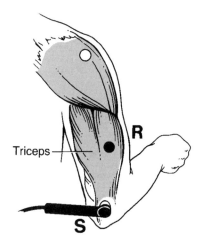

STIMULATION: The examiner then rests his thumb lightly on the tendon of the muscle and elicits the reflex response by a tap with an electronic T-reflex hammer. Ten responses are recorded and the force of the taps is increased until maximum amplitude is reached.

MEASUREMENT: Latency is measured following the conventional method. Maximum amplitude is used.

TEMPERATURE: Not controlled.

NORMAL DATA: Number of subjects: 31. Age range: 20–82 yr.

Measurement	Biceps tendon reflex		Triceps tendon reflex	
	Mean ± SD	Normal limit	Mean ± SD	Normal limit
Latency (msec)	11.4 ± 1.4	14.2	10.7 ± 1.0	12.7
Side-difference (msec)	0.7 ± 0.5	1.7	0.7 ± 0.6	1.9
Amplitude				
Side-difference (%)	0–50	20	5–75	37

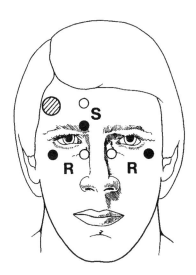

Figure 17.29. Kimura's method of the blink reflex test.

INTERPRETATION: Koenig defined the abnormality as follows: side-difference of latency > 2 msec and side difference of maximum amplitude > 50% in the biceps tendon reflex, and > 75% in the triceps reflex.

COMMENTS: Latencies of the T-reflex response correlated with the upper arm length (C7 to olecranon) in the biceps muscle but not in the triceps muscle. No correlation was found with age. Using the aforementioned criteria of abnormality, he found an abnormal T-reflex latency in 10 (66%) and amplitude reduction in nine (60%) of 15 patients with unilateral C6 or C7 radiculopathy. Overall, the T-reflex response was abnormal in 11 (73%) patients.

Blink Reflex

Stimulation of the supraorbital nerve produces the blink reflex, which consists of two components: an early R1 and a late R2. The R1 component is elicited unilaterally on the side of stimulation and the R2 component bilaterally with unilateral stimulation. Kimura's method (61) is described here (Fig. 17.29).

RECORDING: A two-channel recording is needed to obtain responses from both orbicularis oculi muscles. The active surface electrode is placed on the belly of the orbicularis oculi below the lateral canthus. The reference electrode is placed on the side of the nose or on the temple. Because the R2 latency is normally around 30 msec, the sweep velocity should be at least 5 msec per division.

STIMULATION: The supraorbital nerve, which is in the groove at the medial third of the superior orbit, is stimulated with the active surface electrode. The intensity is increased slowly to a level above which the evoked potential remains constant.

MEASUREMENT: Latency is measured from the stimulus onset to the shortest initial deflection of the eight R1 or R2 components. Amplitude is not important.

TEMPERATURE: Not controlled.

NORMAL DATA: Number of subjects: 30. Age range: 7–67 yr.

Measurement	Mean ± SD	Normal limit
R1 component (msec)	10.6 ± 0.8	12.2
Ipsilateral R2 (msec)	31.3 ± 3.3	37.9
Contralateral R2 (msec)	31.6 ± 3.8	39.2

The difference between R1 latencies on each side is 1.2 msec.

The difference between R2 latencies on each side is 5.0 msec.

INTERPRETATION: The afferent arc of the blink reflex is provided by sensory fibers of the trigeminal nerve, whereas the efferent arc is provided by the facial nerve. Thus, a prolonged latency or the absence of the R1 and R2 responses on the ipsilateral side and of the R2 on the contralateral side suggests a lesion of the afferent arc, in the ipsilateral trigeminal nerve (Fig. 17.5). On the other hand, unilateral delay in the latency or absence of the R1 and R2 responses, regardless of the side of stimulation, suggests a lesion of the efferent arc, the facial nerve.

COMMENTS: In general, the latency measurement of R2 is not as useful as that of R1 because of the wider range of variability. The R2 component, which correlates with eyelid blinking, habituates quickly with repetitive stimulation.

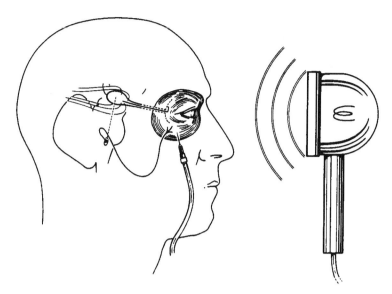

Figure 17.30. Light stimulus-evoked blink reflex. (From Brown W. The physiological and technical basis of electromyography. Boston: Butterworth, 1984:447.)

Light Stimulus-Evoked Blink Reflex

Yates and Brown described a technique of recording the blink reflex using stroscopic light stimuli (Fig. 17.30) (114).

POSITION OF SUBJECT: Patients are tested in the supine position and look downward at an angle of 15–20° to eliminate background EMG activity in the orbicularis oculi muscle. All tests are carried out in a room that is dark except for the low background illumination provided by the test instrumentation. Subjects are given 5 min to adapt to darkness.

RECORDING: The blink response is recorded with concentric needle electrodes inserted into the inferior-lateral quadrant of the orbicularis oculi. At least 10 responses are obtained.

STIMULATION: A Grass PS 22 Photic Stimulator is employed. The light intensity is fixed at ×16. The lamp is located 200 mm in front of the eyes, and the lamp parabola at right angles to the eyeball axis. Light stimuli are delivered at random intervals (smallest interval, 3 sec). Light stimuli are delivered to both eyes together, or to the right and left eyes independently, with the other eye covered by an eye patch.

MEASUREMENT: Latency is measured to the earliest EMG discharges of both orbicularis oculi muscles.

TEMPERATURE: Not controlled.

NORMAL DATA: Number of subjects: 22. Age range: 19–50 yr.

Measurement	Mean ± SD	Normal limit[a]
Right and left eye stimulation		
Right eye recording (msec)	50.8 ± 4.5	64.3
Left eye recording (msec)	50.6 ± 4.7	64.7
Right eye stimulation		
Right eye recording (msec)	51.7 ± 4.0	63.7
Left eye recording (msec)	51.4 ± 4.0	63.4
Left eye stimulation		
Right eye recording (msec)	50.8 ± 4.1	63.1
Left eye recording (msec)	51.0 ± 4.0	63.0

[a]Mean + 3 SD.

INTERPRETATION: The latency is abnormal if the value is above the 3 SD from the normal mean for controls.

COMMENTS: The light-evoked blink reflex was present in all controls, but habituation was observed if the stimuli were delivered at fixed intervals. In some controls, inter-stimulus periods of up to 15 sec were required to prevent habituation (114). No significant difference was observed in the latency of the right or left orbicularis oculi responses to bilateral or unilateral eye stimulation.

Corneal Reflex

Ongerboer de Visser et al. described a technique of recording the corneal reflex using a specially designed metal sphere (115).

RECORDING: The reflex response is recorded from the orbicularis oculi muscle with active surface electrodes over both lower eyelids and with reference electrodes on each side of the nasal bone.

STIMULATION: A metal sphere (2 mm in diameter) is used as a stimulator. Successive manual applications of the metal sphere to the cornea or sclera inside a 2-mm zone around the limbus evokes the corneal reflex. At the moment of touch, contact is established between the subject and an electronic circuit, causing a shift in the electrical potential and producing a trigger pulse in the pulse generator.

MEASUREMENT: The latency of the R2 response is measured from the stimulus onset to the initial deflection of the evoked responses. Two or more responses are superimposed.

TEMPERATURE: Not controlled.

NORMAL DATA: Number of subjects: 32. Age range: 10–82 yr.

Measurement	Mean ± SD	Normal limit	Number of subjects
10–40 yr			
Direct (msec)	44.3 ± 3.9	52.1	12
Consensual (msec)	44.8 ± 3.9	52.6	12
41–60 yr			
Direct (msec)	46.6 ± 7.4	61.4	10
Consensual (msec)	47.4 ± 7.6	62.4	10
61–80 yr			
Direct (msec)	51.4 ± 6.0	63.4	10
Consensual (msec)	51.7 ± 6.0	63.7	10

INTERPRETATION: There was a wide range of normal values among normal controls, ranging from 36–64 msec. Thus, an interindividual comparison was of little practical value. However, a comparison of R2 response latencies in a single subject was found to be of great value. A difference of 10 msec or more in the latencies of direct and consensual R2 responses between right and left corneal stimuli was regarded as abnormal, demonstrating an afferent delay. A delay difference of 8 msec or more between the direct and consensual R2 responses was considered as abnormal, demonstrating an efferent delay.

COMMENTS: Ongerboer de Visser concluded that the lower postcentral region had an excitatory influence upon interneurons of the lateral reticular formation of the lower brainstem mediating the trigeminofacial connections of the corneal reflex (116).

Masseter Reflex (Jaw Jerk)

Ongerboer de Visser and Goor's Method

Ongerboer de Visser and Goor described a technique of recording the masseter reflex with surface electrodes (Fig. 17.31) (68).

RECORDING: The reflex responses are recorded with active surface electrodes on the

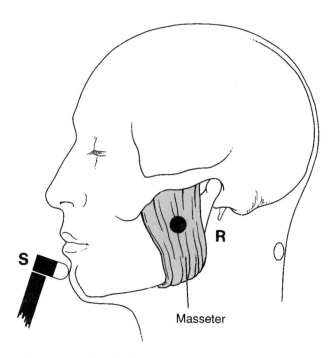

Figure 17.31. Ongerboer de Visser and Goor's method for the masseter reflex.

belly of both masseter muscles and a reference surface electrode on the neck. Two or more recordings are superimposed.

STIMULATION: The examiner's finger is placed on the subject's chin and tapped with an electronic T-reflex hammer.

MEASUREMENT: Latency is measured from the stimulus onset to the initial deflection of the reflex response.

TEMPERATURE: Skin temperature is not controlled.

NORMAL DATA: Number of subjects: 51. Age range: 20–80 yr.

Age group (yr)	Mean	Normal range	Number of subjects
20–30	7.0	6.4–7.8	9
31–40	7.0	6.4–8.0	7
41–50	7.4	6.6–9.2	10
51–60	7.8	6.4–9.2	10
61–70	8.4	8.4–8.4	6
71–80[a]	7.8	7.2–8.6	4

[a]Bilateral absent masseter reflex in five of nine subjects in this age group.

INTERPRETATION: Persistent unilateral absence of reflexes, a difference of more than 0.5 msec between the latencies in the two sides, and bilateral absence of the reflex up to the age of about 70 yr, are considered to be abnormal findings.

COMMENTS: McIntyre and Robinson showed that the masseter reflex is monosynaptic through the motor root of the trigeminal nerve (83).

Yates and Brown's Method

Yates and Brown described a technique of recording the masseter reflex with a concentric needle (84) (Fig. 17.32).

RECORDING: The reflex response is recorded with concentric needles from both masseter muscles.

STIMULATION: The subject's chin is tapped with an electronic hammer. The taps are delivered with the jaw partially open.

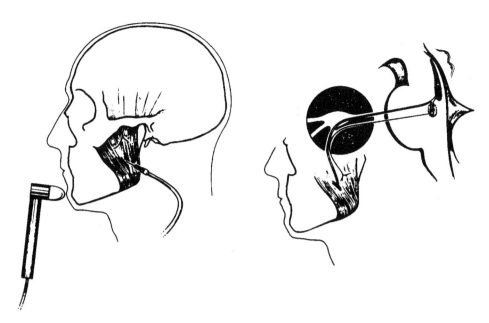

Figure 17.32. Yates and Brown's method for the masseter reflex (jaw jerk). On the right is the reflex pathway. The cell bodies of the primary afferents of the spindle receptors in the masseter are located in the mesencephalic nucleus of the midbrain, and these neurons are monosynaptically connected to the trigeminal motor neurons in the pons. (From Brown W. The physiological and technical basis of electromyography. Boston: Butterworth, 1984:430.)

MEASUREMENT: Latency is measured from the stimulus onset to the initial deflection of reflex response.

TEMPERATURE: Skin temperature is not controlled.

NORMAL DATA: Number of subjects: 22. Age range: 15–69 yr.

Measurement	Mean ± SD	Normal limit
Latency (msec)	8.7 ± 1.0	10.7
Difference between sides (msec)	0.1 ± 0.2	0.5

COMMENTS: Yates and Brown stated that the measurement of the jaw jerk was both simple to carry out and required a little extra time to test (79). In cases of definite multiple sclerosis, the most common abnormality was lack of reflex response on one side in 15% of cases or on both sides in 15%. In 10% of cases, the latency was longer than the longest control.

Sacral Reflexes

Bulbocavernosus Reflex

Tackmann et al.'s Method

Tackmann et al. described a method of BC reflex in males with recording electrodes in each side of the BC muscle (Fig. 17.33) (103). *In our laboratory this method is used for males with a concentric needle in the middle of the BC muscle* (Fig. 17.34).

EMG MACHINE SET-UP: Filter: 200 Hz–3kHz.

RECORDING: Two concentric needles are inserted into each side of the BC muscles. Ten consecutive responses were recorded.

STIMULATION: Stimulating ring electrodes are used with the reference electrode at the corona glandis and the cathode 2 cm proximal to the anode. Stimulus duration is 0.2 msec. Stimulus intensity is 6–8 times higher than the sensory threshold, ranging from 7–16 mA. Stimulation is given at random intervals of 40–60 sec.

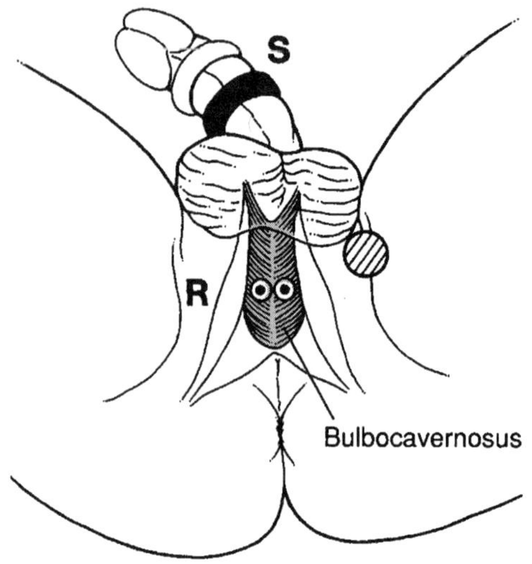

Figure 17.33. Tackmann's method for the bulbocavernosus reflex in males.

Figure 17.34. Method for the bulbocavernosus reflex in males.

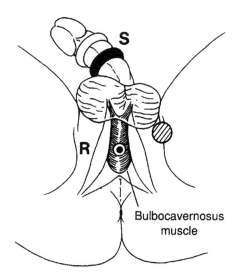

Bulbocavernosus

Bulbocavernosus muscle

MEASUREMENT: The latency of each response is measured following the conventional method. The minimal latency is the shortest latency among the 10 latencies from the right and left BC muscles and the maximal latency, the longest latency among 10 latencies. "Temporal dispersion" is the difference between the minimal and maximal latencies. The difference between the minimal and maximal latencies on each side is also measured.

NORMAL DATA: Number of subjects: 39 males. Age range: 17–69 yr.

Measurement	Mean ± SD	Range	Normal limit
Minimal latency (msec)	31.4 ± 3.4	22–38	38.2
Maximal latency (msec)	34.6 ± 4.7	24–48	44.0
Mean latency (msec)	32.7 ± 3.8	23–39	40.3
"Temporal dispersion"		0–10	
Side difference in minimal latency		0–2	2.0
Side difference in maximal latency		0–5	5.0

COMMENTS: BC reflex responses consisted of two components, the second of which was found to be rather variable in latency and amplitude. Therefore, only the first response was evaluated. Usually, the absence of reflex or prolonged minimal latency were used as criteria of abnormality. However, Tackmann et al. also advocated the use of other minor criteria in judging the reflex as abnormal; abnormality was found in 50% of 130 cases with erectile dysfunction (103).

Bilkey et al.'s Method

Bilkey et al. described a method of the BC (pudendourethro or anal) reflex using a monopolar needle recording in the urethral or anal external sphincter muscles in male and female subjects (98). *In our laboratory we prefer this method for the bulbocavernosus reflex in females with the concentric needle in the EAS and the BC muscles.*

RECORDING: The monopolar needle electrode is used as an active recording electrode.

For the external urethral sphincter (EUS) muscle, the needle is inserted via the vagina or perineum following Chantraine's method (117). The position is different for male and female patients. For the male, the subject lies prone with the legs slightly apart (Fig. 17.35). The examiner palpates the prostate with a finger in the rectum, and the needle (6.5-cm needle) is inserted through the floor of the perineum 2 or 3 cm in front of the anus at the midline. A slight resistance is felt at the moment when the needle penetrates the sphincter, coinciding with the appearance of EMG activity on the oscilloscope. For the female, the lithotomy position is considered to be the best. The EUS muscle is only a short distance from the urethral meatus, and identifying it is no problem. It is simple to pass the needle (37-mm gauge) into the sphincter along the ventral wall lateral or dorsal to the urethra, which is about 1 cm from the mucous membrane (Fig. 17.36).

For the EAS muscle, the needle is inserted diagonally 2–3 cm lateral to the anus toward the midline to a depth of 3–5 cm until electromyographic activity is encountered (Fig. 17.35). Jesel et al. inserted the needle on any side of the anal sphincter about 1–1.5 cm from the center (114). A reference surface electrode is placed on the medial aspect of the thigh close to the needle. Four recordings are made in the raster mode.

STIMULATION: A two-prong stimulating electrode is applied to the glans penis or clitoris with the cathode in the proximal position (Fig. 17.37). A stimulus duration of 0.2 msec is used with gradually increasing intensity until a consistent reflex response is

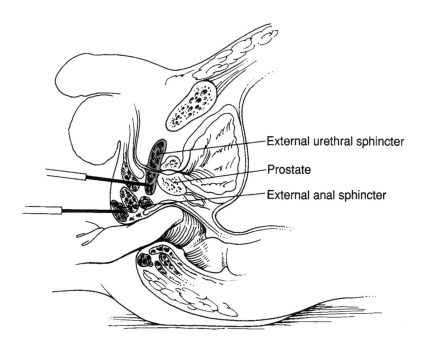

Figure 17.35. Needle EMG insertion into the external urethral sphincter and anal sphincter in males.

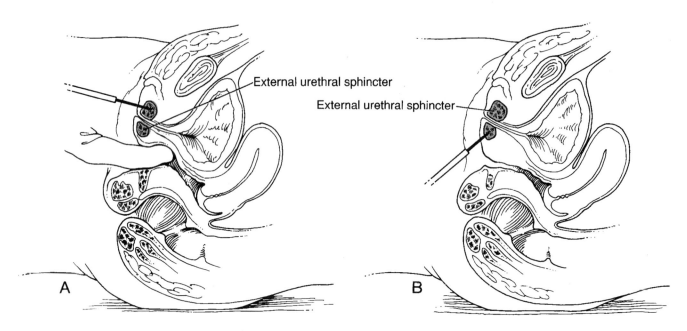

Figure 17.36. Needle EMG insertion into the external urethral sphincters for females through the (**A**) nonvaginal and (**B**) vaginal routes.

noted on the oscilloscope. In women, the stimulating and recording electrodes are so close that a lower stimulus intensity (½ or ⅓ that in men) is required.

MEASUREMENT: Latency is measured following the conventional method.

NORMAL DATA: Number of subjects: 108. Age: 16–98 yr.

Measurements	Mean ± SD	Normal limit
External urethral sphincter		
Males[a]	34.6 ± 5.2	45.0
<40 yr	31.7 ± 3.3	38.3
40–60 yr	32.4 ± 2.7	37.8
>60 yr	39.0 ± 4.5	48.2
Females[a]	37.4 ± 5.5	48.4
>40 yr	33.8 ± 5.8	45.4
40–60 yr	39.0 ± 5.0	49.0
>60 yr	39.0 ± 4.8	48.6
External anal sphincter		
Males[a]	36.0 ± 5.2	47.4
<40 yr	35.4 ± 6.8	49.0
40–60 yr	33.4 ± 3.1	39.6
>60 yr	39.9 ± 5.9	51.7
Females[a]	38.6 ± 4.0	46.6
<40 yr	35.7 ± 2.9	41.5
40–60 yr	38.8 ± 4.6	48.0
>60 yr	40.9 ± 2.5	45.9

[a]The number of male or female subjects is not specified.

COMMENTS: In older subjects, the latency was increased. In 44 patients with upper motor neuron lesions, a significantly shorter latency was found. This was in contrast to the normal mean reflex latency found in such patients by Ertekin and Reel (97). Bilkey claimed that decreased latency resulted from the loss of the inhibitory influence of the higher neural centers on the BC reflex and from increased excitability of the motor neurons at the level of S1–S4.

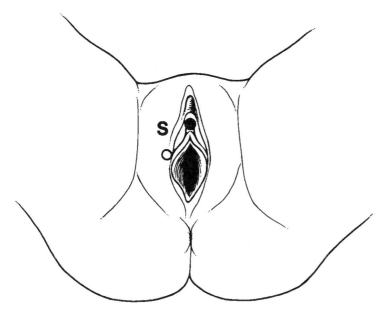

Figure 17.37. Stimulation of the dorsal cutaneous nerve of the clitoris with bipolar surface electrode.

Ertekin and Reel's Method

Ertekin and Reel described a technique of BC reflex in males with recording electrodes in the BC and EAS muscles (Fig. 17.34) (97).

RECORDING: A concentric needle is used as the recording electrode in the BC and EAS muscles. The BC muscle is easily reached behind the scrotum, near the midline in the perianal region. To facilitate location of this muscle, *the patient is asked to cough gently or to attempt to erect the penis, or the glans penis is squeezed slightly by the examiner.* Both procedures clearly produce the MUP response. In the resting position, the BC muscle is completely silent. The EAS muscle is even easier to locate and when the needle is introduced into the sphincter, abrupt and continuous tonic EMG activity appears. Ten to 20 responses are superimposed.

STIMULATION: Velcro "ring" electrodes are placed on the glans penis. Stimulus duration was 0.1–0.2 msec. When the stimulus intensity is increased two to four times above the sensory threshold, a reflex response appears in the BC muscle. A stimulus intensity 1.5–2.5 times stronger than the reflex threshold produces stable and constant responses.

MEASUREMENT: Latency is measured following the conventional method.

NORMAL DATA: Number of subjects: 14. Age range: 16–56 yr.

Measurement	Mean ± SD	Normal limit
Latency to BC muscle	36.1 ± 4.6	38.5

COMMENTS: The reflex response had the shape of either a single motor unit response or a polyphasic response with a few units firing together. In four of 14 normal cases, the reflex consisted of double components, as seen in other flexor polysynaptic reflexes. Stimulation of the glans penis did not constantly evoke a reflex response from the EAS muscle, and only 21% of cases showed such a reflex response.

Vodusek et al.'s Method

Vodusek et al. described a technique for the BC reflex in male and female subjects with recording electrodes in three pelvic floor muscles (119).

RECORDING: Concentric needles are inserted into the BC muscle, the EAS, and the anal sphincter following Jesel et al.'s method (118). Male subjects are placed in the supine position with legs flexed, and a needle electrode is inserted at the midline of the perineum at a point midway between the anal orifice and the bulb of the corpus spongiosum (Fig. 17.35). Location of the urethral sphincter is aided by insertion of the index finger into the rectum, which enables the examiner to feel the median lobe of the prostate gland where the sphincter lies. Guidance is also obtained from the MUPs recorded on insertion of a needle into the sphincter muscles. In females, a needle is inserted through the vaginal route around the urethral meatus to a depth of 15 mm. Local mucosal anesthesia by xylocaine gel may facilitate the examination (Fig. 17.36). Usually, 128 (less frequently up to 256) responses are averaged.

STIMULATION: A bipolar surface electrode is used to stimulate the penis or clitoris. The electrodes are applied to the dorsal aspect of the penis with the reference lying at the base of the glans and the active electrode proximal to the reference. Stimulus duration used is 0.2 msec. Stimulation is given at the rate of 0.2–5 Hz, or randomly. For female subjects, Vodusek recommended the use of ear-clip EEG electrodes (e.g., Nihon-Koden BE301A) as stimulating electrodes (Fig. 19.18) (89). An active electrode is placed over the clitoris and its perputium, and a reference electrode on the labia majora or minora. Contact is assured by using electrode gel, and care is taken that there is no hair between the electrode and skin/mucosa. Stimulus duration is 0.3 msec. Stimulus intensity is four times the sensory threshold.

MEASUREMENT: The response with the shortest latency is accepted. Latency is measured following the conventional method.

TEMPERATURE: Not controlled.

NORMAL DATA: Number of subjects: 82 males; 9 females. Age range 5–72 yr. for males; 18–55 yr for females.

Measurement	Mean ± SD	Normal limit	Number of subjects
External anal sphincter			
Males	35.2 ± 4.6	44.4	14
External urethral sphincter			
Males	33.0 ± 3.9	40.8	14
Females	33.6 ± 3.5	40.6	8
Bulbocavernosus			
Males	32.3 ± 3.9	40.1	60

COMMENTS: With ear-clip electrodes on the clitoris, the threshold for the reflex was between 4–12 mA (94). The responses must be averaged at a sensitivity of 10 or 20 μV. The BC reflex was absent in three of 10 women. Vodusek et al. believed that this may have been because of their reluctance to use strong stimuli. Thus, it is their practice to record the reflex response with a single stimulus of higher intensity.

Varma et al.'s Method

Varma et al. described a method of BC or pudendoanal reflex test using a noninvasive anal plug electrode in male and female subjects (Fig. 17.38) (85).

EMG MACHINE SET-UP: Filter: 2 Hz–10 kHz. Sensitivity: 10 or 20 μV. Sweep velocity: 10 msec. Stimulus duration: 0.1 msec.

RECORDING: The response is recorded with a bipolar surface stainless-steel anal plug electrode—Dantec 13K78 (Dantec Medical, Inc., Santa Clara, CA). Electrode gel is used to improve electrical contact between the plug electrode and the sphincter. This anal plug electrode can be easily replaced by a disposable sphincter electrode (Dantec 13L81). More than 100 responses are averaged.

STIMULATION: The dorsal nerve of the glans or clitoris is stimulated with a felt bipolar surface stimulating electrode (Fig. 17.37). Stimulus intensity is approximately three times the intensity of the sensory threshold. Stimulus duration is 0.2 msec, and stimulation rate is 2/sec.

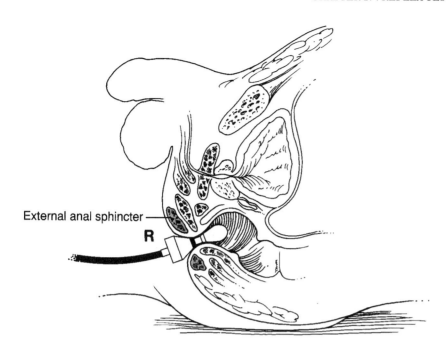

External anal sphincter

R

Figure 17.38. An anal plug electrode (Dantec 13K78) as the recording electrode for the bulbocavernosus reflex. This anal plug electrode can easily be replaced by a disposable sphincter electrode (Dantec 13L81).

MEASUREMENT: Latency is measured from the stimulus artifact to the clearly defined reflex response at the EAS.

NORMAL DATA: Number of subjects: 25 females, 13 males. Age: 23–75 yr.

Measurements	Mean ± SD	Normal limit
Latency (msec)	38.5 ± 5.8	50.1
Amplitude (µV)	4.5 ± 5.4	
Duration (msec)	16.9 ± 7.0	

Galloway et al.'s Method

Galloway et al. described a method of the BC reflex in males and females with recording electrodes in the EAS and on the internal urethral sphincter muscles (120).

EMG MACHINE SET-UP: The sensitivity should be 2–5 µV, since the amplitude of response is less than 5 µV.

RECORDING: For the urethral sphincter recording, a urethral ring electrode (Dantec 21L11) is mounted in a 14F Foley catheter 1 cm below the balloon for females (Fig. 17.39) and 2.5 cm below, depending on the length of the prostatic urethra, in men. A catheter with its electrode is then placed after anesthesia and the balloon inflated. It is gently withdrawn until the balloon is at the internal meatus and the bladder is drained. For the EAS recording, a plug electrode is passed into the anal canal (Fig. 17.38). The response is averaged 120 times.

STIMULATION: A bipolar surface stimulator is placed on the dorsum of the base of the penis for males and at the clitoris for females in the midline overlying the dorsal nerve. Using a stimulus of 0.1 msec duration and a frequency of 2/sec, a stimulus intensity three times the sensory threshold is used for the stimulation.

MEASUREMENT: The latency is measured to the peak of response. The amplitude is measured from peak to peak.

NORMAL DATA: Number of subjects: 18. Age range: not given.

Measurement	Mean ± SD	Normal limit
Latency	38 ± 4	42

COMMENTS: Extremely small (<5 μV) responses were recorded even in normal subjects. If no anal response was noted, it was essential to check the electrical contacts and confirm that the anal electrode had not been displaced (120). Excessive lubrication of the anal plug, a very lax anal canal, or gross obesity contributed to poor contact and gave a false-negative response. If no urethral response was found, the resting EMG pattern was measured and a slight change in position of the electrode was made to enhance the signal.

Dykstra et al.'s Method

Dykstra et al. described a technique for a mechanical BC reflex using a specially designed mechanical "microswitch" hammer in male and female subjects (121).

POSITION OF SUBJECT: Subjects are placed in the dorsal lithotomy position.

RECORDING: A monopolar needle electrode is inserted into the external urethral sphincter via the vagina or perineum.

STIMULATION: A specially designed hammer is used, consisting of a microswitch mounted at the end of a 20-cm tube. The microswitch is connected to the external trigger of the EMG machine to trigger the EMG oscilloscope. Activation of the microswitch is accomplished by tapping the penis or clitoris.

To evoke the mechanical response in male patients, the examiner holds the penis loosely and taps the midline dorsal shaft briskly so that a reflex response is observed on the oscilloscope. The penis is tapped every 2 sec. To evoke a mechanical response in the female patient, the labia are spread gently and the midline dorsal shaft of the clitoris is tapped briskly.

MEASUREMENT: Latency is measured following the conventional method.

TEMPERATURE: Not controlled.

NORMAL DATA: Number of subjects: 18. Age range: Not given.

Measurement	Mean ± SD	Normal limit
Latency	39.1 ± 4.0	47.1

COMMENTS: The electrical reflex latency was shorter than the mechanical reflex latency, the latency with the mechanical hammer was longer: mean difference as 3.9 msec. This difference was significant.

Vesicourethral or Vesicoanal Reflex

This reflex is induced by stimulating the internal urethral sphincter area and recording the response in the external anal sphincter.

Galloway et al.'s Method

Galloway et al. described a method of the vesicoanal reflex using a catheter mounted ring electrode as a stimulating electrode and a bipolar hourglass plug as a recording electrode (Figs. 17.38 and 17.39) (120).

RECORDING: An anal plug recording electrode in the anal canal, as described for the BC reflex.

STIMULATION: A urethral ring electrode (Dantec 21L11), which is used as a recording electrode for the reflex, is used for stimulation. The stimulus intensity is three times the sensory threshold of the urethra.

MEASUREMENT: Latency is measured from the peak to peak.

TEMPERATURE: Not controlled.

NORMAL DATA: Number of subjects: Not given. Age range: Not given.

Measurement	Mean ± SD	Normal limit	Number of subjects
Latency	65 ± 10	85	

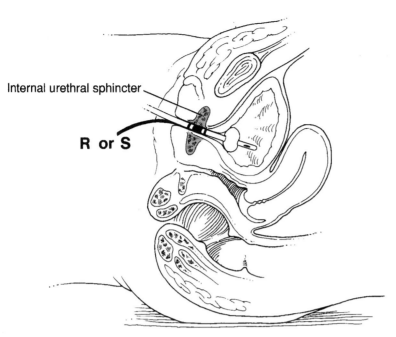

Internal urethral sphincter

R or S

Figure 17.39. Urethral ring electrode as the stimulating electrode for the internal urethral sphincter muscle.

COMMENTS: The reflex latency following stimulation of the bladder mucosa or bladder neck was significantly longer compared with that of the BC reflex. Sarica and Karacan proposed that this is because the innervation of this region is provided by the pelvic and hypogastric nerves, which are small myelinated or unmyelinated fibers (122). Vereecken et al. suggested that the more highly polysynaptic pathway of the reflexes may also contribute to the longer latency (123).

Desai et al.'s Method

Desai et al. described a method of the vesicoanal reflex using a catheter-mounted ring electrode as a stimulating electrode and a bipolar hourglass plug as a recording electrode (Figs. 17.38 and 17.39) (124).

EMG MACHINE SET-UP: Filter frequency: 5 Hz–2 kHz. Signal averaging: 56–200 averagings. Analysis time: 200 msec. Stimulus intensity: Two to three times the sensory threshold. Sensitivity: 5 µV.

RECORDING: The EAS response is recorded with a bipolar hourglass plug electrode (Dantec 13K78).

STIMULATION: A 14F catheter-mounted ring electrode (Dantec 21L11), positioned 2.5 cm below the balloon so as to lie in opposition to the external sphincter, is used as a stimulating electrode. The catheter is lubricated with a 50% mixture of sterile KY jelly and normal saline.

MEASUREMENT: Latency to the first peak (P1) is measured following the conventional method.

TEMPERATURE: Not controlled.

NORMAL DATA: Number of subjects: 19 males. Age range: 22–62 yr.

Measurement	Mean ± SD	Normal limit
Latency to P1 peak (msec)	69.6 ± 8.8	87.2

COMMENTS: Desai et al. found prolonged latency in two and absent response in six of 17 patients with impotence due to diabetic neuropathy and thus concluded that this test was not a reliable indicator of neuropathy.

Anal Sphincter Response

The anal reflex is the reflex contraction of the anal sphincter, which can be elicited by pricking the anal mucosa or scratching the perianal skin.

Vodusek et al.'s Method

Vodusek et al. described a method of anal sphincter response (119).

RECORDING: A concentric needle is inserted into the external anal sphincter following the standard percutaneous approach (Fig. 17.35).

STIMULATION: The perineal region about 2 cm anteriorly to the anal aperture is stimulated with surface electrodes. Stimulus intensity usually has to be stronger than for the BC reflex.

MEASUREMENT: The response with the shortest latency is accepted. Latency is measured to the first deflection of the response from the baseline.

TEMPERATURE: Not controlled.

NORMAL DATA: Number of subjects: 29. Age range: Not given.

Measurement	Mean ± SD	Normal limit
Early response (R1)	4.9 ± 1.1	7.1
Intermediate (R2)	13.2 ± 0.8	14.8
Late (R4)	56.0 ± 8.5	73.0

COMMENTS: Authors stated that the early response could usually be elicited in the EAS with perineal or perianal stimulation. Applying this technique to two patients with myelomeningocele who had no sensation in the perineal area as well as signs of partial denervation in the pelvic floor muscle, authors were able to detect a small amplitude R1 and no R3 (BC reflex) or R4 in the EAS.

REFERENCES

1. Hoffmann P. Über die Beziehungen der Sehnenreflexe zur Willkurlichen Bewegung und zum Tonus. Zeitschrift für Biologie (München) 1918;68:351–370.
2. Verhagen WIM, Schrooten GJM, Schiphof PR, Van Ammers V: The H-reflex of the medial vastus muscle: a study in controls and patients with radiculopathy. EMG Clin Neurophysiol 1988;28:421–425.
3. Cruz Martinez A, Perez Conde MC, Ferrer MT. Motor conduction velocity and H-reflex in infancy and childhood. I. Study in newborns, twins and small-for-dates. EMG Clin Neurophysiol 1977;17:492–505.
4. Hugon M. Methodology of the Hoffman reflex in man. In JE Desmedt, ed. New developments in EMG and clinical neurophysiology. Basel: Karger, 1973;3:277–293.
5. Panizza M, Nilsson J, Hallett M. Optimal stimulus duration for the H reflex. Muscle Nerve 1989;12:576–579.
6. Milner Brown HS, Stein RB, Yemm R. The contractile properties of human motor units during voluntary isometric contraction. J Physiol (London) 1973;228:285–306.
7. Hodes R. Effects of age, consciousness, and other factors on human electrically induced reflexes (EIRs). EEG Clin Neurophysiol 1967;Supp 25:80–91.
8. Tavborikova H, Sax DS. Conditioning of H-reflexes by preceding subthreshold H-reflex stimulus. Brain 1969;92:203–212.
9. Kameyama O, Hayes KC, Wolfe D. Methodological considerations contributing to variability of the quadriceps H-reflex. Am J Phys Med Rehabil 1989;68:277–282.
10. Verrier MC. Alterations in H reflex magnitude by variations in baseline EMG excitability. EEG Clin Neurophysiol 1985;60:492–499.
11. Landau WM, Clare MH. Fusimotor function. Part 4. Reinforcement of the H-reflex in normal subjects. Archives Neurology 1964;10:117–122.
12. Schimsheimer RJ, Ongerboer De Visser BW, Kemp B, Bour LJ. The flexor carpi radialis H-reflex in polyneuropathy: relations to conduction velocities of the median nerve and the soleus H-reflex latency. J Neurol Neurosurg Psychiatry 1987;50:447–452.
13. Lachman T, Shahani BT, Young RR. Late responses as aids to diagnosis in peripheral neuropathy. J Neurol Neurosurg Psychiatry 1980;43:156–162.
14. Oh SJ. Clinical electromyography: nerve conduction studies. Baltimore: University Park Press, 1984.
15. Braddom RI, Johnson EW. Standardization of H reflex and diagnostic use in S1 radiculopathy. Arch Phys Med Rehabil 1974;55:161–166.
16. Schimsheimer RJ, Ongerboer De Visser BW, Kemp B: The flexor carpi radialis H-reflex in lesions of the sixth and seventh cervical nerve roots. J Neurol Neurosurg Psychiatry 1985;48:445–449.
17. Bell KR, Lehmann JF. Effect of cooling on H- and T-reflexes in normal subjects. Arch Phys Med Rehabil 1987;68:490–493.
18. Halar EM, DeLisa JA, Brozovich FV. Nerve conduction velocity: relationship of skin, subcutaneous and intramuscular temperature. Arch Phys Med Rehabil 1980;61:199–203.
19. Jabre JF. Surface recording of the H-reflex of the flexor carpi radialis. Muscle Nerve 1981;4:435–438.

20. Dhand UK, Das SK, Chopra JS. Patterns of H-reflex abnormality in patients with low back pain. EMG Clin Neurophysiol 1991;31:209–213.
21. Aiello I, Rosati G, Serra G, Manca M. The diagnostic value of H-index in S1 root compression. J Neurol Neurosurg Psychiatry 1981;44:171–172.
22. Sabbahi MA, Kahlil M. Segmental H-reflex studies in upper and lower limbs of patients with radiculopathy. Arch Phys Med Rehabil 1990;71:223–227.
23. Schuchmann JA. H-reflex latency in radiculopathy. Arch Phys Med Rehabil 1978;59:185–187.
24. Rico RE, Jonkman EJ: Measurement of the Achilles tendon reflex for the diagnosis of lumbosacral root compression syndromes. J Neurol Neurosurg Psychiatry 1982;45:791–795.
25. Deschuytere J, De Keyser C, Rosselle N, Deschuytere M. Monosynaptic reflexes in the flexor carpi ulnaris muscle in man. EMG Clin Neurophysiol 1981;21:213–222.
26. Ongerboer de Visser BW, Schimsheimer RJ, Hart AAM. The H-reflex of the flexor carpi radialis muscle; a study in controls and radiation-induced brachial plexus lesion. J Neurol Neurosurg Psychiatry 1984;47:1098–1101.
27. Mayer RF. Nerve conduction studies in man. Neurology 1963;13:1021–1030.
28. Blackstock E, Rushwirth G, Guth D. Electrophysiological studies in alcoholism. J Neurol Neurosurg Psychiatry 1972;35:326–334.
29. Mawsley C, Mayer RF. Nerve conduction in alcoholic polyneuropathy. Brain 1965;88:335–356.
30. Guiheneuc P, Bathien N. Two patterns of results in polyneuropathies investigated with the H reflex. J Neurol Sci 1976;30:83–94.
31. Lefebvre d'Amour M, Shahani BT, Young RR, Bird KT. The importance of studying sural nerve conduction and late responses in the evaluation of alcoholic subjects. Neurology 1979;29:1600–1604.
32. Teasdall RO, Park AM, Languth HW, Magladery JW. Electrophysiological studies of reflex activity in patients with lesions of the nervous system. II. Bull Johns Hopkins Hosp 1959;91:245–256.
33. Norris FH. Adult spinal motor neuron disease. In: Vinken PJ, Bruyn GW, eds. Handbook of Clinical Neurology. Amsterdam: North Holland, 1975;22:1–56.
34. Miyasaki JM, Ashby P, Sharpe JA, Fletcher WA. On the cause of hyporeflexia in the Holmes-Adie syndrome. Neurology 1988;38:262–265.
35. Harriman DG, Garland H. The pathology of Adie's syndrome. Brain 1968;91:401–418.
36. Ulrich J. Morphological basis of Adie's syndrome. Eur Neurol 1980;19:390–395.
37. Donofrio P, Walker FO. Tabes dorsalis: electrodiagnostic features. J Neurol Neurosurg Psychiatry 1988;51:1097–1099.
38. Greenfield JG. Infectious diseases of the central nervous system. In: Blackwood W, McMenemey WH, Meyer A, Norman RM, Russel DS, eds. Greenfield's Neuropathology. 2nd ed. Baltimore: Williams & Wilkins, 1963;164–181.
39. Bishop B, Machover S, Honston R, Anderson M. A quantitative assessment of gamma-motor neuron contribution to the Achilles tendon reflex in normal subjects. Arch Phys Med Rehabil 1968;49:145–154.
40. Landau WM, Clare MH. Fusimotor function. Part IV. Reinforcement of the H-reflex in normal subjects. Arch Neurol 1964;10:117–122.
41. Dietrichson P, Sorbye R. Clinical method for electrical and mechanical recording of the mechanically and electrically elicited ankle reflex. Acta Neurol Scand 1971;47:1–21.
42. Koenig SK. T-wave response in cervical root lesions. Acta Neurol Scand 1991;84:273–276.
43. Kuruoglu R, Oh SJ. Tendon-reflex testing in chronic demyelinating neuropathy. Muscle Nerve 1992;15:1178–1179.
44. Malcolm DS. A method of measuring reflex times applied in sciatica and other conditions due to nerve-root compression. J Neurol Neurosurg Psychiatry 1951;14:15–24.
45. Koenig SK. T-wave response in cervical root lesions. Acta Neurol Scand 1991;84:273–276.
46. Weintraub JR, Madalin K. Wong M, Wilbourn AJ, Mahdaa M. Achilles tendon reflex and the H response: their correlation in 400 limbs. Muscle Nerve 1988;11:972.
47. Gassel MM, Ott KH. An electrophysiological study of the organization of innervation of the tendon jerk in humans. In: Desmedt JE, ed. New developments in EMG and clinical neurophysiology. Basel: Karger, 1973;3:308–316.
48. Stam J. The tibialis anterior reflex in healthy subjects and in L5 radicular compression. J Neurol Neurosurg Psychiatry 1988;51:397–402.
49. De Weerd AW, Joost Jonkman E. Measurement of knee tendon reflex latencies in lumbar radicular syndromes. Eur Neurol 1986;25:304–308.
50. Eisen AA, Woods JF, Sherwin AL. Peripheral nerve function in long-term therapy with diphenylhydantoin: a clinical and electrophysiologic correlation. Neurology 1974;24:411–417.
51. Shahani BT, Young RR. Human orbicularis reflexes. Neurology 1972;22:149–154.
52. Kugelberg E. Facial reflexes. Brain 1952;75:385–396.
53. Kaplan PE, Kaplan C. Blink reflex: review of methodology and its application to patients with stroke syndrome. Arch Phys Med Rehabil 1980;61:30–33.
54. Kimura J. Alteration of the orbicularis oculi reflex by pontine lesions: study in multiple sclerosis. Arch Neurol 1970;22:156–161.
55. Kimura J, Lyon LW. Orbicularis oculi reflex in the Wallenberg syndrome: alteration of the late reflex by lesions of the spinal tract and nucleus of the trigeminal nerve. J Neurol Neurosurg Psychiatry 1972;35:228–233.

56. Ongerboer de Visser BW, Kuypers HGJM. Late blink reflex changes in lateral medullary lesions.: an electrophysiological and neuro-anatomical study of Wallenberg's syndrome. Brain 1978;101:285–294.

57. Kimura J. The blink reflex as a test for brain-stem and higher central nervous system function. In Desmedt JE, ed. New Developments in EMG and Clinical Neurophysiology. Basel: Karger, 1973;3:682–691.

58. Ongerboer de Visser BW, Melchelse K, Megens PHA. Corneal reflex latency in trigeminal nerve lesions. Neurology 1977;27:1164–1167.

59. Gandiglio G, Fra L. Further observations on facial reflexes. J Neurol Sci 1967;5:272–285.

60. Penders CA, Delwaide PJ. Physiologic approach to the human blink reflex. In: Desdmedt JE, ed. New developments in electromyography and clinical neurophysiology. Basel: Karger, 1973;3:649–657.

61. Kimura J, Rodnitsky RL, Van Allen MW. Reflex response of orbicularis oculi muscle to supraorbital nerve stimulation: study in normal subjects and peripheral facial palsies. Arch Neurol 1969;21:193–199.

62. Fisher MA, Shahani BT, Young RR. Assessing segmental excitability after acute rostral lesions. II. The blink reflex. Neurology 1979;29:45–50.

63. Auger RG. Hemifacial spasm: clinical and electrophysiologic observations. Neurology 1979;29:1261–1272.

64. Eisen A, Danon J. The orbicularis oculi reflex in acoustic neuromas: a clinical and electrodiagnostic evaluation. Neurology 1974;24:306–311.

65. Ashworth B, Tait GBW. Trigeminal neuropathy in connective tissue disease. Neurology 1971;21:609–614.

66. Hess K, Kern S, Schiller H. Blink reflex in trigeminal sensory neuropathy. EMG Clin Neurophysiol 1984;24:185–190.

67. Lecky B, Hughes R, Murray N. Trigeminal sensory neuropathy. Brain 1987;110:1465–1485.

68. Ongerboer de Visser BW, Goor C. Electromyographic and reflex study in idiopathic and symptomatic trigeminal neuralgias: latency of the jaw and blink reflexes. J Neurol Neurosurg Psychiatry 1974;37:1225–1230.

69. Kimura J, Rodnitzky R, Van Allen M. Electrodiagnostic study of trigeminal nerve. Neurology 1970;20:574–583.

70. Kimura J, Giron LT Jr., Young SM. Electrophysiological study of Bell's palsy: electrically elicited blink reflex in assessment of prognosis. Arch Otolaryngol 1976;102:140–143.

71. Kimura J, Rodnitzky RL, Okawara SH. Electrophysiologic analysis of aberrant regeneration after facial nerve paralysis. Neurology 1975;25:989–993.

72. Nielsen VK. Pathophysiology of hemifacial spasm. I. Ephatic transmission and ectopic excitation. Neurology 1984;34:418–426.

73. Nielsen VK. Pathophysiology of hemifacial spasm. II. Lateral spread of the supraorbital nerve flex. Neurology 1984;34:427–431.

74. Nielsen VK. Electrophysiology of the facial nerve in hemifacial spasm: ectopic/ephatic excitation. Muscle Nerve 1985;8:545–555.

75. Jannetta PJ, Abbasy M, Maroon JC, Ramos FM, Albin MS. Etiology and definitive microsurgical treatment of hemifacial spasm: operative techniques and result in 47 patients. J Neurosurg 1977;47:321–328.

76. Auger RG, Piepgras DG, Laws ER, Miller RH. Microvascular decompression of the facial nerve for hemifacial spasm: clinical and electrophysiologic observations. Neurology 1981;31:346–350.

77. Kim P, Kukushima T. Observations on synkinesis in patients with hemifacial spasm. J Neurosurg 1984;60:821–827.

78. Nielsen VK, Jannetta PJ. Pathophysiology of hemifacial spasm: III. Effect of microsurgical decompression of the facial nerve. Neurology 1984;34:891–897.

79. Kimura J. Electrically elicited blink reflex in diagnosis of multiple sclerosis: review of 260 patients over a seven-year period. Brain 1975;8:413–426.

80. Lacquanti F, Benna P, Gilli M, et al. Brain stem auditory evoked potentials and blink reflex in quiescent multiple sclerosis. EEG Clin Neurophysiol 1979;47:607–610.

81. Khoshbin S, Hallett M. Multimodality evoked potentials and blink reflex in multiple sclerosis. Neurology 1981;31:138–144.

82. Kimura J. An evaluation of the facial and trigeminal nerves in polyneuropathy: electrodiagnostic study in Charcot-Marie-Tooth disease, Guillain-Barré syndrome, and diabetic neuropathy. Neurology 1971;21:745–752.

83. McIntyre AK, Robinson RG. Pathway for the jaw-jerk in man. Brain 1959;82:468–474.

84. Yates SK, Brown WF. The human jaw jerk: electrophysiologic methods to measure the latency, normal values, and changes in multiple sclerosis. Neurology 1981;31:632–634.

85. Goor C, Ongerboer de Visser B. Jaw and blink reflexes in trigeminal nerve lesions. Neurology 1976;26:95–97.

86. Risk WS, Bosch EP, Kimura J, Cancilla PA, Fischbeck KH, Layzer RB. Chronic tetanus: clinical report and histochemistry of muscle. Muscle Nerve 1981;4:363–366.

87. Ricker K, Eyrich K, Zwirner R. Seltenere Formen von Tetanuser-Krankung: klinische und electromyographische Untersuchung. Arch Psychiatr Nervenkr 1971;215:75–91.

88. Struppler A, Struppler E, Adams RD: Local tetanus in man. Arch Neurol 1963;8:162–178.

89. Goodwill C, O'Tuama L. Electromyographic recording of the jaw reflex in multiple sclerosis. J Neurol Neurosurg Psychiatry 1969;32:6–10.

90. Varma JS, Smith AN, McInnes A. Electrophysiological observations on the human pudendo-anal reflex. J Neurol Neurosurg Psychiatry 1986;49:1411–1416.

91. Bors E, Blinn KA. Bulbocavernosus reflex. J Urol 1959;82:128–130.

92. Rushworth G. Diagnostic value of the electromyographic study of reflex activity in man. EEG Clin Neurophysiol 1967 (Suppl);25:65–73.
93. Krane RJ, Siroky MB. Studies on sacral-evoked potentials. J Urol 1980;124:872–876.
94. Vodusek DB. Pudendal SEP and bulbocavernosus reflex in women. EEG Clin Neurophysiol 1990;77:134–136.
95. Fowler CJ. Pelvic floor neurophysiology. Methods in clinical neurophysiology. Skolunde, Denmark: Dantec, 1991;2:1:1–24.
96. Blaivas JG, Zayed AAH, Labib KB. The bulbocavernosus reflex in urology: a prospective study of 299 patients. J Urol 1981;126:197–199.
97. Ertekin C, Reel F. Bulbocavernosus reflex in normal men and in patients with neurogenic bladder and/or impotence. J Neurol Sci 1976;28:1–15.
98. Bilkey WJ, Awad EA, Smith AD. Clinical application of sacral reflex latency. J Urol 1983;129:1187–1189.
99. Vodusek DB, Zidar J. Pudendal nerve involvement in patients with hereditary motor and sensory neuropathy. Acta Neurol Scand 1987;76:457–460.
100. Galloway NT, Chisholm GD, McInnes A. Patterns and significance of the sacral evoked response (the urologist's knee jerk). Brit J Urol 1985;57:145–147.
101. Galloway NTM, Tainsh J. Minor defects of the sacrum and neurogenic bladder dysfunction. Br J Urol 1985;57:154–155.
102. Fidas A, Galloway NTM, Varma J, McInnes A, Chisholm GD. Sacral reflex latency in acute retention in female patients. Br J Urol 1987;59:311–313.
103. Tackmann W, Porst H, Van Ahlen H. Bulbocavernosus reflex latencies and somatosensory evoked potentials after pudendal nerve stimulation in the diagnosis of impotence. J Neurol 1988;235:219–225.
104. Lin JT, Bradley WE. Penile neuropathy in insulin-dependent diabetes mellitus. J Urol 1985;133:213–215.
105. Mehta AJ, Viosca SP, Korenman SG, Davis SS. Peripheral nerve conduction studies and bulbocavernosus reflex in the investigation of impotence. Arch Phys Med Rehabil 1986;67:332–335.
106. Henry M, Swash M. Assessment of pelvic floor disorders and incontinence by electrophysiological recording of the anal reflex. Lancet 1978;1:1290–1291.
107. Bartolo DCC, Jarratt JA, Read MG, Donnelly TC, Read NW. The role of partial denervation of the puborectalis in idiopathic fecal incontinence. Br J Surg 1983;70:664–667.
108. Wright AL, Williams NS, Gibson JS, Neil DE, Morrison JE. Electrically evoked activity in the human external anal sphincter. Br J Surg 1985;72:38–41.
109. Deschuytere J, Rosselle N, De Keyser C: Monosynaptic reflexes in the superficial forearm flexors in man and their clinical significance. J Neurol Neurosurg Psychiatry 1976;39:555–565.
110. Garcia HA, Fisher MA, Gilai A. H reflex analysis of segmental reflex excitability in flexor and extensor muscles. Neurology 1979;29:984–991.
111. Magladery JW, Porter WE, Parle AM, Teasdall HD. Electrophysiological studies of nerve and reflex activity in normal man. IV. The two neuron reflex activity and identification of certain action potentials from spinal roots and cord. Bull Johns Hopkins Hosp 1951;88:499–519.
112. Deschuytere J, Rosselle N: Diagnostic use of monosynaptic reflexes in L5 and S1 root compression. In: Desmedt JE, ed. New Developments in EMG and Clinical Neurophysiology. Basel: Karger, 1973;3:360–366.
113. Wager EW, Buerger AA. A linear relationship between H-reflex latency and sensory conduction velocity in diabetic neuropathy. Neurology 1974;24:711–714.
114. Yates S, Brown W. Light-stimulus-evoked blink reflex: methods, normal values, relation to other blink reflexes and observations in multiple sclerosis. Neurology 1981;31:272–281.
115. Ongerboer de Visser BW, Melchelse K, Megens PHA. Corneal reflex latency in trigeminal nerve lesions. Neurology 1977;27:1164–1167.
116. Ongerboer de Visser BW. Corneal reflex latency in lesions of the lower postcentral regions. Neurology 1981;31:701–707.
117. Chantraine A. EMG examination of the anal and urethral sphincters. In: Desmedt JE, ed. New developments in electromyography and clinical neurophysiology. Basel: Karger, 1973;2:421.
118. Jesel M, Isch-Treussard C, Isch F. Electromyography of striated muscle of anal and urethral sphincters. In: Desmedt JE, ed. New developments in EMG and clinical neurophysiology. Basel: Karger, 1973;2:406–420.
119. Vodusek DB, Janko M, Lokar J. Direct and reflex responses in perineal muscles on electrical stimulation. J Neurol Neurosurg Psychiatry 1983;46:67–71.
120. Galloway NT, Chisholm GD, McInnes A. Patterns and significance of the sacral evoked response (the urologist's knee jerk). Brit J Urol 1985;57:145–147.
121. Dykstra D, Sidi A, Cameron J, Magness J, Stradal L, Portugal J. The use of mechanical stimulation to obtain the sacral reflex latency: a new technique. J Urol 1987;137:77–79.
122. Sarica Y, Karacan I. Cerebral responses evoked by stimulation of the vesico-urethral junction in normal subjects. EEG Clin Neurophysiol 1986;65:440–446.
123. Vereecken RL, Van Mulders J. Techniques and values of sphincter electromyography in urological problems. Urol Int 1982;37:152–159.
124. Desai KM, Dembny K, Morgan H, Gingell JC, Prothero D. Neurophysiological investigation of diabetic impotence: are sacral response studies of value? Brit J Urol 1988;61:68–71.

18

Magnetic and High-Voltage/Low-Impedance Electrical Stimulation Tests

During the past two decades, the clinical value of the evoked potential study has been well established (1, 2). The evoked potentials that are recorded at the scalp or at various sites along the sensory pathways are elicited by stimulating the respective receptors or nerves. These evoked potential studies test the physiological integrity of the sensory pathways and are able to detect abnormalities that may not be clinically obvious. The visual evoked potential (VEP), brainstem auditory evoked potential (BAEP), and somatosensory evoked potential (SEP) tests are most commonly used in clinical practice. However, until recently it has not been possible to assess the physiological integrity of motor pathways in the central nervous system by stimulating the motor cortex through the scalp in conscious human subjects.

The major study of brain stimulation in human patients began with Penfield and Jasper, who studied the cortical functions systematically by stimulating the cortex in patients undergoing brain surgery (3). In 1954, Gualtierotti and Paterson reported that the motor cortex could be stimulated by scalp electrodes with 20–70 mA of "rectangular or sawtooth current" having a frequency of 20–150/sec (4). The movement of contralateral limbs was evoked. Their technique of cortical stimulation, somewhat modified, is still used. Direct electric cortical stimulation in humans has become a standard diagnostic tool during surgery for epilepsy to help the neurosurgeon decide which functional brain areas to remove and which to spare (5–7). Routinely, 5–7 mA of stimulation with 0.3 msec duration applied at 30–60 Hz for 5–15 seconds is used for this purpose. Muscle twitching can be documented by recording the motor evoked potential (MEP) by the cortical stimulation over the exposed motor cortex (5–7). This technique has not been used in conscious human patients.

In 1980, Merton and Morton developed an ingenious high-voltage and low-output impedance (HVLI) electrical stimulator capable of stimulating the underlying cortical motor neurons through the skull (8). They stimulated the motor cortex with a single high-voltage (2000 V) stimulus with a time constant of discharge less than 10 μsec and observed the twitching of the fingers or foot. They claimed that this stimulation was without undue discomfort to the patient. From 1980 to 1985, this device was used to study the central motor conduction in both normal subjects and neurological patients (9–11). Unfortunately, this device proved to be too painful to be of widespread clinical use, contrary to the original claim.

In 1985, Barker et al. developed a magnetic stimulator that induces sufficient current in conductive tissues to stimulate the motor cerebral cortex painlessly through the intact skull in humans (12). The magnetic stimulator has several advantages over the electrical technique, the major one being the lack of pain (13). Since then, this device has largely replaced HVLI electrical stimulation in studying the integrity of the central motor pathways and has been extensively used in normal and diseased individuals (14).

Physiology of the Magnetic and HVLI Electrical Stimulation Tests

The motor cortex has been stimulated in human and animal subjects. In experimental animals, a brief single electrical stimulus to the exposed motor cortex produces a descending series of positive waves recordable from the ipsilateral medullary pyramidal tract and the central pyramidal tract in the spinal cord (15, 16). There are two kinds of waves—the direct (D-) wave and the indirect (I-) wave (Table 8.1; Fig. 18.1). The latency of the D-wave is too short for an interposed synapse, suggesting that conduction takes place in the fast-conducting pyramidal tract axons, and is elicited by stimulation of subcortical white matter after cortical ablation. On the other hand, the I-wave has a longer latency than the D-wave, suggesting one or more interposed synapses. The I-wave appears at higher intensities of stimulation and requires gray matter, suggesting that I-waves are probably caused by synaptic activation of the same cortical pyramidal

Table 18.1.
Physiological Characteristics of Direct and Indirect Waves

Direct (D-) Wave	Indirect (I-) Wave
Early wave: 0.4–0.6 msec	Later wave
No synapse is involved	One or more interposed synapses is involved
Proximal nodes of axons of larger pyamidal neurons°	Cortical excitory interneurons°
Can be induced even after cortical ablation	Intact gray matter is needed

°Site of origin.

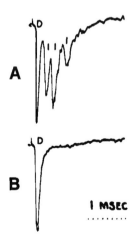

Figure 18.1.   Pyramidal and corticospinal responses from the ipsilateral medullary pyramid to surface stimulation of the motor cortex of the monkey. **A**, Normal direct (D) and periodic indirect (I) waves after a brief stimulus. **B**, Response with stimulation of exposed white matter after ablation of the motor cortex. (From Patton HD, Amassian VE. The pyramidal tract: its excitation and functions. In: Handbook of physiology: Neurophysiology. Washington DC: American Physiology Society, 1960; Sect 1, Vol II:837–861.) (Figure 1 Neurophysiology 1987;20:75.)

neurons but through intracortical neural elements. However, there is only minimal dispersion between the D- and I-waves, suggesting that both D- and I-waves utilize the same fast conduction pathways.

In human subjects, following a single electrical scalp stimulus, the descending D- and I-waves were recorded with epidural electrodes over the spinal cord. It is assumed that these fast-conducting descending pathways have monosynaptic connections with α-motor neurons, and that the descending D- and I-waves produce excitatory postsynaptic potentials that summate to cause them to fire the α-motor neurons. Excitation of the α-motor neuron cells of the spinal cord requires temporal and spatial summation of stimuli (17). Thus, a single stimulus to the pyramidal tract, producing a D-wave alone, is ineffective for this purpose in the anesthesized animal (18). A stimulus to the cortex, however, will produce a volley of I-waves, possibly preceded by a D-wave according to the stimulus characteristics, which will fire anterior horn cells with the final outcome of muscle contraction.

At present it is uncertain which neural elements are excited by scalp stimulation: dendrites, presynaptic terminals, cell bodies, efferent axons, or some combination of these (19). From single motor unit recordings from the small hand muscles, it is thought that *the site of stimulation with weak magnetic stimuli is probably the presynaptic terminals, with stronger stimuli exciting cell bodies or axons or both* (13). Electrical stimuli may act partially on the axons distal to the cell body (13).

HVLI electrical stimulation over the cervical vertebral column has indicated that the site of the excitation is the exit foramina of the motor roots from the spinal canal (20). If the stimulus intensity is increased beyond that required to produce maximal compound muscle action potentials (CMAPs) in small hand muscles, *then responses are seen in the legs clearly due to activation of the descending spinal cord motor pathways* (20).

Magnetic stimulation *cannot be used to stimulate the spinal cord directly* (21). Thus, over the cervical area, the coil was positioned as close as possible to the motor nerve exit foramina in the neck, indicating that the site of excitation with magnetic stimulation is *most likely distal to the site of excitation with HVLI electrical stimulation*. This is also seen in the longer central motor conduction time (CMCT) in magnetic stimulation compared with HVLI electrical stimulation (13).

The CMCT from cortex to cervical area of about 6 msec leaves sufficient time for only one or two synapses to be interposed. The pathway must involve fast myelinated fibers, and for the small hand muscles it is likely to be the corticomotor neuronal tract known to make monosynaptic connection with skeletomotor neurons in primates (13).

Compared with the peripheral nervous system, there are *two distinct characteristics for the brain: (a) anodal cortical stimulation, and (b) facilitation effects*. It has been well established that anodal stimuli to the motor cortex are more effective than cathodal stimuli since the time of Ferrier (22). Rothwell found that the motor cortex was activated preferentially by anodal stimulation with HVLI electrical stimulation (Fig. 18.2) (23). This finding is in accord with surface stimulation studies of the exposed cortex in acute animal experiments: the threshold for anodal stimulation was always lower than for cathodal stimuli (22, 24, 25). Anodal stimulation most likely depolarizes the proximal segments of the Betz cell axons and hyperpolarizes the superficial dendrites, causing a D-wave. Subsequent I-waves may be due to activity in vertically oriented corticocortical projections (26).

The facilitation phenomenon was noted in an early study with HVLI electrical stimulation (8). A similar facilitation phenomenon was observed by Hess with magnetic brain stimulation (27). With minimal voluntary contraction of a muscle during brain stimulation, there was a pronounced increase in the CMAP amplitude and shortening of the latency (Figs. 18.3 and 18.4) (28). This is termed *"facilitation phenomenon" and is peculiar to the brain*. The relationship between background force and CMAP amplitude is approximately linear with electrical stimulation, whereas a small background contraction of the order of 5% of maximum has a striking facilitation effect with magnetic stimulation (26). The facilitation phenomenon can also be induced by minimal contraction of nearby muscles or contralateral muscles. Murray proposed that facilita-

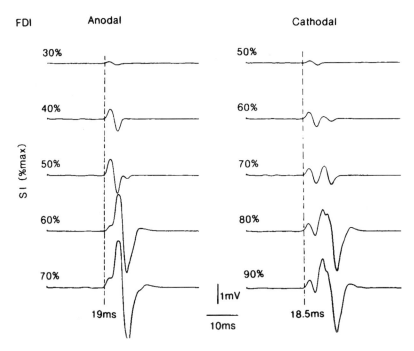

Figure 18.2. Anodal and cathodal difference in cortical stimulation. Comparison of the MEPs from the first dorsal interosseous muscle after anodal and cathodal stimulation of the brain at different intensities. Note the difference in threshold (anodal 30%, cathodal 50%) and the more polyphasic nature of the cathodal responses at just-suprathreshold intensities (compare 50% anodal with 70% cathodal). (From Thompson P, Rothwell J, Day B, Dressler D, Maertens de Noordhout A, Marsden C. Mechanisms of electrical and magnetic stimulation of human motor cortex. In: Chokroverty S, ed. Magnetic stimulation in clinical neurophysiology. Boston: Butterworth, 1990;134.)

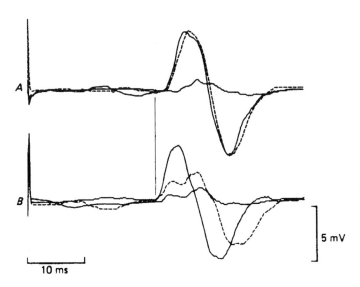

Figure 18.3. Facilitation phenomenon. MEPs from the ADQ muscle with magnetic (**A**) and HVLI electrical (**B**) brain stimulation at an intensity 20% above threshold in relaxed muscle (small response, *continuous lines*), with voluntary background contraction of 10% maximum *(dashed curves),* and with voluntary contraction of 25% maximum (larger responses, *continuous lines*) by each method. The responses of corresponding background contraction are 1.4–3 msec earlier using the electrical method. Note the marked differences in the MEP shapes and amplitudes between the two methods with voluntary background contraction of 10% *(dashed curves).* (From Hess C, Mills K, Murray N. Responses in small hand muscles from magnetic stimulation of the human brain. J Physiol 1987;388:408.)

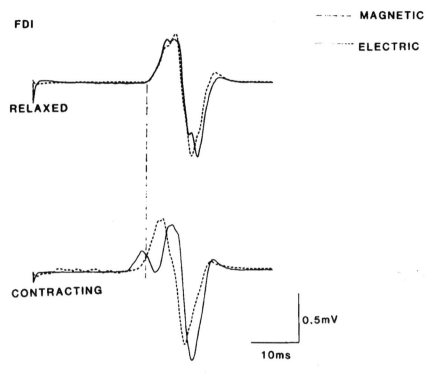

Figure 18.4. Facilitation phenomenon. Effect of voluntary contraction on the latency of MEPs in the first dorsal interosseous (FDI) muscle after HVLI electric *(solid lines)* and magnetic *(dashed lines)* stimulation over the motor cortex. Top tracings were obtained with the subject completely relaxed; bottom tracings were obtained with the subject exerting a small (5–10%) background voluntary contraction. The *vertical dotted lines* correspond to a latency of 24 msec. Shortening of the latency of the MEPs (3.6 msec) with voluntary activation is obvious and much greater after HVLI electrical stimulation. (From Thompson PD, Rothwell JC, Day BL, Dressler D, Maertens de Noordhout A, Marsden CD. Mechanisms of electrical and magnetic stimulation of human motor cortex. In Chokroverty S, ed. Magnetic stimulation in clinical neurophysiology. Boston: Butterworth, 1990;135.)

tion occurs both at spinal and cortical levels: the spinal mechanism occurs with electrical brain stimulation and, during magnetic stimulation, with contralateral facilitation (26). When attention is focused on accurate force production, this is likely to involve the cortical mechanism. At the spinal level, during voluntary activity, there are likely to be motor neurons near enough to threshold for activation to occur with the D-wave causing a shorter latency with voluntary contraction (23, 29).

High-Voltage/Low-Impedance Electrical Stimulation

The electrical stimulator used for motor cortical stimulation (Digitimer Type D 180: Digitimer Ltd, Welwyn Garden City, England) has a high-output voltage and a low-output impedance. It is capable of delivering stimuli of up to 750 V, thus reducing the resistance. The shape of the stimulus is a spike with a fast rise time and then an exponential decay with a time constant of either 50 or 100 μsec. It is capable of delivering stimuli of up to 500 or 900 mA in different subjects. The stimulation is applied through saline-soaked pad electrodes with an approximate area of 1 cm². Unlike the peripheral nerve, where the cathode is used as an active stimulating electrode, *the anode is used as the active stimulating electrode for motor cortex stimulation (Fig. 18.2)*. For HVLI electrical stimulation, there is a somatopical localization that corresponds well to the somatopical localization of the motor cortex (23). Rothwell found that for the muscles in the arm, the anode was placed 7 cm lateral to the vertex and the cathode at the vertex along a line between C_z and A or A_2, and for the leg muscles, the anode was placed at the vertex and the cathode placed 6 cm anteriorly.

Magnetic Stimulation

In 1896, D'Arsonval was the first investigator to describe flickers of light reported by volunteers when their heads were placed within a time-varying magnetic field (30). He labeled this phenomenon "magnetophosphophenes." In 1910, Thompson also reported "faint flickering illumination" when the volunteers' heads were exposed to peak fields of up to 140 mT at 50 Hz of alternating current, probably from stimulating the retina rather than the cortex (31). In 1965, Bickford and Fremming developed a magnetic stimulator that effectively depolarized peripheral nerves (32). However, they were unable to stimulate the cortex. According to Dr. Bickford, each stimulus produced smoke and fire (33). In 1982, Polson et al. developed a smokeless magnetic stimulator, which achieved the first transcortical stimulation (34). In 1985, Barker et al. reported the first clinical trial of the magnetic stimulator in human subject.

Magnetic stimulation is a method of stimulating the neural tissue that *does not depend on the passage of electrical current through electrodes or skin.* In principle, *magnetic current itself does not stimulate the neural tissue directly.* Thus, the name "magnetic stimulation," although a convenient and established description of the technique, is a slight misnomer (35). *The magnetic stimulator generates a pulsed magnetic current that induces an electrical current which, in turn, stimulates the neural tissue lying within its path (Fig. 18.5).* The mechanism of stimulation of the neural tissue is the same for magnetic and electrical stimulation; i.e., the electrical current passes across a nerve membrane and into the axon, resulting in depolarization and the initiation of action potentials that then propagate by the normal method of nerve conduction (36).

The magnetic stimulator has a high energy storage capacitor, which can discharge a brief pulse of strong current through a stimulating coil (Fig. 18.6). The energy storage capacitor C is charged up to a high voltage by the power supply when switch $S1$ is closed. To fire the stimulator, switch $S1$ is opened and switch $S2$ is closed. Current (5000 A at maximal output) then flows from the capacitor as it discharges, through the stimulating coil generating the magnetic field, which approaches *2 Tesla* and a peak at about 150 μsec (13). Diode D and resistor R can be used to control the subsequent rate of decay of the magnetic field. When the pulse of current is discharged through the coil, a magnetic field is induced that, unlike an electric field, can pass easily through all biological structures, including the skull. The magnetic field then induces a small electric current that can be used to stimulate neural tissue.

The direction of the induced electrical currents in the tissue is determined by using the "right hand rule" (37): When the right thumb is placed along the direction of electrical current flow, the natural curl of the fingers points in the direction of the associated magnetic field (Fig. 18.7). The orientation of the magnetic field is perpendicular to the induced electrical current. When the induced currents are in the proper orientation

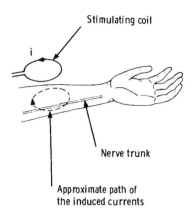

Figure 18.5. Principle of magnetic stimulation. A nearby magnetic coil induces electrical currents in the forearm. (From Barker AT, Freeston IL, Jalinous R, Jarratt JA. Magnetic stimulation of the human brain and peripheral nervous system: an introduction and the results of an initial clinical evaluation. Neurosurgery 1987;20:101.)

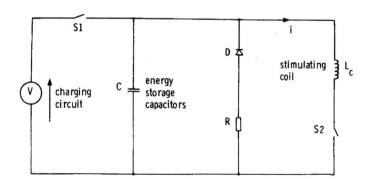

Figure 18.6. Simplified circuit diagram of a magnetic stimulator (From Barker AT, Freeston IL, Jalinous R, Jarratt JA. Magnetic stimulation of the human brain and peripheral nervous system: an introduction and the results of an initial clinical evaluation. Neurosurgery 1987;20:101.)

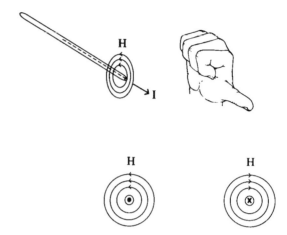

Figure 18.7.   Orientation and direction of the magnetic field (*H*) due to the current (*I*) flowing in the wire can be determined by using the "right-hand rule." When the right thumb is placed along the direction of current flow, the natural curl of the fingers points in the direction of the associated magnetic field. Note that the intensity of the magnetic field diminishes with increasing distance from the wire. End-on views of the wire show the reversal of the magnetic field with reversal of current direction in the wire. o = current flowing from the plane of the page. x = current flowing into the plane of the page. (From Chokroverty S, Spire JP, DiLullo J, Moody E, Maselli R. Magnetic stimulation of the human peripheral nervous system. In: Chokroverty S, ed. Magnetic stimulation in clinical physiology. Boston: Butterworth, 1990:250.)

and of sufficient magnitude, they initiate depolarization of the neural fibers and produce sufficient depolarization to trigger the action potentials. Therefore, theoretically, the proper coil orientation relative to the testing of neural tissue is essential for the best results. In fact, Hess et al. found that *the human motor cortex has a lower threshold in an induced electrical current flow from back to front, i.e., clockwise for left hemisphere stimulation and counterclockwise for right hemisphere stimulation,* with the coil centered at the vertex (28). *This physiological directional specificity is seen with the magnetic stimulator with one polarity,* e.g., the Magstim 200 (Magstim Company, Ltd, Whitland, UK), but not with those of changing polarity, such as the Cadwell magnetic stimulator (Cadwell World Headquarters, Kennewick, WA). Thus, it appears to be important to know the direction of coil current flow when a magnetic stimulator with one polarity is used. *In practice, this does not seem to be an important requirement for a technically satisfactory magnetic stimulation test,* because only three papers have described the coil orientation in detail in their methods (26, 27, 38).

Location of Stimulation with a Magnetic Round Coil

Common sense suggests that stimulation occurs at the center of the coil. However, the center of the coil is the only place where the induced electrical stimulus is exactly zero because the magnetic stimulator induces current most effectively directly under the coil (Fig. 18.8). Thus, *the maximum electrical current is located at the edge of the coil,* indicating that the edge of the coil, rather than its center, should be aligned with the neural structure under stimulation (Fig. 18.9). This also indicates that the electrical field of the magnetic round coil is wider and deeper than that of the electrical stimulator (Table 18.2). For these reasons, magnetic stimulation has several advantages; namely, the neural tissue can be stimulated through the clothing, neural tissue can be stimulated to a greater depth, and the field of stimulation is wider. On the other hand, a crucial disadvantage has been the ill-defined site of stimulation in contrast to that of electrical stimulation. The magnetic stimulator appears to stimulate the motor cortex lateral to the point at which an electrical stimulator produces a given response (13). To achieve the same response, the magnetic coil has to be moved medially. This may be because of the insulating effect of the falx cerebri (Fig. 18.10).

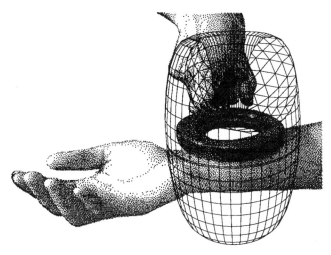

Figure 18.8. Three-dimensional projection illustrates absence of stimulation at center of coil. (From Cadwell J. Principles of magnetoelectric stimulation. In: Chokroverty S, ed. Magnetic stimulation in clinical neurophysiology. Boston: Butterworth, 1990:22.)

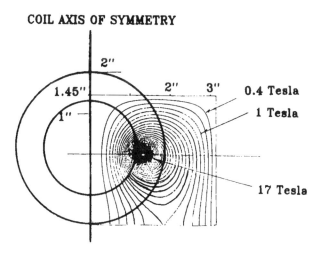

Figure 18.9. Computer-generated plot of magnetic flux density. The 9-cm (outside dimension) coil of the magnetic stimulator is represented by the *two concentric circles.* At maximum power, this stimulator produces a nominal 2-T field at the insulator surface that surrounds the copper coil. (From Edmonds HL, Paloheimo MPJ, Backman MGH, Johnson JR, Holt RT, Shilds CB. TC magnetic motor evoked potentials (tc MMEP) for functional monitoring of motor pathways during scoliosis surgery. Spine 1989;14:684.)

Because of the peculiar nature of the magnetic stimulator, it is possible to observe *paradoxical stimulation in the lumbar area* (Fig. 18.11) (33). If the coil is placed on the midline of the lower back, the response to stimulation is observed in both anterior tibialis muscles because the outer edge of the round coil is stimulating the right and left L5 roots. If the coil is moved off midline toward the side, the contralateral L5 root is still stimulated, whereas the ipsilateral L5 root is not stimulated because it is outside the effective electrical field. For best results, *it is important to place the edge of the coil, rather than its center, closer to the neural tissue to be stimulated.*

To improve focal stimulation, Cadwell made two technical innovations: (*a*) a sharp-cornered coil, and (*b*) a butterfly coil stimulator (Fig. 18.12). The sharp corners of the coil allow precision in determining where a peripheral nerve is depolarized because the current ceases to flow in the nerve at the sharp corner. With the butterfly coil, a "hot spot" (the most effective spot for the induced electrical current) is created at the joint

Table 18.2.
Comparison of the HVLI Electrical and Magnetic Stimulators

	HVLI Electrical Stimulator	Magnetic Stimulator (MS)
Common features		
Stimulating current	Electrical	Electrical
Cortical stimulation	(+)	(+)
Facilitation effect	(+)	(+)
Safety	Safe	Safe
Different features		
Equipment	Simpler and cheaper	Relatively bulky and costly
Physiological features		
Pain	Painful	Painless
Stimulation site	Clearly defined	Not well defined
Stimulation field	Narrow: anode at the cortex; cathode at the spinal cord	Wide
CMAP	Complex waveform, longer duration, lower amplitude, less reproducible	Simpler waveform, shorter duration, larger amplitude, more reproducible
Latency	Shorter than MS by 2 msec	
Absent response	Present	Rare
Spinal cord stimulation	Possible	Not always possible
Leg muscle response	Difficult	Possible
Multiple muscle recording	Less possible	Possible

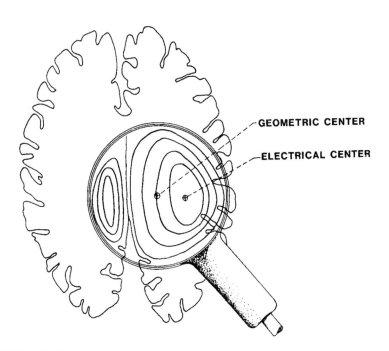

Figure 18.10.   Displacement of geometric and electrical centers due to nonuniform conductivity of the brain. Site of stimulation in the cortex in magnetic stimulation. (From Cadwell J. Principles of magnetoelectric stimulation. In: Chokroverty S, ed. Magnetic stimulation in clinical neurophysiology. Boston: Butterworth, 1990:27.)

where two coils meet. Whether these two innovations will overcome the lack of exact focal stimulation of the magnetic stimulator remains to be seen.

Comparison Between the HVLI Electrical Stimulator and the Magnetic Stimulator

The common feature between these two stimulators is that electrical current is responsible for the final depolarization of neural tissue, regardless of whether the primary cur-

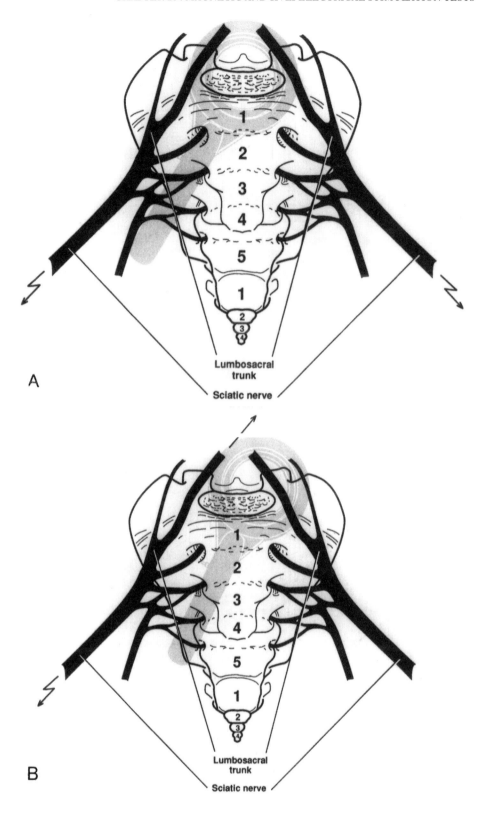

Figure 18.11. Paradoxical stimulation at the lumbar roots. (**A**) Edges of coil overlying both L5 nerve roots producing responses from the muscles in the right and left leg muscles. (**B**) Moving the coil to *the left* from the center produces a response from the muscles innervated by the *right L5 root*. (From Cadwell J. Principles of magnetoelectric stimulation. In: Chokroverty S, ed. Magnetic stimulation in clinical neurophysiology. Boston: Butterworth, 1990:25–26.)

rent is electrical or magnetic. Both stimulating techniques are known to be safe, but there are some other differences between their use in patients (Table 18.2). The most notable difference is the considerable discomfort caused by the HVLI electrical stimulator in comparison with the painlessness of magnetic stimulation (13, 39). HVLI electrical stimulation has to be applied to a clearly defined anatomical site to evoke the MEP from a specific part of body; this is not the case with magnetic stimulation.

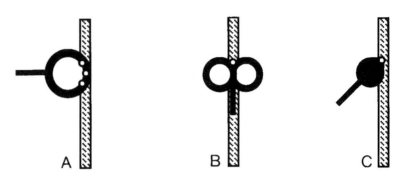

Figure 18.12. Different kinds of magnetic stimulators: **A**, Conventional round coil. **B**, Butterfly coil. **C**, Round coil with sharp bend. The *hatched line* represents the nerve. Three *blank dots* in **A** represent a general area of maximum nerve depolarization. One *blank dot* in **B** and **C** represents the site of maximum nerve depolarization.

Another difference is in the capability of stimulating the spinal cord: only the HVLI electrical stimulator is known to stimulate the spinal cord directly (9, 20). Though Mills and Murray have shown that the electrodes over the cervical region actually excite motor roots at their exit from the spinal canal, they were able to record small MEPs from leg muscles, showing that direct electrical stimulation of the spinal cord is possible (20). The inability to stimulate the spinal cord magnetically is thought to be due to its anatomy (39). Another important difference between these methods is in the latency and shape of the MEPs: *with HVLI electrical stimulation, the latency is shorter and the MEP waves are more complex than with the magnetic stimulator (Fig. 18.3).* The latency from the hand muscle is shorter by 2 msec with HVLI electrical stimulation (28), suggesting that magnetic stimulation is able to excite corticospinal neurons only indirectly (13, 28).

Comparison Between the EMG Stimulator and the Magnetic Stimulator

Many physiological differences between the HVLI electrical stimulator and magnetic stimulator apply here since the conventional EMG stimulator and HVLI electrical stimulator are physiologically identical (Table 18.3). However, certain technical differences are pertinent in this section. In the evaluation of peripheral nerve disorders, the magnetic stimulator has distinct disadvantages: it cannot provide the supramaximal stimulation and the repetitive nerve stimulation suitable for the study of the neuromuscular transmission disorders. Further, the magnetic stimulator is not suitable for eliciting electrical current for the H-reflex, F-wave, or compound nerve action potentials (CNAPs) (40). The only advantage of magnetic stimulation is in studying the nerve conduction of the proximal portions of peripheral nerves (41). With the butterfly stimulator, which more accurately localizes the stimulation site, it is possible that the utility of magnetic stimulation in the study of peripheral nerve conduction may improve, but this has not been confirmed as yet.

Motor Evoked Potentials and Central Motor Conduction Time

The CMAPs recorded from the muscles with magnetic or HVLI electrical stimulation on the cortex or spinal cord are called the motor evoked potentials (MEPs). The CMAPs recorded with stimulation of the peripheral nerves are constant in amplitude, form, and latency from stimulus to stimulus, provided supramaximal stimulation is given. In contrast, *the MEPs recorded from the muscles with magnetic or HVLI electrical stimulation on the cortex tend to vary,* reflecting the varying excitability of nerve cell bodies within the cerebral cortex and spinal cord (42). Therefore, *several MEP recordings should be superimposed to measure the shortest latency.*

Latency is measured from the stimulus onset to the shortest take-off of the MEPs from the baseline, and the amplitude is measured from peak to peak of the MEPs. The

Table 18.3.
Comparison of Conventional EMG and Magnetic Stimulators

	EMG Stimulator	Magnetic Stimulator (MS)
Common features	Electrical	Electrical
Different features		
Physiological aspects		
Primary current	Electrical	Magnetic
Depth of electrical field	Shallow	Deeper
Field of stimulation	Narrow	Wide; multiple nerves nearby can be stimulated
Site of stimulation	Clearly defined	Not well defined
Proximal or deep nerve	Stimulation difficult	Stimulation possible
Pain	Painful	Painless
Skin preparation	Direct stimulation over skin Skin preparation often needed	Stimulation possible through clothes
Equipment	Simple and already incorporated into the EMG machine	Relatively bulky and costly
Technical parameters		
Supramaximal stimulation	Possible	Not possible
Repetition rate	Various stimulation rates possible	Low; 0.3 Hz is possible[a]
Sensory CNAP	Possible	Not obtainable
H-reflex	Possible	Not obtainable
Safety precautions	Cardiac pacemaker or cardiac catheter near the stimulating site	Metallic objects

[a]In recent models, 2–8 Hz stimulation is possible.

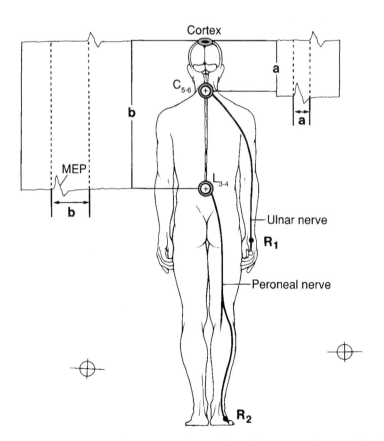

Figure 18.13.   Central motor conduction time (CMCT) from the cortex to the cervical cord (**a**) and from the cortex to the lumbar cord (**b**). R_1 represents the recording electrodes in the ADQ and R_2 in the EDB muscles. MEP refers motor evoked potential.

latency difference between cortical stimulation and cervical or lumbar stimulation is termed *the central motor conduction time (CMCT)* (Fig. 18.13). Every authority agrees that the CMCT is physiologically a better measure than the conduction velocity because part of the time is due to synaptic delay. *The CMCT has become the most commonly used parameter* in the magnetic and HVLI electrical stimulation tests. Physiologically, the CMCT represents a composite of the time needed for depolarization of the intracortical neuron, synaptic transmission before the corticospinal neuron, depolarization of that neuron, transmission of the volleys down the corticospinal tract, synaptic transmission at the α-motor neuron and its depolarization (possibly requiring a summation of descending volleys), and transmission along the lower motor neuron axon to the site of excitation. Thus, the CMCT is not, in the strictest sense, "central motor conduction time." However, in the practical sense, the CMCT represents central motor conduction because the contribution of the peripheral nerves is small. The main advantage of the routine use of CMCT is that most of the peripheral pathway is eliminated as a cause for latency prolongation.

The values of CMCT are different according to the type of stimulator used, the muscle stimulated, and the presence or absence of facilitation (Table 18.4). The CMCT between the cortex and cervical cord when recording MEPs from the hand muscles ranged from 5.0–9.5 msec. In general, *the CMCT is shorter by 2 msec with HVLI stimulation than with magnetic stimulation* (Fig. 18.3). *The CMCT is shorter by 2 msec with facilitation than at rest* (Fig. 18.4). The CMCT between the cortex and lumbar cord when recording MEPs from the pelvic and leg muscles ranged from 15–22.5 msec (Table 18.4).

Table 18.4.
Central Motor Conduction Time (CMCT) in Normal Controls[a]

Muscle	Stimulation	Facilitation	Conduction Time	No. of Subjects	Investigator
CMCT between the cortex and cervical cord					
APB	HVLI ES	+	5.0	11	Cowan et al. (10)
APB	HVLI ES	+	6.8	11	Rossini et al. (87)
APB	HVLI ES (U)	+	6.5	23	Rossini et al. (87)
APB	MS	-	9.5	27	Barker et al. (36)
		+	8.0		
ADQ	HVLI ES	-	8.8	60	Kim and Oh (45)
ADQ	HVLI ES	+	5.0	12	Hess et al. (27)
ADQ	MS-cortex	+	8.4	32	Murray (26)
	HVLI ES-C7				
ADQ	MS	-	9.4	27	Barker et al. (36)
		+	7.4		
ADQ	MS	+	6.8	12	Hess et al. (27)
ADQ	MS	-	8.4	60	Kim and Oh (45)
Forearm flexor	HVLI ES	-	4.1	15	Mills et al. (11)
Biceps brachii	MS	+	6.3	?	Ingram et al. (57)
CMCT between the cortex and lumbar cord					
AH	MS	-	18.8		Barker et al. (36)
		+	16.7		
AH	MS	-	18.2	60	Kim and Oh (45)
EDB	MS	-	17.8	60	Kim and Oh (45)
Anterior tibialis	MS	+	15.0		Ingram et al. (57)
BC	MS	+	17.0	17	Ghezzi et al. (86)
BC	MS	-	22.4	15	Opsomer et al. (84)
		+	15.1		
EAS	MS	-	21.2		
		+	12.4		
EAS	HVLI ES	+	15.3	5	Mathers et al. (60)

[a]*Abbreviations:* HVLI ES, high voltage-low intensity electrical stimulation; MS, magnetic stimulation; APB, abductor pollicis brevis; ADQ, abductor digiti quinti; AH, abductor hallucis; EDB, extensor digitorum brevis; EAS, external anal sphincter.

Considering the strong relationship between the somatosensory latencies and height (43), such a relationship might be expected with the MEP latencies. *Some degree of correlation was found between the MEP latencies and height* (44, 45). Chu found an excellent correlation of the MEP latencies to the abductor digiti quinti (ADQ) and anterior tibialis muscles and a weak correlation between the CMCT from the cortex to the lumbar region with height (44). However, he did not find any correlation of the CMCT from the cortex to the cervical region with height. We found an excellent correlation with height of the MEP latencies from the cervical and lumbar areas but only a weak correlation of the MEP latencies from the cortex to the recording muscles (45). We did not find any correlation of the CMCT from the cortex to the cervical and lumbar cords with height. The difference between these two studies may be due to the use of different types of magnetic stimulators. Chu used a magnetic stimulator with a fixed current direction, whereas we used a magnetic stimulator with alternating current direction.

Prolongation of the CMCT or absent responses may be due to several mechanisms: (*a*) the impairment of cortical stimulation because of a lesion in the motor cortex, as seen in cortical infarction or resulting from anesthetic agents that suppress the excitability of cortical neurons (46, 47); (*b*) slowing or blocking of conduction in the fast-conducting pyramidal tract, as seen in multiple sclerosis, so that the first descending volleys are conducted by slower-conducting, possibly polysynaptic pathways; or the number of descending volleys may be insufficient or dispersed temporally so that additional time may be required for "after-volleys" to summate and discharge the motor neurons; (*c*) there may be complete disruption of the fast-conducting pyramidal tract, as seen in an internal capsule infarction; and (*d*) cortical stimulation may not be capable of firing the anterior horn cells because of decreased excitability of the spinal motor neurons. This may be an example seen in anterior horn cell disease.

Safety Concerns

There is no evidence as yet to suggest that any significant risk exists with transcortical magnetic or HVLI electrical stimulation. The main concern with these procedures has been whether they can induce clinical seizures, or "kindling phenomenon." Goddard et al. have shown that kindling could not be induced at frequencies of less than 10 Hz in experimental animals, regardless of the duration of stimulation (48). The maximum discharge rate of 0.33 Hz in the modern magnetic stimulator is well below this figure. The number of stimuli given to any one subject is not high. Hence, no danger of kindling should exist (39). The relationship between magnetic stimulation and seizure has also been investigated clinically. In one study of 50 seizure patients, magnetic stimulation did not provoke seizures or other EEG changes (49). Another report documented that, in 13 patients with medically intractable complex partial seizures whose anticonvulsant medication had been reduced preparatory to surgery for poorly controlled epilepsy, magnetic stimulation activated previously demonstrated epileptic foci in 12 cases. However, there were no adverse clinical effects. Thus, the authors concluded that the technique is able to activate the epileptic focus in the presurgical evaluation of patients with epilepsy (50).

There have been two reports of patients developing seizures during or soon after magnetic stimulation. One patient with a large ischemic infarction had a first seizure while being examined (51). Two patients with multiple sclerosis developed seizures within 1 month of being tested (52). Considering the large number of patients in Europe who received transcranial (TC) stimulation for an 8–year period, occurrence of seizures was extremely low. Even so, it is safe to regard seizures, or any clinical indications of lowered seizure threshold, as relative contraindications for TC stimulation.

Since it is possible that the magnetic stimulator could induce dangerous currents and voltages in a cardiac pacemaker or other implanted electrical devices, it is prudent not to use magnetic stimulation in individuals with such devices. Any person with metal objects in the head or with a skull defect should not be subjected to TC stimulation.

General Guidelines for Stimulation Technique

The technique is similar to that for the conventional motor nerve conduction test except that stimulation is made over the central nervous system:

1. Recording of the MEP is performed from the target muscle using a surface electrode. Recording surface electrodes should be placed following the tendon-belly method.

2. Though the filter setting for the motor nerve conduction test can be used, some laboratories use a narrower filter setting: 20 Hz–2 Kz.

3. The stimulation is repeated several times at rest and with the recording muscles mildly precontracted.

4. Latency is measured to the shortest latency. The peak-to-peak MEP amplitude should be measured.

5. To stimulate the motor cortex, the following guidelines are used:

   • For magnetic stimulation, a round coil is placed over the scalp with the center of the coil at its vertex. Most studies have shown that the highest MEP amplitudes are achieved when using tangential edge orientation (37, 40). No specific guidelines for localization are needed. In general, *the edge of the coil should be placed near the cortical area corresponding to the target muscle.* In our laboratory at the University of Alabama at Birmingham, we found that the best MEP response with an alternating-direction magnetic stimulator (e.g., the Cadwell magnetic stimulator) is obtained by placing the center of the 9-cm round coil at the C_Z for the hand muscles and at the C_3 or C_4 for the foot muscles. Stimulation is done with an initial intensity of 60%. Depending upon the response, the stimulus intensity is gradually increased to 100%. The angle of the round coil from the scalp should be adjusted to obtain the maximum response. For a stimulator with monopolar direction (e.g., the Magstim 200), for optimum excitation of the left hemisphere, the inducing current travels clockwise when viewed from above; for stimulation of the right hemisphere, the coil is turned over to reverse current direction (counterclockwise) (53). This is not critical for a magnetic stimulator with alternating direction.

   • For HVLI electrical stimulation, the location of the stimulator should be *much more exact over the motor cortex subserving the target muscle:* for the arm muscles, the anode is placed over the motor cortex at a point 7 cm down the interaural (A_1–A_2) line from the vertex and 1 cm anterior to that line (11). The cathode is placed 6 cm anterior to the anode. For the bulbocavernosus (BC) muscle, the anode is placed at C_Z and the cathode 7 cm anterior to the anode (54). *No more than five stimulations are recommended.*

6. For stimulation of the spinal cord, the following guidelines are used:

   • For the magnetic stimulator, the center of the round coil is placed 2–3 cm lateral to the spinal cord.

   • For the HVLI electrical stimulator, the cathode is placed over the spinal cord, and the anode is placed 6 cm lateral to the cathode.

7. For stimulation of the spinal cord, the edge of the magnetic coil should be placed over the tested nerve with the center of the coil at the designated anatomical landmark.

Clinical Applications

Multiple Sclerosis

Multiple sclerosis (MS) is an ideal disease for maximum benefit of the central motor conduction study by magnetic stimulation because of its selective demyelination of the long tract. In fact, in the first published clinical trial of magnetic stimulation, marked prolongation of CMCT was found in patients with MS (55). Barker et al. showed that CMCT was prolonged to the upper and lower limb muscles in a group of 15 patients with MS and that the degree of prolongation was related to the clinical deficit (55). Since then, many studies have confirmed this observation (Table 18.5).

The overall frequency of abnormality in the CMCT ranged from 55–72% of cases. A few studies reported abnormality in 90–100% of cases, but fewer than 10 cases were studied. In Jarratt et al.'s study, the mean CMCT in MS patients was 14.5 msec versus a normal value of 9.8 msec ($P < 0.01$), and the longest CMCT found between head and neck was 34.2 msec (21). The typical CMCT abnormality was a moderate prolongation

Table 18.5.
Diagnostic Sensitivity of Magnetic and HVLI Electrical Stimulation in Multiple Sclerosis[a]

Authors	Stimulator Type	Recording Muscle	Mult Scler Type	No. of Patients	Abnormality	One Side	Both Sides
Central motor conduction time (CMCT)							
Cowan et al. (10)	Cortical HVLI ES	BB, APB	Definite	8	8 (100%)		
	Cervical-HVLI ES						
Mills and Murray (11)	Cortical-HVLI ES	Forearm flexor	Definite	8	8 (100%)		
Hess et al. (27)	Cortical-MS	ADQ	Total	83	60 (72%)	26 (31%)	34 (41%)
	Cervical-HVLI ES		Definite	62[b]	49 (79%)	18 (29%)	31 (50%)
			Probable	11	6 (55%)	4 (36%)	2 (18%)
			Possible	10	5 (50%)	4 (40%)	1 (10%)
Barker et al. (36)	Cortical-MS	ADQ	Definite	16	12 (75%)		
	Cervical-MS						
Ingram et al. (57)	Cortical-MS	BB	Definite	20	12 (60%)	5 (25%)	7 (35%)
	Cervical-MS	APB		20	11 (55%)	3 (15%)	8 (40%)
		AT		20	12 (60%)		12 (60%)
		All three muscles[c]		20	14 (70%)		
Berardelli et al. (58)	Cortical HVLI ES	BB	Definite	29	20 (70%)		
	Cervical ES	Thenar muscle	Probable				
Mathers et al. (60)	Cortical-HVLI ES	EAS	Definite	10	9 (90%)		
Jarratt et al. (21)	Cortical-MS	ADQ	Total	71	36[b] (51%)		
	Cervical-MS		Definite	39	24 (60%)		
			Probable	25	8 (32%)		
			Possible	7	4 (57%)		
Motor conduction velocity in the spinal cord							
Snooks and Swash (56)	Cervical-HVLI ES	Pelvic floor muscle	Definite	5	4 (40%)		
	Lumbar-HVLI ES						

[a]*Abbreviations:* HVLI ES, high-voltage, low-intensity electrical stimulation; MS, magnetic stimulation. Mult scler, multiple sclerosis; APB, abductor pollicis brevis; ADQ, abductor digiti quinti; BB, biceps brachii; AT, anterior tibialis; EDC, extensor digitorum communis; and EAS, external anal sphincter.
[b]In five patients only one side was tested. One patient with abnormal side-to-side difference but normal absolute latency is included.

of latency; an equal number of responses showed normal and reduced amplitudes (Figs. 18.14 and 18.15) (27). Snooks and Swash calculated the conduction velocity in the spinal cord by stimulating the cervical and lumbar levels with HVLI electrical stimulation, finding a slow conduction velocity in four of five cases of MS (56). This slowing was most likely caused by demyelination of corticospinal tracts. Thus, these studies confirmed that the magnetic stimulation technique can demonstrate an abnormality of motor conduction in MS. Response to the cervical roots was normal in all patients (27). The absence of MEP response was extremely rare, occurring in only 0.6% of 166 tested sides in 83 patients, in striking contrast to 19% of 16 tested sides in eight patients by HVLI electrical stimulation (11, 27). A higher incidence of unobtainable responses was found in studies of the lower limbs than in those of the upper limbs (57).

The frequency of abnormality of the CMCT in patients with definite MS was higher (62–79%) than in the groups with probable or possible MS (Table 18.5) (21, 27). This implies that the frequency of abnormality increases with the degree of diagnostic certainty. In patients with progressive spastic paraplegia, Jarratt et al. found abnormalities in 57% of cases, a higher percentage than was found in the early probable and possible groups (21).

There is no consensus on the sensitivity of the CMCT test compared with other evoked potential tests. Hess et al. found an abnormality in a higher percentage of cases by the CMCT (72%) than by the VEP (67%), the SEP (59%), or the BAEP (39%) (27). Berardelli et al. found abnormalities in 72% by the CMCT and in 59% by the SEP (58). In contrast, Jarratt et al. found an abnormality in a higher percentage of cases by the VEP (80%) than by the CMCT (54%) (21). Abnormal CMCT tended to be found in patients with abnormal SEP (27, 58), but no such relationship was found between the CMCT and VEP or between CMCT and BAEP (27). In patients with a previous history or current signs of optic nerve involvement, the VEP was abnormal in 88%, whereas in

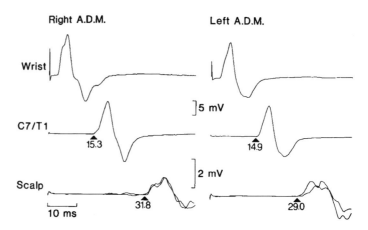

Figure 18.14.   Prolonged CMCT in both sides in a patient with definite MS. MEPs from the abductor digiti minimi (ADM). Electrical stimulation at the wrist and the C7–T1 interspace. Magnetic stimulation over the scalp. (From Hess C, Mills K, Murray N, Schriefer T. Magnetic brain stimulation: central motor conduction studies in multiple sclerosis. Ann Neurol 1987;22:748.)

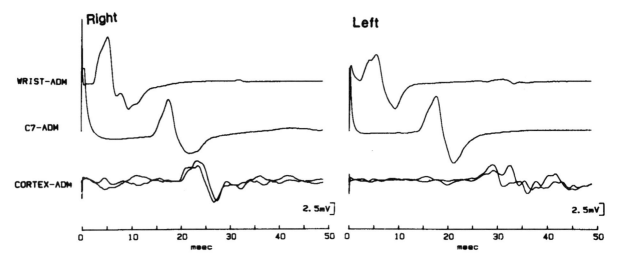

Figure 18.15.   Prolonged CMCT in the left side in a patient with clinically definite MS. MEPs from the abductor digiti minimi (ADM) in a patient with MS. Electrical stimulation at the wrist and the C7–T1 interspace. Magnetic stimulation over the scalp. (From Murray NMF. Magnetic stimulation of cortex: clinical applications. J Clin Neurophysiol 1991;8:67.)

patients with past or current pyramidal tract dysfunction, the CMCT was abnormal in 61%. Thus, both techniques tend to confirm the presence of abnormalities within their own territories, although the VEP appears to be somewhat superior.

With regard to the detection of clinically silent lesions, the VEP and SEP studies are better than the CMCT. The VEP was able to detect a silent lesion in 68% of cases, whereas the CMCT was successful in only 13% (21). The SEP test detected a silent lesion in 67% of cases; the CMCT in only 14% (59). Berardelli et al. found that subclinical impairment in the arms was detected in 61% of cases by the SEP and in 44% by the CMCT test (58).

The MRI is superior to the CMCT in detection of a definite lesion in MS patients. A definite abnormality was found in 83% of cases by the MRI scan and in 65% by the CMCT (27).

In the first study of magnetic stimulation in MS patients, Barker et al. found that the CMCT was longer in chair-bound MS patients than in mobile patients (55). Ingram et al. found the same trend in that increasingly severe disability was correlated with increased CMCT in ambulatory patients (57). The degree of CMCT abnormality in the lower limb muscles was closely correlated with disability on both the Kurtzke Disability Status Scale and the Ambulatory Index (57). Abnormal CMCT is best correlated with pyramidal tract dysfunction (27, 57, 58): hyperreflexia and brisk finger jerks were best correlated with abnormal CMCT (27); abnormal CMCT for the anterior tibialis muscle was invariably associated with extensor plantar response or increased ankle jerk (57). Further, Jarratt et al. found that the CMCT increased with the increasing Kurtzke pyramidal system scale (21). These reports all suggest that *CMCT testing is an effective method of confirming clinical evidence of upper motor neuron dysfunction.* With regard to muscle strength, weakness was associated with increased CMCT for the muscle examined in the lower but not in the upper extremities (57). Mathers et al. found abnormality of the CMCT for the pelvic floor muscles in 46–80% of patients with sphincter trouble (60).

The CMCT test may be potentially useful as a monitoring device in the treatment of MS. In eight patients with acute relapse who were treated with steroids, Jarratt et al. documented a tendency of the CMCT to improve as the patient improved clinically (21).

Cerebrovascular Diseases

In stroke patients, the whole spectrum of CMCT responses, from complete normality through delay to absence of any cortical response, was found (26, 61–63). Absent or small motor responses to cortical stimulation on the 4th day after ictus in seven patients with CVAs correlated well with an incomplete recovery by the 4th week after stroke (61). Murray stated from his preliminary study that the absence of response to cortical stimulation is a bad prognostic sign, whereas a present though delayed response early in the history of the stroke is associated with a better chance of recovery (26). Bridgers found no cortical motor response in six patients with previous stroke who were not able to generate any voluntary motor activity in the affected abductor pollicis brevis muscle (ABP), whereas motor response was normal in four patients who were able to activate the APB voluntarily (62). In 20 patients with stroke occurring 1–22 months before HVLI electrical stimulation of the biceps and APB muscles, no response was noted in 15 cases; the MEP was absent in one muscle in two patients and delayed in one or both muscles in the remaining three patients. In 32 patients with lacunar syndrome, the mean CMCT and the threshold intensity for eliciting the MEP in the relaxed muscle were significantly increased on the affected side. The CMCT for at least one muscle was prolonged in 18 (56%) cases (64). The CMCT abnormality correlated with pyramidal signs and occurred independently of a specific clinical syndrome or a radiologically confirmed lacunar lesion.

Parkinsonism

Parkinsonism is the only disease in which *the amplitude of the MEP was found to be larger* and the CMCT to be shorter in some patients (Fig. 18.16) (65, 66) Both investigators used magnetic stimulation for the study. Kandler et al. reported that the mean amplitude of the MEP was significantly larger and the CMCT was significantly shorter in 56 patients with parkinsonism (65). Eisen et al. found that the maximum amplitude of MEP was increased for the patient's age in seven of 18 patients with parkinsonism (66). These changes were not related to the duration of disease or patients' ages, but were greater in patients with severe clinical disability (65). Kandler et al. found no significant difference between treated and untreated groups. In 13 patients who were followed after the introduction of treatment, there was no significant change in the CMCT. There was no clinical improvement in bradykinesia or rigidity in this group either, although tremor did improve after treatment. Despite these initial negative results, these measurements may prove to be of clinical value in the monitoring of treatment in more severe cases. Dick et al. reported normal CMCT by HVLI electrical stimulation in three patients with parkinsonism (67).

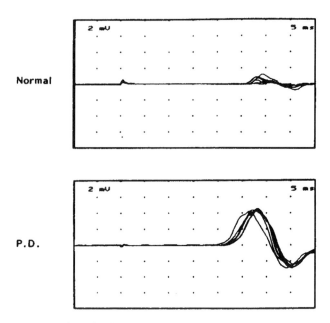

Figure 18.16.   An increased amplitude of the MEPs in a patient with Parkinson's disease (PD) compared with the normal control. Sweep velocity, 5 msec; Sensitivity, 2 mV. Note stimulus artifact of 10 msec after start of sweep. (From Kandler RH, Jarratt JA, Sagar HJ, Cumpert EJW, Venables GS, Davies-Jones GAS. Abnormalities of central motor conduction in Parkinson's disease. J Neurol Sci 1990;100:96.)

Degenerative Cerebellar Ataxic Disorders

Friedreich's ataxia is characterized by early onset of ataxia, autosomal recessive inheritance, pes cavus, absent reflexes, Babinski toe responses, loss of proprioception, scoliosis, and cardiomyopathy. Early-onset cerebellar ataxia (EOCA) is different from Friedreich's ataxia in the preservation of reflexes, absence of cardiomyopathy or scoliosis, and better prognosis (68). Late-onset autosomal dominant cerebellar ataxia (LOCA) is often pathologically associated with olivopontocerebellar atrophy and clinically with pyramidal signs, ophthalmoplegia, dementia, and myoclonus.

The highest incidence of prolonged CMCT was observed in Friedreich's ataxia (82% of 11 cases compared with 60% of 10 cases of EOCA, and 38% of 13 cases of LOCA). When amplitude abnormality was included, the CMCT test was abnormal in 91% of patients with Friedreich's ataxia, 70% with EOCA, and 38% with LOCA (69). These abnormalities were indistinguishable from those encountered in multiple sclerosis or motor neuron disease. One striking feature in Friedreich's ataxia was the much greater duration and apparent temporal dispersion of responses to cortical stimulation compared with the other two groups. The degree of abnormal CMCT was related to the duration of disease and the severity of disability in Friedreich's ataxia and EOCA. The high incidence of abnormal CMCT in Friedreich's ataxia is consistent with the invariable degeneration of pyramidal tract in this disorder. This change is marked enough for the authors to counsel against making a diagnosis of Friedreich's ataxia in a patient with a normal CMCT.

Amyotrophic Lateral Sclerosis (ALS)

A wide spectrum of CMCT findings was noted in this disease: normal through prolonged CMCT to absent responses (Table 18.6; Figs. 18.17 and 18.18) (55, 70–72). The frequency of CMCT abnormalities varied from 0–98% (55, 73). The CMCT changes, when present, were not different from those in multiple sclerosis, although a higher incidence of absent responses to brain stimulation was reported by Murray (26). Barker et al. reported normal CMCT from the cortex to the cervical and lumbar regions in five

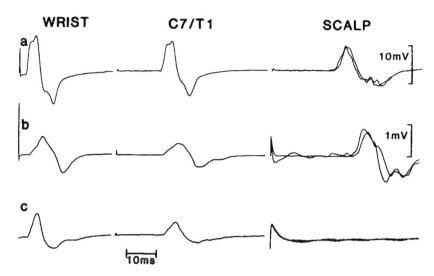

Figure 18.17. MEPs from the ADQ in normal individuals (***a***) and in patients with amyotrophic lateral sclerosis (***b***) and (***c***). Electrical stimulation at the wrist and the C7–T1 interspace. Magnetic stimulation over the scalp. All calibration marks represent 10 mV except the scalp response in (***b***). CMCT in (***a***) is 5.6 msec and is prolonged (11.3 msec) in (***b***), whereas (***c***) shows absent response to scalp stimulation. (From Murray NMF. Magnetic stimulation of the brain: clinical applications. In: Chokroverty S, ed. Magnetic stimulation in clinical neurophysiology. Boston, Butterworth: 1990:219.)

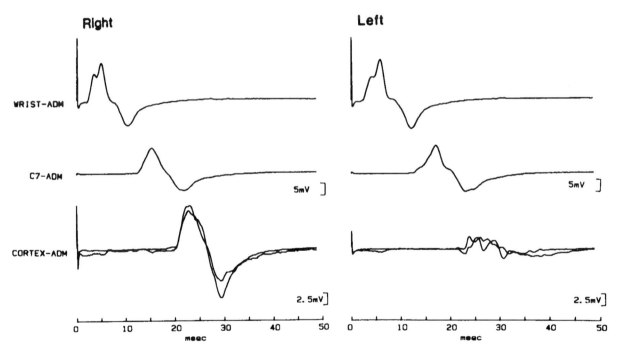

Figure 18.18. A reduced MEP amplitude from the abductor digiti minimi (ADM) muscle in a patient with ALS. CMCT is normal bilaterally (right, 7.3 msec; left, 8.1 msec), but cortical response is small on the left. (From Murray NMF. Magnetic stimulation of cortex: clinical applications. J Clin Neurophysiol 1991;8:71.)

patients with ALS (55). Chiappa and Cros found an abnormal CMCT in 25% of 20 cases: prolonged CMCT in one and no response in four (74). In a larger series of 22 patients, the CMCT to the ADQ muscle was abnormal in 14 patients (64%) and involved 52% of the 42 sides tested: absent response in seven patients and prolonged CMCT in nine patients. In one-half the cases with delayed responses, there were also pathologically small amplitudes (70). A fairly weak correlation was found between abnormal CMCT and brisk finger jerks. Of 11 patients with ALS, Berardelli et al. found absent response or delayed CMCT in eight cases by TC and transcervical HVLI electrical stimulation (72). In 58% of 12 cases, Ingram and Swash, using HVLI electrical stimulation of the cortex and spinal cord, found slowing of CMCT, most marked in the spinal cord, which correlated well with the clinical features of corticospinal involvement (75). They found it more difficult to excite motor pathways in the central nervous system in patients with motor neuron disease than in control subjects. In 40 patients, Eisen et al. reported abnormality in 98% of cases: absent response or prolonged CMCT in 93% and low amplitude (< 15% of the CMAP) in 5% (73). The high incidence of abnormalities in Eisen et al.'s series is due partly to recording from three muscles, the APB, extensor digitorum communis (EDC), and biceps muscles. Hugon et al. reported prolonged CMCT using electrical cortical stimulation in all of 13 patients with motor neuron disease, even those without clinical pyramidal signs (71). In all of 12 patients with severe pseudobulbar palsy, Eisen et al. found that the MEP response was absent, but in other forms of ALS, an MEP was elicted in at least one muscle (73). Some investigators have suggested that the CMCT study can be used reliably to detect physiological abnormalities in the central motor pathways early in the course of motor neuron disease when the EMG study is not yet definite (71, 73, 75). However, this view is not shared by Chiappa and Cros, who found no case in which pathological central motor conduction studies revealed upper motor neuron pathway involvement that was not suspected clinically (74).

Cervical Spondylotic Myelopathy

A prolonged CMCT with recording electrodes in the ADQ muscle was observed in 11 (55%) of 20 examined limbs and only in patients with cord compression at or above the C4–C5 disc interspace (76). On the other hand, normal CMCT was observed in three examined limbs with no compression and in 10 limbs with root compression. Analyzed in terms of patients rather than limbs, 65% of patients with cord compression had an abnormality on one or both sides. These findings suggest that the magnetic stimulation test is of value in identifying a cord compression as well as in identifying the level of compression (76). Postoperative studies have shown changes in the CMCT that correlate with the clinical outcome (77).

Hereditary Spastic Paraplegia

In 10 cases of hereditary spastic paraplegia, a characteristic pattern was reported: the CMCT to the lower limb responses was abnormal in all cases, either absent or very small and with modest prolongation, while responses in the upper limbs were normal in eight cases and mildly prolonged in two cases (78). This observation is consistent with the known pathological findings in this disorder. Murray stated that upper limb sparing in this order is in good contrast to multiple sclerosis (59).

HTLV-I Myelopathy

In HTLV-I myelopathy, the CMCT to the lower limbs is usually abnormal, often with sparing of upper limb responses despite clinical abnormality (79).

Lumbar Radiculopathy and Plexopathy

Using the magnetic stimulator over the lumbar spine and recording the response from the anterior tibialis and soleus muscles, a prolonged latency (more than 1 msec in the affected side compared with the normal side) to the appropriate muscle was found in all of four patients with L5 and/or S1 radiculopathy and in one patient with L5 and S1 plexopathy. The CMAP amplitude was reduced in the affected side in three cases (80).

Peripheral Neuropathy

The CMCT was studied in 49 patients with hereditary sensorimotor peripheral neuropathy (HMSN) (78). The CMCT was normal in all 20 cases of HMSN type I and in 12 cases of HMSN type II. In four patients with HMSN type I with extensor plantar responses, there was marked prolongation of CMCT bilaterally, whereas in five of 10 patients with HMSN type II with pyramidal features, the CMCT was abnormal but only mildly prolonged. These results may reflect an associated involvement of the central motor pathways in some patients with HMSN.

This study indicates that central nervous system impairment can be identified by the magnetic stimulation test in patients with peripheral neuropathy. A markedly prolonged CMCT was reported in one patient with demyelinating neuropathy and multiple sclerosis, as expected (81).

In the Guillain-Barré syndrome (GBS), Mills and Murray found that the HVLI electrical stimulator was of considerable value in demonstrating conduction block in the proximal segments of peripheral nerves and roots in 21 patients in the early stages: only one had a CMAP area decrease below the normal limit from the elbow, seven were abnormal from the axilla, and 15 showed a significant decrease in area from the cord (82). Of these 15 patients with GBS showing abnormal changes between the spinal cord and wrist, five had normal NCV and normal duration. In 29 patients with chronic demyelinating neuropathy, Kim and Oh found slowing of the proximal segments in 60% of cases, which was unrecognizable by the conventional nerve conduction study (41). In addition, Kim and Oh found that the conduction block could not be identified by the magnetic stimulation test because of its inherent limitations.

Focal Neuropathy

Theoretically, focal neuropathy of deeply seated nerves that is not easily accessible to conventional electrical stimulation should be identifiable by magnetic stimulation. In fact, Jarratt et al. reported cases of proximal radial nerve and sciatic nerve lesions that showed low CMAP amplitudes (compared with the normal side) from the innervating muscle upon stimulation of the brachial plexus and the lumbar plexus, respectively (21). Unfortunately, normal values for nerve conduction by magnetic stimulation techniques are rather limited for the peripheral nerves.

The most extensive work has been done in Bell's palsy (38). In 15 of 16 patients with this disorder, no response was recorded with TC magnetic stimulation, whereas stylomastoid stimulation induced a low-amplitude response in 11 cases, thereby localizing the lesion to the labyrinthine segment of the facial canal and documenting a conduction block over the geniculate portion of the facial canal, the alleged site of the lesion. In the prediction of the prognosis of Bell's palsy, authors found that magnetic stimulation was not reliable: in two patients with considerable clinical recovery, they detected no response to magnetic stimulation in the presence of normal electrical distal responses.

Functional Weakness

Normal CMCT was reported in three patients with functional weakness, as expected (Fig. 18.19) (83). In this situation, the more important finding was a prolonged CMCT, indicative of organic dysfunction in the central motor pathways and ruling out functional weakness.

Patients with Sphincter Problems

The CMCT study can identify upper motor neuron defects in patients with sphincter problems. Using HVLI electrical stimulation at the cortex and L1 levels with MEPs from the urinary striated sphincter and EAS muscles, Mathers et al. studied the CMCT in 23 patients with multiple sclerosis and sphincter disturbance (60). They found abnormalities in the CMCT in 19 of 21 tested cases: no MEPs in eight, and prolonged CMCT

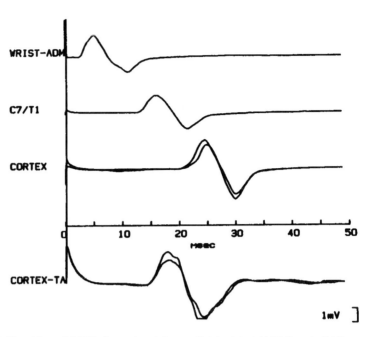

Figure 18.19. Normal MEPs from the abductor digiti minimi (ADM) and tibialis anterior (TA) muscles in a patient with probable functional hemiparesis. (From Murray NMF. Magnetic stimulation of the brain: clinical applications. In: Chokroverty S, ed. Magnetic stimulation in clinical neurophysiology. Boston: Butterworth, 1990:226.)

in 11 patients, confirming that upper motor neuron defects are responsible for the sphincter problems in a majority of these patients. There was no correlation with the severity of upper motor neuron signs in the legs and a prolonged CMCT in these cases. In 16 patients, there was additional evidence of damage to the lower motor neuron pathways. A possible reason for these abnormalities, other than multiple sclerosis, was found in 12 of these cases. Opsomer et al. also reported a prolonged CMCT in a patient with MS and impotence (84).

Magnetic stimulation at the sacral roots can identify lower motor neuron defects in patients with sphincter problems. Opsomer et al. reported a prolonged sacral latency in a patient with partial resection of the presacral nerves for perineal pain associated with bladder cancer (84).

Techniques and Normal Values

Central Motor Conduction Time (CMCT)

Kim and Oh's Method

Kim and Oh measured the CMCT and peripheral nerve conduction by stimulating the cortex, the spinal cord, and the peripheral nerves with a magnetic stimulator while recording the MEPs from the ADQ, APB, abductor hallucis (AH), and extensor digitorum brevis (EDB) muscles (Fig. 18.20–18.24).

POSITION OF SUBJECT: For cortical, cervical, lumbar, and knee stimulation, subjects are placed prone with a soft pillow under the chin. For Erb's point and elbow stimulation, subjects are supine with the arm extended and in approximately 45° abduction from the body.

EMG MACHINE SET-UPS: Filters: 20 Hz–10 KHz. Sweep velocity: 5 msec for the ADQ and APB and 10 msec for the AH and EDB muscles. Sensitivity: start with 0.2 mV. Stimulation rate: one every 3 sec.

RECORDING: For the CMCT from the cortex to the cervical cord, surface recording electrodes are placed on the ADQ (ulnar nerve) and APB (median nerve) muscles following the belly-tendon method. For the CMCT from the cortex to the lumbar cord,

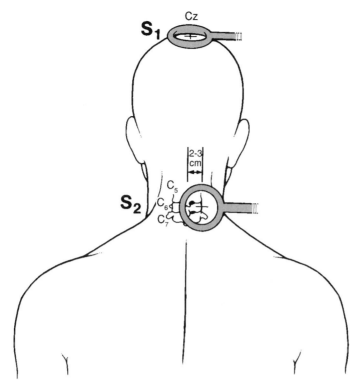

Figure 18.20. Position of the magnetic stimulating coil for the hand muscles. For stimulation on the cortex (S₁), the center of the coil is at C_z. For stimulation on the cervical cord (S₂), the center is 2–3 cm lateral from the midline at the C5–C6 intervertebral space.

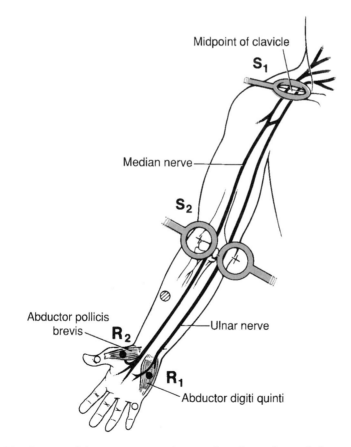

Figure 18.21. Position of the magnetic stimulating coil on the median and ulnar nerves at Erb's point (S₁) and at the elbow (S₂). R₁ represents the recording electrodes in the ADQ and R₂ in the APB muscles.

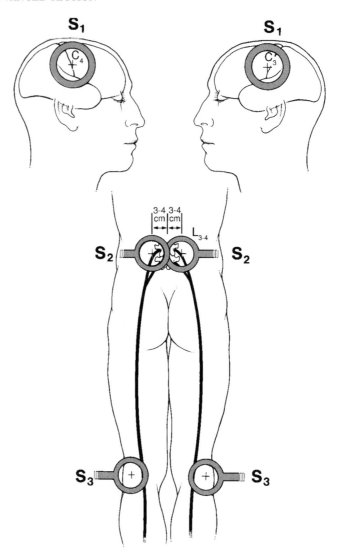

Figure 18.22.   Position of the magnetic stimulating coil for the foot muscles. For stimulation on the cortex (S$_1$), the center of the coil is at C$_3$ (right foot) or C$_4$ (left foot). For stimulation on the lumbar area (S$_2$), the center of the coil is 3–4 cm lateral from the midline at the L3–L4 intervertebral space. S$_3$ represents stimulation of the posterior tibial nerve on the popliteal fossa.

surface recording electrodes are placed on the AH (posterior tibial nerve) and EDB (peroneal nerve) muscles. Two to four recordings should be superimposed.

STIMULATION: The magnetic stimulator with the changing polarity (the Cadwell magnetic stimulator) is used. Cortical stimulation: For the ADQ and APB muscles, the center of the 9-cm coil is placed at C$_z$. For the AH and EDB muscles, the center of the coil is placed at C$_3$ or C$_4$. For cervical stimulation, the center of the coil is placed at the C5–C6 intervertebral space 2–3 cm laterally from the midline toward the side of the recording muscles. For lumbar stimulation, the center of the stimulating coil is placed at the L3–L4 intervertebral space 3–4 cm laterally from the midline toward the side of the recording muscles. For Erb's point stimulation of the median and ulnar nerves, the coil is placed over the supraclavicular area with its center along the upper border of the clavicle. For stimulation of the median and ulnar nerves at the elbow, the edge of the coil is placed over the nerves with its center at the level of the elbow crease. The median and ulnar nerves can often be stimulated simultaneously with the stimulating coil placed between the two nerves at the elbow. For stimulation of the posterior tibial nerve at the knee, the edge of the coil is placed over the posterior tibial nerve in the popliteal fossa with the center of the coil at the level of the posterior fossa crease. For stimulation of the peroneal

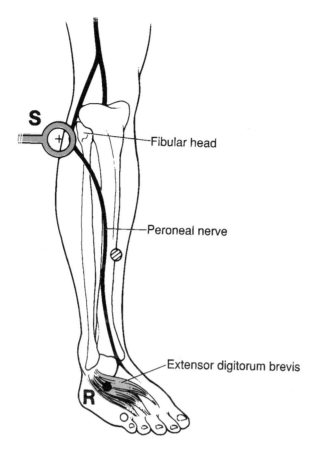

Figure 18.23.　Position of the magnetic stimulating coil for the peroneal nerve at the fibular head.

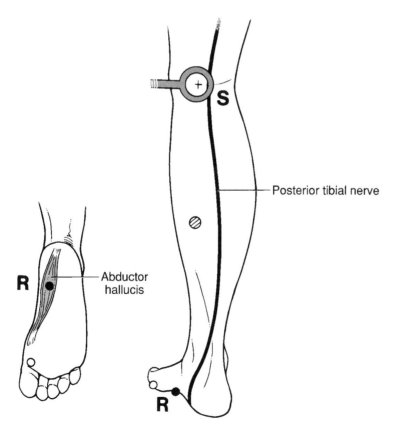

Figure 18.24.　Position of the magnetic stimulating coil for the posterior tibial nerve at the popliteal fossa.

nerve at the knee, the edge of the coil is placed over the peroneal nerve at the fibular head with its center at the level of the fibular head.

MEASUREMENT: Latency is measured from the stimulus onset to the shortest beginning of the initial deflection of the MEP or CMAP. Duration is measured from the beginning of the initial deflection to the end of the last deflection of the MEP or CMAP.

TEMPERATURE: Skin temperature of the elbow and knee is above 32°C.

NORMAL DATA: Number of tests: 60. Number of subjects: 30. Age range: 19–54 yr (Table 18.7).

COMMENTS: In all normal subjects, cortical, lumbar, and peripheral nerve stimulation was possible. However, it was not possible to record MEPs from the ADQ in three cases and from the APB in four cases in cervical stimulation. Latencies to the Erb's point, cervical, and lumbar cord were highly correlated with height. Latencies to the cortex were moderately correlated with height. The CMCT between the cortex and cervical cord was not correlated with height, but the CMCT between the cortex and lumbar cord was weakly correlated with height.

Barker et al.'s Method

Barker et al. measured the CMCT by stimulating the cortex and the spinal cord with a magnetic stimulator while recording the MEP from the ADQ, APB, and AH muscles (36).

POSITION OF SUBJECT: Subjects are usually reclining in a chair.

Table 18.7.
Normal Values of the Latencies and Duration of MEP or CMAP in the EMG Laboratory of the University of Alabama at Birmingham[a]

	Latency (msec)		Duration (msec)	
	Mean ± SD	Normal Limit	Range	Normal Limit
Median nerve				
Elbow	8.01 ± 0.71	9.43	11–30	30
Erb's point	12.74 ± 1.12	14.93	15–30	30
Cervical cord	14.02 ± 1.30	16.62	10–30	30
Cortex	22.94 ± 1.59	26.12	10–30	30
Erb's point-elbow	4.75 ± 0.92	6.59		
CC-Erb's point	1.40 ± 1.30	3.12		
CMCT	8.76 ± 1.30	11.36		
Ulnar nerve				
Elbow	7.11 ± 0.77	8.65	13–30	30
Erb's point	12.49 ± 1.01	14.51	13–30	30
Cervical cord	13.84 ± 1.51	16.86	13–30	30
Cortex	22.19 ± 1.71	25.91	10–30	30
Erb's point-elbow	6.67 ± 0.62	7.91		
CC-Erb's point	1.40 ± 1.30	3.12		
CMCT	8.35 ± 1.35	11.05		
Peroneal nerve				
Popliteal fossa	12.20 ± 1.55	15.30	10–30	30
Lumbar cord	24.28 ± 2.69	29.56	10–30	30
Cortex	43.19 ± 5.08	52.35	10-40	40
LC-popliteal fossa	12.07 ± 2.14	16.35		
CMCT	17.84 ± 4.17	26.18		
Posterior tibial nerve				
Popliteal fossa	13.08 ± 1.59	16.26	10–35	35
Lumbar cord	23.91 ± 2.95	29.81	10–40	40
Cortex	42.12 ± 4.85	51.82	10–50	50
LC-popliteal fossa	10.83 ± 2.51	15.85		
CMCT	18.21 ± 3.63	25.47		

[a]*Abbreviations:* CC, cervical cord. LC, lumbar cord.

RECORDING: The MEP is recorded with surface electrodes from the ADQ and APB muscles in the hand and from the AH muscle in the foot. The MEP is recorded from each muscle in both a relaxed and a slightly contracted state. Several recordings are made.

STIMULATION: For cortical stimulation, the stimulating coil is placed over the head such that a potential of maximal amplitude could be recorded. This is usually achieved with the center of the coil in the region of the vertex (Figs. 18.20 and 18.22). The dominant hemisphere is usually chosen for study.

For cervical stimulation, the stimulating coil is placed just lateral to the lower cervical spine (C7–T1 intervertebral space) as close to the exit foramina as possible (Fig. 18.20).

For lumbar stimulation, the stimulating coil is placed over the lower lumbar area (Figs. 18.22).

MEASUREMENT: Latency is measured to the onset of the initial deflection from the baseline.

NORMAL DATA: Number of subjects: 27. Age range: 21–61 yr.

Measurement	Relaxed state (msec)		Contraction state (msec)	
	Mean ± SD	Normal limit	Mean ± SD	Normal limit
Abductor digiti quinti				
Latency from cortex	22.5 ± 1.5	25.5	20.5 ± 1.7	23.9
Latency from cervical area	13.1 ± 1.1	15.3	13.1 ± 1.1	15.3
CMCT	9.4 ± 1.0	11.4	7.4 ± 1.2	8.8
Abductor pollicis brevis				
Latency from cortex	22.6 ± 1.2	25.0	21.1 ± 1.5	24.1
Latency from cervical area	13.1 ± 1.0	15.1	13.1 ± 1.0	15.1
CMCT	9.5 ± 1.1	11.7	8.0 ± 1.2	10.4
Abductor hallucis				
Latency from cortex	43.3 ± 3.0	49.3	41.2 ± 3.4	48.0
Latency from lumbar area	24.5 ± 2.1	28.7	24.5 ± 2.1	28.7
CMCT	18.8 ± 2.0	22.8	16.7 ± 2.4	21.5

COMMENTS: Authors stated that it was not possible to stimulate the spinal cord at the cervical level. However, by placing the coil just lateral to the spine as close to the exit foramina as possible, potentials corresponding to those obtained during stimulation at the head could be recorded. The CMCT between the latency measurements corresponding to the two stimulation sites was mainly within, but not entirely confined to, the central nervous system.

Ingram et al.'s Method

Ingram et al. measured the CMCT by stimulating the cortex and spinal cord with the magnetic stimulator with the recording electrodes in the biceps brachii, APB, and anterior tibialis muscles (57).

POSITION OF SUBJECT: For cortical and cervical stimulation, subjects remain semirecumbent on a couch, and for lumbar stimulation they are in the left lateral position.

MACHINE SET-UP: Filter band: 3.2 Hz–3.2 KHz.

RECORDING: The MEPs are recorded with surface electrodes from the biceps brachii, APB, and anterior tibialis muscles. At least six recordings are made.

STIMULATION: For cortical stimulation, the stimulating coil is placed over the vertex of the skull (Fig. 18.20). This position is found to be optimal for excitation of upper limb muscles in most subjects. For leg muscles, the optimal site is usually slightly anterior to this position. By inverting the coil, the direction of current flow can be reversed, and this permits preferential stimulation of the opposite cortex. During the stimulation, subjects are asked to make a slight sustained voluntary contraction of at least 5% maximal isometric tension of the tested muscle, which is monitored by the surface EMG signal.

For cervical stimulation, the stimulating coil is placed over the lower cervical vertebral spine (approximately C5–C6) (Fig. 18.20).

For lumbar stimulation, the stimulating coil was placed over the lower lumbar vertebral spine (approximately L4–L5) (Fig. 18.22).

MEASUREMENT: The latency is measured to the onset of the initial negative deflection of the CMAP with the shortest latency.

NORMAL DATA: Number of subjects: Not mentioned. Age range: 24–53 yr.

Measurement	Mean ± SD (msec)	Normal limit (m/sec)
Biceps brachii		
Latency from the cortex	11.6 ± 1.17	13.9
Latency from the C5–C6	5.3 ± 0.42	6.1
CMCT	6.3 ± 1.08	8.5
Right-left difference	0.50 ± 0.34	1.2
Abductor pollicis brevis		
Latency from the cortex	20.6 + 1.21	23.0
Latency from the C5–C6	13.0 ± 0.96	14.9
CMCT	7.6 ± 0.79	9.2
Right-left difference	0.45 ± 0.44	1.3
Anterior tibialis		
Latency from the cortex	27.4 ± 1.56	30.5
Latency from the L4–L5	12.3 ± 1.20	14.7
CMCT	15.0 ± 1.53	18.1
Right-left difference	0.44 ± 0.30	1.0

COMMENTS: According to the authors, simultaneous recordings could be made from these muscles with cortical stimulation in many cases.

Murray's Method

Murray measured the CMCT by stimulating the cortex with a magnetic stimulator and the motor root at C7–T1 with an HVLI electrical stimulator to obtain the CMCT (26, 27).

EMG MACHINE SET-UP: Filter band: 20–2 KHz.

RECORDING: The MEP is recorded from the ADQ muscle with surface electrodes using the belly-tendon method. Four responses are recorded.

STIMULATION: For wrist stimulation of the ulnar nerve, the HVLI electrical stimulator (Digitimer D180) is used.

For C7–T1 stimulation, the HVLI electrical stimulator is used with the cathode placed over the C7–T1 interspace and with the anode 6 cm laterally on the ipsilateral side (Fig. 18.25).

For cortical stimulation, a magnetic stimulator is used with the center of the coil placed on the vertex. For optimum excitation of the left hemisphere, the inducing current travels clockwise when viewed from above; to stimulate the right hemisphere the coil is turned over to reverse the current direction. Magnetic stimuli are given at the vertex at increasing intensities while the patient maintains a slight voluntary abduction of the 5th finger.

MEASUREMENT: The latency is measured to the onset of the initial negative deflection of the MEP with the shortest latency. The amplitude is measured from the baseline to the negative peak of the MEP with the largest amplitude. No attempt is made to obtain maximal MEP from scalp stimulation. The amplitude of the scalp evoked MEP is calculated as a percentage of the amplitude of the MEP from supramaximal wrist stimulation.

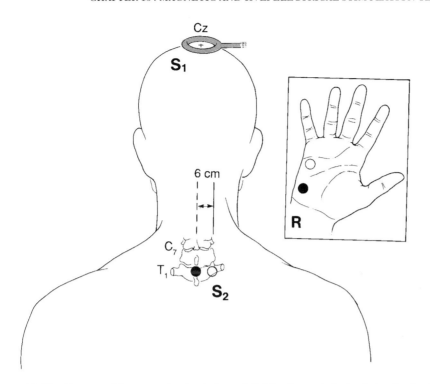

Figure 18.25. Position of the magnetic stimulating coil (S_1) for the cortical stimulation for the ADQ (R) muscle and position of the HVLI ES electrode (S_2) on the cervical cord.

NORMAL DATA: Number of subjects: 32. Number of tests: 36. Age range: 21–78 yr.

Measurement	Mean ± SD	Normal limit	Range
Conduction time to C7–T1 (msec)	13.6 ± 1.4	17.1	10.9–16.9
Conduction time to scalp (msec)	19.7 ± 1.3	23.0	17.5–23.1
Conduction time from wrist to C7–T1 (msec)	11.2 ± 1.2	14.9	8.7–13.8
CMCT (msec)	6.1 ± 0.9	8.4	4.7–7.7
Side-to-side difference in CMCT (msec)	0.7 ± 0.6	2.2	0–1.8[a]
Amplitude as % of amplitude from wrist			18.7–96.6

[a]N = 17

INTERPRETATION: For latency, the level of abnormality is 2.5 SD beyond the mean latency. The criteria for an abnormal side-to-side difference in onset latency is also 2.5 SD beyond the mean. For the scalp amplitude, a level of less than 15% of the wrist amplitude is considered abnormal.

Mills and Murray's Method

Mills and Murray measured the central motor conduction by stimulating the cortex and C7 spinal cord with the HVLI electrical stimulator (11).

POSITION OF SUBJECT: Subjects are tested on an examination couch, sitting at an angle of about 45° with the legs extended.

MACHINE SET-UP: Filter band: 20 Hz–2 KHz.

RECORDING: The MEP is recorded with bipolar surface electrodes (interelectrode distance 3.5 cm) from the forearm flexor muscles.

STIMULATION: The peripheral nerve, the spinal cord, and the cortex are stimulated with the HVLI electrical stimulator (D180 digitimer).

For peripheral nerve stimulation, the nerve is stimulated at the axilla.

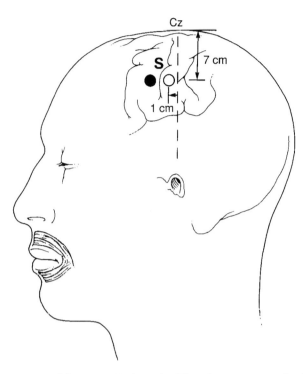

Figure 18.26.   Position of the HVLI ES electrodes (S) on the motor cortex for the arm muscles.

For spinal cord stimulation, the cathode is placed between the C6–C7 vertebrae with the anode 6 cm lateral to the cathode (Fig. 18.25).

For cortical stimulation, the anode is placed over the motor area for the arm, a point 7 cm down the interaural line from the vertex and 1 cm anterior to that line (Fig. 18.26). The cathode is placed 6 cm anterior to the anode. Subjects are asked to relax as fully as possible and then to perform a moderate wrist flexion by lifting a 1-kg weight while a cortical shock is given. No more than five shocks are given on any one side. Voltage is increased until the latency of the response does not change.

MEASUREMENT: Latency is measured to the onset of the initial deflection of the CMAP from the baseline.

NORMAL DATA: Number of subjects: 15. Age range: 19–37 yr.

Measurement	Mean ± SD	Normal limit
Conduction time from the C7 to the axilla (msec)	4.1 ± 0.6	5.3
CMCT from the cortex to the C7 (msec)	4.4 ± 0.8	6.0

COMMENTS: Apparently, this method is not favored any longer. Later studies from the same institution used magnetic stimulation for cortical stimulation (26).

Motor Conduction Velocity in the Spinal Cord

Snooks and Swash described a technique of calculating the motor conduction velocity (MCV) in the spinal cord by stimulating the cervical and lumbar areas with the HVLI electrical stimulator (56).

POSITION OF SUBJECT: The subject lies in the left lateral position.

RECORDING: The MEP is recorded from the pelvic floor muscles, using intra-anal surface electrodes. The intra-anal recording electrode consists of an anal plug electrode (Dantec 13K78) placed in the anal canal adjacent to the EAS muscle, a disposable sphincter electrode (Dantec 13L81), or a pair of electrodes mounted on the tip of a rubber finger stall held digitally in the anal canal against the puborectalis bar (see Fig. 11.93). The latter technique gives a better result.

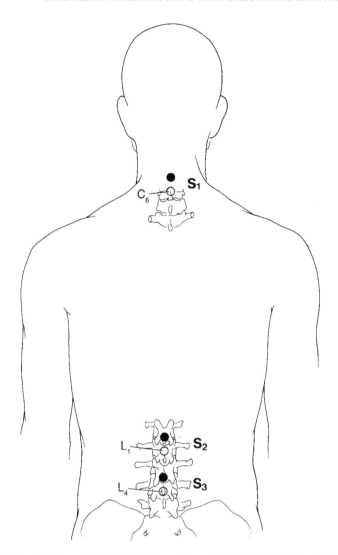

Figure 18.27. Position of the HVLI ES electrodes at the C6 (S$_1$), L1 (S$_2$), and L4 (S$_3$) levels.

STIMULATION: The spinal cord is stimulated with the HVLI electrical stimulator with the anode at the C6, L1, and L4 levels in the midline and the cathode 5 cm cranially (60) (Fig. 18.27).

MEASUREMENT: Latency is measured by the conventional method. Distances between the distant stimulating electrodes between the C6, L1, and L4 levels are measured. The MCVs of the cord (C6–L1) and cauda equina (L1–L4) are determined.

NORMAL DATA: Number of subjects: 21. Age range: 22–75 yr.

Measurement	Mean ± SD (m/sec)	Normal limit (m/sec)
C6–L1 Motor conduction velocity	67.4 ± 9.1	49.2
L1–L4 motor conduction velocity	57.9 ± 10.3	37.3

COMMENTS: The CMAPs recorded after C6 stimulation were more complex than those recorded after L1 and L4 stimulation. Mean MCV in the spinal cord was about 10 m/sec faster than in the cauda equina. Although there was a tendency for MCV to decrease with age in both the spinal cord and the cauda equina, there was no statistical difference. In four patients with MS and one with radiation-induced myelopathy, the spinal cord MCV was slower, though the cauda equina MCV was normal. In one patient with MS with lesions in the brainstem and optic nerve, the spinal cord and cauda equina MCVs were normal. No difference in motor latency was observed following spinal cord or cauda equina stimulation when the stimulus was applied with the anode, or the cathode, placed caudally on the spinal cord (56).

Magnetic Stimulation of the Facial Nerve

Schriefer et al. described a technique of direct transcutaneous stimulation of the intracranial portion of the facial nerve (Fig. 18.28) (38).

EMG MACHINE SET-UP: Filter bands: 20 Hz–2 KHz.

RECORDING: An active surface recording electrode is placed on the superior orbicularis oris and a reference electrode is placed in the midline of the upper lip. If the latency of the subsequently recorded MEP could not be measured with certainty, the position of the reference electrode is altered so as to produce a waveform with a sharp, initially negative deflection.

STIMULATION: For stimulation of the intracranial portion of the facial nerve, the magnetic stimulator is used. The center of the stimulating coil is placed 3 cm posterior and 6 cm lateral to C_z, so that the coil lies ipsilateral to the facial nerve being stimulated. The coil is moved as necessary to produce an optimal response. As viewed from above, a clockwise-inducing current proves preferable for right facial nerve stimulation and a counter-clockwise-inducing current for left facial nerve stimulation. Four responses to supramaximal stimulation are recorded.

For stimulation of the facial nerve at the stylomastoid foramen, an HVLI electrical stimulator (Digitimer D180) is used. The cathode (active electrode) is placed anterior to the mastoid process, and the anode is positioned so as to minimize stimulus artifact and inadvertent masseter stimulation. Two responses to supramaximal electrical stimuli are recorded.

MEASUREMENT: Latency is measured to the onset of the initial negative deflection. Amplitude is measured from the point of the initial negative deflection to the negative peak of the MEP.

TEMPERATURE: Not controlled.

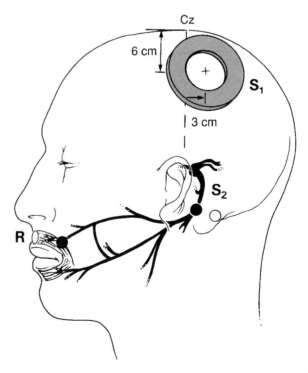

Figure 18.28. Techniques for intracranial magnetic stimulation (S_1; the center of the coil is 3 cm posterior and 6 cm lateral to C_z), and for extracranial HVLI electrical stimulation (S_2) of the facial nerve.

Normal Data: Number of subjects: 15. Number of tests: 30. Age range: 19–60 yr.

Measurement	Latency (msec)		Amplitude (mV)
	Mean ± SD	Normal limit	Range
Styloid stimulation (S)	3.8 ± 0.8	5.4	0.5–2.8
Transcranial stimulation (TC)	5.1 ± 0.8	6.7	0.4–2.2
Intratemporal conduction time (TC-S)	1.3 ± 0.2	1.7	
TC-S amplitude difference			-0.4 to 0.7
Right-left TC-S conduction time difference	0.1 ± 0.1	0.3	
Right-left amplitude difference at S			0–2.8
Right-left amplitude difference at TC			0–1.2

Comments: For TC stimulation, a supramaximal response was obtained by magnetic stimulation at only 50% of its maximal strength. In the majority of cases, the initial stimulation site proved adequate. Occasionally, supramaximal responses were obtained only after the coil had been moved 3–4 cm posterolaterally from its original site. Voluntary contraction of the orbicularis oris during magnetic stimulation produced no changes in the amplitude of the MEP. Authors concluded that the magnetic stimulation of the facial nerve occurred between the root entry zone and the beginning of the facial canal. In 15 of 16 patients with Bell's palsy, no response was recorded with TC magnetic stimulation, whereas stylomastoid stimulation induced low-amplitude responses in 11 cases, localizing the lesion to the labyrinthine segment of the facial canal. In predicting the prognosis of Bell's palsy, the authors found that magnetic stimulation was not reliable.

Magnetic Stimulation of the Phrenic Nerve

Similowski et al. described a technique of phrenic nerve stimulation with the magnetic stimulator (Fig. 18.29) (85).

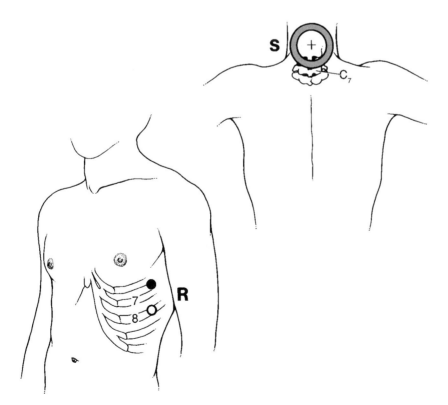

Figure 18.29. Technique for magnetic stimulation of the phrenic nerve. The central hole of the magnetic stimulating coil (S) is at the midline above the C7 spinous process.

POSITION OF SUBJECT: Subjects are studied in a semirecumbent posture, with abdomen unbound and head bent forward, 30° ahead of the vertical plane and, for convenience, the hands over the head.

RECORDING: Active surface electrodes are placed in the 6th and 7th right and left intercostal spaces, approximately on the anterior axillary line, with the reference electrode positioned on the corresponding lower rib. For esophageal recording, an esophageal probe (Dantec 13K63) including two platinum rings (width 3 mm, surface area 19 mm², interval 21 mm) cast in a resin support, is connected to the EMG machine via an isolated cable.

STIMULATION: The magnetic coil is placed on the center back of the neck, parallel to the frontal plane of the subject, with the central hole above the spinous process of the 7th cervical vertebra (C7). In each subject, the intensity of the stimulus and the exact position of the coil are chosen to obtain maximal stimulation.

MEASUREMENT: Latency is measured from the stimulus onset to the onset of initial deflection of the MEP. Amplitude is measured from peak to peak of the MEP.

TEMPERATURE: Not controlled.

NORMAL DATA: Number of subjects: 4. Age range: 24–38 yr.

Measurement	Mean ± SD	Normal limit	Number of subjects
Right phrenic nerve			
Latency (msec)	6.4 ± 0.55	7.5	4
Amplitude (µV)	273.9 ± 79.6		
Left phrenic nerve			
Latency (msec)	7.0 ± 0.72	8.4	4
Amplitude (µV)	233.8 ± 66.1		
Phrenic nerve conduction with esophageal electrodes			
Latency (msec)	7.9 ± 0.73	9.4	3
Amplitude (µV)	752 ± 337		

Motor Evoked Potentials from the Bulbocavernosus Muscle after Transcranial and Lumbar Magnetic Stimulation or HVLI Electrical Stimulation

Ghezzi et al.'s Method

Ghezzi et al. described a technique of obtaining the motor response from the BC muscle with the magnetic stimulation on the cortex and lumbar magnetic stimulation (86).

POSITION OF SUBJECT: Subjects are asked to relax and then to contract the perineal muscles slightly.

EMG MACHINE SET-UP: Filter band: 2–2 KHz. Sensitivity: 200–300 µV.

RECORDING: The MEP is recorded with an active surface electrode from the BC muscle and with a reference electrode at the S1 area. At least eight responses are recorded.

STIMULATION: Cortical stimulation: A magnetic stimulating coil is placed over the vertex, or slightly anterior to it (Fig. 18.20).

Lumbar stimulation: The coil is placed over the L1 spinous process (Fig. 18.22). The intensity of stimulation is increased, starting from 70% of the maximal output of the device. For cortical stimulation, an intensity of 90–100% and a slight contraction of the pelvic floor muscles are necessary. For lumbar stimulation, an intensity of 70–80% of the maximal output is sufficient to obtain a reliable response, and muscle contraction is not necessary.

MEASUREMENT: For cortical stimulation, latency is measured to the first deflection of the potential from the baseline (onset latency) and to the first negative peak (peak latency) of the MEP. For lumbar stimulation, latency is measured to the positive deflection of the MEP. Amplitude is measured from peak to peak.

NORMAL DATA: Number of subjects: 17 males. Age range: 22–80 yr.

Measurement	Mean ± SD	Normal limit
Cortical stimulation		
Onset latency (msec)	22.9 ± 1.8	26.5
Peak latency (msec)	27.7 ± 3.6	34.9
Amplitude (μV)	353 ± 205	
Lumbar stimulation		
Latency (msec)	5.9 ± 0.4	6.7
CMCT (msec)	17.0 ± 2.5	22.0

COMMENTS: The authors stated that the MEP of the BC muscle could be easily recorded with surface electrodes during mild pelvic muscle contractions. Notice that the MEP amplitude was relatively low (86).

Opsomer et al.'s Method

Opsomer et al. measured the CMCT for the EAS and BC muscles by stimulating the cortex and sacral roots with magnetic stimulation (84).

EMG MACHINE SET-UP: Filter band: 1.6–1600 Hz.

RECORDING: The MEPs are recorded with a concentric needle in the right BC and EAS muscles. For cortical stimulation, the MEPs are recorded at rest and during contraction, but for sacral stimulation, the MEPs are obtained at rest. Final MEPs are the average of five recordings.

STIMULATION: For cortical stimulation, the magnetic stimulating coil is placed with the posterior edge of the coil applied 2 cm behind C_z. This is somewhat anterior to the placement of coil in Figure 18.20.

For sacral root stimulation, the center of the coil is placed 3 cm lateral to the spine at the level of the right iliac crest (Fig. 18.30). Stimulation is delivered at a rate of 0.2/sec.

MEASUREMENT: Latency is measured to the onset of the first steady deflection from the baseline.

NORMAL DATA: Number of subjects: 15 males. Age range: 22–60 yr.

Measurement	Bulbocavernosus muscle		External anal sphincter	
	Mean ± SD	Normal limit	Mean ± SD	Normal limit
CMCT from the sacral root (msec)	7.2 ± 1.0	9.2	7.9 ± 2.1	12.1
CMCT from the cortex				
At rest (msec)	28.8 ± 2.6	34.0	30.0 ± 4.4	38.8
With contraction (msec)	22.5 ± 2.7	27.9	22.8 ± 3.6	30.0
CMCT				
At rest (msec)	22.4 ± 1.7	25.8	21.2 ± 4.6	30.4
With contraction (msec)	15.1 ± 3.1	21.3	12.4 ± 2.9	18.2

Mathers et al.'s Method

Mathers et al. described a technique of measuring the CMCT with recording electrodes in the EAS muscle by stimulating the cortex and lumbar cord with an HVLI electrical stimulator (60).

POSITION OF SUBJECT: The subject lies in the flexed left-lateral position.

RECORDING: The MEP is recorded from the EAS using a glove- or anal plug-mounted surface bipolar electrode while the subject is asked to weakly contract the EAS muscle.

STIMULATION: For cortical stimulation, the anode is placed over the vertex in the median sagittal plane (C_z) with the cathode 5 cm anterior to this (Fig. 18.31). For lumbar stimulation, the anode is placed at the L1 level with the cathode 5 cm cranially in the midline (Fig. 18.27).

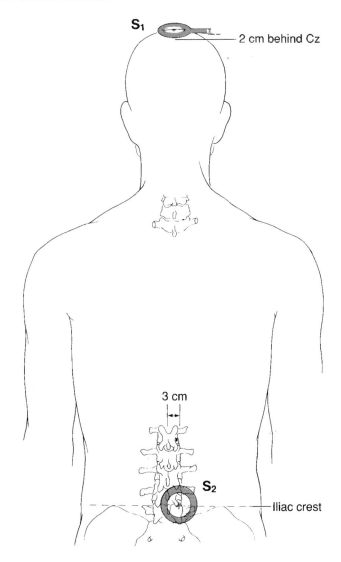

Figure 18.30.   Position of the magnetic stimulating coil at the cortex (S_1) and at the sacral roots (S_2) for the pelvic muscles.

MEASUREMENT: The shortest latency of the MEPs is measured following the conventional method. The CMCT is calculated by subtracting the L1 spinal latency from the cortical latency to the EAS muscle.

TEMPERATURE: Not controlled.

NORMAL DATA: Number of subjects: 5. Age range: ? yr.

Measurement	Mean ± SD	Normal limit
Spinal latency (msec)	4.7 ± 0.4	5.5
Cortical latency (msec)	20.0 ± 3.9	27.8
CMCT (msec)	15.3 ± 3.5	22.3

COMMENTS: In 23 patients with MS and sphincter disturbance, the CMCT was significantly increased compared with normal controls (60).

Ertekin et al.'s Method

Ertekin et al. described a method of measuring the conduction latency with the recording electrodes in the BC and EAS muscles by stimulating the cortex with a HVLI electrical stimulator (54).

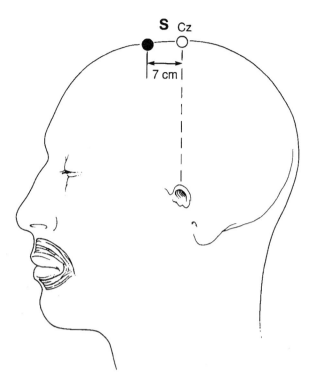

Figure 18.31. Position of the HVLI ES electrode on the motor cortex for the pelvic muscles.

RECORDING: A concentric needle is inserted into the EAS and BC muscles following the standard approach. At least two recordings are made.

STIMULATION: The cortex is stimulated with the anode at C_z and the cathode 7 cm anterior to this (Fig. 18.31). The interval between stimuli varies from 1–3 min. Supramaximal stimulation is given with the patient in a relaxed state.

MEASUREMENT: The shortest latency of the MEPs is measured following the conventional method.

NORMAL DATA: Age range: 23–73 yr.

Measurement	Mean ± SD	Normal limit	Number of subjects
External anal sphincter (msec)	36.1 ± 6.1	48.3	13
Bulbocavernosus (msec)	31.1 ± 3.5	38.1	15

REFERENCES

1. Holliday A. Evoked potentials in clinical testing. Edinburgh: Churchill Livingstone, 1982.
2. Chiappa K. Evoked potentials in clinical medicine. New York: Raven Press, 1983.
3. Penfield W, Jasper H. Epilepsy and the functional anatomy of the human brain. Boston: Little Brown & Co, 1954.
4. Gualtierotti T, Paterson A. Electrical stimulation of the unexposed cerebral cortex. J Physiol 1954;125:278–291.
5. Gates JR. Epilepsy: presurgical evaluation in the era of neurodiagnostic monitoring. In: Gumnit RJ, ed. Advances in neurology. Intensive neurodiagnostic monitoring, vol. 46. New York: Raven Press, 1986.
6. Engel J. Surgical treatment of the epilepsies. New York: Raven Press, 1987.
7. Lesser RP, Lüder H, Klem G, Morris HH, Hahn JF, Wyllie E. Extraoperative cortical functional localization in patients with epilepsy. J Clin Neurophysiol 1987;4:27–53.
8. Merton P, Morton H. Stimulation of the cerebral cortex in the intact human subject. Nature 1980;285:22.
9. Merton P, Morton H. Scope of a technique for electrical stimulation of human brain, spinal cord and muscle. Lancet 1982;2:597–600.
10. Cowan JMA, Dick JPR, Day BL, Rothwell JC, Thompson PD, Narsdeb CD. Abnormalities in central motor pathways conduction in multiple sclerosis. Lancet 1984;2:304–307.
11. Mills KR, Murray NMF. Cortical tract conduction time in multiple sclerosis. Ann Neurol 1985;18:601–605.
12. Barker A, Jalinous R, Freeston I. Non-invasive magnetic stimulation of the human motor cortex. Lancet 1985;1:1106–1107.

13. Mills KR, Murray NMF, Hess C. Magnetic and electrical transcranial brain stimulation: physiological mechanism and clinical applications. Neurosurgery 1987;20:164–168.
14. Chokroverty S. Magnetic stimulation in clinical neurophysiology. Boston: Butterworth, 1990.
15. Patton HD, Amassian VE. Single- and multiple-unit analysis of cortical stage of pyramidal tract action. J Neurophysiol 1954;17:345–363.
16. Patton HD, Amassian VE. The pyramidal tract: its excitation and functions. In: Handbook of physiology/neurophysiology. Washington DC: American Physiology Society, 1960;Sect 1, 11:837–861.
17. Amassian V, Stewart M, Quirk G, Rosenthal J. Physiological basis of motor effects of a transient stimulus to cerebral cortex. Neurosurgery 1987;20:74–93.
18. Adrian E, Moruzzi G. Impulses in the pyramidal tract. J Physiol 1939;388:397–419.
19. Young R, Cracco R. Clinical neurophysiology of conduction in central motor pathways. Ann Neurol 1985;18:606–610.
20. Mills KR, Murray NMF. Electrical stimulation over the human vertebral column: Which neural elements are excited? EEG Clin Neurophysiol 1986;63:582–589.
21. Jarratt J, Barker A, Freeston I, Jalinous R, Kandler R, Jaskolski D. Magnetic stimulation of the human nervous system: clinical applications. In: Chokroverty S, ed. Magnetic stimulation in clinical neurophysiology. Boston: Butterworth, 1990;185–203.
22. Ferrier D. The function of the brain. London: Smith Elder, 1886.
23. Rothwell J, Thompson P, Day B. Motor cortical stimulation in intact man. I. General characteristics of EMG responses in different muscles. Brain 1987;110:1173–1190.
24. Kernel D, Wu C. Responses of the pyramidal tract to stimulation of the baboon's motor cortex. Physiol 1967;191:653–672.
25. Thompson P, Rothwell J, Day B, Dressler D, Maertens de Noordhout A, Marsden C. Mechanisms of electrical and magnetic stimulation of human motor cortex. In: Chokroverty S, ed. Magnetic stimulation in clinical neurophysiology. Boston: Butterworth, 1990;121–143.
26. Murray NMF. Magnetic stimulation of the brain: clinical application. In: Chokroverty S, ed. Magnetic stimulation in clinical neurophysiology. Boston: Butterworth, 1990;205–231.
27. Hess C, Mills KR, Murray NMF, Schriefer T. Magnetic brain stimulation: central motor conduction studies in multiple sclerosis. Ann Neurol 1987;22:744–752.
28. Hess C, Mills KR, Murray NMF. Responses in small hand muscles from magnetic stimulation of the human brain. J Physiol 1987;388:397–419.
29. Day B, Rothwell J, Thompson P. Motor cortex stimulation in intact man. II. Multiple descending volleys. Brain 1987;110:119–120.
30. D'Arsonval A. Dispostitifs pour la mesure des courants alternatifs de toutes fréquences. C R Soc Biol 1896;3:450–451.
31. Thompson S. A physiological effect of an alternating magnetic field. Proc R Soc Lond (Biol), 1910;82:396–398.
32. Bickford R, Fremming B. Neuronal stimulation by pulsed magnetic fields in animals and man. Digest 6th Int Conf Med Electronics Biol Eng, 1965.
33. Cadwell J. Principles of magnetoelectric stimulation. In: Chokroverty S, ed. Magnetic stimulation in clinical neurophysiology. Boston: Butterworth, 1990;13–32.
34. Polson M, Barker A, Freeston I. Stimulation of nerve trunks with time varying magnetic fields (Shieffiel method). Med Biol Eng Comput 1982;20:243–244.
35. Barker A. An introduction to the basic principles of magnetic nerve stimulation. J Clin Neurophysiol 1991;8:26–37.
36. Barker A, Freeston I, Jalinous R, Eng B, Jarratt J. Magnetic stimulation of the human brain and peripheral nervous system: an introduction and the results of an initial clinical evaluation. Neurosurgery 1987;20:100–109.
37. Chokroverty S, Spire JP, DiLullo J, Moody E, Maselli R. Magnetic stimulation of the human peripheral nervous system. In: Chokroverty S, ed. Magnetic stimulation in clinical neurophysiology. Boston: Butterworth, 1990;249–295.
38. Schriefer TN, Mills KR, Murray NMF, Hess CW. Evaluation of proximal facial nerve conduction by transcranial magnetic stimulation. J Neurol Neurosurg Psychiatry 1988;51:60–66.
39. Barker A, Freeston I, Jarratt J, Jalinous R. Magnetic stimulation of the human nervous system: an introduction and basic principles. In: Chokroverty S, ed. Magnetic stimulation in clinical neurophysiology. Boston: Butterworth, 1990;55–72.
40. Evans B. The utility of magnetic stimulation for routine peripheral nerve conduction studies. Muscle Nerve 1988;11:1074–1078.
41. Kim DE, Oh SJ. Proximal slowing in chronic inflammatory demyelinating neuropathy. Muscle Nerve 1990;13:880.
42. Jarratt J. Magnetic stimulation: a new method of investigating the nervous system. Advanced Hospital Technology. December 1990;28–32.
43. Sunwoo IN, Cho HK, Oh SJ. Height, an important factor in the latency of somatosensory evoked potentials. EMG Clin Neurophysiol 1990;30:169–174.
44. Chu N. Motor evoked potentials with magnetic stimulation: correlations with height. EEG Clin Neurophysiol 1989;74:481–485.
45. Kim DE, Oh SJ. Unpublished data.
46. Bridgers S. Magnetic cortical stimulation in stroke patients with hemiparesis. In: Chokroverty S., ed. Magnetic stimulation in clinical neurophysiology. Boston: Butterworth, 1990;233–247.

47. Shields C, Paloheimo M, Backman M, Edmonds HJ, Johnson J. Intraoperative use of transcranial magnetic motor evoked potentials. In: Chokroverty S, ed. Magnetic stimulation in clinical neurophysiology. Boston: Butterworth, 1990;173–184.

48. Goddard G, McIntyre D, Leech C. A permanent change in brain function resulting from daily electrical stimulation. Exp Neurol 1969;25:295–330.

49. Tassinari C, Michlucci R, Forti A, et al. Transcranial magnetic stimulation in epileptic patients; usefulness and safety. Neurology 1990;40:1132–1133.

50. Hufnagel A, Elger C, Durwen H, Böker D, Entzian W. Activation of the epileptic focus by transcranial magnetic stimulation of the human brain. Ann Neurol 1990;27:49–60.

51. Homberg V, Netz J. Generalized seizures induced by transcranial magnetic stimulation of motor cortex. Lancet 1989;2:1223.

52. Kandler R. Safety of transcranial magnetic stimulation. Lancet 1990;1:469.

53. Chiappa KH, Cros D, Cohen D. Magnetic stimulation: determination of coil current flow direction. Neurology 1991;41:1154–1155.

54. Ertekin C, Hansen MV, Larsson LE, Sjödahl R. Examination of the descending pathway to the external anal sphincter and pelvic floor muscles by transcranial cortical stimulation. EEG Clin Neurophysiol 1990;75:500–510.

55. Barker AT, Freeston IL, Jalinous R, Jarratt JA. Clinical evaluation of conduction time measurements in central motor pathways using magnetic stimulation of human brain. Lancet 1986;1:1325–1326.

56. Snooks S, Swash M. Motor conduction velocity in the human spinal cord: slowed conduction in multiple sclerosis. J Neurol Neurosurg Psychiatry 1985;48:1135–1139.

57. Ingram D, Thompson A, Swash M. Central motor conduction in multiple sclerosis: evaluation of abnormalities revealed by transcutaneous magnetic stimulation of the brain. J Neurol Neurosurg Psychiatry 1988;51:487–494.

58. Berardelli A, Inghilleri M, Cruccu G, Fornarelli M. Stimulation of motor tracts in multiple sclerosis. J Neurol Neurosurg Psychiatry 1988;51:677–683.

59. Murray NMF. Magnetic stimulation of cortex: clinical applications. J Clin Neurophysiol 1991;8:66–76.

60. Mathers S, Ingram D, Swash M. Electrophysiology of motor pathways for sphincter control in multiple sclerosis. J Neurol Neurosurg Psychiatry 1990;53:955–960.

61. Kandler RH, Jarratt JA, Gumpert EJW, Davies-Jones GAB, Venables GS, Sagar HJ. Magnetic stimulation as a quantifier of motor disability. J Neurol Neurosurg Psychiatry 1989;52:1205.

62. Bridgers SL. Magnetic cortical stimulation in stroke patients with hemiparesis. In: Chokroverty S. ed. Magnetic stimulation in clinical neurophysiology. Boston: Butterworth, 1990;233–247.

63. Beradelli A, Inghilleri M, Manfred M, Zamponi A, Cecconi V, Dolce G. Cortical and cervical stimulation after hemispheric infarction. J Neurol Neurosurg Psychiatry 1987;50:861–865.

64. Abbruzzese G, Morena M, Dall'Agata D, Abbruzzese M, Favale E. Motor evoked potentials (MEPs) in lacunar syndromes. EEG Clin Neurophysiol 1991;81:202–208.

65. Kandler RH, Jarratt JA, Sagar HJ, Cumpert EJW, Venables GS, Davies-Jones GAS. Abnormalities of central motor conduction in Parkinson's disease. J Neurol Sci 1990;100:94–97.

66. Eisen A, Siejka S, Schulzer M, Calne D. Age-dependent decline in motor evoked potential amplitude, with a comment on changes in Parkinson's disease. EEG Clin Neurophysiol 1991;81:209–215.

67. Dick J, Cowan J, Day B. The corticomotoneuron connection is normal in Parkinson's disease. Nature 1984;310:407–409.

68. Harding AE. The hereditary ataxias and related disorders. London: Churchill Livingstone, 1984.

69. Claus D, Harding AE, Hess CW, Mills KR, Murray NMF, Thomas PK. Central motor conduction in degenerative ataxic disorders: a magnetic stimulation study. J Neurol Neurosurg Psychiatry 1988;51:790–795.

70. Schriefer TN, Hesse CW, Mills KR, Murray NMF. Central motor conduction studies in motor neuron disease using magnetic brain stimulation. EEG Clin Neurophysiol 1989;74:431–437.

71. Hugon J, Lubear M, Tabaraud F, Chazot F, Vallat JM, Dumans M. Central motor conduction in motor neuron disease. Ann Neurol 1987;22:544–546.

72. Berardelli A, Inghilleri M, Formisano R, Accornero N. Stimulation of motor tracts in motor neuron disease. J Neurol Neurosurg Psychiatry 1987;50:732–737.

73. Eisen A, Shybel W, Murphy K, Hoirch M. Cortical magnetic stimulation in amyotrophic lateral sclerosis. Muscle Nerve 1990;13:146–151.

74. Chiappa KH, Cros D. Transcranial magnetic stimulation of the human motor cortex for evaluation of central motor pathways. Neurology Chronicle 1991;1:1–5.

75. Ingram DA, Swash M. Central motor conduction is abnormal in motor neuron disease. J Neurol Neurosurg Psychiatry 1987;50:159–166.

76. Jaskolski DJ, Jarratt JA, Jakubowski J. Clinical evaluation of magnetic stimulation in cervical spondylosis. Br J Neurosurgery 1989;3:541–548.

77. Jaskolski DJ, Laining RJ, Jarratt JA, Jakubowski J. Pre- and postoperative motor conduction times, measured using magnetic stimulation, in patients with cervical spondylosis. Br J Neurosurg 1990;4:187–192.

78. Calus D, Waddy HM, Harding AE, Murray NMF, Thomas PK. Hereditary motor and sensory neuropathies and hereditary spastic paraplegia: a magnetic stimulation study. Ann Neurol 1990;28:43–49.

79. Waddy H, Calus D, Murray NMF, Rudge P. Central motor conduction studies in tropical spastic paraparesis TSP. EEG Clin Neurophysiol 1990;75:S159–160.

80. Chokroverty S, Sachdeo R, Dilullo J, Dovoisin RC. Magnetic stimulation in the diagnosis of lumbosacral radiculopathy. J Neurol Neurosurg Psychiatry 1989;52:767–772.

81. Mills KR, Murray NMF. Neurophysiological evaluation of associated demyelinating peripheral neuropathy and multiple sclerosis: a case report. J Neurol Neurosurg Psychiatry 1986;49:320–323.

82. Mills KR, Murray NMF. Proximal conduction block in early Guillain-Barré syndrome. Lancet 1985;2:659.

83. Schriefer TN, Mills KR, Murray NMF. Magnetic brain stimulation in functional weakness. Muscle Nerve 1987;10:643.

84. Opsomer RJ, Caramia MD, Zarola F, Pesce F, Rossini PM. Neurophysiological evaluation of central-peripheral sensory and motor pudendal fibers. EEG Clin Neurophysiol 1989;74:260–279.

85. Similowski T, Fleury B, Launois S, Cahtahla HP, Bouche P, Derenne JP. Cervical magnetic stimulation: new painless method for bilateral phrenic stimulation in conscious humans. J Appl Physiol 1989;67:1311–1318.

86. Ghezzi A, Callea L, Zffaroni M, Montanini R, Tezzera G. Motor potentials of bulbocavernosus muscle after transcranial and lumbar magnetic stimulation: comparative study with bulbocavernosus reflex and pudendal evoked potentials. J Neurol Neurosurg Psychiatry 1991;54:524–526.

87. Rossini PM, Marciani MG, Caramia M, Roma V, Zarola F. Nervous propagation along "central" motor pathways in intact man: characteristics of motor responses to "bifocal" and "unifocal" spine and scalp non-invasive stimulation. EEG Clin Neurophysiol 1985;61:272–286.

19

Somatosensory Evoked Potentials in Peripheral Nerve Lesions

Somatosensory evoked potentials (SEPs) are the potentials elicited by stimulation of peripheral nerves and recorded at various sites along the sensory pathway. The cortically recorded SEPs are usually impossible to recognize against the continuous background of electroencephalography (EEG) activity because the SEPs are small in amplitude. Therefore, a signal-averaging technique should be used to cancel the randomly occurring "signals" (EEG waves) and to record the summated "time-locked signals," SEPs. To record these small time-locked evoked potentials, the evoked potential system has special components that are quite different from those of the EEG machine (Table 19.1). Because of greater similarities between the evoked potential system and the electromyography (EMG) machine, in recent years many EMG machines have been modified to record the evoked potentials and are available commercially.

Differences Between SEPs and CNAPs

In general, SEPs are smaller in amplitude and longer in latency than compound nerve action potentials (CNAPs) (Table 19.2), but there are more important physiological dif-

Table 19.1.
Evoked Potential System Compared with EEG and EMG Machines[a]

Parameter	Evoked Potential System	EMG Machine	EEG Machine
Stimulator	Yes	Yes	No
Signal averager	Yes	Yes	No
Artifact rejection	Yes	Yes	No
Voltage range	0.1–5 μV	0.5–10 mV	1.0–100 μV
Frequency range	1–5,000 Hz	1–30,000 Hz	0.1–100 Hz

[a]Modified from Oh (116).

447

Table 19.2.
SEPs Versus CNAPs

Parameter	SEPs	CNAPs
Stimulation of nerve	Yes	Yes
Sites of recording	Over the spinal cord and cerebrum	Over the peripheral nerve
Latency	Long: 10–100 msec	1–13 msec
Amplitude	0.1–5 μV	0.5–100 μV
Shape	Early components are constant; shape different on each recording site	Constant (diphasic or triphasic[a]); shape same on each recording site
Specific generator	Some components generated from the recording site but others not	Potential generated from the recording site

[a]Diphasic with surface electrodes and triphasic with the near-nerve technique.

ferences between these two potentials. Basically, the CNAPs are traveling potentials with a constant triphasic or diphasic shape along the peripheral nerve. In contrast, SEPs are characterized by different shapes at different recording sites along the sensory pathway in the central nervous system (CNS) because they are generated from the recording (near-field) site as well as from distant (far-field) areas. Because of the complexity of the generators of SEPs, their shape and polarity are heavily dependent on the recording montage.

Technical Differences Between SEP and CNAP Recordings

Two technical factors distinguish SEP recording from CNAP recording: filter selection and signal averaging.

Filter Selection

The concept of filter selection in EMG is discussed fully in Chapter 3. For the short-latency SEP components (those with latencies of under 25 msec when stimulating an arm and less than 45 msec when stimulating a leg), a wider high-frequency limit is needed. Desmedt et al. (1) observed several distortions in the latencies and amplitudes of the SEPs for the high-frequency limit below 1 KHz, and recommended that the overall system filter range be extended to 3 KHz when studying the early components. In fact, El-Negamy and Sedgwick (2) used a frequency range of 10 Hz to 10 KHz for cervical SEPs. On the other hand, for late components a narrow frequency range can be used, e.g., 1–100 Hz for cortical SEPs. Unlike with sensory or mixed nerve conduction, a change of filter influences the latency of the SEP substantially. Desmedt et al. (1) observed about 4-msec delay in the latency of the N1 component of the cortical SEP with the 100-Hz high filter compared with the 3-KHz filter. This substantial delay is due to the longer latency of the SEP and emphasizes the importance of comparing the patient's result with the normal values collected with the same filter ranges.

Signal Averaging

More extensive signal averaging is used for SEP recording than for sensory or mixed nerve conduction because SEPs are much smaller than CNAPs. For the sensory and mixed nerve conduction, we usually use fewer than 256 signal averagings. On the other hand, 500 averagings are minimal for the median nerve evoked cortical SEPs. The rule of signal averaging is that, *as the averaging proceeds, the signal/noise ratio increases by the square root of the number (N) of times averaged* (Fig. 19.1), or:

$$\frac{\text{Signal}}{\text{Noise}} = \frac{\text{signal amplitude}}{\text{noise amplitude}} \times \sqrt{N}$$

There is only a twofold increase in signal size when the number of responses averaged is increased by a factor of four (e.g., 4000 versus 1000 stimuli). In general, the

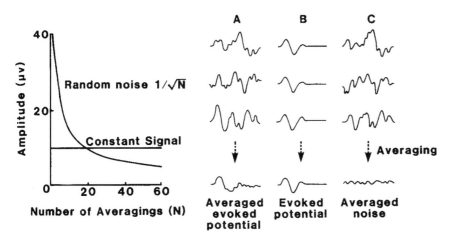

Figure 19.1. Rule of signal averaging. The signal/noise ratio increases by the square root of the number (*N*) of times averaged. (Modified from Picton TW, Hink RF. Evoked potentials: how? what? and why? Am J EEG Technol 1975;14:23.) (132).

more averaging that is done, the better the record will be. Obviously, it is not very helpful to double the number of sweeps above 2000, but it is not unusual to perform averaging beyond 2000 to obtain the SEP in some pathological cases.

Polarity, Nomenclature, and Electrode Montage of SEPs

In clinical neurophysiology it has been traditional to label the downward deflection "positive." This is the case for EEGs and EMGs. For the SEP a majority of laboratories label the downward deflection of the potential "positive," although some laboratories (3, 4) label the upward deflection of the potential "positive." The SEP consists of a sequence of positive and negative components that have been variously designated by different authors. A nomenclature was recently proposed that signifies a component's polarity—positive (P) and negative (N)—and latency in msec (P14, N20). This system has several drawbacks. The same component can have a different polarity depending on the recording montage used. Generally, far-field (subcortical) potentials are positive in polarity when a noncephalic reference is used, whereas these same components have a negative polarity when the reference is on the scalp (5). In addition, use of absolute latencies in terminology can cause confusion with abnormal SEPs since the N20 component in a normal subject may be located at 30 msec.

In this regard, Donchin et al. (6) suggested the use of an overlined latency terminology (e.g., 30 msec to $\overline{N20}$) indicating that, although in this person the latency of the scalp SEP was in fact 30 msec, it corresponded to the normal mean, usually at 20 msec. This system, though imperfect, is widely used at this time and is recommended by the American EEG Society (7). The picture is further complicated by the lack of consensus among authorities regarding electrode montage. To record the short-latency SEP, many have used a noncephalic referential recording method in which the reference electrode is placed over the shoulder, arm, hand, or knee. As discussed in the section on technical factors in nerve conduction, this recording montage has a disadvantage in that EMG and other interference becomes formidable, necessitating the averaging of several thousand potentials. In addition, all components may not be universally recordable in normal subjects. On the other hand, scalp bipolar recordings, in which the reference electrode is placed on the scalp, are technically much easier to achieve. Averaging of 256 or 512 signals is often sufficient. The cephalic reference may produce a cancellation effect, however, so that identification of all the subcortical components is not always possible.

Currently, there is no consensus among authorities regarding the designation of the components of the SEPs and in the recording montage. Thus, it is imperative to indicate the recording montage being employed and to compare the patient's result with the normal data that have been collected using the same technique.

Physiology of SEPs

Short-latency components are remarkably stable within the normal milieu of the laboratory, being unaffected by drowsiness, sleep, or light anesthesia (8, 9). They are, however, affected by deeper anesthesia, especially barbiturates (10). Medium- and long-latency components are much less stable.

The SEP is largely mediated via large-diameter IA sensory fibers in the peripheral nerve and the dorsal column-medial lemniscal system in the CNS (Fig. 19.2). Mixed nerve stimulation evokes a cortical SEP having a latency that is about 5 msec shorter

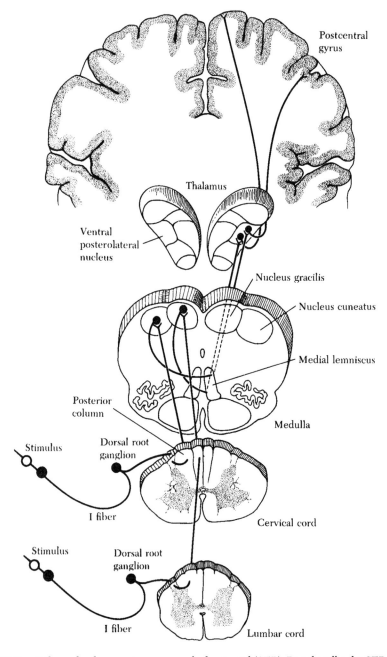

Figure 19.2.   Pathway for the somatosensory evoked potential (SEP). Peripherally, the SEP is mediated by large IA sensory fibers and centrally by the dorsal column-medial lemniscal system.

than that evoked by cutaneous nerve stimulation using comparable stimulation sites (11, 12). The difference is probably due to activity of the faster group I muscle afferents compared with group II cutaneous afferents (11). Various clinical and experimental observations support the finding that the SEP is mediated centrally via the dorsal columns. An abnormal SEP is particularly associated with position sense loss (13–15), and the SEP is markedly attenuated or abolished after experimental selective destruction of these tracts (16). Conversely, isolated segmental dorsal column preservation keeps the SEP intact (16).

Accurate identification of the neural generators of SEP components is paramount for optimal clinical usefulness. For median or ulnar nerve evoked SEPs, the most popular method is to record the response at three locations along the sensory pathway: Erb's point, the lower cervical area, and the contralateral sensory cortex (Fig. 19.3). By using this method, the interwave latency can be measured and a central dysfunction can be differentiated clearly from a peripheral dysfunction. At Erb's point, a typical CNAP is obtained with the initial positive and prominent negative (EP; N9) peaks, indicating that the potential is originating at the recording site (17). In the cervical area, the most commonly used recording montage is to place the active electrode at the lower cervical spine (C7–C4 depending on the laboratory) and the reference electrode at the frontal area (either F_Z or F_{pZ}). With this montage, five negative components may be identified in normal individuals. *The first negative peak (N9) corresponds well with the EP,* reflecting activity in the brachial plexus. *The last negative peak reflects arrival of impulses at the somatosensory cortex (N20).* There are three components that represent the subcortical structures. *The first peak (N11) is a traveling wave within the dorsal columns* (18, 19). *The second peak (N13), the most consistent and prominent component in the cervical SEP, has a fixed generator, reflecting activity in the higher cervical cord. The third negative peak (N14) is another fixed generator, reflecting activity in the medial lemniscus* (3, 18–21). Even in normal individuals, the first (N11) and third peaks (N14) are not consistently obtainable. Thus, the cervical SEP has more often one prominent negative peak (N13). The characteristic cortical SEPs recorded at the somatosensory area (C_3' or C_4', 2 cm behind C_3 or C_4 consist of a primary short-latency

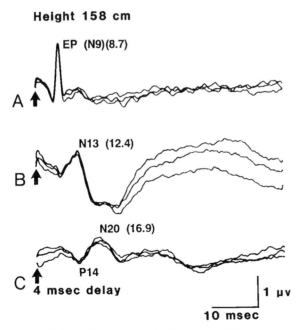

Figure 19.3. Designations of the median nerve evoked SEP in our laboratory. *A*, Erb's CNAP: The most prominent peak is EP (N9). *B*, Cervical SEP: The most prominent peak is N13. *C*, Cortical SEP. The most prominent peak is N20. The numbers in parentheses indicate the latency in a short individual (height, 158 cm).

response and a diffuse secondary long-latency response. The primary short-latency response is characterized by a first positive peak (P14) followed by negative (N20) and positive peaks. *The P14 represents subcortical activity, corresponding well to the third negative cervical SEP component. The N20 and next positive peak are maximally recorded near the primary somatosensory area and are of opposite polarity on either side of the central sulcus (20). They thus represent a dipolar generation in the primary somatosensory cortex.* Chiappa et al. disagree with this view, claiming that these components reflect thalamic activity (22, 23). The primary response is followed by a late response, a series of waves. Unlike the primary response, the secondary response is not highly localized to the sensory cortex. It appears diffusely over most of the ipsilateral and contralateral cortex.

For peroneal and posterior tibial nerve evoked SEPs, the most popular method is to record the response at two locations along the sensory pathway: the lumbar area (LP; N16) and the midline somatosensory cortex (C_Z', 2 cm behind C_Z). By using this method, the interwave latency can be measured and a central dysfunction can be differentiated from a peripheral dysfunction (Fig. 19.4). For the cortical SEP, Cruse et al. (24) recorded a substantially higher amplitude and at times opposite polarity of the SEPs at the hemisphere ipsilateral to the stimulated posterior tibial nerve. An explanation of this *paradoxical lateralization* is that the cortical generators of the evoked potentials to posterior tibial nerve stimulation are located in the mesial surface of the cortex, adjacent to the interhemispheric fissure, and therefore project transversely or parallel (not perpendicular) to the scalp surface. A similar paradoxical lateralization is reported in the peroneal nerve evoked SEP (22). The wave pattern of the peroneal nerve evoked SEP is almost identical to that evoked by median and ulnar nerve stimulation, but the positive peaks are more consistent and better recognizable than the negative peaks in the peroneal SEP. Thus, many laboratories use the positive peaks as the point of reference for the latency measurement. *The presumed neural generators of the various components in the peroneal SEP with the stimulation at the fibular head are also similar to those in the median SEP, P27 reflecting subcortical activity and N30 and P37 reflecting primary somatosensory cortical activity (25).*

The earlier subcortically generated peaks (gracile nucleus and dorsal columns) have recently been recorded using noncephalic references (26) and bipolar cephalic montages (27). However, the peroneal and posterior tibial SEP are notoriously variable in shape even in normal individuals according to our experience. *The most consistently observed components are the first positive peak (P37 or P40) and second positive peak (P60) in the posterior tibial and peroneal SEPs with the stimulation at the ankle (Fig. 19.4).* Thus, the absence of one or more components is not uncommon in peroneal SEPs. A lumbar SEP that has maximum amplitude over the lower thoracic-upper lumbar spine can be recorded by use of either a common (iliac crest) reference or a bipolar (T12–T10) derivative (28–33). The potential is triphasic. The initial negative peak (the cauda potential) is a traveling wave that reflects conduction through the cauda equina

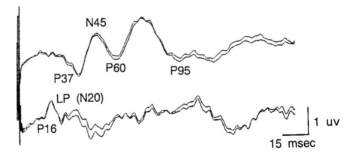

Figure 19.4. Designations of the posterior tibial nerve evoked cortical SEP in our laboratory. LP represents the lumbar potential. P37, P60, and P95 are the cortical potentials. The most constant peaks are P37 and P60.

and root (33). The second negative peak is of larger amplitude and has a fixed latency over the lower thoracic and upper lumbar cord. It represents volume-conducted post-synaptic activity in the dorsal columns. An approximation of spinal transit time can be obtained by calculating the interwave latency between the simultaneously recording lumbar and cortical SEPs.

Evaluation of Sensory or Mixed Nerve Conduction

Sensory or mixed nerve conduction can be evaluated by the SEP technique in three ways: (*a*) measuring the latency and amplitude of Erb's potential; (*b*) measuring the latency between Erb's potential and the cervical SEP; and (*c*) calculating the mixed and sensory nerve conduction velocities (NCVs).

The median and ulnar nerve evoked SEPs record the response at Erb's point, the lower cervical area, and the contralateral sensory cortex. In peripheral nerve lesions distal to Erb's point, the amplitude and latency of the Erb's potential (EP) are abnormal: The amplitude is reduced and the latency is prolonged. In proximal peripheral nerve lesions of sciatic nerve, the amplitude and latency of the lumbar potentials (LP) in the peroneal and posterior tibial SEPs are abnormal: The amplitude is reduced and/or the latency is prolonged.

Mixed and sensory nerve conduction in the extreme proximal segment of peripheral nerves can be evaluated by measuring the interpeak latency between Erb's potential (EP) and the cervical SEP (N13) and between the lumbar potential (LP) and popliteal fossa potentials. Because these segments cannot be evaluated by routine nerve conduction techniques, the SEP technique is definitely useful.

Sensory or mixed NCVs can also be calculated by using the SEP technique. Desmedt and Noel (34) compared sensory NCVs using the conventional method and the SEP method over the finger-axilla segment in normal individuals (Fig. 19.5). They measured the latency to the first positive peak in the CNAP from the axilla with finger stimulation. Using the SEP method, cortical SEPs were recorded after stimulation at the finger and axilla. The latency was measured to the onset and the peak of N1 and also to the peak of the P1 component. Conduction times were calculated by subtracting the axilla-stimulated SEP latency from the finger-stimulated SEP latency. The distance between the finger and the axilla was divided by the conduction time between the two stimulating sites to obtain the NCVs. The latency difference was roughly the same for the onset and the peak of N1 as well as the peak of the P1 component. This is not surprising because the two components are "primary" in nature, as discussed earlier, and fairly well localized to the parietal projection for the contralateral hand. *There was good correlation between the conventional and SEP methods in the calculated sensory NCVs.* Robertson and Lambert (35) also measured sensory NCV in 16 children 3–16 years of age with the SEP method. Using the latencies to the N1 and P1 components, the sensory NCVs for the wrist-elbow segment of the median nerve were in a range of 58–74 m/sec. These figures were compared with a range of 58–70 m/sec for the sensory NCVs obtained by the conventional antidromic method. There was no significant difference between the two techniques. In individual subjects, values obtained with the two techniques differed by 0–9 m/sec when using the N1 component and by 0–11 m/sec when using the P1 component of the cortical SEP. Mean values when using N1 and P1 were not significantly different. Thus, it is possible, by stimulating the different sites along the nerve, to record cortical SEPs, which can be reliably compared and the latency difference of which can be a basis for an evaluation of sensory or mixed NCVs. Most likely the sensory or mixed NCV can be measured by using the cervical as well as the lumbar SEP. No comparable studies have yet been published.

A sizable, often fairly normal-looking SEP can be recorded even when the peripheral sensory or mixed CNAPs are too small and presumably too desynchronized to be recognizable. *The possibility of recording an SEP in the absence of a CNAP is due to central amplification of the incoming peripheral volley* (36). Central amplification is a normally occurring phenomenon that doubles the response when stimulus intensities

Figure 19.5. Evaluation of the maximum peripheral sensory NCV from the latency of the cortical SEP in normal adults. *A* and *B*, Cortical SEPs from the contralateral parietal projection of the hand with stimulation of the median nerve at the fingers (*B*) and the axilla (*A*). The latency of *N1* is indicated. *C*, Averaged CNAP at the axilla while stimulating the fingers. Abscissa: time in milliseconds. The vertical calibration is in microvolts. *D*, Pooled data of the maximum sensory NCV of the median nerve from finger to axilla in 11 normal young adults. This shows the linear relationship between the maximum NCV estimated by the two methods illustrated in *A–C*, i.e., by the conventional method of NCV calculation and by the latency difference of the cortical SEPs. (From Desmedt JE, Noel P. Average cerebral evoked potential in the evaluation of lesions of the sensory nerves and of the central somatosensory pathway. In: Desmedt JE, ed. New developments in EMG and clinical neurophysiology, vol. 2. Basel: Karger, 1973:354.)

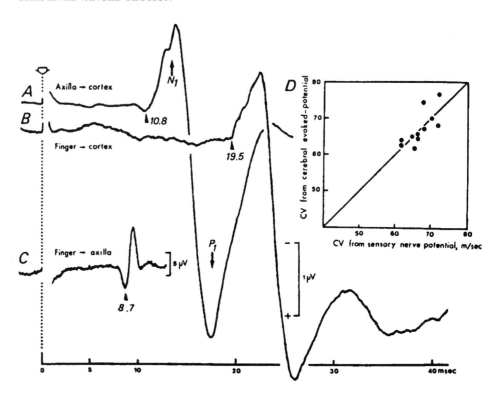

used to evoke SEPs and sensory CNAPs are 50–70% above the threshold. This central amplification phenomenon is unique in the SEP system and renders a technical advantage over the routine sensory and mixed nerve conduction methods in providing quantitative NCVs.

Desmedt (37) described a patient with metachromatic leukodystrophy in whom the CNAP was unobtainable but whose sensory NCV by the SEP technique was 18 m/sec. Robertson and Lambert (35) were also able to measure a mixed NCV of 16 m/sec for the wrist-elbow segment of the median nerve by using the SEP technique in a patient with a diagnosis of Charcot-Marie-Tooth disease. Parry and Aminoff measured the mixed NCV in the wrist-elbow segments by the SEP technique in 15 median or ulnar nerves in eight CIDP patients whose sensory CNAP in the finger-wrist segment was either absent or less than 1 μV (38). In 11 nerves, the mixed NCV was slow; in 10, there was relatively equal slowing in sensory and motor NCVs, whereas in one nerve there was a disproportionate slowing in mixed NCV (CNAPs were absent, and median motor NCV was 11 m/sec). In four nerves, the mixed NCV by the SEP technique was normal despite slowing of motor nerve conduction. Unfortunately, the mixed NCV by the conventional nerve conduction technique was not performed in these cases. Thus, it is possible to calculate mixed or sensory NCVs by the SEP technique in patients with peripheral neuropathy even when the CNAPs are not recordable by the conventional technique. However, there is no advantage in obtaining the quantitative NCV using the SEP in patients in whom peripheral nerve lesions have already been diagnosed by conduction tests on the basis of the absence of the CNAPs. In fact, this method of estimation of the mixed NCV may produce "false normal NCV values" because of the amplification effect of the central nervous system, even when the EP or N13 was not recordable (38). Accordingly, this author does not recommend this method of estimation of the mixed NCV.

SEP Abnormalities in Peripheral Nerve Lesions

Neuropathy without CNS Involvement

Various authors have reported abnormal latencies in cortical SEPs or absent SEPs in cases of neuropathy without CNS involvement (12, 13, 37, 39). These abnormalities are not unexpected in view of the long contribution of peripheral nerves along the pathway of the sensory impulse. The peripheral contribution in the abnormal SEP can easily be detected by Erb's and lumbar potentials. These potentials invariably show abnormalities in diffuse neuropathies. For this reason, it is essential to monitor Erb's and lumbar potentials routinely in the SEP study. Because the diagnosis can be made by a routine nerve conduction study in this group of patients, the SEP study does not provide any additional diagnostic information.

On the other hand, there is a definite advantage of the SEP technique when evaluating proximal neuropathies, e.g., the Guillain-Barré syndrome (GBS), chronic inflammatory demyelinating neuropathy (CIDP), brachial or lumbosacral plexus neuropathies, and diabetic amyotrophy.

In the GBS, four studies have shown conflicting results (Table 19.3). A median SEP abnormality at Erb's point and the cervical cord was documented in 48–91% of cases: absent EP or N13 potentials or prolonged EP–N13 interwave latency (40–43). Ropper and Chiappa detected an SEP abnormality in 75% of cases in the peroneal/posterior tibial SEPs: LP was either absent or the latency to LP was prolonged (42). However, there is no consensus with regard to the diagnostic value of the SEP in comparison with the conventional nerve conduction study including F-wave. Ropper and Chiappa found that the F-wave response was more sensitive than SEPs (42) whereas Walsh et al. found the SEP to be more sensitive (41). Brown and Feasby found an abnormal SEP in 10 cases in contrast to abnormal proximal ulnar motor conduction in 4 and abnormal sensory nerve conduction up to the axilla in one case (40). The F-wave latency was not discussed in Brown and Feasby's cases. In three of Walsh et al.'s patients in whom median nerve conduction was normal, the test in other nerves showed abnormalities (41). From this review, it seems that *there is no advantage of the SEP over an extensive nerve conduction study which includes the F-wave testing in GBS.*

In chronic acquired demyelinating peripheral neuropathy, Parry and Aminoff reported no potential at Erb's point or in the cervical cord in eight cases but a consistent SEP over the contralateral "hand area" of the scalp (38).

In five cases of polyneuropathy with pigmentation, hypertrichosis, edema, and plasma dyscrasia, a prolonged Erb's N9 latency and prolonged N9–N13 interwave latency indicated a proximal neuropathy (44). In all cases, the conventional nerve conduction showed a definite abnormality.

Table 19.3.
SEP Abnormality in GBS

Investigator	SEP Abnormality	NCV/F-Wave Abnormality	Comments
Median nerve evoked SEP			
Walsh et al. (41) (N = 17)	12 (71%)	11 (65%)	Normal median NCS in three; abnormal F-wave and SEP[a]
Brown and Feasby (40) (N = 11)	10 (91%)	6 (60%)[b]	Normal ulnar motor NCS in four
Ropper and Chiappa (42) (N = 21)	10 (48%)	16/18 (89%) F-wave	Abnormal SEP and F-wave in all 10
Ganji and Frazier (43) (N = 11)	9 (82%)		Prolonged EP–N13 latency in 9 Reduced N13 amplitude in all cases Prolonged EP latency in 2
Gilmore and Nelson (117) (N = 19)	10 (53%)	11/16 (84%)	Prolonged EP–P13 in 0 Absent or delayed EP: main abnormality
Peroneal/posterior tibial nerve evoked SEP			
Ropper and Chiappa (42) (N = 12)	9 (75%)		
Gilmore and Nelson (117) (N = 19)	17 (90%)	12 (63%)	Absent or prolonged N22 in 17

[a]In three cases, all tests were normal. In three cases with normal median NCS, there was some other nerve conduction abnormality.
[b]In six of 10 cases with abnormal SEP, slow motor NCV was noted in the Erb's point-axilla segment in the ulnar nerve.

Diabetic subjects without any obvious neurological deficits were found to have a defect in the posterior column of the spinal cord in 19% of juvenile diabetics (45) and in 40% of adult diabetics (46).

In neuropathy associated with chronic renal failure, two studies showed a delay in the EP, N13, and N20 latencies, but no prolongation in the interpeak latencies (47, 48). Studies on patients undergoing dialysis did not show any significant change in the peak or interpeak latencies (48).

Rossi et al. documented a significant increase in the EP-N13 interpeak latency but no defect in the central conduction in nine patients with the Charcot-Marie-Tooth disease (49), while Jones et al. found additional central conduction in about one-third of 14 cases (50).

Peripheral Neuropathies with CNS Involvement

Another area where the SEP is helpful in the diagnostic process is in diseases that involve the peripheral nerves together with the CNS. These diseases include vitamin B_{12} deficiency, Friedreich's ataxia, adrenoleukodystrophy, metachromatic leukodystrophy, Krabbe's disease, and infantile neuroaxonal dystrophy. The SEP method has an advantage in that it evaluates the entire somatosensory pathway, and it is possible to distinguish between lesions located in the peripheral nerve, in the dorsal column pathway, or both.

Three patients with vitamin B_{12} deficiency were studied with SEPs and nerve conduction tests (51). In all three cases, the N20 in the scalp SEP was moderately prolonged, and in two cases, the N9 (EP) was at the upper border of normal. Thus, it was concluded that in two cases there was a slight axonal loss in the peripheral nerve and severe demyelination in the posterior columns of the spinal cord, and in the other case myelopathy was predominant. The nerve conduction study confirmed these findings with regard to the peripheral nerve. Jones et al. studied the median SEP in seven patients with sensory impairments due to vitamin B_{12} deficiency, noting prominent abnormality in the cervical N13 components in all cases and prolonged N9–20 interwave latency in six cases (52). On the other hand, Erb's N9 latency was normal in six cases and the N13–N20 interwave latency was prolonged in four cases. These studies indicate a predominantly central lesion without marked peripheral nerve involvement in vitamin B_{12} deficiency.

In Friedreich's ataxia, Jones et al. (53) studied the SEPs in 22 patients and found these characteristic SEP features: (a) loss of amplitude of peripheral (N9, EP) and cervical (N13) potentials without evidence of markedly delayed peripheral nerve conduction; (b) dispersed and delayed cortical potentials with a prolongation of N20 onset-to-peak separation; and (c) a normal shift in the latency of temporal dispersion, when the stimulus was delivered to the wrist rather than to the elbow (Fig. 19.6). They interpreted this to mean that the major pathological process causing loss of SEP amplitude is the axonal degeneration of the peripheral nerve, whereas the delay and dispersion of N20 is a central effect caused by degeneration of the posterior columns of higher structures. They concluded that the pattern of SEPs in Friedreich's ataxia is sufficiently characteristic to distinguish this condition from: (a) peripheral neuropathy (axonal or demyelinating) without CNS involvement; (b) degenerative diseases of the CNS without peripheral sensory nerve involvement; and (c) multiple sclerosis. In a study of 44 patients with hereditary ataxias, Nuwer et al. concluded that the SEP abnormalities in Friedreich's ataxia are so characteristic that they can be used as a differential tool among the various hereditary ataxic syndromes (54). A single case of Friedreich's ataxia was described by Desmedt and Noel (34), in which sensory CNAPs were absent and the cortical SEPs were delayed in onset latency. The difference in SEP latency with stimulation at the fingers and the axilla was 14–15 msec, which is markedly increased compared with the normal values (approximately 6 msec). In later investigations of six patients (55), the onset latency of the cortical SEP was found to be normal or near-normal, but the initial cortical negative peak (N20) was split into two or three compo-

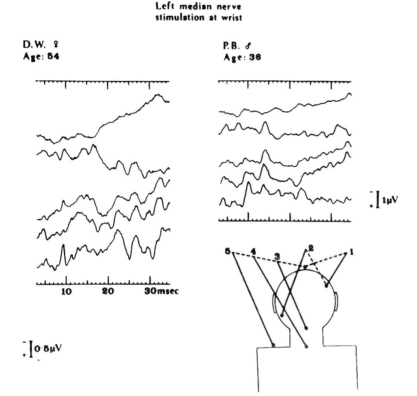

Figure 19.6. SEPs in two patients with Friedreich's ataxia. N9 (EP) and N13 are apparent in both cases, with very low amplitude but normal latency. N14 is present for D.W. (channel 2) but slightly delayed. N20 shows a characteristically delayed peak (just visible at 34 msec for P.B.), although the onset is much less delayed. (From Jones SJ, Baraistser M, Halliday AM. Peripheral and central somatosensory nerve conduction defects in Friedreich's ataxia. J Neurol Neurosurg Psychiatry 1980;43:498.)

nents. These wavelets were present with finger as well as axilla stimulation. They concluded that the pattern of SEP abnormality could not be entirely accounted for by the peripheral neuropathy, and therefore that central conduction must have been delayed also, either in the dorsal columns or elsewhere in the dorsal column/medial lemniscal pathway. These SEP abnormalities are compatible with the pathological findings in this disorder: primary degeneration of the dorsal root ganglia and secondary dorsal column degeneration in the SEP pathway.

In metachromatic leukodystrophy, three SEP studies confirmed peripheral neuropathy as well as central demyelination (37, 56, 57). Desmedt (37) reported a marked delay in latency and low amplitude (0.2 μV) of the cortical SEP in a 2.5-year-old child with metachromatic leukodystrophy. The sensory CNAP was absent in the peripheral nerves, but the sensory NCV by the SEP technique was 18 m/sec, in contrast to 11 m/sec for the median motor NCV. Carlin et al. also reported a prolonged latency to the Erb's potential and a prolonged N13–N20 interwave latency in a case of metachromatic leukodystrophy (56). Markand et al. reported absent or inconsistent response at N9 in two cases and absent responses at N13 and N20 in three cases of metachromatic leukodystrophy (57).

In adrenoleukodystrophy, Vercruyssen et al. reported minimal abnormality at EP in one of five cases, prolonged latency of N13 in four cases, and markedly prolonged latency to N20 in the median SEP and markedly abnormal shape in the posterior tibial SEP in all of five cases (58). Nerve conduction studies showed slow NCV in the peroneal nerve in all five cases.

In giant axonal neuropathy, no recognizable potentials at the EP, N13, or N20 in the median SEP were detected in three cases, indicating possible peripheral and central abnormalities (59).

Compression and Traumatic Lesions of the Peripheral Nerves

There is no need for the SEP test in the diagnosis of most compression neuropathies because the conventional nerve conduction study can identify them and no added information is obtained from the SEP test. Nonetheless, a few of these cases have been studied by the SEP technique. In contrast to the neuropathies, in which the SEP waveform is frequently broadened as well as prolonged in latency, delayed responses with a preserved waveform were described in two cases of carpal tunnel syndrome, the stimuli being delivered to the distal phalanx of the third finger (37). Stimuli delivered to the 5th finger or to the proximal phalanx of the 3rd finger gave rise to cortical SEPs of normal latency, presumably mediated by fibers of the unaffected ulnar and radial nerves. In one patient with a partial ulnar nerve lesion, the motor NCV across the elbow was 32 m/sec, and no CNAP across the elbow was recorded. In this case there was a cortical SEP delay across the elbow.

Synek and Synek showed a prolonged latency of the first cortical negative potential of the lateral femoral cutaneous cortical SEP in five of six patients with meralgia paresthesica (60, 61). Synek and Cowan also reported abnormal saphenous SEP in four cases of intraabdominal femoral neuropathy (60, 62). Ito et al. reported prolongation of the P27–P30 (popliteal fossa-fibular neck stimulation) in all of 11 cases of peroneal nerve palsy at the fibular head and prolongation of the P27–P37 (dorsum of the foot stimulation) in three cases of superficial peroneal neuropathy (63). Dumitru and Marquis reported an attenuation of amplitude in the posterior femoral cutaneous cortical SEP compared with the opposite side in a case of posterior femoral cutaneous neuropathy (64). Dumitru et al. reported prolonged latency and attenuation of amplitude in the medial plantar SEP compared with the normal side in two cases of tarsal tunnel syndrome (65). Tranier et al. found absence of the saphenous cortical SEP in one case and prolonged latency compared with the normal side in three cases of saphenous neuropathy (66).

In metastatic brachial plexus neuropathy, SEP testing can localize the tumor infiltrating the brachial plexus. Synek and Cowan reported absent EP and attenuated, delayed, or absent cervical N13 in the median and ulnar SEPs in two patients with diffuse lesions; they also found absent EP and N13 in the ulnar SEP in two patients with lower trunk lesions (67). According to Synek, median nerve SEPs are most often altered after radiation damage to the brachial plexus (68). This is understandable because radiation-induced brachial plexopathy usually involves the whole plexus, while metastatic brachial plexopathy involves the lower trunk selectively.

There is a need for the SEP study in a few compression or plexus neuropathies in which the conventional nerve conduction study is not able to identify or localize the lesion. This is especially true in the proximal neuropathy involving the legs due to an intraabdominal lesion (61, 62). Synek stated that the SEP study is essential in sciatic nerve lesions because the sensory nerve conduction in the proximal segment of the sciatic nerve is not possible with the conventional technique (68). Synek reported abnormal SEP (latency delay and amplitude reduction compared with the normal side) in the posterior tibial or peroneal SEP in five of seven patients with a proximal sciatic neuropathy, including a case of "pyriformis syndrome" (60, 68). He also reported an abnormal SEP in a patient with "obturator neuropathy" (68).

The SEP technique does have potential value for evaluating the regeneration of sutured nerves. Desmedt (37) demonstrated evidence of regeneration in the hand after traumatic section of the median nerve at the wrist by the presence of delayed SEPs to digital nerve stimulation. There were signs of returning sensation in the distal phalanges of the 2nd and 3rd fingers 5 months after surgical suture of the median nerve, as reflected by a markedly delayed cortical SEP (57.5 msec to the peak of N20) of very small amplitude. No CNAP could be recorded from the median nerve in response to distal stimulation of the 3rd finger. Thus, the cortical SEP provided the sole confirmation of sensory fiber regeneration. Assmus (69) recorded 106 cortical SEPs in 37 patients with sutured median and ulnar nerves during various follow-up periods. The first major positive peak in the late response was the first component of the SEP detected after sensory reinnervation, before the primary potential N20 appeared. At this stage of reinnervation, no CNAP of the peripheral nerve was detected in any patient. A small and delayed primary potential could, in most cases, be detected only when some kind of spatial differentiation was evident. The grade of clinical recovery was paralleled by improvement in the SEP. The authors concluded that this method may be useful in forensic cases for supplying data for the evaluation of patients' claims of sensory loss after nerve suture. Potential value of the SEP in the evaluation of sensory loss in forensic medicine is also discussed by Debecker et al. (70).

Brachial Plexus Injury

The most extensive study of the SEP has been done in brachial plexus injuries. Jones (71, 72) investigated the peripheral, cervical, and cortical SEPs in 26 patients with unilateral traction injuries of the brachial plexus (Fig. 19.7). He stimulated the median nerve at the wrist and recorded the SEPs at Erb's point, C2 and the parietal somatosensory cortex. He stressed the importance of comparison with the intact side. The largest latency difference between the right and left sides was less than 6% of the latency of the earlier response in all three SEPs. The largest amplitude difference between the right and left sides was 40% in N9 (EP), 50% in N13, and 60% in N20 of the amplitude of the larger response. Jones (71, 72) was able to predict the site of a lesion distal or proximal to the dorsal root ganglia with reasonable validity. He predicted a *brachial plexus lesion distal to the dorsal root ganglion when the EP was either absent, more*

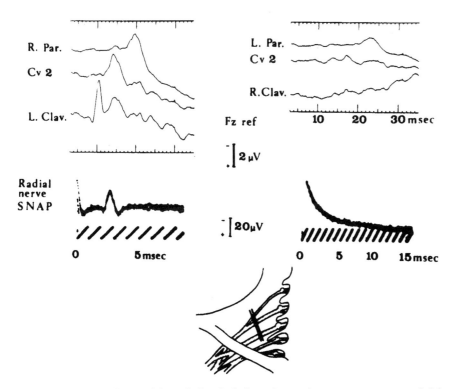

Figure 19.7. Traction lesion of the right brachial plexus (C5–C7) causing attenuation and delay of N13 or N20 but abolition of EP (N9) and radial nerve CNAP. At operation, the upper roots were found to be damaged distal to the dorsal root ganglia, although anatomical continuity was preserved. (From Jones SJ. Somatosensory evoked potentials: the abnormal waveform. In: Halliday AM, ed. Evoked potentials in clinical testing. Edinburgh: Churchill Livingstone, 1982:440.)

attenuated, or equally attenuated compared with the N13 (73). Attenuation of Erb's potential is proportional to the severity of the lesion in the trunk and cord of the brachial plexus (68). He predicted a root lesion, proximal to the dorsal root ganglion, when the EP was normal or less attenuated compared with the N13 (Fig. 19.8). His prediction was correct in eight of 10 surgically confirmed cases. In one case the avulsion was not detectable because of an extensive distal lesion. This distinction is important in traction injuries of the brachial plexus (74) because there is as yet no capacity for restoring axonal continuity between the spinal cord and a root that has been avulsed at the point of entry, whereas with a more distal lesion, regeneration of sensory and motor axons may take place, either spontaneously when anatomical continuity is preserved or aided by surgical reconstruction of ruptured nerves.

Synek and Cowan (75) studied 12 patients with traumatic lesions of the brachial plexus by SEPs upon stimulation of the median, radial, and ulnar nerves at the wrist and recording at the arm, Erb's point, cervical spinal cord, and contralateral cortex. Their findings are essentially the same as those in Jones's study. They stressed that it is important to stimulate nerves having roots near the anatomical site of the lesion as determined clinically and electromyographically, and that *at least two different nerves traversing separate entries to the cervical spinal cord should always be tested.* Synek recommended the following program: for the C8 and T1 roots, the ulnar nerve SEP should be included; for the C7 root, the radial SEP is essential; and for the C5 and C6 roots, the musculocutaneous nerve SEP should be performed in addition to radial nerve stimulation (68). Eisen claimed that it is possible to roughly distinguish the different trunks or cords of the brachial plexus by selecting particular nerves to stimulate, as noted in Table 19.4 (76). This is *extremely helpful* when the needle EMG test is not able to delineate the lesion anatomically, as happens shortly after trauma before fibrillations or positive sharp waves have time to develop.

Zalis et al. (77) and Warren et al. (78) reported normal sensory CNAPs and the absence of cortical SEPs in the presence of total anesthesia in the involved dermatomes in patients with root avulsion; and Rosen et al. (79) reported normal sensory CNAPs

Figure 19.8. C6–T1 root avulsion causing abolition of cervical and cortical SEPs but with EP (N9) preserved. At operation, C5 root was found to be ruptured distal to the dorsal root ganglion but C6–T1 were avulsed from the spinal cord. (From Jones SJ. Somatosensory evoked potentials: the abnormal waveform. In: Halliday AM, ed. Evoked potentials in clinical testing. Edinburgh: Churchill Livingstone, 1982:436.)

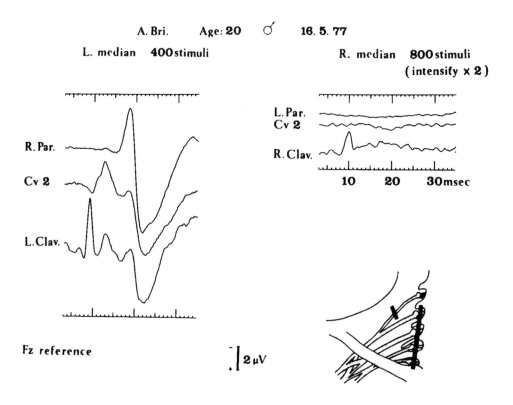

Table 19.4.
Nerves Stimulated to Elicit SEPs in the Evaluation of Brachial Plexopathy

Nerve	Cord	Trunk	Roots
Musculocutaneous	Lateral	Upper	C5, **6**
Radial	Posterior	Middle	C6, **7**, 8
Medial	Lateral	Upper	C6, **7**
	Medial	Lower	**C8**, T1
Ulnar	Medial	Lower	**C8, T1**

and abnormal cervical SEPs. Zverina and Kredba (80) studied seven patients with brachial plexus injuries by recording antidromic CNAPs from the 1st, 2nd, and 5th digits, and cortical SEPs in response to stimulation of the median nerve at the wrist, elbow, and axilla. They concluded that the preservation of antidromic sensory CNAP with absent cortical SEP was a reliable indicator of a root lesion proximal to the dorsal root ganglia. These studies are consistent with Jones's study (32). Thus, the diagnostic value of the SEP in brachial plexus injuries is well proved: *This test is essential in the diagnosis of a root avulsion. Characteristic findings are a normal sensory CNAP and EP in the presence of clinical sensory impairment and markedly abnormal cervical and cortical SEPs.*

Thoracic Outlet Syndrome (TOS)

In 1981, Glover et al. (81) reported abnormal ulnar nerve evoked SEPs in 13 (68.4%) of 19 new cases of thoracic outlet syndrome (TOS). Seven of the nine with abnormal preoperative SEPs had normal repeat studies 2–6 weeks after surgery (Table 19.5). Unfortunately, Glover et al. (81) did not describe the nature of the SEP abnormalities, although their articles seem to indicate that they found abnormal Erb's potentials. This can be tested easily by the routine NCV test using segmental mixed nerve conduction and sensory nerve conduction (see Chapter 21). The latter test has an advantage in that a distal ulnar compression neuropathy can be well ruled out. If the SEP study alone is performed, the abnormality of the EP, as observed in a paper by Glover et al. (81), can be seen in patients with ulnar compression neuropathy at the elbow, which can clinically mimic thoracic outlet syndrome. As discussed in Chapter 21, Glover et al.'s finding is consistent with an absent or a reduced amplitude of the CNAP in the ulnar nerve in patients with cervical rib syndrome (82), which is caused by wallerian degeneration distal to the lesion. Theoretically, there should be a low amplitude in the N13 and a delay in the EP–N13 interwave latency in patients with thoracic outlet syndrome because the most common lesions are located proximal to Erb's point. In fact, our study showed such abnormalities in the SEPs in three patients with neurogenic thoracic outlet syndrome who had neurological abnormalities: lower amplitude of Erb's potential (N10) and cervical SEP (N13) and prolonged interwave (EP–N13) latency. In one case the SEP was absent at all three recording sites. In three patients with nonneurogenic thoracic outlet syndrome, the SEPs were normal.

Yiannikas and Walsh (83) studied SEPs in 12 patients with this disorder. In seven patients with no neurological signs, this test was completely normal. In five patients with neurological signs, two types of abnormalities were observed in the ulnar nerve evoked SEPs: (*a*) a normal Erb's potential and an abnormal or absent cervical SEP, which was observed in two patients (Fig. 19.9); and (*b*) an attenuation and prolongation of the latency of Erb's potential (N9) with the cervical SEP (N13) affected to an equal or a lesser extent and/or an increase in the N13–N9 conduction time (Fig. 19.10). These authors found abnormal SEPs in two patients with normal EMGs and nerve conduction studies, indicating greater sensitivity to the conventional electrophysiological studies.

Since these studies, there have been many reports of SEP abnormalities in TOS (Table 19.5). Two strongly opposing views are apparent from a review of these studies.

Table 19.5.
SEP and Other Electrophysiological Abnormalities in Thoracic Outlet Syndrome

Investigator	No of Cases	SEP	F-Wave	Ulnar Sensory NCS	EMG	Comments
Glover et al. (81)	19	13 (68%) (abnormal N9?)				
Morales-Blanquez and Delwaide (118)	31	No difference from controls				Significantly low ulnar and median sensory CNAP amplitude in patients
Silvola et al. (119)	13	9 (69%) (low amplitude)[a]				Abnormality in median nerve in six, in ulnar nerve in five; low NCV in 2
Yiannikas and Walsh (83)	12	5 (42%)[b]		3	3	
Nonneurogenic	7	0		0	0	
Neurogenic	5	5		3	3	
Jaeertt et al. (120)[c]	18	12 (67%) (low N9 amplitude)	6 (33%)	2	5 (28%)	Abnormal SEP or F-wave in 17 (94%) Prolonged N9–N13 in seven; four had neurogenic TOS
Neurogenic	4	2	2		1	
Chodoroff et al. (121)	14	6 (43%)	1 (7%)	0	1 (7%)	Dynamic maneuver: absent N13 in six; absent N9 in one; normal SEP in anatomic position
Synek (122)	14	9 (64%)[d]				
Nonneurogenic	5	0	0	0	0	
Neurogenic	9	9	0	0	9 (100%)	Normal median SEP; abnormal ulnar SEP
Veilleux et al. (123)[e]	20	3 (15%)[f]	0	4 (20%)	5 (25%)	No cases of neurogenic TOS
Machleder et al. (124)	80	59 (74%)[g]				Abnormal ulnar SEP in anatomic position in 48 Abnormal median SEP in 12
Oh	6	3 (50%)		2	3	
Nonneurogenic	3	0		0	0	
Neurogenic	3	3[h]		2	3	

[a]This is a mixed NCV with stimulation at the elbow in the median nerve and above-the-elbow in the ulnar nerve and with recording at Erb's point.
[b]All had neurogenic TOS.
[c]Four cases of neurogenic TOS.
[d]N9, N13, N20 low amplitude in three; low amplitude and prolonged latency in four; absent in one; absent N9 and low and delayed response in N13 and N20 in one.
[e]No cases of neurogenic TOS.
[f]Reduced N9 amplitude in one; reduced N13 amplitude in one; absent N13 and prolonged N9–12 interpeak latency in one. SEP was normal in all seven patients with nonneurogenic TOS.
[g]N9 amplitude abnormality: either absolute low amplitude or relative low amplitude compared with median or normal side.
[h]Absent SEP in one case; low amplitude and N9 and N13 with prolonged N9–N13 interwave latency in two cases.

Synek maintained that SEP testing is more sensitive than the EMG and nerve conduction study, and it should be included in the assessment of this condition (68). His view is based on his findings that an SEP abnormality was identified in nine (64%) of 14 cases of TOS and a prolonged F-wave latency or abnormal ulnar sensory nerve conduction in one of 14 cases (84). On the other hand, Veilleux et al. took the opposing view that the routine use of ulnar SEPs is of little value in the assessment of patients with TOS (85). Their view is based on their findings that an abnormal SEP was found in only 15% of 20 cases, an abnormal ulnar sensory nerve conduction in 20%, and an abnormal EMG in 25%.

The diagnostic sensitivity of the SEP in TOS was found to range from 15% (85) to 69% (86). Silvola et al. observed a low amplitude of mixed CNAP in the elbow-Erb's point segment of the median nerve and in the above elbow-Erb's point segment of the ulnar nerve in nine (69%) of 13 cases of TOS (86). Their finding is unusual in that abnormal CNAPs were more often observed in median nerve conduction. This is in contrast to other findings that the SEP abnormality is confined to the ulnar nerve evoked SEPs (83, 84). Considering that the SEP abnormality was usually absent in nonneurogenic TOS, the low diagnostic sensitivity in Veilleux et al.'s series is understandable since they did not include any case of neurogenic TOS (85). On the other hand, Jaeertt et al. observed an abnormal SEP in 67% of 18 cases of mostly nonneurogenic TOS (87). The most dramatic SEP abnormality was reported by Chodoroff et al., who observed an absent N13 potential in the dynamic position (abduction and external rotation) of the arm in six patients in whom the anatomic position showed normal SEP findings (88). Though they claimed that there was no change in the amplitude of the N13 potential between the anatomic and dynamic positions among 14 normal controls,

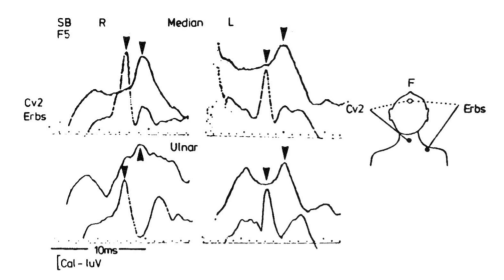

Figure 19.9. SEP upon median and ulnar nerve stimulation in a patient with neurogenic thoracic outlet syndrome. The responses on stimulating the asymptomatic left arm are shown for comparison. When stimulating the ulnar nerve on the symptomatic side, the amplitude of the cervical (N13) SEP is reduced. (From Yiannikas C, Walsh JC. Somatosensory evoked responses in the diagnosis of thoracic outlet syndrome. J Neurol Neurosurg Psychiatry 1983;46:238.)

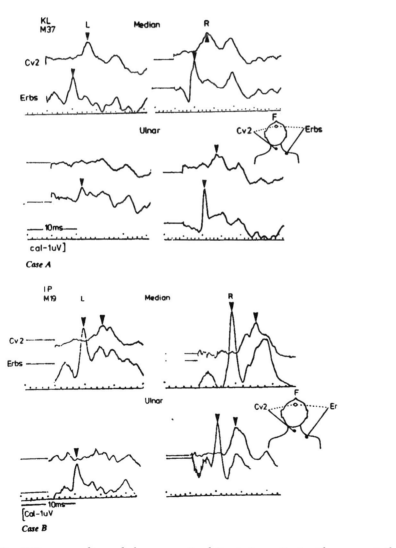

Figure 19.10. SEP upon median and ulnar nerve stimulation in two patients with neurogenic thoracic outlet syndrome. The SEPs upon stimulation of the asymptomatic side are shown for comparison. On stimulation of the ulnar nerve, the cervical SEP (N13) is absent for the affected left arm and EP is reduced in case A. Note the low amplitude of the cervical SEP and normal Erb's CNAP for the affected right arm in case B. (From Yiannikas C, Walsh JC. Somatosensory evoked responses in the diagnosis of thoracic outlet syndrome. J Neurol Neurosurg Psychiatry 1983;46:237.)

Veilleux et al. observed a more than 50% reduction in the amplitude of the N13 potential in four normal controls in the dynamic position. Thus, there is some doubt that the SEP recording in the dynamic position is technically valid. The diagnostic sensitivity of the SEP in TOS seems to vary depending on the frequency of neurogenic TOS among the studies (83, 84, 89). *In nonneurogenic TOS cases, the SEP was not abnormal, while almost all patients with neurogenic TOS showed abnormal SEPs.*

Based on our review, we conclude with the following points:

1. In nonneurogenic TOS, the SEP abnormality is extremely rare;
2. In neurogenic TOS, the SEP abnormality is more common;
3. In neurogenic TOS, the SEP is more diagnostically sensitive than the F-wave or sensory nerve conduction of the ulnar nerve;
4. In TOS, there are two patterns of SEP abnormalities; (*a*) normal EP potential and abnormal N13 potentials or prolonged EP–N13 interwave latency; and (*b*) abnormal EP potentials and N13 potentials with or without EP–N13 interwave latency; and
5. It seems reasonable that the SEP study should be included in the diagnostic assessment of TOS, especially for the neurogenic form.

Intraoperative SEP Test in Brachial Plexus Injuries

Landi et al. (90) used cortical SEP recording and distal CNAP recordings during surgery to evaluate brachial plexus injuries. We have already discussed the value of intraoperative nerve conduction in the repair of a peripheral nerve injury (see Chapter 16). The functional integrity of the root proximal to the stimulating site can be ascertained by adding the SEP study. Landi et al. (90) used this technique during surgery in 15 patients with brachial plexus injuries (Fig. 19.11). They found this test useful in three ways: (*a*) a proximal lesion in the apparently normal looking root can be detected

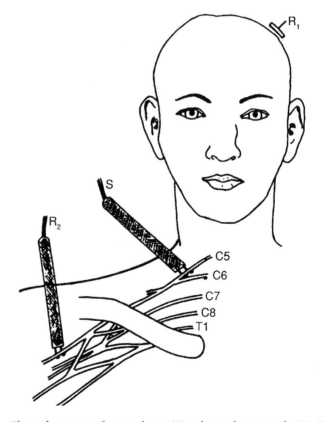

Figure 19.11.   Electrode positions for stimulation (*S*) and recording cortical SEPs (*R1*) and CNAPs (*R2*) intraoperatively. (From Landi SA, Copeland SA, Wynn Parry CB, Jones SJ. The role of somatosensory evoked potentials and nerve conduction studies in the surgical management of brachial plexus injuries. J Bone Joint Surg 1980;62B:403.)

by the absence of the cortical response to stimulation of the proximal stump, which was observed in three patients; (*b*) the presence of a cortical SEP in the apparently damaged roots showed functional continuity, indicating the suitability of the C5 root for grafting and predicting subsequent recovery in other roots; and (*c*) complete root avulsions could be confirmed by the absence of cortical SEPs, thus preventing any further unnecessary dissection. Thus, Landi et al. (90) demonstrated the value of the intraoperative SEP study in the rational surgical management of brachial plexus injury. It should be noted that the absence or presence of the SEPs is judged to be more important than abnormalities of SEP latency or amplitude in this situation. Celli and Rovesta used this technique to determine the integrity of the sensory tract proximal to the root, especially in the intraforaminal area (91). Intraoperative stimulation was accomplished by means of a bipolar stimulating electrode directly on the root with a frequency of 10/sec, an intensity of 7–10 mA (40–60 V), and a duration of 0.1 msec. The scalp SEP was obtained with 100 signal averagings, using a filter range of 2–100 Hz. They normally obtained an initial negative peak at approximately 7–10 msec with an amplitude of 0.3–2 μV.

Van Beek et al. (92) used the SEP system in the operating room during peripheral nerve repair. The cervical SEP and Erb's CNAP are recorded percutaneously after stimulation of the exposed nerve below and above the neuroma. These authors claimed that the technique has an advantage over Kline's technique (see Chapter 16) in that general nerve dissection is not needed. In Kline's technique, the generous separation between the stimulating and recording electrodes is needed to record the CNAP without distortion by the stimulus artifact. He recommended simple neurolysis in the presence of a cervical SEP and Erb's CNAP across the lesion in continuity and neurorrhaphy in the absence of the potentials. We believe that the same information can be obtained before surgery, employing the same technique with an ordinary EMG machine. Thus, the intraoperative SEP recording technique does not seem to provide any advantage over the detailed preoperative CNAP study.

Radiculopathy and Spondylosis

Radiculopathy may be difficult to evaluate by electrophysiological means. The F-wave and needle EMG abnormalities, including those encountered in paraspinal muscles, reflect only dysfunctions of the motor roots. The routine H-reflex abnormalities are limited to diseases of the S1 sensory root. Thus, the SEP may provide valuable information on the physiological status of the sensory roots and aid in the diagnosis of disc disease involving the common cervical and lumbosacral levels, with predominant or even isolated sensory abnormalities. Eisen (5) claimed that a good correlation between the SEP and myelographic and clinical abnormalities (or absence of these) has been demonstrated by "segmental sensory stimulation."

Cortical responses can be evoked by stimulating any accessible cutaneous nerve. In this way, segmental specificity can be achieved, which was not possible by stimulating a mixed nerve trunk such as the median or posterior tibial nerves (5). This is called "segmental sensory stimulation." *According to Eisen's scheme (5), the cutaneous branch of the musculocutaneous nerve, the thumb, adjoining surfaces of the 2nd and 3rd fingers, and the 5th finger are representative of the 5th, 6th, 7th, and 8th cervical dorsal roots, respectively. The saphenous, superficial peroneal, and sural nerves at the ankle are representative of the 4th and 5th lumbar and 1st sacral roots, respectively.* The cutaneous nerve is stimulated at two to three times the sensory threshold at a rate of 3–5/sec. When relating clinical cutaneous sensory deficits to abnormal SEPs, cutaneous stimulation is more relevant than is mixed nerve stimulation, which also excites faster conducting muscle afferents (11). The cutaneous nerves referred to contain relatively few axons compared with a mixed nerve, and many more responses must be summated to record adequate subcortical SEP components (5). The cortical SEP is, however, comparable to that obtained using mixed nerve stimulation requiring the same amount of averaging.

However, the latencies of the different dermatomal SEP components are slightly longer than those of a corresponding SEP evoked by mixed nerve stimulation at a site that is equidistant from the cortex (93). Keep in mind that it is not possible to stimulate a single dermatomal representation in this way because most peripheral cutaneous nerves contain fibers from two or more roots (76).

Another technique to improve the stimulation of a single root is "dermatomal stimulation" (94). According to Scarff et al. (94), the SEP evoked by peripheral nerve stimulation is of little value in the diagnosis of lumbar herniated disc disease. Because of this, they stimulated the L5 or S1 dermatomes: *the median aspect of the foot along the side of the big toe for the L5 dermatome and the lateral aspect of the foot adjacent to the little toe for the S1 dermatome.* They recorded the SEP at the scalp (P_z–F_z) and termed this SEP the dermatomal somatosensory evoked potential. The representative area of skin is stimulated preferably with a large active electrode against a small anode at two to three times the sensory threshold (94). The nerve terminals are of small diameter, relatively few in number, and of variable conduction. Because of this, the volley that is initiated is desynchronized, and the resulting SEP is usually small and dispersed (76). This makes it difficult to measure the latencies and virtually impossible to measure other SEP characteristics.

There are a few isolated case reports of abnormal SEPs in cervical radiculopathy (5, 95). Silvola et al. described one patient with a C6 herniated disc who showed total loss of the N13 in the median cervical SEP (95). Eisen described a patient with a C8 herniated disc who had no recordable N13 when the 5th finger was stimulated, despite a normal peripheral sensory action potential (5). However, a larger series showed abnormal SEP in a few patients with cervical radiculopathy (Table 19.6). The cervical SEP abnormality, when present, consisted of either low amplitude or absence of N13. Ganes found normal cervical SEPs in patients with pure sensory symptoms caused by cervical spondylosis (96). In patients with objective neurological radicular signs, the most conspicuous findings were a reduced amplitude of N13 and an increased N9–N13 latency on the involved side in the median SEP.

Markedly abnormal cervical SEPs are consistently reported in all studies in patients with cervical spondylotic myelopathy (Table 19.6). Though Yu and Jones reported an abnormal median SEP in only 18% of cases (97), a majority of studies showed an abnormal median SEP in more than 69% of patients with cervical spondylotic myelopathy.

Table 19.6.
SEP Abnormality in Cervical Radiculopathy and Spondylotic Myelopathy[a]

Investigator	Diseases	No. of Cases	Abnormal SEP	Comments
Ganes (96)	Cervical radiculopathy without deficit	6	0	Normal median SEP
	Cervical radiculopathy with deficit	12	?	Prolonged EP–N13 with reduced N13 amplitude as a group
	Cervical spondylotic myelopathy	3	2	Prolonged EP–N14 in one; prolonged N13–N20 in one
Silvola et al. (95)	1 disc; 2 CSM; spondylosis 9	12	6	Median SEP: EP–N13 delay in one; absent N13 in one; Reduced amplitude in the remainders
El-Negamy and Sedgwick (99)	Radiculopathy and/or myelopathy	14	10 (71%)	
	Cervical spondylotic myelopathy	10	9 (90%)	Absent N13 in four, low N13/increased EP–N13 in five
	Cervical radiculopathy	4	1	
Tackmann and Radü (125)	Cervical radiculopathy	20	8 (40%)	N13 abnormality in 35% of cases
Oh et al. (98)	Cervical spondylotic myelopathy	20	26 (90%)	N13 abnormality in 74% of cases
Yu and Jones (97)[b]		34	22 (65%)	Median SEP in 18% of cases; ulnar 41%; posterior tibial in 56% of cases
	Radiculopathy	6	2	SEP abnormality is correlated with myelopathy but not with radiculopathy
	Myelopathy alone	15	13 (87%)	
	Radiculopathy/myelopathy	6	5 (83%)	
	Neck pain alone	7	2	
Synek (26)	Cervical radiculopathy	13	1	Median SEP
Perlik (127)[c]	Cervical spondylotic myelopathy	13	13 (100%)	Abnormal median SEP in nine (69%) cases
	Cervical radiculopathy	8	0	

[a]Unless stated, median SEP was performed.
[b]Median, ulnar, and posterior tibial SEPs were performed.
[c]Median and posterior tibial SEPs were performed.

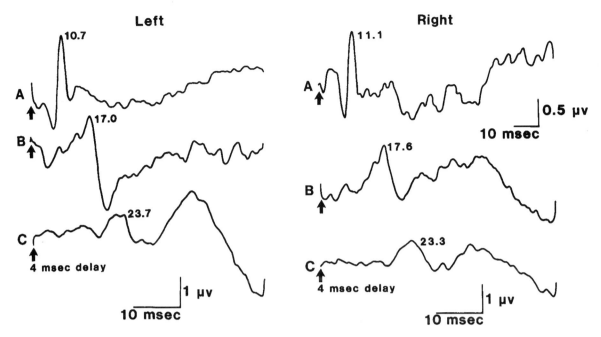

Figure 19.12. The median nerve evoked SEP abnormalities in cervical spondylotic myelopathy. *A*, EP (N9). *B*, Cervical SEP (N13). *C*, Cortical SEP (N20). Left indicates the left median nerve evoked SEPs and right, the right median nerve evoked SEPs. Latencies to EP are normal. EP–N13 interpeak latencies are prolonged bilaterally (normal, 4.3 msec) while N13–N20 interpeak latencies are normal (normal, 7.1 msec). Number at the peak of potentials refers to latency in milliseconds.

The SEP abnormalities are characterized either by a low N13 amplitude with prolonged EP–N13 latency or an absent N13. In a small number of patients with higher cervical lesions, there was prolongation in the N13–N20 (96, 98, 99). Compared with the median SEP, the posterior tibial SEP was abnormal more frequently: In 65–100% of cases of cervical spondylotic myelopathy, P40 was either absent or prolonged in latency. *In short, in cervical spondylotic myelopathy, cervical SEPs are abnormal in most patients, with a prolonged EP–N13 interwave latency and low amplitude of N13 (Fig. 19.12); the posterior tibial SEP is also markedly abnormal in most patients. We have found these tests extremely helpful in differentiating between cervical spondylotic myelopathy and amyotrophic lateral sclerosis* (100).

The diagnostic value of the SEP in lumbar radiculopathy has been studied extensively in the past decade, and the results are confusing. Initially, hope was high on the basis of Feinsold et al.'s report that the peroneal SEP was able to identify all types of lumbar radiculopathy in 100% of 76 cases (101). However, subsequent studies showed extremely confusing results (Table 19.7). It is beyond common sense to believe that the peroneal SEP can identify L4, L5, and S1 radiculopathy in 100% of cases, because the mixed nerve SEP entails multisegmental activation, precluding the detection of abnormality in a single root lesion. Their high rate of abnormality was based on erroneous criteria of abnormality, e.g., the absence of various components in the peroneal SEP. It is not unusual for one component not to be clearly visible, even in normal SEPs. The rate of abnormal peroneal SEPs in lumbar radiculopathy has been found to range from 0% (102) to 100% (103). With the segmental stimulation technique, the rates of abnormal SEPs were 48–70%. These varying rates of abnormality are most likely due to the use of different criteria of SEP abnormality. Many authors have relied on rather liberal criteria of abnormality, such as side-to-side comparison of the latency and amplitude or above-and-below-segment comparison, to increase the diagnostic yield rather than the traditional criteria based on the absolute latency and absence of potentials. This was well illustrated by Aminoff et al. (102), who found a dermatomal SEP abnormality in 32% of cases by the conventional criteria but who would have found abnormal SEPs in

Table 19.7.
Diagnostic Value of SEP in Lumbar Radiculopathy

Investigator	No. of Cases	Stimulation Method	Abnormal SEP	Abnormal EMG	Comments
Scarff et al. (94)[a]	38	Dermatomal SEP	35 (92%)	<50%	
Feinsold et al. (101)[b]	76	Peroneal SEP	76 (100%)		L4 in five cases; L5 in 30; S1 in 32
Eisen et al. (128)[c]	36	Segmental	21 (57%)	27 (75%)	F-wave abnormal in 43% of cases
Cassvan and Park (129)[d]	28	Peroneal SEP	20 (71%)	64%	L5 radiculopathy
Aminoff et al. (130)[e]	28	Peroneal SEP	0 (0%)	21 (75%)	
		Dermatomal SEP	7 (25%)		
Aminoff et al. (102)[f]	19	Dermatomal SEP	6 (32%)		In one, abnormality at different level
		Peroneal SEP	0		58% by Scarff's criteria
Perlik et al. (105)[g]	30	Segmental	21 (70%)	6 (20%)	14 (82%) of 17 cases with definite definite CT abnormality
Seya et al. (131)[h]	21	Segmental	10 (48%)	8/17 (47%)	Spinal SEP abnormality in 48% Scalp SEP abnormality in 19%
Rodriquez et al. (103)[i]	31	Dermatomal SEP	11 (35%)	19 (60%)	
Katifi and Sedgwich (104)[j]	20	Dermatomal SEP	19 (95%)		
Walk et al. (106)[k]	38[l]	Segmental SEP	32 (84%)	11 (29%)[m]	

Criteria of abnormalities:
[a]Side latency difference >3 msec; amplitude <25% of normal side.
[b]Prolonged latency; distortion of the wave shape; absence of various components.
[c]Latency >mean +3SD; amplitude reduction >50% of contralateral SEP or a segment above or below; a poor morphology compared with the contralateral SEP or the SEP above or below segment.
[d]P35 latency >40 msec; >2 msec on the normal side.
[e]DSEP: absent or <25% of the amplitude on the other side. Peroneal SEP: latency difference >3 msec for P30 or 0.6 msec for N11.
[f]DSEP: absent or delayed latency.
[g]Absent P40; latency and difference between two sides >95% confidence normal limit.
[h]Four criteria of abnormality were used.
[i]Absent response.
[j]Five criteria of abnormality were used.
[k]Used Perlik's criteria of abnormality.
[l]Myelogram/CT scan indicative of or consistent with root compression.

58% of cases if Scarff et al.'s looser criteria had been used. Rodriquez found the side-to-side amplitude difference to be too variable as criteria of abnormality (103). Katifi and Sedgwich, who found abnormalities in 95% of cases in the dermatomal SEP, used five different criteria (104).

In comparison with the needle EMG, divergent conclusions were also drawn: three studies showed the needle EMG to be better in identifying a lumbar radiculopathy than the SEP, while three studies showed the opposite results. In this regard, Perlik's series was unique in that the conventional EMG was abnormal in only 20% of cases, an extremely low figure for the needle EMG in lumbar radiculopathy (105). This low figure reflects the absence of patients with clear EMG abnormality from the SEP study according to the later study from the same laboratory (106).

The role of SEP in the diagnosis of lumbar radiculopathy can be summarized as follows:

1. There has been no consensus of opinion regarding the role of the SEP in the diagnosis of lumbar radiculopathy. This is true for both the stimulation technique and the diagnostic sensitivity and is most likely due to the different criteria applied by various investigators.

2. If the strict conventional criteria for SEP abnormalities are used, it seems that the rate of SEP abnormality is relatively small in lumbar radiculopathy and that the SEP study contributes little to the diagnosis of this entity.

In our laboratory, the needle EMG study was able to identify lumbar radiculopathy in 86% of patients with neurological deficits. We did not feel any necessity for additional SEP studies in lumbar radiculopathy. This author concurs with Eisen, on the basis of personal experience, that all methods of eliciting the SEP using segmental sensory stimulation have thus far had a disappointing diagnostic yield in radiculopathies (76). Eisen's viewpoint is remarkable considering that he was the first advocate for the segmental stimulation technique in the workup of radiculopathy and reported abnormal SEPs in 57% of cases in his previous study (5).

Pudendal Somatosensory Evoked Potentials

A cortical SEP can be easily obtained with stimulation of the pudendal nerve. The latency and waveform of the pudendal SEP are remarkably similar to those of the posterior tibial SEP (107, 108). In both tests the first positive peak (P40) response is the easiest to identify, and the amplitude is maximal over the sensory cortex in the midline (C_Z': 2 cm behind C_Z). Haldeman et al. were also able to record the lumbar potentials, although they are of much lower amplitude and much earlier latency than the posterior tibial lumbar potentials (108). As with the posterior tibial SEP, there is a good correlation between height and latency of the P40 response in the pudendal SEP (109).

The similarities in the shapes and latencies of the pudendal and posterior tibial SEPs suggest similar pathways for the neural impulse for both SEPs. Considering the distance between the stimulating and recording electrodes, *the pudendal SEP is clearly slower* than the posterior tibial SEP. Fowler stated that this slowing can be explained by the relative slowing of spinal conduction of the pudental SEP, since the lumbar potential latency is approximately 9 msec in contrast to 20 msec for the posterior tibial lumbar potential (110). On the other hand, Ertekin et al. attributed this slowing to the slower NCV in the fastest afferent nerve fibers of the pudendal nerves (111).

Technical Aspects

The same method of stimulation for the bulbocavernosus reflex (BCR) can be used for the pudendal SEP, but the stimulus intensity required for the pudendal SEP is much less, and a faster rate of stimulation can thus be employed. The recommended stimulus intensity is two to four times that of the sensory threshold, and the recommended stimulation rate ranges from 2–5/sec. The best recording of the pudendal SEP is made in the midline, 2 cm posterior to C_Z. The lumbar potential can be recorded with a recording electrode at the upper lumbar area.

Clinical Aspects

The pudendal SEP is useful in the investigation of impotence and neurogenic bladder when the causes are not known. Impotence of spinal origin is more likely to be confused with impotence of psychogenic origin because it may be possible to stimulate reflex erections although voluntary erections are poor (110). In such cases the pudendal SEP has become an essential test. It has been recommended that the pudendal SEP and the BCR test be performed routinely in the workup for impotence (107, 109, 111, 112). Abnormalities in the BCR or pudendal SEP were found in 66% of 130 patients with erectile dysfunction by Porst et al. (112), in 35% of 17 impotent patients by Haldeman et al. (107), and in 35% of 97 impotent patients by Ertekin et al. (111). A higher diagnostic sensitivity was noted in the pudendal SEP than in the BCR in two studies: Among 246 impotent men in whom both tests were done, the SEP alone was abnormal in 21 patients in Tackmann et al.'s series (109), whereas Ertekin et al. found prolonged BCR in 16% and SEP abnormalities in 21% of 97 patients (111). Ertekin et al. clarified further the indications for the BCR and pudendal SEP. In patients with diabetes mellitus, the BCR showed a higher diagnostic yield; in those with spinal cord lesions, the BCR and pudendal SEP showed an equal diagnostic yield; and for patients with multiple sclerosis or Parkinson's disease, the pudendal SEP was more productive (111).

The pudendal SEP was abnormal in 21–31% of patients with erectile dysfunction (109, 112). In Tackmann et al.'s series, no etiology was found in 40% of patients with abnormal SEP (109). Abnormalities in the pudendal SEP consisted of absent or delayed response (Fig. 19.13). Ertekin et al. (111) compared the peroneal with the pudendal SEP in 29 patients with either known spinal cord lesions or multiple sclerosis and found the same proportion of abnormalities with each response. Whether this observation will

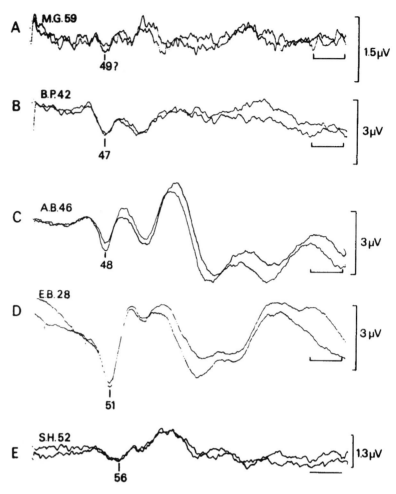

Figure 19.13.   Pudendal SEPs in males. *A* and *B*, Patients 59 and 42 years of age with erectile dysfunction but clinically without neurological symptoms or signs. *C*, Patient aged 46 years, suffering from insulin-dependent diabetes mellitus for 16 years. *D* and *E*, Patients 28 and 52 years old suffering from multiple sclerosis. Figures below or above the first peak of the potentials indicate the latency. (From Tackmann W, Porst H, Van Ahlen H. Bulbocavernosus reflex latencies and somatosensory evoked potentials after pudendal nerve stimulation in the diagnosis of impotence. J Neurol 1988;235:223.)

be true in cases of unknown etiology is not yet settled. Eardley et al. found an abnormal pudendal SEP in 88% of 24 patients with multiple sclerosis and urethrovesical dysfunction, and there was a good correlation between the pudendal SEP abnormality and hyperreflexic bladder (113).

Techniques and Normal Values

Median and Ulnar Nerve Cervical and Cortical SEPs

The technical details and normal values given below are used in the EMG and Evoked Potential Laboratory at the University of Alabama at Birmingham:

Evoked Potential Machine Set-up: Filter frequency: 10 Hz–2 KHz. Sweep time (analysis time): 50 msec. Sensitivity: 25–50 μV. Duration of stimulus: 0.1 msec. Rate of stimulation: 5.5 Hz. Number of averagings: (*a*) 750 for the median nerve at the wrist; (*b*) 1000 for the ulnar nerve at the wrist; (*c*) 1000 or 1500 for digit 3; (*d*) 1500 or 2000 for digit 5.

Recording: Surface recording electrodes are used. For the Erb's potential (EP), an active electrode is placed at the ipsilateral Erb's point and a reference electrode over the ipsilateral ear (A₁ or A₂) (Fig. 19.14). For the cervical SEP, an active recording electrode is placed midline on the cervical 5 (C5) spinous process and a reference electrode over the F_Z. For the cortical SEP, an active recording electrode is placed at the contralateral "hand" area (C_3': 2 cm behind the C_3 or C_4': 2 cm behind the C_4), and a reference electrode is placed at the contralateral ear (A_1 or A_2).

STIMULATION: Stimulating electrodes are placed on either the median or ulnar nerve at the wrist when stimulating the mixed nerve, or on the 3rd or 5th finger when stimulating the pure sensory nerve. Wrist stimulation is done with bar surface electrodes, and digit stimulation is done with ring electrodes. The active stimulating electrode (cathode) is placed proximally. For wrist stimulation, the stimulus intensity is increased to show minimal twitching of the fingers. For finger stimulation, the stimulus intensity is three times the sensory threshold.

TEMPERATURE: Skin temperature at the wrist is above 31°.

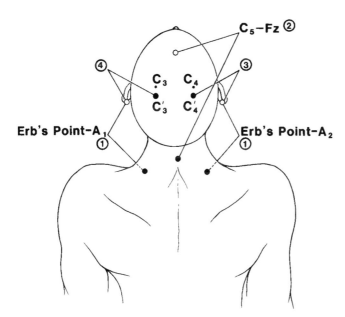

Figure 19.14. Montage of the recording electrode arrangement in the median and ulnar nerve evoked SEPs.

Table 19.8.
Normal Values for Median and Ulnar Nerve Evoked SEPs[a]

Nerve	Latency (msec)			Interpeak Latency (msec)			Amplitude (μV)		
	EP (N9)[b]	N13	N20	EP–N13	N13–N20	EP–N20	EP	N13	N20
Median nerve									
Mean ± SD	9.80 ± 0.62	13.10 ± 0.73	18.64 ± 1.13	3.30 ± 0.39	5.54 ± 0.63	8.85 ± 0.76	4.58 ± 1.82	2.04 ± 0.48	2.34 ± 0.62
Normal limit	11.35	15.13	21.47	4.28	7.12	10.75	0.94	1.08	1.10
Ulnar nerve									
Mean ± SD	10.25 ± 0.78	14.04 ± 1.02	19.02 ± 1.31	3.85 ± 0.34	4.91 ± 0.75	8.70 ± 0.87	1.53 ± 0.78	0.93 ± 0.30	1.00 ± 0.33
Normal limit	12.20	16.59	22.30	4.70	6.77	10.87	0.20	0.33	0.34
Thumb digital nerve									
Mean ± SD	12.31 ± 0.93	15.92 ± 1.09	21.28 ± 1.46	3.60 ± 0.54	5.42 ± 0.71	9.02 ± 0.94	0.96 ± 0.52	0.58 ± 0.23	0.98 ± 0.40
Normal limit	14.64	18.65	24.92	4.96	7.20	11.36	0.20	0.13	0.19
Middle finger digital nerve									
Mean ± SD	12.50 ± 0.94	15.94 ± 1.03	21.50 ± 1.56	3.44 ± 0.55	5.57 ± 0.92	9.00 ± 1.11	0.78 ± 0.38	0.66 ± 0.23	0.86 ± 0.29
Normal limit	14.85	18.51	25.41	4.82	7.88	11.77	0.19	0.20	0.28
Little finger digital nerve									
Mean ± SD	12.93 ± 1.25	16.49 ± 1.32	21.74 ± 1.66	3.55 ± 0.44	5.26 ± 0.73	8.81 ± 0.96	0.41 ± 0.22	0.40 ± 0.14	0.56 ± 0.23
Normal limit	16.05	19.79	25.89	4.66	7.07	10.74	0.04	0.12	0.11

[a]Number = 40. Age range: 20–50 years. Skin temperature: >31°C.
[b]EP (N10), Erb's potential; N13, cervical potential; N20, cortical SEP.

A

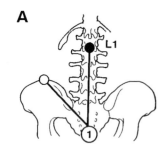

B

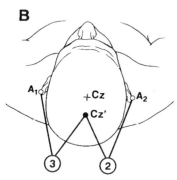

Figure 19.15. Montage of the recording electrode arrangement in the lumbar (**A**) and cortical (**B**) areas in the posterior tibial SEP.

MEASUREMENT: Latency is measured to the negative peak at the Erb's point (EP), to the major negative peak of cervical SEP (N13), and the first major negative peak of the cortical SEP (N20). Then, three interpeak latencies are measured: EP–N13, N13–N20, and EP–N20.

NORMAL DATA: Number of subjects: 40. Age range: 20–50 years.

Table 19.8: Normal Values for Median and Ulnar Nerve Evoked SEPs

Posterior Tibial Nerve Lumbar and Cortical SEPs

The technical details and normal values given below are used in the EMG and Evoked Potential Laboratories at the University of Alabama at Birmingham:

EVOKED POTENTIAL MACHINE SET-UP: Filter frequency: 10 Hz–2 KHz. Sweep time (analysis time): 150 msec. Sensitivity: 50–100 μV (50 μV is recommended if possible). Duration of stimulus: 0.2 msec. Rate of stimulation: 4.5 Hz. Number of averagings: 1000.

RECORDING: Surface recording electrodes are used. For the spinal SEP, an active electrode is placed midline at the L1 spinous process and a reference electrode over the spine at the ipsilateral iliac crest (Fig. 19.15). For the cortical SEP, an active recording electrode is placed at C_z' (2 cm behind the C_z) and a reference electrode at the contralateral ear (A_1 or A_2).

STIMULATION: Stimulating electrodes are placed on the posterior tibial nerve at the ankle. The intensity of the stimulus is increased to show minimal but brisk twitching of the toe flexion.

TEMPERATURE: Skin temperature at the ankle is above 31°.

MEASUREMENT: Latency is measured to the first positive and negative peaks of the lumbar potential (LP; N20), and the first, second, and third positive peaks (P37, P60, and P95) of the scalp SEP. Interpeak latency is measured between LP (N20) and the first positive peak of the scalp SEP (P37) (Fig. 19.4).

NORMAL DATA: Number of subjects: 40. Age range: 20–50 years.

	Latency (msec)		Amplitude (μV)	
Measurement	Mean ± SD	Normal limit	Mean ± SD	Normal limit
Lumbar SEP (LP)				
P16	16.5 ± 1.9	20.2	0.4 ± 0.3	0.1
N20	20.8 ± 1.5	23.8	1.6 ± 5.9	0.2
Cortical SEP				
P37	38.1 ± 2.9	43.9	2.0 ± 1.4	0.4
P60	58.4 ± 3.0	64.4	2.9 ± 2.0	0.7
P95	94.6 ± 7.9	110.4	3.3 ± 2.7	0.8
N20–P37 interpeak latency	17.2 ± 2.4	22.0		

COMMENTS: It is very important to relax the lower back muscles. In obese individuals or individuals whose backs are not relaxed, the lumbar potential is often not obtained. Rarely, the first positive peak (P37) is not clearly identifiable even in normal individuals. In this case, the second positive peak (P60) should be used as the latency measurement.

Pudendal SEP

Tackmann et al.'s Method

Tackmann et al. described a method of obtaining the cortical pudendal SEP in male subjects (109).

EVOKED POTENTIAL MACHINE SET-UP: Filter frequency: 2 Hz–3 kHz. Sensitivity: 20 μV. Averaging: 1024 times. Analysis time: 200 msec. Stimulus duration: 0.2 msec. Stimulus intensity: three times the sensory threshold. Stimulus frequency: 3/sec.

RECORDING: A platinum-iridium needle is inserted subcutaneously on the scalp. An active recording electrode is 2 cm behind C_z, and a reference electrode is on the forehead at F_{pz}.

STIMULATION: The dorsal nerves of the penis are stimulated with a ring electrode around the penis with an anode (reference) at the corona glandis and a cathode (active) electrode 3 cm proximal. Stimulus intensity used for the pudendal SEP is much less than that required for the BCR study (Fig. 19.16). The stimulus intensity is three times the sensory threshold.

MEASUREMENT: Latency is measured to the first positive (P1) and negative (N1) peaks. Amplitude is measured from the P1 peak to N1 peak.

NORMAL DATA: Number of subjects: 30 males. Age range: 17–69 years.

Measurement	Mean ± SD	Normal limit
P1 latency (msec)	41.7 ± 2.8	47.3
N1 latency (msec)	53.1 ± 3.0	59.1
Amplitude (P1–N1) (μV)	2.4 ± 1.3	0.6–5.4

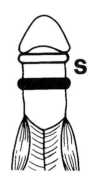

Figure 19.16. Location of the stimulating electrode for the pudendal SEP in males.

COMMENTS: SEPs consisted of 3-4 positive and 3-4 negative components during the first 200 msec. In three of 30 control subjects, the second positive peak was not clearly discernible from the neighboring peaks N1 and N2. The P1–N1 amplitude is too variable to be a dependable parameter for clinical use. P1 and N1 latencies show a linear relationship between the latencies and height (Fig. 19.17).

Vodusek's Method

Vodusek described a method of cortical pudendal SEP in females using an ear-clip electrode for stimulating the pudendal nerve at the clitoris (114).

EVOKED POTENTIAL MACHINE SET-UP: Filter frequency: 8 Hz–3.2 KHz. Signal averaging: 128. Stimulus duration: 0.3 msec. Stimulus intensity: four times the sensory threshold. Stimulus frequency: 1/sec.

RECORDING: Surface electrodes are used to record the cortical SEP. An active recording electrode is placed 2 cm behind the C_Z and a reference electrode at F_Z.

STIMULATION: Ear clip EEG electrodes are attached to the vulva: an active electrode is over the clitoris, and a reference electrode is on the labia major or minora (Fig. 19.18). Good contact should be assured by the use of electrode jelly and the removal of any hair between the electrode and the skin or mucosa.

MEASUREMENT: Latency to the onset of P1 and the peak of P1, N1, and P2 waves. Amplitude is measured from the P1 peak to N1 peak.

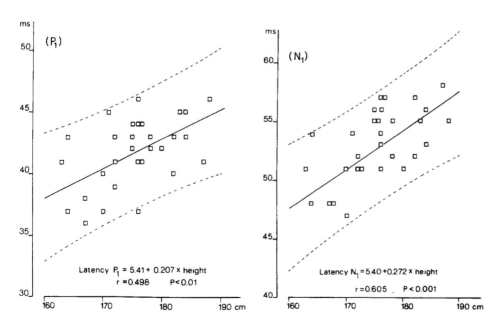

Figure 19.17. Normal P1 and N1 latency in relation to height. Equations for the regression lines are given in each diagram. The *broken lines* indicate the 95% range. (From Tackmann W, Porst H, Van Ahlen H. Bulbocavernosus reflex latencies and somatosensory evoked potentials after pudendal nerve stimulation in the diagnosis of impotence. J Neurol 1988;235:222.)

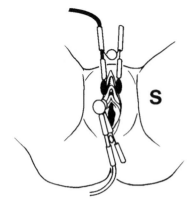

Figure 19.18. Location of stimulating electrodes over the pudendal nerve in the perineum using the ear clip EEG electrodes for the pudendal SEP in females.

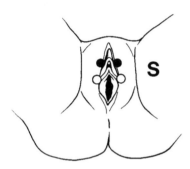

Figure 19.19. Location of stimulating electrodes over the pudendal nerve in the perineum for the pudendal SEP in females.

NORMAL DATA: Number of subjects: 12. Age range: 18–76 years.

Measurement	Mean ± SD	Normal limit	Number of subjects
Onset of P1 (msec)	32.3 ± 2.1	36.5	12
P1 peak (msec)	40.2 ± 2.2	44.6	12
N1 peak (msec)	52.1 ± 3.6	59.3	12
P2 peak (msec)	62.3 ± 2.9	68.1	10

COMMENTS: Instead of a cup electrode adjacent to the clitoris and hand-held surface electrodes on the clitoris, Vodusek used an earclip electrode to minimize embarrassment. He found the application of this "clip" electrode to be easy and quick and thus practical for stimulation of the dorsal clitoral nerve. *We also found this "clip" electrode extremely practical.*

Haldeman et al.'s Method

Haldeman et al. described a method for the pudendal SEP at the L1 level and the cortex (107, 108, 115).

EVOKED POTENTIAL MACHINE SET-UP: Filter frequency: 3 Hz–250 Hz. Signal averaging: 1,000. Stimulus duration: 0.3 msec duration. Frequency of stimulation: 4.7/sec.

RECORDING: Surface recording electrodes are used. For the spinal SEP, an active electrode is placed midline at the L1 vertebral level and a reference electrode over the spine at the L5 level. For the cortical SEP, an active recording electrode is placed 2 cm behind C_z and a reference electrode at FP_z.

STIMULATION: For male subjects the dorsal branch of the penis is stimulated with two ring electrodes placed at the base of the penis approximately 1 cm apart (Fig. 19.16). For female subjects, the clitoral branches of the pudendal nerve are stimulated simultaneously with 5-mm cup electrodes. The active stimulating electrode is placed adjacent to the clitoris, and the reference electrode is placed in the groove between the labia minora and labia majora 2 cm posterior to the active stimulating electrode (Fig. 19.19). The stimulus intensity is increased gradually to above the threshold for sensation but well below the level of discomfort.

MEASUREMENT: Latency is measured to the peak of the major waves. Amplitude is measured from peak to peak. The central conduction time is calculated between the spinal N1 and the cortical P1 latencies.

NORMAL DATA: Number of subjects: 13 males, 7 females. Age range: 20–40 years.

Measurement	Males		Females	
	Mean ± SD	Normal limit	Mean ± SD	Normal limit
Spinal SEP				
N1	12.9 ± 0.8	14.5		
Cortical SEP				
P1	42.3 ± 1.9	46.1	39.8 ± 1.3	42.4
P2	64.9 ± 3.4	71.7	59.4 ± 2.8	65.0
P3	96.6 ± 4.7	106.0	90.1 ± 5.8	101.7
Central conduction time				
N1–P1	30.0 ± 3.2	36.4		

COMMENTS: In overweight subjects it was often difficult or impossible to discern reproducible spinal SEPs. Consistent spinal SEPs could not be recorded in female subjects. The easiest identifiable peaks were the spinal N1 and cortical P1 peaks. Thus, the central conduction time is arbitrarily defined between these two peaks.

REFERENCES

1. Desmedt JE, Brunko E, Debecke J, Carmeliet J. The system bandpass required to avoid distortion of early components when averaging somatosensory evoked potentials. EEG Clin Neurophysiol 1974;37:407–410.

2. El-Negamy E, Sedwick EM. Delayed cervical somatosensory potentials in cervical spondylosis. J Neurol Neurosurg Psychiatry 1979;42:238–241.
3. Kritchevsky M, Wiederholt WC. Short-latency somatosensory evoked potential. Arch Neurol 1978;35:706–711.
4. Starr A. Sensory evoked potentials in clinical disorders of the nervous system. Ann Rev Neurosci 1978;1:103–127.
5. Eisen A. The somatosensory evoked potentials. AAEE Minimonograph #19. Rochester, Minnesota: AAEE, 1982.
6. Donchin E, Callaway E, Cooper R, et al. Publication criteria for studies of evoked potentials (EP) in man: Report of a Committee. In: Desmedt JE, ed. Progress in clinical neurophysiology, vol. 1. Basel, Switzerland: Karger, 1977:9–11.
7. American EEG Society. American EEG Society guidelines for clinical evoked potential studies. J Clin Neurophysiol 1984; 1:3–53.
8. Abrahamian HA, Allison T, Goff WR, et al. Effects of theopental on human cerebral somatic evoked responses. Anesthesiology 1963;24:650–657.
9. Goff, WR, Allison T, Shapiro A, et al. Cerebral somatosensory responses evoked during sleep in man. EEG Clin Neurophysiol 1966;21:1–9.
10. Shaw NA, Cant BR. The effect of pentobarbital on central somatosensory conduction times in the rat. EEG Clin Neurophysiol 1981;51:674–677.
11. Burke D, Skuse NF, Lethlean AK. Cutaneous and muscle afferent components of the cerebral potential evoked by electrical stimulation of human peripheral nerve. EEG Clin Neurophysiol 1981;51:579–588.
12. Eisen A, Ellenke G. Sensory nerve stimulation and evoked cerebral potentials. Neurology 1980;30:1097–1105.
13. Giblin DR. Somatosensory evoked potentials in healthy subjects and in patients with lesions of the nervous system. Ann NY Acad Sci 1964;122:93–142.
14. Halliday AM. Changes in the form of cerebral evoked responses in man associated with various lesions of the nervous system. EEG Clin Neurophysiol 1967;25:178–192.
15. Namerow NS. Somatosensory evoked responses in multiple sclerosis patients with varying sensory loss. Neurology 1968;18:1197–1204.
16. Cusik JF, Myklebust JB, Larson SJ, Sanges A. Spinal cord evaluation by cortical evoked responses. Arch Neurol 1979;36:140–143.
17. Emerson RG, Pedley TA. Generator sources of median somatosensory evoked potentials. J Clin Neurophysiol 1984;1:203–218.
18. Desmedt JE, Cheron G. Central somatosensory conduction in man: neural generators and interpeak latencies of the far-field components recorded from neck and right or left scalp and earlobe. EEG Clin Neurophysiol 1980;50:382–403.
19. Desmedt JE, Cheron G. Prevertebral (oesophageal) recording of subcortical somatosensory evoked potentials in man: the spinal P13 component and the dual nature of the spinal generators. EEG Clin Neurophysiol 1981;52:257–275.
20. Allison T, Goff WR, Williamson PD, et al. On the neural origin or early components of the human somatosensory evoked potential. In: Desmedt JE, ed. Progress in clinical neurophysiology, vol 7. Basel, Switzerland: Karger, 1980:51–68.
21. Anziska B, Cracco RQ, Cook AW, et al. Somatosensory far-field potentials: studies in normal subjects and patients with multiple sclerosis. EEG Clin Neurophysiol 1978;45:602–610.
22. Chiappa KH. Short latency somatosensory evoked potentials (SLSEP). Paper presented at the American Academy of Neurology, April 27, 1982. Washington, DC.
23. Chiappa KH, Choi SK, Young RR. Short latency somatosensory evoked potentials following median nerve stimulation in patients with neurological lesions. In: Desmedt JE, ed. Progress in clinical neurophysiology, vol. 7. Basel, Switzerland: Karger, 1980:264–281.
24. Cruse R, Klem G, Lesser RP, Lueders H. Paradoxical lateralization of cortical potentials evoked by stimulation of posterior tibial nerves. Arch Neurol 1982;39:222–225.
25. Beric A, Prevec TW. The early negative potential evoked by stimulation of the tibial nerve in man. J Neurol Sci 1981;50:299–306.
26. Vas GA, Cracco JB, Cracco RQ. Scalp-recorded short latency cortical and subcortical somatosensory evoked potentials to peroneal nerve stimulation. Electroencephalogr Clin Neurophysiol 1981;52:1–8.
27. Leandri M, Favale E, Ratto S. Conducted and segmental components of the somatosensory cervical response. J Neurol Neurosurg Psychiatry 1981;44:718–722.
28. Cracco RQ. Spinal evoked response: Peripheral nerve stimulation in man. EEG Clin Neurophysiol 1973;35:379–386.
29. Dimitrijevic MR, Larsson LE, Lehmkuhl D, et al. Spinal cord and nerve root potentials in humans using a non-invasive recording technique. EEG Clin Neurophysiol 1978;44:331–340.
30. Eisen A, Odusote K. Central and peripheral conduction times in multiple sclerosis. Electroencephalogr Clin Neurophysiol 1980;48:253–265.
31. El-Negamy E, Sedgwick EM. Properties of a spinal somatosensory evoked potential recorded in man. J Neurol Neurosurg Psychiatry 1978;41:762–768.
32. Jones SJ. Investigation of brachial plexus traction lesions by peripheral and spinal somatosensory evoked potentials. J Neurol Neurosurg Psychiatry 1979;49:107–116.
33. Phillips LH II, Daube JR. Lumbosacral spinal evoked potentials in humans. Neurology 1980;30:1175–1183.
34. Desmedt JE, Noel P. Average cerebral evoked potential in the evaluation of lesions of the sensory nerves and of the central somatosensory pathway. In: Desmedt JE, ed. New developments in EMG and clinical neurophysiology, vol. 2. Basel: Karger, 1973:352–371.

35. Robertson WC, Lambert EB. Sensory nerve conduction velocity in children using cerebral evoked potentials. Arch Phys Med Rehabil 1978;59:1–4.

36. Eisen A, Purves S, Horrch M. Central nervous system amplification: its potential in the diagnosis of early multiple sclerosis. Neurology 1982;32:359–364.

37. Desmedt JE. Somatosensory cerebral evoked potentials in man. In: Cobb WA, ed. Somatic sensation. Handbook of electroencephalography and clinical neurophysiology, vol. 9. Amsterdam: Elsevier, 1971:55–82.

38. Parry GJ, Aminoff MJ. Somatosensory evoked potentials in chronic acquired demyelinating peripheral neuropathy. Neurology 1987;37:313–316.

39. Bergamini L, Bergamasco B, Fra L, Gangdiglio G, Mombelli AM, Mutanti R. Somatosensory evoked cortical potentials in subjects with peripheral nervous lesions. Electromyography 1965;5:121–130.

40. Brown WF, Feasby TE. Sensory evoked potentials in Guillain-Barré polyneuropathy. J Neurol Neurosurg Psychiatry 1984;47:288–291.

41. Walsh JC, Yiannikas C, McLeod JG. Abnormalities of proximal conduction in acute idiopathic polyneuritis: comparison of short latency evoked potentials and F-waves. J Neurol Neurosurg Psychiatry 1984;47:197–200.

42. Ropper AH, Chiappa KH. Evoked potentials in Guillain-Barré syndrome. Neurology 1986;36:587–590.

43. Ganji S, Frazier E. Somatosensory evoked potential studies in acute Guillain-Barré syndrome. EMG Clin Neurophysiol 1988;28:313–317.

44. Shibasaki H, Ohnisha, Kuroiwa Y. Use of SEPs to localize degeneration in a rare polyneuropathy: studies on polyneuropathy associated with pigmentation, hypertrichosis, edema, and plasma cell dyscrasia. Ann Neurol 1982;12:355–360.

45. Cracco J, Castells S, Mark E. Spinal somatosensory evoked potentials in juvenile diabetes. Ann Neurol 1984;15:55–58.

46. Gupta PR, Dorfman LJ. Spinal somatosensory conduction in diabetes. Neurology 1981;31:841–845.

47. Rossini PM, Treviso M, DiStefano E, DiPaolo B. Nervous impulse propagation along peripheral and central fibers in patients with chronic renal failure. EEG Clin Neurophysiol 1983;56:293–303.

48. Ganji S, Mahajan S. Changes in short-latency somatosensory evoked potentials during hemodialysis in chronic renal failure. Clin EEG 1983;14:202–206.

49. Rossi A, Paradiso C, Dell'Anna P, Mondell M. Short latency somatosensory evoked potentials in Charcot-Marie-Tooth disease. Acta Neurol Scand 1985;71:156–163.

50. Jones SJ, Carroll WM, Halliday AM. Peripheral and central sensory nerve conduction in Charcot-Marie-Tooth disease and comparison with Friedreich's ataxia. J Neurol Sci 1983;61:135–148.

51. Fine EJ, Hallett M. Neurophysiological study of subacute combined degeneration. J Neurol Sci 1980;45:331–336.

52. Jones SJ, Yu YL, Rudge P, et al. Central and peripheral SEP defects in neurologically symptomatic and asymptomatic subjects with low vitamin B12 levels. J Neurol Sci 1987;82:55–65.

53. Jones SJ, Baraistser M, Halliday AM. Peripheral and central somatosensory nerve conduction defects in Friedreich's ataxia. J Neurol Neurosurg Psychiatry 1980;43:495–503.

54. Nuwer MR, Perlman SL, Packwood JW, Kark RAP. Evoked potential abnormalities in the various inherited ataxias. Ann Neurol 1983;13:20–27.

55. Noel P, Desmedt JE. Cerebral and far-field somatosensory evoked potentials in neurological disorders involving the cervical spinal cord, brainstem, thalamus and cortex. Clinical uses of cerebral, brainstem and spinal somatosensory evoked potentials. In: Desmedt JE, ed. Progress in clinical neurophysiology, vol 7. Basel: Karger, 1980:205–230.

56. Carlin L, Roach SE, Riela A, Spudis E, McLean WT. Juvenile metachromatic leuko-dystrophy: evoked potentials and computed tomography. Ann Neurol 1983;13:105–106.

57. Markand ON, Garg BP, DeMyer WE, Warren C, Worth RM. Brainstem auditory, visual and somatosensory evoked potentials in leukodystrophies. EEG Clin Neurophysiol 1982;54:39–48.

58. Vercruyssen A, Martin JJ, Mercelis R. Neurophysiological studies in adrenomyeloneuropathy. A report of five cases. J Neurol Sci 1982;56:327–336.

59. Majnemer A, Rosenblatt B, Watters G, Andermann F. Giant axonal neuropathy: central abnormalities demonstrated by evoked potentials. Ann Neurol 1986;19:394–396.

60. Synek VM. Assessing sensory involvement in lower limb nerve lesions using somatosensory evoked potential techniques. Muscle Nerve 1985;8:511–515.

61. Synek VM, Synek BJL. Intractable meralgia paresthetica after repeated abdominal surgery. EMG Clin Neurophysiol 1986;26:103–106.

62. Synek VM, Cowan JC. Saphenous nerve evoked potentials and the assessment of intraabdominal lesions of the femoral nerve. Muscle Nerve 1983;6:453–456.

63. Ito J, Yamao S, Kameyama M. Analysis of somatosensory evoked potentials in peroneal nerve palsy. Acta Neurol Scand 1987;75:385–390.

64. Dumitru D, Marquis S. Posterior femoral cutaneous nerve neuropathy and somatosensory evoked potentials. Arch Phys Med Rehabil 1988;69:44–45.

65. Dumitru D, Kalantri A, Dierschke B. Somatosensory evoked potentials of the medial and lateral plantar and calcaneal nerves. Muscle Nerve 1991;14:665–671.

66. Tranier S, Durey A, Chevallier B, Liot F. Value of somatosensory evoked potentials in saphenous entrapment neuropathy. J Neurol Neurosurg Psychiatry 1992;55:461–465.

67. Synek VM, Cowan JC. Somatosensory evoked potentials in patients with metastatic involvement of the brachial plexus. EMG Clin Neurophysiol 1983;23:545–551.

68. Synek VM. Role of somatosensory evoked potentials in the diagnosis of peripheral nerve lesions: recent advances. J Clin Neurophysiol 1987;4:55–73.
69. Assmus H. Somatosensory evoked cortical potentials in peripheral nerve lesions. In: Barber C, ed. Evoked potentials. Baltimore: University Park Press, 1980:437–442.
70. Debecker J, Noel P, Desmedt JE. The use of averaged cerebral evoked potentials in the evaluation of sensory loss in forensic medicine. Electromyography 1971;11:131–135.
71. Jones SJ. Investigation of brachial plexus traction lesions by peripheral and spinal somatosensory evoked potentials. J Neurol Neurosurg Psychiatry 1979;42:107–116.
72. Jones SJ. Somatosensory evoked potentials: the abnormal waveform. In: Halliday AM, ed. Evoked potential in clinical testing. Edinburgh: Churchill Livingstone, 1982:429–470.
73. Bonney G, Gilliatt RW. Sensory nerve conduction after traction lesion of the brachial plexus. Proc Royal Soc Med 1958;51:365–367.
74. Drake DG. Diagnosis and treatment of lesions of the brachial plexus and adjacent structures. Clin Neurosurg 1964;11:93–142.
75. Synek VM, Cowan JC. Somatosensory evoked potentials in patients with supraclavicular brachial plexus injuries. Neurology 1982;32:1347–1352.
76. Eisen A. The use of somatosensory evoked potentials for the evaluation of the peripheral nervous system. Neurol Clin 1988;6:825–838.
77. Zalis AW, Oester YT, Rodriquez AA. Electrophysiologic diagnosis of cervical root avulsion. Arch Phys Med Rehab 1970;51:709–710.
78. Warren J, Gutmann L, Figueroa AE, Bloor BM. Electromyographic changes of brachial plexus root avulsions. J Neurosurg 1969;31:137–140.
79. Rosen I, Sornas R, Elmquist D. Cervical root avulsion—electrophysiological analysis with electrospinogram. Scand J Plast Reconst Surg 1977;11:247–250.
80. Zverina E, Kredba J. Somatosensory cerebral evoked potentials in diagnosing brachial plexus injuries. Scand J Rehabil Med 1977;9:47–54.
81. Glover JL, Worth RM, Bendrick PJ, Hall PV, Markand OM. Evoked responses in the diagnosis of thoracic outlet syndrome. Surgery 1981;89:86–93.
82. Gilliatt RW, Willison RG, Dietz V, Williams IR. Peripheral nerve conduction in patients with a cervical rib and band. Ann Neurol 1978;4:124–129.
83. Yiannikas C, Walsh JC. Somatosensory evoked responses in the diagnosis of thoracic outlet syndrome. J Neurol Neurosurg Psychiatry 1983;46:234–240.
84. Synek VM. Diagnostic importance of somatosensory evoked potentials in the diagnosis of thoracic outlet syndrome. Clin EEG 1986;17:112–116.
85. Veilleux M, Stevens JC, Campbell JK. Somatosensory evoked potentials: lack of value for diagnosis of thoracic outlet syndrome. Muscle Nerve 1988;11:571–575.
86. Silvola J, Sulg I, Pokela R. Somatosensory evoked responses as a diagnostic aid in thoracic outlet syndrome. Acta Chir Scand 1982;148:647–652.
87. Jaeertt SA, Cuzzone LJ, Pasternak BM. Thoracic outlet syndrome. Electrophysiological reappraisal. Arch Neurol 1984;41:960–963.
88. Chodoroff G, Lee DW, Honet JC. The diagnosis of thoracic outlet syndrome using somatosensory evoked potentials. Arch Phys Med Rehab 1985;66:3–6.
89. Oh SJ. Clinical electromyography: nerve conduction studies. Baltimore: University Park Press, 1984:339.
90. Landi SA, Copeland SA, Wynn Parry CB, Jones SJ. The role of somatosensory evoked potentials and nerve conduction studies in the surgical management of brachial plexus injuries. J Bone Joint Surg 1980;62B:482–496.
91. Celli L, Rovesta C. Electrophysiologic intraoperative evaluations of the damaged root in tractions of the brachial plexus. In Terzis JK, ed. Microreconstruction of nerve injuries. Philadelphia: WB Saunders, 1987:473–482.
92. Van Beek A, Hubble B, Kinkead L, Torro S, Suchy H. Clinical use of nerve stimulation and recording techniques. Plast Reconstr Surg 1983;71:225–240.
93. Eisen A, Aminoff MJ. Somatosensory evoked potentials. In Aminoff MJ, ed, Electrodiagnosis in clinical neurology. 2nd ed. New York: Churchill Livingstone, 1986:532–573.
94. Scarff TB, Dallmann DE, Toleikis JR, Bunch WH. Dermatomal somatosensory evoked potentials in the diagnosis of lumbar root entrapment. Surgical Forum 1981;32:489–491.
95. Silvola J, Sulg I, Heiskavi M. Somatosensory evoked potentials in diagnosis of cervical spondylosis and herniated disc. EEG Clin Neurophysiol 1981;51:674–677.
96. Ganes T. Somatosensory conduction times and peripheral cervical and cortical evoked potentials in patients with cervical spondylosis. J Neurol Neurosurg Psychiatry 1980;43:683–689.
97. Yu YL, Jones SJ. Somatosensory evoked potentials in cervical spondylosis. Correlation of median, ulnar and posterior tibial nerve responses with clinical and radiological findings. Brain 1985;108:273–300.
98. Oh SJ, Sunwoo IN, Lee KW, Kim HS, Cho HK. Median nerve somatosensory evoked potentials in cervical spondylotic myelopathy. Electroencephalograph Clin Neurophysiol 1990;75:S 107.
99. El-Negamy E, Sedgwick EM. Delayed cervical somatosensory potentials in cervical spondylosis. J Neurol Neurosurg Psychiatry 1979;42:238–241.
100. Oh SJ, Kim HS, Faught E. Cervical and cortical somatosensory evoked potentials differentiate cervical spondylotic myelopathy from amyotrophic lateral sclerosis. Neurology 1985;35:S 147–148.

101. Feinsold M, Balu D, Findler G, Hadani M, Beller AJ. Somatosensory evoked potential to peroneal nerve stimulation in patients with herniated lumbar disc. Neurosurgery 1982;11:506–511.

102. Aminoff MJ, Goodin DS, Barbaro NM, Weinstein PR, Rosenblum ML. Dermatosomal somatosensory evoked potentials in unilateral lumbosacral radiculopathy. Ann Neurol 1985;17:171–176.

103. Rodriquez AA, Kanis L, Rodriquez AA, Lane D. Somatosensory evoked potentials from dermatomal stimulation as an indicator of L5 and S1 radiculopathy. Arch Phys Med Rehabil 1987;68:366–368.

104. Katifi HA, Sedgwick EM. Evaluation of the dermatomal somatosensory evoked potentials in the diagnosis of lumbo-sacral root compression. J Neurol Neurosurg Psychiatry 1987;50:1204–1210.

105. Perlik S, Fisher MA, Patel DV, Slack C. On the usefulness of somatosensory evoked responses for the evaluation of lower back pain. Arch Neurol 1986;43:907–913.

106. Walk D, Fisher MA, Doudoulakis SH, Hemmati M. Somatosensory evoked potentials in the evaluation of lumbosacral radiculopathy. Neurology 1992;42:1197–1202.

107. Haldeman S, Bradley W, Bhatia N. Evoked responses from the pudendal nerve. J Urol 1982;128:974–980.

108. Haldeman S, Bradley WE, Bhatia NN, Johnson BK. Pudendal evoked responses. Arch Neurol 1982;39:280–283.

109. Tackmann W, Porst H, Van Ahlen H. Bulbocavernosus reflex latencies and somatosensory evoked potentials after pudendal nerve stimulation in the diagnosis of impotence. J Neurol 1988;235:219–225.

110. Fowler CJ. Pelvic floor neurophysiology. Methods in Clinical Neurophysiology 1991;2:1–24.

111. Ertekin C, Akyurekli O, Gurses AN, Turgut H. The value of somatosensory evoked potentials and bulbocavernosus reflex in patients with impotence. Acta Neurol Scand 1985;71:49–53.

112. Porst H, Tachmann W, Van Ahlen H. Neurophysiological investigation in potent and impotent men. Brit J Urol 1988;61:445–450.

113. Eardley I, Nagendran K, Lechy B, Chapple CR, Kirby RS, Fowler J. Neurophysiology of the striated urethral sphincter in multiple sclerosis. Brit J Urol 1991;68:81–88.

114. Vodusek DB. Pudendal SEP and bulbocavernosus reflex in women. EEG Clin Neurophysiol 1990;77:134–136.

115. Haldeman S, Bradley W, Bhatia N, Johnson B. Cortical evoked potentials on stimulation of pudendal nerve in women. Urology 1983;21:590–593.

116. Oh SJ. Cerebral evoked potentials: their clinical applications. Ala J Med Sci 1980;17:308–314.

117. Gilmore RL, Nelson KR. SSEP and F-wave studies in acute inflammatory demyelinating polyradiculoneuropathy. Muscle Nerve 1989;12:538–543.

118. Morales-Blanquez G, Delwaide PJ. The thoracic outlet syndrome: an electrophysiological study. EMG Clin Neurophysiol 1982;22:255–263.

119. Silvola J, Sulg I, Pokela R. Somatosensory evoked responses as a diagnostic aid in thoracic outlet syndrome. Acta Chir Scand 1982;148:647–652.

120. Jaeertt SA, Cuzzone LJ, Pasternak BM. Thoracic outlet syndrome. Electrophysiological reappraisal. Arch Neurol 1984;41:960–963.

121. Chodoroff G, Lee DW, Honet JC. The diagnosis of thoracic outlet syndrome using somatosensory evoked potentials. Arch Phys Med Rehab 1985;66:3–6.

122. Synek VM. Diagnostic importance of somatosensory evoked potentials in the diagnosis of thoracic outlet syndrome. Clin EEG 1986;17:112–116.

123. Veilleux M, Stevens JC, Campbell JK. Somatosensory evoked potentials: lack of value for diagnosis of thoracic outlet syndrome. Muscle Nerve 1988;11:571–575.

124. Machleder HI, Moll F, Nuwer M, Jordan S. Somatosensory evoked potentials in the assessment of thoracic outlet compression syndrome. J Vasc Surg 1987;6:177–184.

125. Tackmann W, Radü EW. Observations on the application of electrophysiological methods in the diagnosis of cervical root compressions. Eur Neurol 1983;22:397–404.

126. Synek VM. Validity of median nerve somatosensory evoked potentials in the diagnosis of supraclavicular brachial plexus lesions. EEG Clin Neurophysiol 1986;65:27–35.

127. Perlik SJ, Fisher MA. Somatosensory evoked response evaluation of cervical spondylotic myelopathy. Muscle Nerve 1987;10:481–489.

128. Eisen A, Hoirch M, Moll A. Evaluation of radiculopathies by segmental stimulation and somatosensory evoked potentials. Can J Neurol Sci 1983;10:178–182.

129. Cassvan A, Park SY. Cortical somatosensory evoked potentials following peroneal nerve stimulation in lumbosacral radiculopathies. EMG Clin Neurophysiol 1983;23:393–402.

130. Aminoff MJ, Goodin DS, Parry GJ, Barbaro NM, Weinstein PR, Rosenblum ML. Electrophysiologic evaluation of lumbosacral radiculopathies: electromyography, late responses, and somatosensory evoked potentials. Neurology 1985;35:1514–1518.

131. Seyal M, Sandhu LS, Mack YP. Spinal segmental somatosensory evoked potentials in lumbosacral radiculopathies. Neurology 1989;39:801–805.

132. Picton TW, Hink RF. Evoked potentials: how? what? and why? Am J EEG Technol 1975;14:9–44.

20

Interpretation of Nerve Conduction Data

Almost all parameters of the nerve conduction study are helpful in the diagnosis of the diseased nerve because each represents a particular physiological function.

Motor Nerve Conduction

Latency

Latency is a measure of the combined time for conduction of the nerve impulse from the point of stimulation to the axonal terminal, the neuromuscular transmission, and the depolarization of muscle fibers.

Amplitude

Amplitude is the rough estimation of the number of muscle fibers that are activated to nerve stimulation and, subsequently, of the number of nerve fibers that become excitable to nerve stimulation when neuromuscular transmission is normal. The amplitude of the compound muscle action potential (CMAP) is an insensitive measure of mild impairment because of its wide variation among normal subjects (1).

Duration

The duration reflects the synchrony of discharge of the individual muscle fibers. When the muscle fibers are activated in near synchrony, the duration of the CMAP becomes short. If the conduction velocities vary widely among different nerve fibers, some muscle fibers are activated earlier than others, producing a longer-duration CMAP. Thus, the duration of the CMAP is related to the range of conduction velocities of the large-diameter motor nerve fibers. Unless the CMAP is split into numerous phases producing *a long-duration abnormal temporal dispersion (dispersion phenomenon)*, the shape and duration are not a reliable gauge of the impairment of the slower fibers, since they vary according to the locations of the active and indifferent electrodes (2).

"Repetitive discharges" can mimic the CMAP with abnormal temporal dispersion because one or more repetitive discharges may follow the main CMAP (Fig. 20.1).

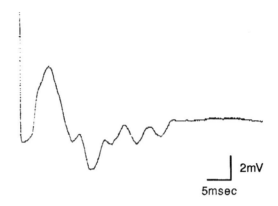

Figure 20.1. Repetitive discharge of the CMAP from the abductor digit quinti muscle in a patient with myokymia-fasciculation syndrome.

Repetitive discharges are caused either by repetitive muscle contractions after a single nerve stimulation or by repetitive nerve discharges originating from peripheral nerves. In the case of the former, repetitive discharges are seen in patients with anticholinesterase overtoxicity, organophosphate poisoning, Types A and B congenital myasthenic syndrome, and in myasthenia gravis patients treated with germine acetate (3). Repetitive nerve discharges have been reported in the acquired and familial forms of continuous muscle activity causing myokymia (4). To distinguish between these types of discharges, the peripheral nerve may be tapped lightly with a reflex hammer or finger. If the repetitive discharge originates from the peripheral nerve, this maneuver can produce a repetitive discharge with identical amplitude and latency to that caused by electrical stimulation at that site (4).

Area

The area represents the combination of the amplitude and duration of the CMAP and is thus the rough sum of the number as well as a synchrony of the activated muscle fibers to nerve stimulation. It is consequently influenced by a change in the amplitude or duration of the CMAP. A decrease in the amplitude of the CMAP may simply result from the prolonged duration of the CMAP. This means that *abnormal temporal dispersion alone produces a decrease of the CMAP amplitude, possibly mimicking a genuine "conduction block."* In this case, there is no change in the area, and area measurement thus reflects more accurately the number of activated muscle fibers to nerve stimulation. This assumes that the phase cancellation of the components of the CMAP is not operative.

Nerve Conduction Velocity

Nerve conduction velocity (NCV) represents the maximum NCV of the fastest nerve fibers. So long as one motor fiber exists with a normal conduction velocity, normal values for motor conduction velocity may be obtained (5). Almost all motor nerve fibers must be slowed for the NCV to be diminished. Thus, the presence of a few intact motor fibers may yield an entirely normal NCV in patients with neuropathy (1). According to Gilliatt (6), it is necessary that about 75% of the large-diameter, fast-conducting fibers be lost before there is any noticeable effect in the overall maximal NCV of the nerve.

Sensory Nerve Conduction

Latency

Latency is a measure of the time required for conduction of the nerve impulse from the point of stimulation to the point of recording. A normal latency to the initial positive peak of the sensory compound nerve action potential (CNAP) requires about 200 normally conducting nerve fibers 10 μm or more in diameter, one-fourth of the fibers in the normal sural nerve are of this caliber (1). *The negative peak latency includes the rise-time of the action potential and may therefore give an indication of temporal dispersion.*

Amplitude

Amplitude is the rough estimation of the number of nerve fibers more than 9 μm in diameter that are activated by nerve stimulation (7). With surface electrodes, the amplitude is heavily influenced by the distance of the recording electrode from the nerve. Thus, the amplitude is a less sensitive measure of mild impairment with surface electrodes (8). With near-nerve needle electrodes, the amplitude is a more sensitive index of impairment (2, 9). However, even with this technique, the lower limit of normal is 30–40% below the average amplitude, indicating a wide variation among normal subjects (1). A loss of about one-third of the fibers of a diameter in excess of 7 μm is necessary before a significant drop in potential can be measured (10).

Duration

The duration is the range of NCVs of the various sensory fibers. In the normal sural nerve, this is predominantly determined by fibers 3–14 μm in diameter (11). The duration of the CNAP is thus an index of temporal dispersion. Prolonged temporal dispersion is called *abnormal temporal dispersion ("dispersion phenomenon").* It is difficult or impossible to document abnormal temporal dispersion with surface electrodes because the varying degrees of slowing in different fibers spread out by the CNAP and lower its amplitude to the point where it is no longer discernible (Fig. 20.9) (5). However, with the near-nerve needle technique, *abnormal temporal dispersion* can easily be documented and is *typically observed in the presence of segmental demyelination* (Fig. 20.10). According to Ludin and Tackmann (10), the duration of the CNAPs and the number of their components are the most sensitive single parameters of abnormalities in patients with mild nerve lesions.

Nerve Conduction Velocity

The NCV represents *the maximum NCV of the fastest sensory fibers* when the latency is measured to the first positive peak. The conduction velocity can be roughly calculated from the class of fibers of the largest diameter that contains at least 10 fibers. In the human sural nerve, the conversion factors for the NCV (meters per second) from the fiber diameter (micron) have been found to be *4.3* and *4.55* (12). *With the surface electrode and without the aid of a signal averager, an NCV slower than 20 m/sec is seldom seen* because beyond this point the CNAP is too small to be registered (5).

When the latency is measured to the negative peak with the surface electrode technique, it provides an estimate of conduction of the slower fibers.

When the latency is measured to the smallest recognizable component with the near-nerve needle technique, the slowest NCV can be calculated. With photographic superimposition, the slowest velocity is 28–30 m/sec, corresponding to 6 micron fibers. Using signal averaging, 0.1–0.15 μV amplitude potential is recognizable with an average NCV of 19 m/sec. This potential is generated by 3–4 micron fibers (11). In some diseased nerves, the minimum NCV is slowed while the maximum NCV and the amplitude and shape of the main components are still unchanged (9, 13).

Mixed Nerve Conduction

The physiological functions of the various parameters in mixed nerve conduction are similar to those in sensory nerve conduction, except that the CNAPs are generated from mixed motor and sensory nerves.

Electrophysiological Responses in Diseased Nerves

Electrophysiological responses in diseased nerves are limited. Responses can be classified into three groups: (*a*) conduction slowing; (*b*) conduction block; and (*c*) reduced or absent excitability of the nerves.

Nerve conduction slowing is the most important parameter in the nerve conduction study and is seen as prolonged latency or conduction time. This slowing is attributed to three factors: (*a*) segmental demyelination; (*b*) loss of large-diameter fibers; and (*c*) metabolic abnormalities.

With segmental demyelination, nerve conduction slowing occurs because of lengthened conduction time in the two demyelinated nodes of Ranvier and the loss of saltatory conduction in the relatively thin demyelinated fibers (14, 15). *Slowing of the NCV parallels the degree of demyelination.*

Because the NCV is proportional to the outer fiber diameter of myelinated fibers, it is not difficult to understand that the loss of large-diameter fibers is responsible for the slow nerve conduction. However, total loss of the large-diameter fibers slows the NCV, usually not more than 20% below the normal mean (7). This may be the pathological basis of the minimal slowing seen in axonal neuropathy.

Physiological and metabolic changes are also responsible for the slowing of the NCV. The effect of lowered skin temperature on the NCV has been discussed previously (see Chapter 13). In human uremic neuropathy, rapid improvement in the NCV after renal transplantation is explained on the basis of metabolic improvement (16).

Conduction block occurs with physiological alteration, as with a local anesthetic block, and segmental demyelination. Slowing of conduction is a typical electrophysiological manifestation with mild segmental demyelination, but in more serious demyelination some demyelinated fibers fail to conduct the nerve impulse, producing a conduction block. Conduction block is manifested in the reduction of amplitude of the CMAP and CNAP. *This is best recognized when there is a dramatic reduction of amplitudes of the CMAP or CNAP across the site of the block,* such as in the case of entrapment neuropathy.

Reduced or absent excitability of the nerve is observed when conduction block or axonal degeneration becomes severe. This is measured by the need for an increase in duration and intensity of the stimulus to generate the muscle or nerve action potential. *If the conduction block or axonal degeneration is complete, the nerve eventually becomes inexcitable.* This is best observed in cases of wallerian degeneration of all the nerve fibers distal to the lesion when the nerve is severed. A few days after total severance of the nerve, the excitability is totally extinguished distal to the site of severance, and no further CMAP or CNAP can be recorded. The exception is in cases of root avulsion because the sensory nerve fibers continue to conduct quite normally distally, as the axon is not severed from its nerve cell.

Electrophysiological Characteristics in Axonal Degeneration and Segmental Demyelination

The pathology of the diseased nerve can be classified into two basic processes: axonal degeneration and segmental demyelination. Although it is true that the matter is not that simple because in human diseased nerves both processes may be present together, this classification is useful in recognizing the diseased nerve by the nerve conduction abnormalities (Table 20.1).

Axonal Degeneration

The hallmark of nerve conduction abnormalities is *the diminution of the amplitude of the CMAP and CNAP in the presence of normal or near-normal maximal NCVs and a normal or diminished temporal dispersion of the responses* (8, 11, 17) *(Figs. 20.2–20.5).*

Table 20.1.
Electrophysiological Characteristics in Axonal Degeneration and Segmental Demyelination

Characteristic	Axonal Degeneration[a]	Segmental Demyelination[a]
Motor Nerve Conduction (with surface electrodes)		
Amplitude	↓↓	N or ↓; conduction block
Duration	N	Dispersion phenomenon
Shape	N	N or multiphasic
Terminal latency	N or ↑ (<150%)	↑↑ (>150%)[b]
Conduction velocity	N or ↓ (>60%)	↓↓ (<60%)
Sensory Nerve Conduction		
With surface electrodes		
Amplitude	↓↓ or often absent	N, ↓, or absent
Duration	N	↑ or rarely dispersion phenomenon
Shape	N	Rarely multiphasic
Conduction velocity	N or ↓ (>60%)	↓↓ (<60%)
With near-nerve needle technique		
Amplitude	↓↓	N or ↓; conduction block
Duration	N	Prominent dispersion phenomenon
Shape	N	Multiphasic with many components
Conduction velocity	N or ↓ (>60%)	↓↓ (<60%)
F-wave	↑<150% or absent	↑>150% or absent
H-reflex	↑<150% or absent	↑>150% or absent

[a]↑, Increased. ↓, Decreased. N, Normal.
[b]Percentage of normal means.

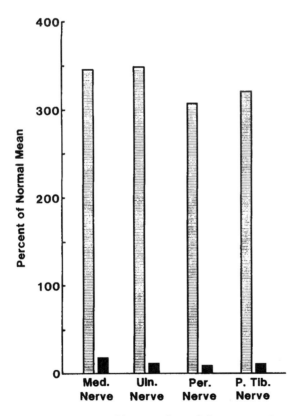

Figure 20.2.   Comparison of the terminal latency of axonal degeneration (arsenic neuropathy) and segmental demyelination (subacute demyelinating neuropathy). The *hatched bar* represents mean terminal latencies from 18 cases of subacute demyelinating neuropathy, and the *solid bar* from eight cases of arsenic neuropathy. The normal mean is at 0%. Markedly prolonged terminal latencies are noted in the presence of segmental demyelination, whereas with axonal degeneration terminal latencies are still within normal limits (30% of the mean) (20, 47).

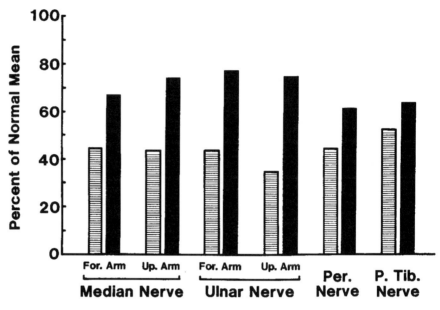

Figure 20.3. Comparison of the motor NCVs of axonal degeneration (arsenic neuropathy) and segmental demyelination (subacute demyelinating neuropathy). The *hatched bar* and *solid bar* represent segmental demyelination and axonal degeneration, respectively. The normal mean is at 100%, and the lower normal limit at 80% of the mean. With segmental demyelination, the motor NCVs are below 60% of the normal mean, whereas with axonal degeneration they are above 60% of the normal mean.

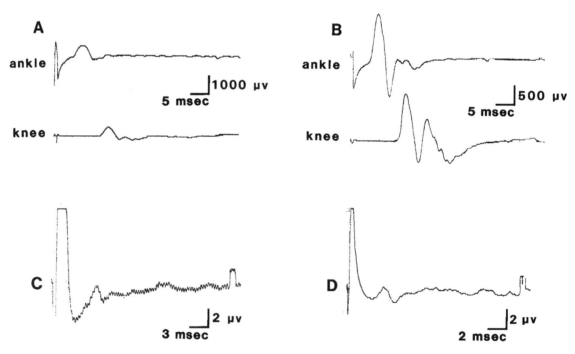

Figure 20.4. Motor and sensory nerve conduction in axonal degeneration (arsenic neuropathy). *A*, The amplitude of the CMAP in the peroneal nerve is markedly reduced. Terminal latency and motor NCV are minimally abnormal. *B*, Improved CMAP in the peroneal nerve 2 years later. *C*, Markedly reduced amplitude and mild slowing of the sensory NCV (34.3 m/sec) over the finger-wrist segment of the median nerve. *D*, Reduced amplitude and mild slowing in the sensory NCV (33.3 m/sec) over the finger-wrist segment of the ulnar nerve.

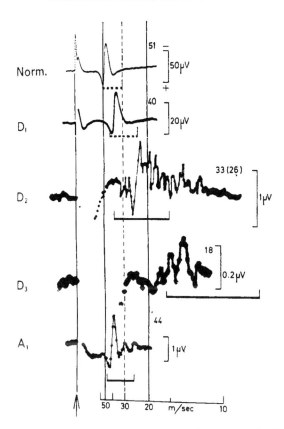

Figure 20.5.   Sensory CNAP with the near-nerve needle technique over the digit I-wrist segment of the median nerve. **D_1**, Segmental demyelination without fiber block. **D_2**, Segmental demyelination with block of an unknown number of fibers. **D_3**, Segmental demyelination with block of most fibers. **A_1**, Axonal degeneration with normal velocity of the fastest fibers. The recordings are normalized to the scale of conduction velocities given below. The figures above each potential indicate the velocity of the fastest fibers; the figure in parentheses (**D_2**) refers to the velocity of the main component. *Vertical lines* (from left to right) represent onset of stimulus; velocity of fastest fibers in normal nerve; velocity of slowest fibers in normal nerve recorded by photographic superimposition *(broken line)* and recorded by electronic averaging. *Horizontal lines* represent average range of velocities determined by photographic superimposition *(broken lines)* and by electronic averaging. (From Buchthal F, Rosenfalck A. Sensory potentials in polyneuropathy. Brain 1971;94:248.)

The following findings are typically found in the presence of axonal degeneration. In motor conduction:

1. *Unequivocal reduction of the amplitude of the CMAP in proportion to the clinical severity of the diseased nerve;*

2. *Normal shape and duration of the CMAP.* Exception has been seen rarely when the muscle is atrophied following axonal degeneration. The shape of the CMAP becomes minimally abnormal, sometimes mimicking abnormal temporal dispersion, but *the duration of the CMAP is invariably normal.*

3. *Minimal prolongation of the terminal latency by not more than 50% of the normal mean;*

4. *Normal or near-normal NCV. The NCV is hardly altered because conduction in individual nerve fibers generally remains normal until they cease functioning with axonal degeneration.* If many of the large diameter fibers are lost because of axonal degeneration, there may be mild slowing in the NCV, but not more than 40% below the normal mean. The motor NCV in the median nerve is usually above 40 m/sec and in the peroneal nerve above 35 m/sec (17–19); and

5. *In severe cases, the nerve becomes inexcitable to elicit any CMAPs.*

In sensory conduction, the following findings are typical of axonal degeneration:

1. *Unequivocal reduction of the amplitude of the CNAP* (11). *With surface electrodes and without any help from signal averaging, the amplitude is so small that the CNAP is often*

unrecordable. With near-nerve needle electrodes and the use of the signal averager, a significantly low amplitude is recorded, which is proportional to the severity of involvement of the diseased nerve. However, it is difficult to discriminate between some of the later slow components and noise;

2. The shape and duration of the CNAP are normal unless the regeneration takes place together with axonal degeneration;

3. The NCV is normal or near-normal. Slowing of the NCV is less than 40% below the normal mean. The sensory NCV is usually above 35 m/sec in the median nerve and above 30 m/sec in the sural nerve using the negative peak latency method. With surface electrodes, the CNAP is often unobtainable for calculating the NCV if signal averaging is not used; and

4. In severe cases the nerve is inexcitable to obtain any CNAP, even with the near-nerve technique and the signal averager.

Segmental Demyelination

The hallmarks of nerve conduction abnormalities in segmental demyelination are:

1. *Conduction block that is more common and more severe in acute than chronic disorders;*
2. *Abnormal temporal dispersion (dispersion phenomenon); and*
3. *Marked slowing in the NCV.*

The following findings are typically found in the presence of segmental demyelination (Figs. 20.2, 20.3, 20.5, and 20.6–20.10). In motor conduction:

1. *Normal or reduced amplitude of the CMAP. Substantial slowing of the NCV in the presence of a normal amplitude is indicative of segmental demyelination when the large-diameter fibers are*

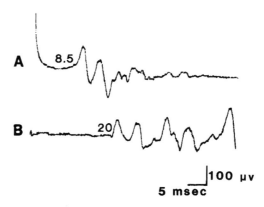

Figure 20.6. CMAP in segmental demyelination. This is from the posterior tibial nerve at the ankle (**A**) and the popliteal fossa (**B**) in a case of hypertrophic neuropathy. The reduced amplitude of the CMAP is due to a marked dispersion phenomenon (duration of the CMAP is 30 msec). Terminal latency is 8.5 msec. Motor NCV is 35.8 m/sec.

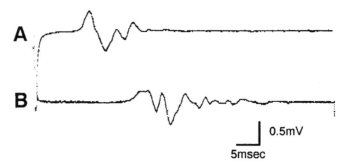

Figure 20.7. Abnormal temporal dispersion in the CMAP from the posterior tibial nerve at the popliteal fossa (**B**) compared with the CMAP at the ankle (**A**). NCV in this segment was 40.0 m/sec. No essential change is noted in the CMAP amplitude. There was a 35% increase in the negative-duration and a 90% increase in the total-duration in the proximal CMAP compared with the distal CMAP. The NCV in this segment is 40.0 m/sec.

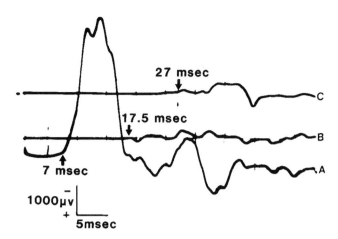

Figure 20.8. Conduction block in segmental demyelination. Median motor nerve conduction in a case of subacute demyelinating neuropathy. *A*, Normal amplitude of the CMAP with wrist stimulation. *B*, A dramatic reduction in amplitude of the CMAP with elbow stimulation. *C*, CMAP with axillary stimulation. Conduction block is clearly seen between wrist and elbow stimulation. The dispersion phenomenon is also observed. The motor NCV is 21.9 m/sec over the wrist-elbow segment and 15.8 m/sec over the elbow-axilla segment.

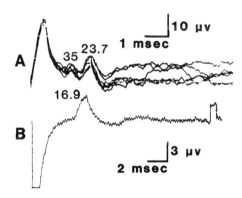

Figure 20.9. Dispersion phenomenon in the sensory CNAP recorded with a surface electrode in cases of carpal tunnel syndrome. *A*, Double-peaked CNAP over the palm-wrist segment. The first peak NCV is 35.0 m/sec. The higher second peak NCV is 23.7 m/sec. *B*, Note the long duration of the sensory CNAP (3.7 msec) over the finger-wrist segment. The NCV is 16.9 m/sec.

preferentially impaired. When the amplitude is reduced, this reduction is proportional to the degree of temporal dispersion of the CMAP and the conduction block.

2. *The shape of the CMAP is abnormal, with multiple phases and prolonged duration. This is compared either with the duration of normal CMAPs or with the duration of CMAPs at distal sites. This is called abnormal temporal dispersion or "dispersion phenomenon," which is typical of segmental demyelination* (20). The shape of the CMAP is dispersed because there is wide variation of nerve conduction at the time of arrival of the impulses traveling along demyelinated nerve fibers.

3. *Marked prolongation of the terminal latency. The terminal latency is prolonged by more than 50% of the normal mean.* In the median nerve, a terminal latency longer than 6 msec and in the peroneal nerve longer than 10 msec, are indicative of segmental demyelination (18–20).

4. *The NCV is unequivocally slow. Slowing of the NCV depends on the degree of segmental demyelination. However, to recognize the slow NCV as being caused by segmental demyelination, the NCV should be slowed by more than 40% below the normal mean* (18–20). The motor NCV in the median nerve is usually below 35 m/sec and in the peroneal nerve below 30 m/sec. A motor NCV of 6–7 m/sec has been documented in some cases of demyelinating neuropathy.

5. *The conduction block is characterized by a substantial reduction of the amplitude proximal to the site of the block.* The amplitude is somewhat lower with stimulation at more proximal sites in normal subjects. The degree of amplitude reduction differs among the nerves: 25–30% reduction in the median, ulnar, and peroneal nerves, and 35–41% reduction for the posterior tibial

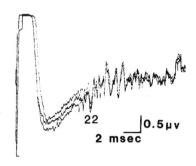

Figure 20.10. The sensory CNAP from the ankle with digits 1–2 interdigital nerve stimulation in a patient with tarsal tunnel syndrome. The maximum NCV is 22 m/sec. The dispersion phenomenon is obvious.

nerve (Table 7.12). *In the past, a reduction of the amplitude by more than 40% was generally accepted as a definite criterion of conduction block* (21). However, in recent years, there has been some modification in these criteria (see below). Moreover, the concept of "interphase cancellation" has been introduced: i.e., when negative and positive phases of different motor unit action potentials overlap, they cancel each other because of temporal dispersion (22). This may be mistakenly identified as conduction block. Using a computer model, Rhee et al. concluded that "maximum interphase cancellations between positive and negative components can result in no more than 50% reduction of negative CMAP area," and that "area reduction greater than 50% indicates at least some degree of conduction block" (22). This may be applicable for the normal nerve. Whether or not this model applies to the diseased nerve is not clear. *Considering the controversy regarding the conduction block, we recommend using the most stringent criteria at this time: a more than 50% reduction of the CMAP amplitude and area with normal duration.*

According to Cornblath et al., a discrepancy in the amplitude or area between proximal and distal stimulation should be regarded at best as "suggestive of partial motor conduction block" (23). Regardless of whether our criteria are indicative or suggestive of "genuine physiological conduction block" or not, we believe that they represent a reasonable compromise because they enable us to confirm the presence of demyelination with a degree of certainty in clinical practice. *The conduction block may be present when the NCV is normal, but in a majority of cases it is associated with abnormal temporal dispersion and a slowed NCV.* The amplitude of the CMAP is smaller across the demyelinated area because of the smaller number of fibers that are capable of responding to the stimulation. If the conduction block is severe, no recordable potential can be obtained across the site of the block.

In sensory conduction:

1. *Normal or reduced amplitude of the sensory CNAP* (11). *Substantial slowing of the NCV in the presence of a normal amplitude is indicative of segmental demyelination.* This is observed when large-diameter fibers of 11 μm or more are preferentially impaired. The amplitude is reduced in severe segmental demyelination. The amplitude of the CNAP is diminished because of: (*a*) an increase in temporal dispersion associated with slowing in conduction; and (*b*) blocked conduction in some fibers because the demyelinated segment has ceased to conduct (18). *Thus, this reduction is in proportion to the degree of temporal dispersion and the conduction block.* With surface electrodes, the sensory CNAP is commonly absent in severe segmental demyelination if signal averaging is not used.

2. *Abnormal temporal dispersion (dispersion phenomenon).* Abnormal temporal dispersion of the sensory CNAP may be seen with surface electrodes in the presence of segmental demyelination. *However, this can best be documented with the near-nerve needle electrode after signal averaging. The sensory CNAP is markedly split and lengthened in duration; numerous smaller potential components follow the main component.*

3. *Unequivocally slow NCV.* Slowing of the sensory NCV depends on the severity of segmental demyelination. *To recognize the NCV slowing as being due to segmental demyelination, the NCV should be less than 60% of the normal mean* (1, 24). The sensory NCV in the median nerve is usually below 30 m/sec and in the sural nerve below 25 m/sec by the negative peak latency measurement. Rarely with the surface electrodes, an NCV below 20 m/sec is obtained in severe segmental demyelination because the sensory CNAP is unobtainable due to the smaller amplitude (5).

4. *Conduction block. This can be demonstrated when the sensory fibers are orthodromically stimulated and the recording electrodes are placed distal and proximal to the site of the block. Recognition of a conduction block is difficult with surface electrodes unless the sensory CNAP is absent proximal to the block. However, the conduction block can easily be demonstrated with the near-nerve needle electrodes when this technique is combined with signal averaging.* Across the block there is a substantial reduction in amplitude and dispersion phenomenon. If the conduction block becomes severe, no sensory CNAP can be obtained across the block.

Other criteria of demyelination have been proposed by different investigators (Table 20.2). For the NCV, Cornblath (25) and Albers et al. (26) recommended a finding less than 70–95% of the lower limit of normal, which they did not specifically define. Since a value two standard deviations below the mean is usually used as the lower normal limit, 80% of this figure equals 60% of the normal mean. Kelly also used an NCV less than 60% of the normal mean as his criterion of demyelination (27). Thus, *an NCV less than 60% of the normal mean or less than 80% of the lower limit of normal is widely accepted as an electrophysiological criterion of demyelination.* An NCV less

Table 20.2.
Different Criteria for Segmental Demyelination

Investigator	Cornblath (25, 45)	Albers et al. (26)	Feasby et al. (30)	Bromberg (46)	Oh
Nerve conduction velocity	1. <80% of LLN[a] if amplitude >80% of LLN; 2. <70% of LLN if amplitude <80% of LLN	<95% of LLN if amplitude >50% of LLN; <85% of LLN if amplitude <50% of LLN		<75% of LLN	<60% of normal means
Conduction block					
Definite	>20% drop in N-P area or P-P amplitude and <15% change in N-P duration	>30% drop in amplitude	>20% drop in the P-P amplitude and <15% change in N-P duration	>30% drop in the amplitude	>50% drop in the amplitude and area
Possible or probable	Possible: >20% drop in N-P area or P-P amplitude and >15% change in N-P duration		"Probable": >30% reduction in the P-P amplitude and in the N-P area, when >15% change in duration.		Probable: <24–41% drop in the amplitude and area, when <15–33% change in duration[c]
Abnormal temporal dispersion	>15% change in N-P duration		>15% change in duration.		>15–33% change in duration.
Terminal latency	1. >125% of ULN° if amplitude >80% of LLN; 2. >150% of ULN if amplitude <80% of LLN	>110% of ULN if amplitude normal; >120% of ULN if amplitude < normal		>130% of ULN	>150% of normal means
F-wave	Absent or prolonged F-wave latency 1. >120% of ULN if amplitude >80% of LLN; 2. >150% of ULN if amplitude <80% of LLN	>120% of ULN		>130% of ULN	>150% of normal means
H-reflex[b]	Absent (supportive)				>150% of normal means
Sensory nerve conduction[b]	<80% of LLN				<60% of normal means

[a]Abbreviations: N-P area, negative peak area. P-P amplitude, peak-to-peak amplitude. LLN, lower limit of normal. ULN, upper limit of normal.
[b]These are quoted from (45).
[c]Amplitude, N-P amplitude and P-P amplitude; Area, N-P area and total area; Duration, N-P duration and total duration.

489

than 95% of the lower limit of normal (75% of the normal mean) as a criterion of demyelination is not acceptable because the mean NCVs in axonal neuropathy are within this range (Fig. 20.3). Different values for the criteria of demyelination have been recommended for the low CMAP amplitude: 80% of the lower limit of normal by Cornblath (25) and 50% by Albers et al. (26). The physiological basis for these different figures was not explained.

For the terminal latency and F-wave latency, more than 110–120% of the upper limit of normal is recommended as the criterion of demyelination (25, 26). Thus, *we use a finding of more than 150% of the normal mean (equivalent to 130% of the upper limit of normal) as a reasonable index of demyelination* by which we can clearly differentiate axonal neuropathy from demyelinating neuropathy (Fig. 20.2). Cornblath recommended more than 150% of the upper limit of normal for the lower CMAP (25), although no physiological basis for the different figures was given. An absent F-wave or H-reflex response should not be interpreted as an indication of demyelination because these may be absent in patients with severe axonal neuropathy.

For the conduction block, reductions of the CMAP by more than 20% with normal duration and by 30% with prolonged duration are recommended as the criteria of demyelination by Brown and Feasby (28). This is based on their observation that there was never more than a 20% decline in the CMAP peak-to-peak amplitude or more than a 10% decline in the negative peak area between the most proximal stimulation site at Erb's point and the most distal stimulation site at the wrist in the ulnar nerve conduction. An equivalent decline in the CMAP amplitude and area was observed in the peroneal and median nerves (28). Our figure, *25% for the peak-to-peak amplitude and for the negative area for the median, ulnar, and peroneal nerves* (Table 7.12), is quite close to Brown and Feasby's 20% (28). Our study also showed that these figures are not acceptable *for the posterior tibial nerve: e.g., 36% for the peak-to-peak amplitude and 25% for the negative area* (29).

In abnormal temporal dispersion ("dispersion phenomenon") between proximal and distal sites, a prolongation in the negative-peak duration and peak-to-peak duration of more than 15% is recommended as a criterion for demyelination, based on observation in the ulnar nerve (28). This figure is smaller than ours: i.e., *20% for the negative duration and 27% for the total duration in the median, ulnar, and peroneal nerves.* For the posterior tibial nerve, these figures are much higher: *30% for the negative duration and 33% for the total duration (Table 7.12).*

When an abnormal temporal dispersion is present, it is difficult to make any comment about conduction block because a decline in the CMAP amplitude and area could simply be a product of increased temporal dispersion or phase cancellations between components of biphasic and sometime triphasic motor unit potentials in the summation of CMAPs (28). When an abnormal temporal dispersion is present, the term "possible conduction block" is used by Cornblath to indicate more than a 20% drop in the amplitude or area (25) and Feasby et al. use the phrase "probable conduction block" when there is more than a 30% drop (30). However, nerve teasing in the sural nerve biopsy in cases of "probable conduction block" showed more demyelinated fibers than did cases of "definite conduction block," indicating that "probable conduction block" can be used as an electrophysiological index of demyelination. Any argument regarding the terminology of "possible or probable conduction block" is moot in the practical sense since *an abnormal temporal dispersion alone is indicative of demyelination.*

Cornblath et al. stated that a discrepancy in the amplitude or area between the surface-recorded responses to proximal and distal stimulation does no more than *suggest* the presence of a conduction block in individual fibers (23). To confirm the conduction block further, they recommended three methods. The first method is short-segment stimulation. An abrupt change in area and/or amplitude over 2–4 cm is strong evidence of conduction block. A gradual change is more likely to be caused by temporal dispersion. Unfortunately, this can be applied percutaneously only to a few nerve segments: the ulnar nerve from the elbow to the axilla and the peroneal nerve around the knee. At other locations, the insertion of a monopolar needle electrode as a stimulating cathode near the nerve is required. Use of a coaxial or bipolar needle to record the muscle action potential (MAP) is the second method. It is sometimes possible to establish whether there are individual motor units in the response to distal stimulation that cannot be activated by proximal stimulation. The final recommended method is resynthesis of the evoked MAP using recordings of the surface-recorded recruitment pattern at the same sweep and gain. We believe that these methods are *not practical* in clinical practice and thus recommend the compromised criteria discussed above.

An abnormal temporal dispersion can also be judged in comparison with the normal CMAP duration. It can easily be recognized when *the duration of the CMAP is prolonged with multiple phases* (Figs. 20.6 and 20.7). On the other hand, if the duration of the CMAP is only prolonged, an accurate measurement of the duration is essential for determination of abnormal temporal dispersion. Since this method is *the sole means of identifying abnormal temporal dispersion in the distal CMAP*, it provides *important electrophysiological information*. An abnormal temporal dispersion can be identified by a prolongation of CMAP duration *greater than 20 msec by the manual measurement, 8 msec by the negative duration and 35 msec by the total duration with electronic measurement* (Table 7.12).

Specific Patterns of Nerve Conduction Abnormalities

Though most peripheral neuropathies show mixed motor and sensory nerve conduction abnormalities in the nerve conduction study, there are certain patterns of abnormalities specific enough to be of value to clinicians in localizing the lesions to specific parts of the nerves and in suggesting the nature of a neuropathy (Table 20.3).

With a pure motor neuropathy, the motor nerve conduction is abnormal, whereas the sensory nerve conduction is completely normal. Moreover, the motor nerve conduction abnormalities can be classified into two categories: axonal and demyelinating. The classic pattern of axonal pure motor neuropathy is pathognomonic of anterior horn cell lesions or ventral polyradiculopathy (Table 20.4). This pattern is *characterized by a low CMAP amplitude and mild motor NCV slowing, whereas the sensory and mixed nerve conductions are perfectly normal.* The best examples of this pattern are seen in amyotrophic lateral sclerosis (see Chapter 22) and a few cases of axonal Guillain-Barré neuropathy (31). There are a few other causes. However, this pattern is an ominous finding because in 75% of the cases it was found to be caused by motor neuron disease or neoplasm, either directly or indirectly (remote effect: chemotherapy), in one study (32). *The pattern of demyelinating pure motor neuropathy is characterized by nerve conduction abnormalities typical of demyelination confined to the motor fibers.* This pattern is indicative of a demyelinating neuropathy involving the motor fibers alone and has been

Table 20.3.
The Characteristic Pattern in the Nerve Conduction

Motor NCS	Sensory NCS	Pathology	Typical Diseases
Pure Motor Neuropathy			
Axonal neuropathy	Normal	Anterior horn cell	Motor neuron disease
		Polyradiculopathy	Axonal form of GBS
Demyelination	Normal	Pure motor neuropathy	Multifocal demyelinating neuropathy
		Polyradiculoneuropathy	GBS (early stage)
Pure Sensory Neuronopathy			
Normal	Abnormal	Dorsal root ganglion	Friedreich's ataxia
			Sjögren's syndrome neuropathy
			Paraneoplastic subacute sensory neuropathy
Demyelinating Mixed Neuropathy			
Uniform demyelination	Abnormal	Hereditary neuropathy	HMSN type I
Nonuniform demyelination	Abnormal	Acquired demyelinating N	CIDP, GBS, CSDN
Axonal Mixed Neuropathy			
Axonal	Abnormal	Axonal neuropathy	Alcoholic neuropathy, Vasculitic neuropathy

Table 20.4.
Pure Motor Neuropathy Pattern

Axonal type[a]
  Amyotrophic lateral sclerosis or progressive spinal muscular atrophy
  Dapson-induced neuropathy
  Axonal form of Guillain-Barré syndrome
  Diffuse myelopathy
  Generalized radiculopathy (cervical and lumbar stenosis or metastatic carcinomatosis)
  Lambert-Eaton syndrome
  Myopathy (chronic)
Demyelinating type
  Guillain-Barré syndrome
  Multifocal demyelinating neuropathy

[a]From Wilbourn (32).

Table 20.5.
Pure Sensory Neuronopathy Pattern

Friedreich's ataxia
Ataxia telangiectasia (Louise-Barr syndrome)
Bassen-Kornzweig's syndrome
Carcinomatous (paraneoplastic) sensory neuropathy
Sjögren's syndrome sensory neuropathy
Chronic ataxic sensory neuropathy (idiopathic)
HSAN Type I (hereditary sensory radicular neuropathy of Denny-Brown)
HSAN Type II (congenital sensory neuropathy)
Piridoxin-induced neuropathy
Vitamin E deficiency-induced neuropathy

Table 20.6.
Uniform Demyelinating Polyneuropathy

Hereditary motor sensory neuropathy (HMSN) type I (39)
Metachromatic leukodystrophy (40)
Krabbe globoid leukodystrophy
Cockayne syndrome

described in many reported cases of multifocal demyelinating neuropathy and in some patients with the Guillain-Barré syndrome in the early stage (33, 34). In the majority of our patients with multifocal demyelinating neuropathy or the GBS, sensory nerve conductions were abnormal (34, 35).

With a pure sensory neuronopathy, the sensory nerve conduction is markedly abnormal, but the motor nerve conduction is completely normal. The sensory nerve conduction abnormalities are characterized by the pattern of axonal degeneration: extremely low or absent CNAP with mild slowing of sensory NCV. The pattern of pure sensory neuronopathy is pathognomonic of a sensory neuronopathy involving the dorsal root sensory ganglia (Table 20.5). This pattern is classically observed in Friedreich's ataxia (36), sensory neuropathy associated with Sjögren's syndrome (37), and paraneoplastic subacute sensory neuropathy (38).

Uniform demyelinating neuropathy is a useful concept in differentiating between hereditary motor sensory neuropathy (HMSN) and acquired chronic demyelinating neuropathy (Table 20.6). This distinction is important because many patients with acquired chronic demyelinating neuropathy may respond to immunotherapies. *In uniform demyelinating neuropathy, the NCV is slowed "uniformly" to the same degree over all nerves and nerve segments.* In addition, conduction block or abnormal temporal dispersion is absent because of the "uniform demyelination of all fibers" (39). This pattern has been classically described in HMSN type I and familial neuropathies associated with metachromatic leukodystrophy, globoid leukodystrophy, and Cockayne syndrome (40). On the other hand, in acquired chronic demyelinating neuropathy, the nonuniform slowing of nerve conduction over the different nerves and nerve segments, conduction block, and abnormal temporal dispersion are typically observed. Although this rule is generally true, exceptions are common enough that care must be used in basing a conclusion on the nerve conduction findings alone (41).

Diagnostic Value of Motor and Sensory Nerve Conduction

Studies have repeatedly shown that sensory conduction is a more sensitive indicator of a peripheral nerve lesion than motor conduction (2, 5, 13, 24, 42, 43). Buchthal and Rosenfalck (2) found that motor nerve conduction was normal in about one-half of 25 patients with slight but clear-cut abnormalities in sensory nerve conduction distally (digits to wrist). According to them, the advantage of testing sensory nerve conduction is based on the following factors: (a) sensory fibers are often affected earlier than motor nerves; (b) severe loss of nerve fibers can be discriminated more precisely in sensory than in motor fibers. In sensory fibers, a reduction of $\frac{1}{500}$ of the normal amplitude is the lower limit of measurement. This is a range about 10 times that for the motor response because of interference from other nerves; (c) a response from other than the fastest fibers can be recognized in sensory potentials. An increase in temporal dispersion may be an early sign of impairment when conduction velocity along the fastest fibers and the amplitude of the potential are still within the range of normal (6, 23).

In interpreting the nerve conduction data, one has to answer five questions:

1. Are these data normal or abnormal? This can easily be answered by comparing the obtained data with the normal data and by recognizing of the abnormal electrophysiological responses listed for diseased nerves.

2. Do these abnormalities represent axonal degeneration or segmental demyelination? This question can be answered on the basis of the nerve conduction characteristics described earlier (Table 20.1). This distinction is important because it helps in understanding the disease process and in identifying a definite etiology.

3. Is the disease process focal, multifocal, or diffuse? The nerve conduction study is helpful in identifying and localizing the site of individual nerve compression or entrapment. This information is crucial in the surgical management of many focal or entrapment neuropathies. A distinction can also be made by nerve conduction studies as to whether the neuropathy is multifocal or diffuse. There are two groups of neuropathies that are marked by electrophysiological mononeuropathy multiplex: (a) multifocal demyelinating neuropathy (44), often with sites of persistent conduction block occurring away from the usual loci of entrapment; and (b) multifocal axonal neuropathy. The latter are ischemic in origin, as in cases of vasculitic neuropathy. Diffuse nerve conduction abnormalities are seen in patients with a polyneuropathy.

4. Is there any specific pattern of the nerve conduction abnormalities? This question is answered on the basis of the nerve conduction characteristics described above (Table 20.3). These distinctions are important because they enable the clinician to localize a lesion to a specific part of the nerves and help in identifying a definite etiology.

5. Finally, are the electrophysiological abnormalities relevant to the clinical problems? This is the most important aspect of the interpretation of nerve conduction data. The data must be interpreted in the context of the clinical history and findings. It is in this correlation that the knowledgeable and experienced clinician distinguishes him- or herself.

Once these five questions are answered correctly, the nerve conduction data can provide the clinician with invaluable information about the diseased nerve, which cannot be obtained by any other means.

REFERENCES

1. Buchthal F. Sensory and motor conduction in polyneuropathies. In: Desmedt JE, ed. New developments in electromyography and clinical neurophysiology, vol. 2. Basel: Karger, 1973:259–271.
2. Buchthal F, Rosenfalck A. Sensory potentials in polyneuropathy. Brain 1971;94:241–262.
3. Oh SJ. Electromyography: Neuromuscular transmission studies. Baltimore: Williams & Wilkins, 1988.
4. Auger RG, Daube JR, Gomez MR, Lambert EH. Hereditary form of sustained muscle activity of peripheral nerve origin causing generalized myokymia and muscle stiffness. Ann Neurol 1984;15:13–21.

5. Downie AW. Studies in nerve conductions. In: Walton JN, ed. Disorders of voluntary muscles. Edinburgh: Churchill Livingstone, 1974:973–1002.
6. Gilliatt RW. Nerve conduction in human and experimental neuropathies. Proc Roy Soc Med 1966;58:989–993.
7. Behse F, Buchthal F. Sensory action potentials and biopsy of the sural nerve in neuropathy. Brain 1978;101:473–493.
8. Gilliatt RW, Sears TA. Sensory nerve action potential in patients with peripheral nerve lesions. J Neurol Neurosurg Psychiatry 1958;21:109–118.
9. Rosenfalck A. Early recognition of nerve disorders by near-nerve recording of sensory action potentials. Muscle Nerve 1978;1:360–367.
10. Ludin HP, Tackmann, W. Sensory neurography. New York: Thieme-Stratton, 1981.
11. Buchthal F, Rosenfalck A, Behse F. Sensory potentials of normal and diseased nerves. In: Dyck PJ, Thomas PK, Lambert EH, eds. Peripheral neuropathy. Philadelphia: WB Saunders, 1975:442–464.
12. Tackmann W, Spalke G, Oginszus HJ. Quantitative histometric studies and relation of number and diameter of myelinated nerve fibers to electrophysiological parameters in normal sensory nerves of man. J Neurol 1976;212:71–84.
13. Tackmann W, Minkenberg R. Nerve conduction velocity of small components in human sensory nerve. Eur Neurol 1977;16:270–279.
14. Bostock H, Sears TA. Continuous conduction in demyelinated mammalian nerve fibers. Nature (Lond) 1978;263:786–787.
15. Rasminsky M, Sears TA. Internodal conduction in undissected demyelinated fibers. J Physiol (Lond) 1972;227:323–350.
16. Oh SJ, Clements RS, Lee YW, Diethelm AG. Rapid improvement in nerve conduction velocity following renal transplantation. Ann Neurol 1978;4:369–373.
17. Gilliatt RW. Recent advances in the pathophysiology of nerve conduction. In: Desmedt JE, ed. New developments in EMG and clinical neurophysiology, vol 2. Basel: Karger, 1973:2–18.
18. McLeod JG. Nerve conduction measurements for clinical use. In: Van Duijn H, Donker DNJ, Van Hufflen AC, eds. Current concepts in clinical neurophysiology. The Hague: NV Drukkerij Trio, 1977:83–98.
19. McLeod JG, Prineas JW, Walsh JC. The relationship of conduction velocity to pathology in peripheral nerves. A study of the sural nerve in 90 patients. In: Desmedt JE, ed. New developments in EMG and clinical neurophysiology, vol 2. Basel: Karger, 1973:248–258.
20. Oh SJ. Subacute demyelinating neuropathy responding to corticosteroid treatment: electrophysiological findings. Muscle Nerve 1982;5:562.
21. Gilliatt RW. Nerve conduction in human and experimental neuropathies. Proc R Soc Lond 1966;58:989–993.
22. Rhee EK, England JD, Sumner AJ. A computer simulation of conduction block: effects produced by actual block versus interphase cancellation. Ann Neurol 1990;28:146–156.
23. Cornblath DR, Sumner AJ, Daubet J, et al. Conduction block in clinical practice. Muscle Nerve 1991;14:869–871.
24. Bannister RG, Sears A. The changes in nerve conduction in acute idiopathic polyneuritis. J Neurol Neurosurg Psychiatry 1962;25:321–328.
25. Cornblath DR. Electrophysiology in Guillain-Barré syndrome. Ann Neurol 1990;27 (suppl):S17–S20.
26. Albers JW, Donofrio PD, McGonable TK. Sequential electrodiagnostic abnormalities in acute inflammatory demyelinating polyradiculoneuropathy. Muscle Nerve 1985;8:528–539.
27. Kelly JJ. The electrodiagnostic findings in peripheral neuropathy associated with monoclonal gammopathy. Muscle Nerve 1983;6:504–509.
28. Brown WF, Feasby TE. Conduction block and Guillain Barré polyneuropathy. Brain 1984;107:219–239.
29. Kim DE, Kuruoglu HR, Oh SJ. What is the best diagnostic index of conduction block and temporal dispersion? Muscle Nerve 1991;14:884.
30. Feasby TE, Brown WF, Gilbert JJ, Hahn AF. The pathological basis of conduction block in human neuropathies. J Neurol Neurosurg Psychiatry 1985;48:239–244.
31. Feasby TE, Gilbert JJ, Brown WF, Bolton CF, Hahan AF, Koopman WF, Zochodne W. An acute axonal form of Guillain-Barré polyneuropathy. Brain 1986;109:1115–1126.
32. Wilbourn AJ. Generalized low motor-normal sensory conduction responses: the etiology in 55 patients. Muscle Nerve 1984;7:564–565.
33. Van den Bergh P, Logigian EL, Kelly JJ. Motor neuropathy with multifocal conduction blocks. Muscle Nerve 1989;11:26–31.
34. Thomas T, Oh SJ, Bosse B, Joy J. Diagnostic sensitivity of the initial nerve conduction study in acute inflammatory demyelinating polyneuropathy. Neurology, 1991;41 (Suppl 1):132.
35. Riser E, Joy J, Oh S. Demyelinating mononeuropathy multiplex. Neurology 1988;38 (Suppl 1):225.
36. Oh SJ, Halsey JH. Abnormality in nerve potential in Friedreich's ataxia. Neurology 1973;23:52–54.
37. Malinow K, Yannakakis D, Glusman SM, et al. Subacute sensory neuropathy secondary to dorsal root ganglionitis in primary Sjögren's syndrome. Ann Neurol 1986;20:535–537.
38. Horwich MS, Cho L, Proor L, Posner JB. Subacute sensory neuropathy in patients without carcinoma. Ann Neurol 1977;2:7–19.
39. Lewis RA, Sumner AJ. Electrodiagnostic distinctions between chronic familial and acquired demyelinative neuropathies. Neurology 1982;32:592–596.
40. Miller RG, Gutmann L, Lewis RA, Sumner AJ. Acquired versus familial demyelinative neuropathies in children. Muscle Nerve 1985;8:205–210.

41. Oh SJ, Chang CW. Conduction block and dispersion in hereditary motor and sensory neuropathy. Muscle Nerve 1987;10:656A.

42. Lamontagne A, Buchthal F. Electrophysiological studies in diabetic neuropathy. J Neurol Neurosurg Psychiatry 1970;33:442–452.

43. Shefner JM, Dawson DM. The use of sensory action potentials in the diagnosis of peripheral nerve disease. Arch Neurol 1990;47:341–348.

44. Lewis RA, Sumner AJ, Brown MJ, Asbury AK. Multifocal demyelinating neuropathy with persistent conduction block. Neurology 1982;32:958–964.

45. Ad Hoc Subcommittee of the AAN AIDS Task Force. Research criteria for diagnosis of chronic inflammatory demyelinating polyneuropathy (CIDP). Neurology 1991;41:617–618.

46. Bromberg MB. Comparison of electrodiagnostic criteria for primary demyelination in chronic polyneuropathy. Muscle Nerve 1991;14:968–976.

47. Oh SJ. Abnormality in sensory nerve conduction: a distinct electrophysiological feature of arsenic polyneuropathy. EEG Clin Neurophysiol 1980;49:21.

21

Nerve Conduction in Focal Neuropathies

Focal neuropathies are common diagnostic problems for the clinical electromyographer. For the precise localization of a focal neuropathy, nerve conduction and the needle electromyography (EMG) studies are essential. The electrophysiological changes found by nerve conduction velocity (NCV) studies in these disorders vary according to the rapidity with which the neuropathy develops, the duration and severity of the lesions, and the underlying causes. Among nontraumatic causes, the compression neuropathies (Table 21.1), in which a nerve is compressed at anatomically vulnerable sites, are the most common.

The ulnar, common peroneal, and radial nerves are those most commonly subject to damage by external pressure, in the order named. The median nerve is most frequently affected by constriction by a fascial band at the carpal tunnel. The axillary nerve is commonly affected in an allergic reaction to injection of serum, and the sciatic nerve by direct injection of drugs.

We discuss nontraumatic focal neuropathies in this chapter.

Table 21.1.
Focal Neuropathies

1. Traumatic—peripheral nerve injuries
2. Nontraumatic
   a. Compression neuropathies
      Acute
      Chronic
   b. "Infectious" neuropathies
      Bell's palsy
      Brachial plexus neuropathy (neuralgic amyotrophy)
      Lumbar plexus neuropathy
      Herpes zoster
      Leprosy mononeuropathy
   c. Vasculitic focal neuropathy
   d. Radiation neuropathy
   e. Tumor
      Neurofibroma
      Carcinomatous neuropathy

Acute Compression Neuropathy

Acute compression neuropathy is characterized by the acute onset of neuropathy following a prolonged period of pressure compression on the nerves (Table 21.2). The classical example is "Saturday night palsy," so called because of the number of cases attributable to prolonged resting of the head on the upper arm while the patient was in an alcoholic stupor.

In the past, acute compression neuropathy was thought to be the result of neurapraxia, or conduction block without any structural damage. However, recent studies

Table 21.2.
Acute and Chronic Compression Neuropathies

1. Acute compression neuropathies
   - a. Tourniquet paralysis
   - b. Saturday night palsy (radial nerve palsy)
   - c. Crossed-leg palsy (peroneal nerve palsy)
   - d. Perioperative ulnar nerve palsy
2. Chronic compression (entrapment) neuropathies
   - a. Compression in a fibroosseous tunnel
     - Carpal tunnel syndrome
     - Cubital tunnel syndrome
     - Tarsal tunnel syndrome
   - b. Angulation and stretching
     - Tardy ulnar nerve palsy
     - Thoracic outlet syndrome (including cervical rib syndrome)
   - c. Recurrent compression by external forces
     - Some ulnar compression neuropathy at elbow
     - Deep branch neuropathy of the ulnar nerve
     - Meralgia paresthetica
3. Hereditary compression neuropathies

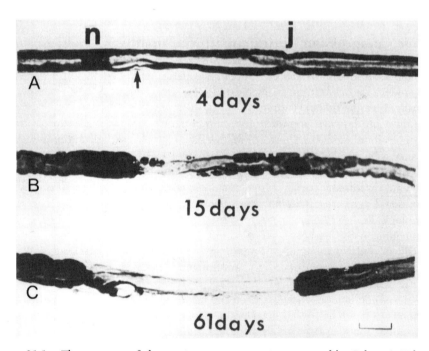

Figure 21.1.   The sequence of changes in acute compression suggested by Ochoa. **A**, Telescoping displacement (n) of the nodes of Ranvier a few days after injury is followed by paranodal demyelination. **B**, Early remyelination. **C**, With the formation of an intercalated segment. (From Gilliatt RW. Acute compression block. In: Sumner AJ, ed. The physiology of peripheral nerve disease. Philadelphia: WB Saunders, 1980:293.)

with animals have revealed the pathological basis for this disorder (1). The telescoping displacement of myelin in the nodes of Ranvier was found to be the earliest change, followed by paranodal demyelination occurring toward the edge of the compression region (Fig. 21.1). These processes seem to affect the larger fibers selectively. In severe cases, wallerian degeneration is also present (2). This mild *focal demyelinating process* is responsible for the conduction block that is the characteristic electrophysiological finding in this disorder and which explains the complete paralysis of the involved muscle.

Tourniquet Paralysis

Tourniquet paralysis is a well-known but rare acute compression neuropathy found as a complication following use of a pneumatic tourniquet to produce a bloodless field during surgery. Clinically, this compression neuropathy produces motor and sensory impairments in multiple nerves distal to the placement of the pneumatic tourniquet. Because of the common application of tourniquet around the upper arm, median, ulnar and radial nerve palsies are common findings in this disorder.

Three studies of human patients with tourniquet paralysis (2–4) demonstrated the typical conduction block, as observed in animals (5). Electrophysiological findings were:

1. Normal amplitude of the compound muscle action potentials (CMAP) and compound nerve action potentials (CNAP) with normal motor and sensory NCVs distal to the site of the block;

2. Across the block, conduction block and slow motor and sensory NCVs; dispersion phenomenon in sensory CNAP;

3. Subsequent gradual electrophysiological and clinical recovery over a period of a few months; and

4. In a single patient with protracted recovery, EMG evidence of additional wallerian degeneration (2).

Saturday night palsy, crossed-leg palsy, and acute ulnar compression neuropathy during surgery are discussed under the sections dealing with the respective involved nerves.

Chronic Compression (Entrapment) Neuropathy

Entrapment neuropathy refers to a mononeuropathy produced by chronic mechanic impingement of a nerve in normally narrow anatomical sites. The best example of this neuropathy is carpal tunnel syndrome.

The most prominent symptoms of an entrapment neuropathy are sensory, ranging from pain to numbness (6). These are followed by motor weakness and muscle wasting in advanced cases. Tinel's sign can pinpoint the site of entrapment if the nerve is located superficially. The primary sensory abnormalities are revealed in the impairment of two-point discrimination, light touch, and pin-prick, in that order. Classically, these symptoms and signs are confined to the territory of the involved nerve.

Pathologically, entrapment neuropathies are characterized by: (*a*) paranodal demyelination in the early stages; (*b*) *complete segmental demyelination* in the full-blown stage; and (*c*) complete degeneration of fibers in the later stage. Wallerian degeneration in the nerve distal to the entrapment is a natural consequence of the late stage (Fig. 21.2).

The nerve conduction study has been the means of definite diagnosis in the entrapment neuropathies. The focal demyelinating process caused by mechanical entrapment is responsible for the electrophysiological evidence of chronic focal demyelination: marked focal slowing of the NCV (6). The presence of conduction block in chronic entrapment neuropathies is less often demonstrable by nerve stimulation than in acute compression neuropathy (7).

To localize the focal demyelinating process, it is imperative to study the involved segment by the segmental nerve conduction study (8, 9). There are a few technical

CHRONIC NERVE COMPRESSION AND ENTRAPMENT

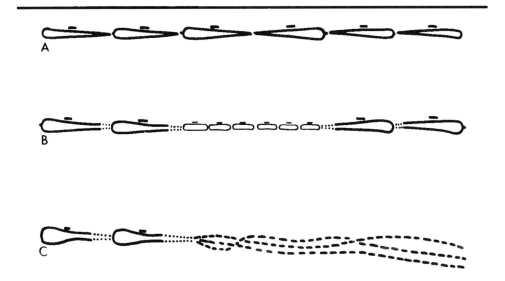

Figure 21.2. The sequence of change in chronic compression and entrapment suggested by Ochoa. *A*, Distorted internodal segments in a minimal entrapment lesion, with reversal of polarity at the center. *B*, A more severe lesion with paranodal demyelination affecting the distorted internodes at the edges and complete demyelination followed by remyelination in the center. *C*, More marked distortion of the internodes on the proximal side of the lesion, with wallerian degeneration distally (255). (From Ochoa J. Nerve fiber pathology in acute and chronic compression. In: Omer GE, Spinner M, eds. Management of peripheral nerve problems. Philadelphia: WB Saunders, 1980:487–501.)

problems we must address in this connection. In human entrapment neuropathy, it has been shown that the primary abnormalities in conduction are confined to the short segments (often 5–10 mm) of the nerve (10–12). The consequence of the discrete nature of these lesions is that when nerve conduction is measured over long segments (80–100 mm), the NCVs could become less abnormal or even normal because of the inclusion of longer normal or near-normal segments in the calculation. Most authorities regard *10 cm as the shortest acceptable distance* for the segmental conduction velocity (see Chapter 12). This distance may be too generous to detect the segmental nerve conduction abnormality in some patients with focal neuropathy.

Despite the inherent technical limitations of the short distance technique, the shorter distance has been used by several investigators in studies of sensory nerve conduction in the palm-wrist segment (10, 11, 13), and in precise localization of the lesion in ulnar and peroneal compression neuropathy (10, 12). In all these studies, the authors were able to pinpoint the lesion better with the shorter distance technique so long as the technique was carefully controlled. Percutaneous stimulation at short intervals along the length of an involved nerve (the "inching" technique) is especially useful for providing the exact localization of the lesion by demonstrating the conduction block and conduction delay (12). This is used as a routine in our laboratory in cases with the ulnar neuropathy at elbow.

The common entrapment neuropathies and their characteristic features are summarized in Table 21.3. The various focal neuropathies are discussed next under the heading of the involved nerve.

Trigeminal Nerve

The trigeminal nerve has two main components—motor and sensory fibers. Motor fibers arise from the trigeminal motor nucleus in the pons and follow the mandibular branch, exiting through the foramen ovale and forming the inferior alveolar branch, which innervates the pterygoid, masseter, and temporalis muscles. Sensory fibers are formed with three main divisions—ophthalmic, maxillary, and mandibular nerves—and have three relay neurons: the spinal trigeminal tract, the main sensory nucleus of the pons, and the mesencephalic nucleus.

Trigeminal neuralgia is the best known trigeminal disorder. In this disorder, the blink and masseter reflexes are normal (14, 15). Trigeminal sensory neuropathy is a rare

Table 21.3.
Compression Site and Typical Clinical Features of the Common Compression Neuropathies

Compression Syndrome	Entrapment Site	Typical Clinical Features
Median nerve		
Carpal tunnel syndrome	Carpal tunnel	Tinel's sign at the wrist. Sensory impairment over the first 3.5 fingers. Motor deficits on thenar muscles.
Anterior interosseous syndrome	At its origin from the median nerve	Pure motor weakness of the flexion of the middle phalanx of the first three fingers.
Pronator syndrome	At the level of pronator teres	Entire motor and sensory neuropathy with pronator teres spared. Pronator muscle tenderness and Tinel's sign on it.
Ulnar nerve		
Tardy ulnar palsy Cubital tunnel syndrome	Elbow	"Claw hand." Motor deficit on hypothenar muscles. Sensory impairment over the dorsal and palmar aspects of the last 1.5 fingers.
Guyon's canal	Wrist	Same as above except sensory impairment over palmar aspects of the last 1.5 fingers.
Thoracic outlet syndrome	Thoracic outlet	Sensory impairment over the ulnar side of the entire arm and hand. Motor deficits of the intrinsic hand muscles.
Radial nerve		
Saturday night palsy	Spiral groove	Wristdrop.
Posterior interosseous syndrome	The tendinous arcade of Frohse	Fingerdrop.
Suprascapular nerve	Suprascapular foramen	Motor deficits of the supra- and infrascapular muscles.
Long thoracic nerve		Scapular winging.
Peroneal nerve		
Crossed-leg palsy	Fibular head	Footdrop.
Posterior tibial nerve		
Tarsal tunnel syndrome	Tarsal tunnel	Sensory impairment over the palmar aspect of the foot. Tinel sign at the ankle.
Morton's neuroma	III–IV interdigital nerve	Sensory impairment over the V-shaped area between the III and IV toes.
Lateral femoral cutaneous nerve		
Meralgia paresthesica	Anterior iliac crest	Sensory impairment over the lateral thigh.
Femoral nerve	Inguinal ligament	Weak knee extension. Absent knee jerk.
Saphenous nerve	Hunter's canal	Sensory impairment in the medial aspect of knee and leg.
Sural nerve		Sensory impairment over lateral aspect of the foot.

disorder that is commonly associated with scleroderma or mixed connective disease. The main clinical features are a slowly evolving unilateral or bilateral facial numbness, which is sometimes associated with pain and paresthesia and commonly accompanied by disturbed taste (16). The blink reflex evoked by glabellar tap in three cases showed a normal response in one, an absent first component in one, and a delayed first component in one case (17). In another study of 17 cases, the blink reflex was abnormal in 11 (65%); the most common abnormality, present in six cases, was an "afferent type" defect, e.g., delay in all components but with normal latencies on stimulation of the contralateral supraorbital nerve (Fig. 21.3) (16). On the other hand, Hess et al. found that the first component was delayed in six of eight cases and the second component delayed in only one case (18).

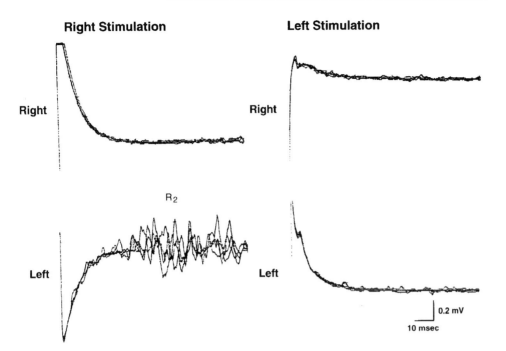

Figure 21.3. Blink reflex in left trigeminal neuropathy (the first branch) and right facial palsy due to carcinomatous meningitis.

Facial Nerve

Facial palsy is probably the most common mononeuropathy. There are many causes of facial palsy, including herpes zoster infection and otitis media. However, the etiology is unknown in a majority of patients. This facial palsy is called Bell's palsy.

Bell's palsy is usually unilateral and of acute onset. It is characterized by the paralysis of all muscles innervated by the facial nerves, including the upper facial muscles. Depending upon the site of the lesion (Fig. 21.4), facial palsy may be accompanied by impaired lacrimation, hyperacusis, and/or a disturbance of taste. This disorder is benign in that the majority of patients recover. In more than half of the patients, recovery is complete within 2–3 months. In the remaining patients, recovery is incomplete, but only about 5–10% of patients are seriously handicapped with permanent disfigurement or sequelae (19). In recent years steroid treatment has increased the proportion of patients who recover completely (20). However, there are a few physicians who advocate surgical decompression of the facial canal within 2 weeks after onset for patients whose expected outcome is poor (21, 22).

Thus, some means of predicting the final outcome at an early stage of the disease is required to select the minority who may require prolonged steroid treatment (23) or surgery (21, 22). Generally, a useful clinical indicator of good prognosis is an incomplete palsy when the patient is first seen. In complete palsy, the clinical findings are of limited value (19). To select the group of patients whose expected outcome is poor, electrophysiological tests are most helpful in Bell's palsy.

Nerve Excitability Test

Campbell et al. (24) compared nerve excitability between the normal and affected sides in 197 patients with complete Bell's palsy. The test was performed as soon as possible after the 3rd day following onset, 50% being done before the 14th day. The patients were followed until their conditions appeared static. The authors found that full recovery occurred in 90% of the patients when there was no difference on the two sides, whereas full recovery occurred in only 20% of patients when the nerve was not excitable on the affected side. On this basis, they concluded that this test is capable of distinguishing between "physiological block" and degeneration of the facial nerve as early as 72 hr after the onset of facial palsy. Since then, the NET has been widely used

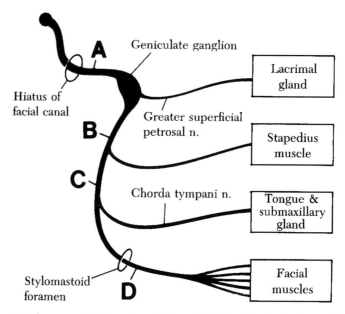

Figure 21.4.   Facial nerve and its branches. **A**, When diminished lacrimation is noted, the lesion is at or proximal to the geniculate ganglion. **B**, When the stapedial reflex is impaired (hyperacusis), the lesion is in the middle ear segment. **C**, When the taste is impaired, the lesion is in the vertical course of the facial nerve in the mastoid bone. **D**, When pure facial paralysis is present, the lesion is at the stylomastoid foramen or distal to it.

Table 21.4.
Nerve Excitability Test: Rate of Full Recovery in Bell's Palsy

Investigator	NET Criteria		
	Unimpaired	Diminished	Absent
Campbell et al. (24)	90[a] (N = 61)	49 (N = 21)	20 (N = 35)
Laumans (26)	96 (N = 24)	20 (N = 15)	0 (N = 71)
Saade and Karam (28)	84 (N = 26)	17 (N = 6)	14 (N = 7)
Alford et al. (25)	95 (N = 21)	24 (N = 5)	
LeClaire et al. (27)	99 (N = 130)	44 (N = 18)	15 (N = 26)
Devi et al. (23)[b]	77 (N = 48)	35 (N = 20)	32 (N = 19)[c]

[a]%: Recovery rate.
[b]Two-thirds of patients were treated with steriod.
[c]All of these patients were treated with steriod.
N = Number of cases.

as an electrophysiological indicator of prognosis in Bell's palsy. Subsequent studies confirmed Campbell et al.'s (24) findings (25–28) (Table 21.4). When there was no significant difference in the NET between two sides, the full recovery rate ranged from 84 to 99%. When the NET was diminished, full recovery rates were between 17 and 49%. On the other hand, when the nerve was inexcitable, full recovery rates dropped to 0–20%. Thus, these studies showed the prognostic value of the NET in facial nerve palsy.

It should be noted that a small proportion of patients in whom nerve excitability was unimpaired initially, and therefore in whom an excellent recovery was anticipated, later lost excitability. Hence, an erroneous good prognosis was made in 11% of the cases (24). This late loss of the NET usually happened after the 10th day, indicating that in a small percentage of patients, degeneration of the facial nerve continues within the first week. In practice, this means that the test should be repeated after the 10th day if the initial NET within a few days showed a normal response before predicting the prognosis of facial palsy.

Recently there have been a few investigators who have questioned the reliability of this test. May et al. (29) reported that the maximal stimulation test becomes abnormal sooner than the NET and is a more reliable guide to prognosis. The maximal stimulation test is identical to the NET test except that the stimulation is slowly increased up to 5 mA or until the patient begins to note discomfort. The response (visual) on the involved side is compared to that on the normal side. Yanagihara and Kishimoto (30) compared the NET, the strength-duration curve, and the CMAP with the concentric needle in the motor conduction test. They concluded that in patients with slight residual paresis (no great handicap to a patient's social activities), the motor conduction test was better able to detect abnormality than the NET, but in patients with moderate or severe residual paresis the NET was dependable in predicting a definitely unfavorable prognosis. Adour et al. (31) compared the maximal NET and the CMAP with the surface electrode in the motor conduction and concluded that the maximal NET is more reliable than the motor conduction for predicting the prognosis of facial paralysis. The maximal NET test is different from the NET test in that the current is increased 2 mA above the threshold to obtain the "maximal nerve excitability threshold," and the degree of visible muscle motion on the affected side is compared with the nonaffected side. It is our opinion that the comparison of "visible muscle twitch" is fraught with subjective errors and that the maximal NET test or the maximal stimulation test is less objective. This may be the reason why these tests are not widely used by others.

Devi et al. (23) did serial NETs in 100 patients with facial palsy, of whom 61 were treated with steroids; they concluded that serial NETs were useful not only for prognosis, but also helpful in regulating the dosage of prednisone. They recommended a higher dose for longer periods until a significant improvement in the NET was noted.

Motor Nerve Conduction

Motor Latency

Gilliatt and Taylor (32) stimulated the facial nerve percutaneously after transection and found the latency unaltered until the response became unobtainable 4–7 days later. Serial tests were performed in patients with Bell's palsy by Langworth and Taverner (33) and Zander Olsen (19). In a study of 167 patients with Bell's palsy, Langworth and Taverner found that the serial latencies were normal (less than 4.0 msec) in patients with needle EMG evidence of no denervation, that the latencies were either normal or increased during the 2nd week in patients with partial denervation, and that the nerve became inexcitable within 7 days after the onset in patients with complete denervation. From these observations, they concluded that a response to electrical stimulation, regardless of whether the latency is increased, more than 5 days after the onset of the paralysis always indicates a good prognosis and that a nonresponse to electrical stimulation within 7 days is indicative of a poor prognosis. Thus nerve excitability is more important than the latency measurement as the indicator of prognosis. Zander Olsen (19) found that a normal latency in some muscles was associated with moderate or severe sequelae and that the latency was not systematically related to the initial severity of the facial palsy. Brown et al. (34) also did not find any evidence that the motor latency is of predictive value in facial palsy.

Amplitude of the CMAP

Because the amplitude of the CMAP evoked by a maximal stimulation to the nerve depends on the number of conducting axons, the reduction in amplitude is a suitable method of assessing the degree of damage and estimating the prognosis. Yanagihara and Kishimoto (30) found that in patients with slight residual paresis the motor nerve conduction test was better than the NET in detecting abnormality, and only amplitudes of less than 200 µV with the concentric needle could be used to indicate partial degeneration of the nerve. Zander Olsen (19) found in a study of 50 patients with facial palsy that, of the electrophysiological parameters (threshold, CMAP, latency, and needle

EMG) early after the onset of the palsy, the amplitude of CMAP evoked by maximal stimuli to the facial nerve was the best way to predict the final outcome. He studied patients initially 5 days to 2.5 months (usually within 3 weeks) after the onset. When the amplitude was reduced to 10% or less of that of the contralateral muscle, recovery took 6 months to 1 year, and sequelae were severe or moderate. It made no difference whether the nerve was inexcitable or responded with a small potential, indicating that degeneration was not total. When the amplitude was reduced to 30–10% of normal, recovery took 2–8 months, and sequelae were mild or moderate. When the amplitude was above 30% of normal, full recovery occurred within 2 months after the onset of the palsy. All of his patients had some reduction in amplitude of CMAP in one or more of the three muscles examined, indicating that nerve fibers had degenerated. The reduction in amplitude was similar in all three muscles (frontalis, triangularis, and orbicularis oculi), proving that one muscle was as solicitable to denervation as another in Bell's palsy.

According to Fisch (21), the serial motor nerve conduction study indicates that the destiny of the facial nerve in Bell's palsy is decided within the first 2–3 weeks after onset of the palsy. All patients having less than 90% maximal degeneration (90% reduction of the amplitude of CMAP recorded with the surface electrode) of facial nerve fibers within 3 weeks of onset of the palsy reach a satisfactory return of facial movements without any form of treatment. On the other hand, 50% of the patients with 95–100% maximal degeneration within 2 weeks of onset of the palsy have a permanent unsatisfactory recovery of facial function. In view of this, he proposed immediate surgical decompression as soon as 90% of the facial nerve fibers have undergone degeneration within 2 weeks after the onset of Bell's palsy. He claimed that surgery performed when degeneration has reached 95–100% within 1–14 days after onset of the palsy significantly improves the recovery of facial movements. Esselen, recording with surface electrodes from the orbicularis oris muscle, found that a reduction of 50% or less of normal was associated with full recovery and that a reduction to 10% of normal was still associated with good recovery (35).

May et al. believed that a 75% axonal loss (as determined by side-to-side amplitude comparison), rather than 90%, was an appropriate cutoff for predicting a good prognosis. Among patients who had a 75% axonal loss or less, complete recovery was achieved in 77%. However, in patients with greater than a 75% loss, 88% had incomplete recovery. They also concluded that neither facial nerve decompression procedures nor systemic corticosteroids benefited most patients with Bell's palsy.

Redhead and Mugliston (36) considered the side-to-side CMAP amplitude comparison to be the best electrical method of objectively formulating a prognosis in patients with acute lesions in the 7th cranial nerve (36). Canter et al., however, failed to find any statistically significant correlation between CMAP measurement and the clinical outcome at 12 months in a prospective study of 23 patients with complete paralysis (37).

Thus, the majority of studies found that *the CMAP amplitude comparison is the most useful test for formulating a prognosis in the acute stage of Bell's palsy and that a reduction of CMAP to 10% or less is usually associated with a poor prognosis.*

Blink Reflexes

The NET and the motor nerve conduction test of the facial nerve measure the degree of wallerian degeneration of the nerve distal to the lesion in Bell's palsy but fail to test the proximal segment of the facial nerve, which is primarily affected in this disorder. The blink reflex, on the other hand, reflects the conduction of the entire length of the facial nerve, including the involved proximal interosseous portion.

In unilateral facial palsy, the classical findings on the blink reflex test are: (*a*) prolongation of latency or complete absence of both components (R1 and R2) of the blink reflex on the involved side after stimulation on either side; (*b*) a normal R2 component appearing on the noninvolved side after stimulation on the side of the lesion; and (*c*) normal R1 and R2 components appearing on the noninvolved side after stimulation on

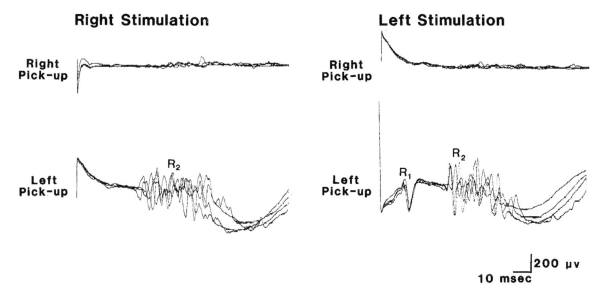

Figure 21.5. Blink reflex in the right Bell's palsy. No response is noted in the right orbicularis oculi (right) with right or left supraorbital stimulation.

the noninvolved side (Fig. 21.5). In general, the latency measurement of R2 is not as useful as that of R1 because of the wider range of variability. Nonetheless, analysis of direct and consensual R2 is essential in determining the affected portion of the reflex arc.

The blink reflex has been of some usefulness for determining the prognosis of this disorder. Schenck and Manz (38) concluded, on the basis of their experience with 30 patients, that the prognosis is favorable if the R1 and R2 components are at all recognizable or reappear during the first 10 days and that the prognosis is unfavorable when both R1 and R2 remain absent during the first 2–3 weeks. On the basis of serial changes in the direct and reflex response, Kimura et al. (39) concluded that in patients with excitability of the distal segments of the facial nerve that was retained until blink reflex responses returned showed a good clinical recovery. Complete recovery was noted in 81% of 21 patients who were followed up beyond 2 months after onset. When the R1 component was present, its latency was substantially greater than normal during the first 2 days after onset, further increased during the latter half of the 1st week, then remained essentially unchanged up to the 4th week. The latency showed a notable reduction during the 2nd month and became essentially normal during the 3rd and 4th months. On the other hand, patients in whom a direct response to facial nerve stimulation became unsolicitable, indicating distal degeneration of the nerve before reflex responses returned, had a prolonged and generally incomplete recovery. None of the 25 patients in this group showed appreciable return of function during the first 2 months.

From this review, it is clear that *the amplitude of the CMAP together with the repeated NET is the most practical and reliable prognostic procedure for Bell's palsy early after onset of symptoms.*

Needle EMG Test

Granger studied the relationship between the MUPs 72 hr after onset of paralysis and a functional prognosis in 90 patients with Bell's palsy (40, 41). When MUPs were present in four of five facial muscles (posterior auricular, frontalis, orbicularis oculi, zygomaticus, and orbicularis oris), a favorable prognosis was seen in 91% of patients. When MUPs were seen in two or three muscles, the outcome was satisfactory in 87% of cases, whereas the prognosis was favorable in only 11% of patients in whom MUPs were absent or present in only one muscle (40). Blom and Ekstrand also observed that the presence or absence of MUPs within 10 days after the onset of paresis correctly indicated a good prognosis in 82% of the patients who recovered completely and a poor prognosis in 67% of those who had an incomplete recovery (42). They concluded that the presence or absence of MUPs in the facial muscles can be used as a guide for the early prediction of prognosis. However, May et al. found that the needle EMG was unreliable for prognostic purposes: their study showed that 75% of patients with no MUPs as well as 38% of those with MUPs in the affected facial muscles had an incomplete recovery at 6 months (43).

Although some earlier studies regarded the presence of fibrillation as a sign of a poor prognosis (44, 45), later studies did not confirm this (46, 47). Krogness showed that fibrillation does not necessarily indicate a poor prognosis as long as the MUPs remain (47). Another drawback is that fibrillation is not detectable during the first 10 days of paresis.

In general, *the needle EMG test is not a reliable indicator of prognosis*. However, it has a definite value in identifying an incomplete lesion by revealing a few remaining MUPs during the acute period of facial palsy and demonstrating reinnervation by recording a few small polyphasic MUPs during the early stage of recovery, despite the clinical absence of facial function.

Accessory Nerve

The accessory nerve, the 11th cranial nerve, arises from the C1–C4 spinal roots and ascends into the intracranial cavity through the foramen magnum, leaves the intracranial cavity through the jugular foramen accompanied by the glossopharyngeal and vagus nerves, and descends into the neck to supply the sternomastoid. It appears at the posterior border of the sternomastoid at the level of the upper edge of the thyroid cartilage, and runs obliquely downward and backward toward the posterior cervical triangle to supply the upper third or upper half of the trapezius muscle.

The accessory nerve lies superficially where it crosses the floor at the posterior cervical triangle and can be damaged by trauma at this point. However, most lesions of the accessory nerve result from surgical procedures on the posterior triangle directed to removing the lymph nodes and other tissues intimately related to the nerve (48). Idiopathic spinal accessory nerve palsy has also been reported (49).

With injury to the accessory nerve, the trapezius muscle is always involved (Fig. 21.6), and if the damage is high the sternocleidomastoid is also affected. Thus, the

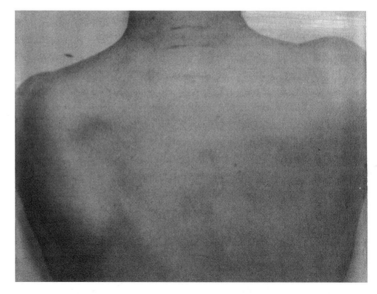

Figure 21.6.   Left accessory nerve palsy. Atrophy of the left trapezius muscle and upper scapular winging are obvious.

Table 21.5.
Clinical Features of Common Neurogenic Causes of Scapular Winging

Clinical Features	Serratus Anterior Palsy (Long Thoracic Nerve)	Trapezius Palsy (Accessory Nerve)
Pain	Localized to scapular region	Localized to supraclavicular fossa
Deformity at rest	Minimal	Shoulder droops
Winging		
At rest	Minimal winging of the lower part of the scapula	Minimal winging of the upper part of the scapula
During activity	Pronounced, accentuated by forward elevation and pushing with outstretched arms	Moderate, accentuated by arm abduction at the shoulder level
Scapular displacement during activity	Inferior angle farther from midline	Inferior angle moved toward midline

Table 21.6.
Nerve Conduction Abnormalities in Accessory Nerve Palsy

Investigator	No. of Cases	Normal	Prolonged Latency	Absent CMAP
Cherington (50)	1		1	
Eisen and Bertrand (49)	4		3	1
Fahrer et al. (51)	8	3	2	3
Krogness (52)	1		1	
Logigian et al. (353)	2	1		1
Petrera and Trojaborg (354)	10	4	6	
Barkhaus et al. (355)	1		1	
Total	27	8	14	5

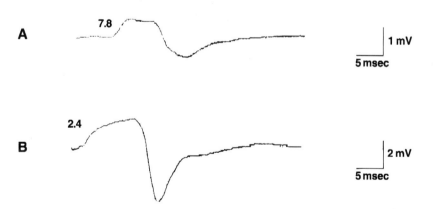

Figure 21.7. **A**, Prolonged latency (7.8 msec) and low CMAP amplitude (1.7 mV) in the left accessory motor conduction compared with normal motor conduction in the right accessory nerve (**B**).

prominent signs and symptoms of accessory nerve injury are due to paralysis of the trapezius muscle. This neuropathy is most commonly confused with paralysis of the serratus anterior muscle. The differential features are presented in Table 21.5.

Nerve conduction tests have been performed in a few cases (49, 50–55). Among 27 cases of accessory nerve palsy, there was no response in five cases and a prolonged terminal latency in 14 cases (Table 21.6). Thus, accessory nerve palsy can be confirmed by the nerve conduction test (Fig. 21.7). The needle EMG shows denervation in the upper and middle trapezius muscles, and additionally in the sternocleidomastoid muscle if the lesion is high.

Greater Auricular Nerve

The greater auricular nerve (C2, C3), a pure sensory nerve and the largest ascending branch of the cervical plexus, emerges along the posterior border of the sternocleidomastoid just proximal to the midpoint between the mastoid process and the clavicle insertions (see Fig. 11.10). It innervates sensation over the mastoid area and the back of the lower part of the auricle. This nerve is easily susceptible to injury and is affected commonly in leprosy and hereditary motor sensory neuropathy (HMSN) type I as a thickened nerve (56).

Palliyath reported a low CNAP in the greater auricular nerve in a patient with this neuropathy that was induced by a central venous line during surgery (56). A 3-mm neuroma was found in the nerve.

Phrenic Nerve

The phrenic nerve is formed from branches of the C3–C5 spinal nerves. It descends in front of the scalenus anterior and then traverses the mediastinum, finally innervating the diaphragm (see Fig. 11.19). Phrenic neuropathy can be caused by a mediastinal mass or injury during thoracic surgery, and may be involved in acute brachial plexus neuropathy (57). Isolated phrenic neuropathy can occur, possibly as a variant of acute brachial plexus neuropathy (58), and is usually unilateral. Unilateral phrenic neuropathy is usually asymptomatic or produces only mild dyspnea. Bilateral phrenic neuropathy produces severe dyspnea and usually represents a more widespread disease such as amyotrophic lateral sclerosis or the Guillain-Barré syndrome (GBS) (Fig. 21.8).

The phrenic nerve conduction study was able to confirm this neuropathy in a few patients with isolated phrenic neuropathy (Oh, unpublished data). Among 30 randomly selected diabetic patients, seven had slowing in the phrenic nerve conduction, with bilateral slowing in five and unilateral slowing in two (59). In 28 patients with GBS, phrenic nerve conduction time was prolonged in 18 cases (60).

Brachial Plexus

The brachial plexus arises from the C5–C8 and T1 spinal nerves and is divided into trunks, divisions, and cords as it passes through the supraclavicular fossa to the axilla (Fig. 5.2). There are three trunks: (a) the upper trunk from the C4, C5, and C6 roots; (b) the middle trunk from the C7 root; and (c) the lower trunk from the C8 and T1 roots. The trunks are located in the supraclavicular fossa, just distal to the scalenes muscle, and are divided into the anterior and posterior divisions which eventually form the cords. The divisions are situated deep to the middle third of the clavicle.

There are three cords: (a) the lateral cord formed by the anterior divisions of the

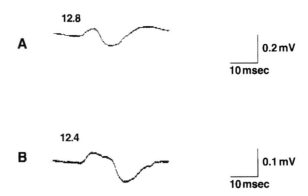

Figure 21.8. Prolonged terminal latency of (**A**) 12.8 msec in the right phrenic nerve and (**B**) 12.4 msec in the left phrenic nerve due to bilateral phrenic neuropathy in a patient who had a difficulty weaning from the ventilator.

upper and middle trunks; (*b*) the posterior cord formed by all posterior divisions of the three trunks; and (*c*) the medial cord formed by the anterior division of the lower trunk. The cords are situated at the axilla. Major peripheral nerves originate from the cords: from the lateral cord, the musculocutaneous nerve and the lateral head of the median nerve; from the posterior cord, the axillary and radial nerves; and from the medial cord, the medial head of the median and ulnar nerves.

There are several nerves branching out at each level of the brachial plexus that are important to remember for the sake of localization of lesions:

1. At the spinal nerve level, *the long thoracic nerve and dorsal scapular nerves;*
2. At the trunk level, *the suprascapular and subclavian nerves from the upper trunk;* and
3. At the division level, *the medial and lateral anterior thoracic nerves.*

The clinical features of brachial plexus lesions are represented by complex motor and sensory deficits depending on the location of the lesions. Thus anatomical knowledge of the brachial plexus is important for the accurate localization of brachial plexus lesions.

Acute Brachial Plexus Neuropathy

Acute brachial plexus neuropathy (ABPN) (neuralgic amyotrophy; Parsonage and Turner syndrome, paralytic brachial neuritis) is characterized by acute severe pain in the shoulder area followed by weakness of the muscles innervated by the brachial plexus. The proximal muscles of the arm and shoulder girdle are most frequently involved. In 65% of patients tested the involvement was unilateral, and in 45% there had been an antecedent infection or other event.

Clinical involvement is usually patchy and not strictly anatomic, in keeping with the scattered foci of demyelination, which is the pathological basis of this condition (61). This latter has not been proved by adequate pathological studies. Although the fact that many patients recover within a few weeks suggests that the lesion is most likely demyelinating, the common needle EMG findings of fibrillation and positive sharp waves in the affected muscles also provide evidence of axonal degeneration. In general, ABPN behaves like a restricted variety of the Guillain-Barré syndrome. It should be also noted that ABPN may present along with a distal mononeuropathy such as anterior interosseous neuropathy, or in various combinations (62). The ultimate prognosis is good, with 80% of patients recovering within two years (61).

Even though this entity is not uncommon, electrophysiological studies have been limited to a few articles. Weikers and Mattson (63) found evidence of widespread slowing of motor NCV in five of their seven patients with this disorder, despite fairly localized signs and symptoms (in most cases the slowing was maximal distally) and suggested that the plexus involvement might be the localized form of a diffuse polyneuropathy. More recent studies have not been able to confirm this finding (64, 65). The cases studied by Weikers and Mattson were different from others in that five of the seven were "immunization"-related.

The following is a summary of the most important electrophysiological findings related to brachial plexus neuropathy:

1. In general, routine motor nerve conduction studies were not particularly useful. Martin and Kraft (65) found no abnormality in the standard distal motor NCV in median, ulnar, radial or peroneal nerves in any of their 18 patients. Flaggman and Kelly (64) found mild abnormality (slowing of NCV or reduced amplitude of CMAP) in median and ulnar motor conductions in three of 16 patients.

2. *Routine sensory nerve conduction showed more abnormalities than the routine motor nerve conduction.* In one-third of cases there were minimal abnormalities (low amplitude of the sensory CNAP with normal or slightly slow NCV) in median and ulnar sensory conductions (64).

3. The motor NCV of ulnar and median nerves from the Erb's point through the brachial plexus was normal (64, 65).

4. *The sensory NCV through the brachial plexus was abnormal in four of six patients* (64). In all four patients the distal sensory conduction was normal.

5. Median and ulnar F-wave latencies are not helpful. They were abnormally prolonged in only three of 16 patients (64).

6. The musculocutaneous motor nerve was studied in 11 patients. Four patients had abnormal findings: no response in one case, reduced amplitude in all cases, slow NCV in one case.

7. *The latency from Erb's point to the shoulder girdle muscle was abnormal in all cases* (65). The latency to affected muscles ranged from slightly greater than normal to more than eight times normal. However, according to Gassell (66), two of four patients had slight to moderate prolongation in the latency in some muscles tested, but latencies were normal in some severely wasted muscles. Reduction in the latency toward normal was usually the first indication of impending clinical improvement (65).

It seems that the latency test to the shoulder girdle muscles and the sensory nerve conduction test from Erb's point through the brachial plexus are the most useful, but even they are of limited value in this disorder.

At present, *the needle EMG is the best means of delineating the anatomic extent and physiological severity of the disease* (64, 67). The needle EMG study shows fibrillations and positive sharp waves and/or MUP changes indicative of denervation in the affected muscles (64). Paraspinal muscles are usually normal. In a small number of patients, the paraspinal EMG shows fibrillation and positive sharp waves (Oh; unpublished data). About 50% of patients with unilateral clinical involvement have bilateral abnormalities on the needle EMG (64).

Tumor-Induced Brachial Plexus Neuropathy

The most common cause of tumor-induced brachial plexus neuropathy is cancer of the lung and breast that has spread via the lymph nodes or bone metastasis (68). Neoplastic invasion of the plexus is seldom the earliest manifestation of cancer except in Pancoast syndrome, which is nearly always caused by a carcinoma at the apex of the lung invading the lower trunk of the brachial plexus and the inferior cervical sympathetic ganglion, producing Horner's syndrome in two-thirds of patients. Clinically, this neuropathy is characterized by subacute progressive painful plexopathy predominantly involving the lower trunk (C8 and T1 roots) and often associated with Horner's syndrome (68). In 63% of patients, a cervical myelogram showed epidural extension of the disease. The CT or MRI scan is very helpful in detecting malignant infiltration of the brachial plexus.

In about one-half of patients tested the sensory nerve conduction was abnormal in median, ulnar, or radial nerves, and in two-thirds of patients the motor nerve conduction was abnormal in median and ulnar nerves, reflecting a predominant lower trunk involvement (69). The needle EMG was most productive, demonstrating fibrillations and "neurogenic MUPs" in almost all cases. Fasciculation was rare and myokymia was absent in this disorder.

Radiation-Induced Brachial Plexopathy

Radiation-induced brachial plexopathy is a well-known entity. This condition is dose-dependent; i.e., if more than 6000 rads are given, plexopathy occurs in up to 73% of patients. Lower doses given over longer periods of time are much safer (68, 70). This plexopathy can occur a few months or up to 26 years following irradiation (68). The distinction between this entity and tumor-induced brachial plexopathy is not easy. In contrast to tumor-induced plexopathy, radiation-induced plexopathy is usually painless, more often involves the upper trunk (affecting the C5, C6, and C7 roots), and is associated with progressive lymphedema (68). Visible fasiculation or myokymia is helpful in recognizing this entity.

Nerve conduction abnormalities in this disorder are not much different from those found in tumor-induced plexopathy, though sensory nerve conduction abnormalities are more common here (69). The needle EMG showed fibrillations and "neurogenic MUPs" in almost all cases (69). *The most typical needle EMG findings for this disorder are fasciculation and myokymia.* In this disorder, fasciculation was observed in two-thirds of patients and myokymia in about half (69). Myokymia and low-frequency complex repetitive discharges have been reported by others as occurring particularly following radiation (71, 72).

Traumatic Plexopathies

The brachial plexus is vulnerable to trauma because of its superficial location. Depending on the location of an injury and the combination of lesions, the clinical presentations are different. However, there are three well-known distinct syndromes: (*a*) root avulsion; (*b*) brachial plexus injury in newborns; and (*c*) intraoperative brachial plexus injury.

Root Avulsion

Avulsion of the spinal nerve roots is a serious complication of trauma because the avulsed root cannot be repaired and does not regenerate spontaneously. Because of this, it is important to distinguish a plexus lesion from a root avulsion. The lower cervical roots are most often involved. Root avulsion is best confirmed by myelogram. However, it is also characterized by a *typical combination* of electrophysiological abnormalities: (*a*) fibrillation and positive sharp waves in the paraspinal muscles; (*b*) normal sensory nerve conduction in the affected area; and (*c*) an absent cervical or cortical SEP in the affected segment. EMG of the paraspinal muscles is abnormal because the root damage is proximal to the dorsal rami (73). Because the damage to the sensory fibers is proximal to the dorsal root ganglia, the distal sensory fibers are viable, thus producing normal sensory nerve potentials in the arms, even though the patient has no feeling in the avulsed root segments (74). For the same reason, the cervical or cortical SEP will be absent in the presence of normal sensory CNAPs or Erb's potentials (see Chapter 19). The histamine skin test is also helpful in determining whether a sensory lesion is proximal or distal to the dorsal root ganglia, because the flare response is abolished if the sensory fibers are damaged distal to the ganglia (75).

Brachial Plexus Injuries in Newborns

There are two well-known syndromes: (*a*) Erb's palsy involving the upper trunk; and (*b*) Klumpke's palsy involving the lower trunk. These are usually stretch injuries caused by manual or forceps traction, although they occur rarely during an uncomplicated delivery (57). In the more common Erb's palsy, the needle EMG shows denervation in the shoulder girdle muscles. In the less common Klumpke's palsy, the needle EMG shows denervation in the lower trunk innervated muscles and motor and sensory nerve conduction abnormalities in the median and ulnar nerves.

Intraoperative Brachial Plexus Injury

Intraoperative injury is particularly frequent after a median sternotomy during coronary artery bypass surgery. One prospective study showed that brachial plexus injury occurred in 5% of these patients (76). It usually involves the lower trunk or medial cord, and its signs can easily be misinterpreted as those of an ulnar neuropathy (76, 77). There are two different opinions regarding the pathogenesis of this injury: traction or compression of the plexus (77), or jugular cannulation (76). EMG studies in 11 patients with clinical lower trunk lesions showed fibrillations in the lower trunk-innervated muscles in all cases and an ulnar sensory, motor, and F-wave abnormality in one-third of patients (78). One patient had an upper trunk lesion and another had a lower trunk lesion with bilateral ulnar neuropathy.

Long Thoracic Nerve

The long thoracic nerve arises directly from the anterior rami of the C5, C6, and C7 spinal nerves shortly after they emerge from the intervertebral foramen, passes laterally behind the brachial plexus, and courses down the lateral aspect of the chest wall, finally innervating the serratus anterior muscle (see Fig. 11.25).

Long thoracic nerve palsy is most commonly of traumatic origin (79). Classically, this disorder produces scapular winging caused by palsy of the serratus anterior muscle (Table 21.5).

Kaplan (80) reported the mean latency of the motor conduction of the long thoracic nerve as 6.3 ± 0.3 msec (normal is less than 5.1 msec) in four patients and as 4.0 ± 0.5 msec in the same patients after recovery. Among 18 patients with long thoracic nerve palsy, Petrera and Trojaborg (79) reported no response in four cases, prolonged latency in nine cases, and normal latency in six cases. These studies showed that the latency measurement is helpful in the diagnosis of long thoracic nerve palsy.

Dorsal Scapular Nerve

The dorsal scapular nerve originates from the C5 spinal nerve and innervates the levator scapulae and rhomboid muscles (Fig. 5.2). Isolated neuropathy of this nerve has not been clearly documented. Fibrillations and absence of MUP in the rhomboid muscles associated with minimal medial scapular winging was reported (81). However, this was as a result of a C5 root injury. Thus, the main value of the needle EMG in the rhomboids is to establish a C5 root injury because these muscles originate directly from the C5 spinal nerve.

Suprascapular Nerve

The suprascapular nerve arises from the upper trunk of the brachial plexus formed by the C5 and C6 spinal nerve roots (Fig. 5.2). It crosses the posterior cervical triangle and then runs under the trapezius muscle and through the suprascapular notch to innervate the supraspinatus muscle. The nerve then twists around the spinoglenoid notch of the scapular spine to innervate the infraspinatus. Suprascapular neuropathy produces selective weakness and wasting of the supra- and infraspinatus muscles.

Suprascapular nerve palsy is a rare disorder. However, the suprascapular nerve can be paralyzed as a manifestation of brachial plexus neuropathy or stretch injuries. Entrapment of this nerve as it passes through the suprascapular notch below the transverse suprascapular ligament is a well-documented syndrome, producing paralysis of the supra- and infrascapular muscles (Fig. 21.9). The entrapment of this nerve at the lateral edge of the scapular spine, in the spinoglenoid notch, is rare, and produces selective paralysis of the infraspinatus muscle. Nerve conduction tests have been performed in 11 cases of suprascapular nerve palsy (82–85). There was a delay of latency (3.3–12.0 msec) to the affected muscles, and in one case (82), the marked prolongation of latency was confined to the infraspinatus muscle, thus pinpointing the distal entrapment.

Subscapular and Thoracodorsal Nerves

The subscapular and thoracodorsal nerves arise from the posterior cord of the brachial plexus (Fig. 5.2). The subscapular nerve innervates the subscapularis and teres major muscles, which rotate the shoulder medially. The thoracodorsal nerve innervates the latismus dorsi, which adduct and rotate the shoulder medially. The needle EMG in these muscles is valuable only in localizing the level of a posterior cord injury.

Medial and Lateral Anterior Thoracic (Pectoral) Nerves

The lateral and medial anterior thoracic nerves (from the C5, C6, and C7, and the C8 and T1, respectively) innervate the pectoralis major and minor muscles, which adduct and rotate the humerus medially (Fig. 5.2). Again, the needle EMG in these muscles can be helpful in localizing a brachial plexus injury. Isolated lateral pectoral nerve injury caused by trauma from a seatbelt was documented by fibrillations and the

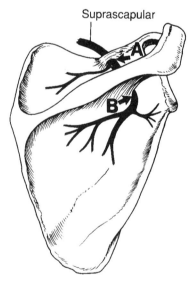

Suprascapular

Figure 21.9. Entrapment sites of suprascapular nerve. **A**, Entrapment at the suprascapular notch produces palsy of the supra- and infraspinatus muscles. **B**, Entrapment at the spinoglenoid notch produces paralysis of the infraspinatus muscle.

absence of MUPs in the clavicular head of the pectoralis major muscle, which was atrophic (86).

Axillary Nerve

The axillary nerve originates from the posterior cord of the brachial plexus formed from the C5 and C6 spinal roots (Fig. 5.2). It innervates the teres minor and deltoid muscles and supplies the sensory fibers to the skin over the deltoid. Axillary neuropathy produces wasting and weakness of the deltoid muscles and sensory loss in a small area over the deltoid muscle.

The most common cause of this neuropathy is trauma (87, 88). The needle EMG showed denervation in the deltoid and teres minor muscles in all patients with this neuropathy (87–89). The terminal latency to the deltoid muscle from the Erb's point can be measured.

Musculocutaneous Nerve

The musculocutaneous nerve arises from the lateral cord of the brachial plexus formed from the C5, C6, and C7 nerve roots (see Fig. 11.29). As it courses down between the biceps and brachialis muscles, it innervates the coracobrachialis, biceps, and brachialis muscles. It emerges at the elbow just lateral to the biceps tendon and then continues as the lateral cutaneous nerve of the forearm, innervating the radial aspect of the forearm flexor surface.

Weakness and wasting of the biceps muscle and sensory impairment on the territory of the lateral cutaneous nerve of the forearm are characteristic of this neuropathy. Isolated musculocutaneous neuropathy is uncommon. The needle EMG showed denervation in the coracobrachialis, biceps, or brachialis muscles, depending on the site of the lesion (90–92). The nerve conduction test of the musculocutaneous nerve with stimulation at Erb's point showed no response from the biceps muscle in one case (90) and prolonged latency with a low CMAP amplitude in one case (92). Trojaborg presented three cases illustrating the usefulness of the motor and sensory nerve conduction tests of this nerve: in two cases of C5 root avulsion, the tests were normal; in one case of isolated musculocutaneous nerve injury, the initial test showed no response in the motor and sensory nerve conduction, whereas a later test showed improvement in the nerve conduction (93).

Felsenthal et al. reported three patients with a sensory neuropathy of the lateral cutaneous nerve of the forearm that was confirmed by prolonged latency or a decrease in the CNAP amplitude on nerve conduction testing of this nerve (94).

Median Nerve

The median nerve is a major nerve formed by the union of the lateral and medial cords (from the C5–C7 and the C8–T1 spinal nerves, respectively) (see Fig. 5.3). It lies first in the lateral wall of the axilla and then in the medial aspect of the upper arm close to the brachial artery and the radial and ulnar nerves. At the elbow, it lies medial to the biceps tendon and brachial artery and then passes between the two heads of the pronator teres muscle. As it emerges from the pronator teres, the anterior interosseous nerve branches from the main median nerve, which passes through the two heads (the "sublimis bridge") of the flexor digitorum superficialis muscle and courses down distally in the forearm between the flexor digitorum superficialis and profundus muscles. The median nerve enters the hand through the carpal tunnel. Distal to the carpal tunnel, the nerve divides into two branches—motor and sensory. The motor branch innervates the APB, opponens pollicis, and superficial head of the flexor pollicis brevis muscles through the recurrent branch, and the 1st and 2nd lumbricalis muscles through the small terminal branch. The sensory fibers innervate sensation over the first 3.5 digits of the hand.

Proximal Median Neuropathy

In proximal median neuropathy the median nerve is usually involved together with the ulnar or radial nerve (Fig. 21.10). Thus, an isolated proximal median neuropathy is rare and characterized by complete motor and sensory median neuropathy. Trauma is the common cause of isolated proximal median neuropathy. Roth et al. reported four cases in which the patients developed an isolated proximal median neuropathy during sleep, probably caused by compression at the "canalis brachialis of Cruveilhier," a narrow fibromuscular space under the inferior border of the pectoralis major (95). In all cases, conduction block was found between Erb's point and the axilla. In two cases, sensory nerve conduction up the wrist was slow. Needle EMG in two cases showed denervation in all median-innervated muscles, including the pronator teres muscle.

Supracondylar Spur/Ligament of Strutcher Syndrome

Supracondylar spurs and/or ligaments under which the brachial artery and median nerve pass are rare causes of median nerve compression (57). The diagnosis is usually confirmed by palpation of the spur or by a simple x-ray. It produces a complete motor and sensory median neuropathy (96). The needle EMG study showed denervation in all median nerve-innervated muscles, including the pronator teres. The median nerve conduction study showed conduction block and slow motor NCV between the "above elbow" and "below-elbow" segments in the motor nerve conduction and absent sensory CNAP at the wrist (96).

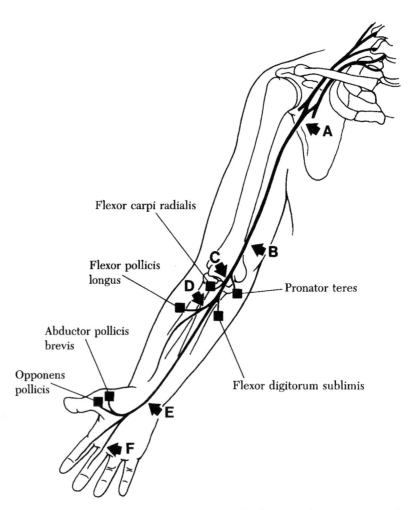

Figure 21.10.   Entrapment sites in median nerve. **A**, At the thoracic outlet. **B**, Ligament of Strutcher syndrome. **C**, Pronator syndrome. **D**, Anterior interosseous neuropathy. **E**, Carpal tunnel syndrome. **F**, Digital neuropathy.

Pronator Teres Syndrome

Pronator teres syndrome (PTS) is thought to result from the compression or irritation of the median nerve as it passes through the pronator teres muscle. Diagnosis of this syndrome is based on characteristic symptoms and signs: (a) aching and pain in the volar aspect of the forearm, worsened by repeated forearm pronation; (b) paresthesias in the median nerve territory when the forearm is pronated forcibly against resistance; (c) tenderness and firmness on the pronator teres muscle; and (d) tenderness and a positive Tinel's sign in the median nerve at the elbow (97). However, objective evidence of median nerve dysfunction has been mild or absent in a majority of cases (97, 98). An exception was reported by Morris and Peters (99), who found some weakness of the median-innervated forearm and hand muscles in all of seven patients and median sensory loss in six (99).

Nerve conduction abnormalities can be divided into two groups, depending on the absence or presence of objective neurological deficits: nonneurogenic PTS, and neurogenic PTS. In nonneurogenic PTS, the routine median motor and sensory nerve conductions are relatively normal (97, 98, 100). Only two of 39 patients had definite evidence of PTS: local slowing or a block at the pronator teres (97). This study also reported segmental "compression" of sensory nerve conduction across the pronator teres in four patients and carpal tunnel syndrome in seven patients. Mysiew and Colachis did not find any abnormality in the median motor NCV in 10 patients (98), nor did Werner et al. in their nine patients (100). On the other hand, in most patients with neurogenic PTS, the median motor nerve conduction was abnormal. Slow motor NCV in the forearm segment with a normal distal latency and sensory latency was observed in six of Morris and Peters' seven patients, indicating a lesion in the forearm. In three of seven cases of median neuropathy at the elbow (probable pronator syndrome), Buchthal et al. found abnormal sensory conduction below and above the entrapment site (101). In studies of two patients, Gessini et al. found slow motor and sensory NCV across the elbow in one and an unexcitable median nerve in the other (102). In Martinelli et al.'s case, there was slow median motor NCV in the forearm segment (103).

To improve the diagnostic sensitivity, Werner et al. tested the median motor nerve conduction before, during, and after forced isometric forearm pronation and found borderline abnormal nerve conduction in three of nine patients with PTS: in one patient, a 0.5 msec prolongation and a 40% reduction of the amplitude, and a 20% reduction in the amplitude in two others (100). However, Mysiew and Colachis compared the median motor and sensory nerve conductions in 10 patients before and after the same dynamic maneuver and did not find any motor nerve conduction abnormality (98). These authors did find a postexercise amplitude change in the median sensory CNAP in one patient. Thus, they concluded that the *dynamic test maneuver does not improve the sensitivity* of conventional nerve conduction studies in the diagnosis of PTS. The intraoperative nerve conduction study in 10 patients showed slow NCV in only one patient (97). In classical PTS, denervation on the EMG study should be confined to the median nerve-innervated superficial and deep forearm and hand muscles except in the pronator teres muscle (97, 100, 103). Buchthal et al. found EMG abnormalities in the superficial and deep flexor muscles in six of seven patients (101). In only six of 39 patients was the needle EMG study able to localize the lesion to the elbow region (97), and in only one of nine patients the needle EMG showed denervation in the thenar and flexor pollicis longus muscles (100). Denervation was found in the pronator teres muscles in at least three cases (97, 102, 104). Contrary to the conventional teaching, Gross and Jones observed fibrillations and positive sharp waves in the pronator teres muscle in 13 of 17 patients with a proximal median neuropathy, probably due to PTS (105). On this basis, they warned that the needle EMG cannot differentiate between a median nerve lesion at the pronator teres and more proximal lesions.

Anterior Interosseous Syndrome

The anterior interosseous nerve arises from the median nerve as it emerges between the two heads of the pronator teres muscle and courses deep in the forearm between

Figure 21.11. "Pinch sign" in anterior interosseous nerve palsy in the left hand. **A**, Normal right hand. **B**, Left hand showing inability to "pinch" with the tips of the thumb and index finger because of paralysis of the flexor pollicis longus and flexor digitorum profundus of the 2nd digit.

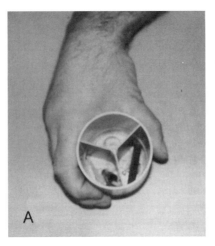
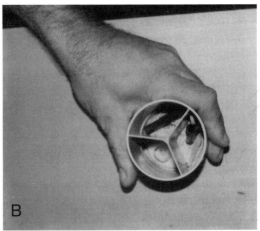

the anterior interosseous membrane and the flexor digitorum profundus muscle. It is entirely motor and innervates the flexor pollicis longus, the II and III flexor digitorum profundus, and the pronator quadratus muscles. The characteristic clinical feature of anterior interosseous neuropathy is the inability to flex the terminal phalanges of the thumb and index fingers. The patient typically forms a triangle with the thumb and index fingers ("*pinch sign*") instead of forming a circle and has difficulty holding a cup tightly between the thumb and index fingers (Fig. 21.11). Weakness of pronation with elbow flexion suggests weakness in the pronator quadratus. There is *no sensory impairment* in this neuropathy.

Anterior interosseous neuropathy is induced by trauma or entrapment at the fibrous bands arising from the pronator teres or the flexor digitorum superficialis muscles (57). It can also be associated with acute brachial plexus neuropathy (106).

The routine median motor and sensory nerve conductions are normal in this neuropathy (107–109). The anterior interosseous nerve conduction demonstrated an abnormal temporal dispersion in all of seven patients, a low CMAP amplitude in four, and prolonged latency from the elbow to the pronator quadratus in five, confirming this neuropathy (107). Rosenberg used the "AIM (anterior interosseous/median) score," which is obtained by dividing the motor latency to the pronator quadratus muscle by the latency to the APB with stimulation of the median nerve at the midhumerus level (110). The AIM score in normal controls was 0.52–0.68. In five patients with anterior interosseous neuropathy, the mean AIM score was 0.76, indicative of a longer latency to the pronator quadratus muscle. However, Rosenberg did not state how many patients had an abnormally high AIM score.

Needle EMG evidence of denervation occurs in the flexor pollicis longus, pronator quadratus, and flexor digitorum profundus I and II, but not in the flexor carpi radialis or flexor digitorum superficialis muscles (107–109, 111).

Other Median Neuropathies of the Forearm

Median neuropathy in the forearm may result from trauma or hematoma. Ischemic neuropathy involving median, ulnar, or radial nerves in the forearm and/or hand was reported after a bovine shunt was inserted between the brachial artery and cephalic vein in the upper arm in a patient undergoing chronic hemodialysis (112, 113). This developed immediately or within a few hours after creation of the fistula. In severe cases, the motor and sensory nerve conduction of all three nerves was abnormal in the hand and forearm (112). In mild cases, sensory nerve conduction was abnormal in all three nerves in the hands (112, 113). The needle EMG usually shows evidence of axonal degeneration in the clinically involved muscles (112, 113). Ischemic neuropathy involving the median and ulnar nerves in the hand and forearm has also been reported after insertion of a bovine shunt between the radial artery and cephalic vein in the forearm (114). In all of seven cases, median and/or ulnar nerve conduction was abnormal: median neuropathy in the hand and forearm in four; median neuropathy at the wrist in two; ulnar neuropathy at the elbow in three (114).

Neuropathy of Recurrent Motor Branch of the Median Nerve

When the median nerve emerges from the carpal tunnel, the terminal motor branch passes laterally to innervate the APB and opponens pollicis muscles. Compression neuropathy of this branch, caused by anomalous branching and producing wasting and weakness of the thenar muscles without sensory abnormality, was reported (115). Electrophysiological studies showed a prolonged terminal latency and denervation in the APB muscle with normal sensory nerve conduction in the finger-wrist segment.

Neuropathy of Palmar Cutaneous Branch

The palmar cutaneous branch of the median nerve arises about 5 cm above the wrist crease, courses down distally, passes through a short tunnel of its own within the transverse carpal tunnel, and innervates sensation over the thenar eminence. Damage to this branch produces paresthesias over the thenar eminence. Detection of sensory loss over the territory of this branch is clinically more important because this is indicative of median neuropathy above the elbow. This nerve can be injured by transverse incisions at the wrist during carpal tunnel decompression and by a ganglion resulting from blunt trauma to the wrist.

Carpal Tunnel Syndrome

Carpal tunnel syndrome (CTS) (Figs. 21.12–21.14) is the most common treatable entrapment neuropathy that can be diagnosed with confidence by the nerve conduction study. It is caused by chronic compression of the median nerve along the carpal tunnel, which is formed on the dorsal, medial, and lateral sides by the carpal bones and on the volar surface by the deep transverse carpal ligaments. The classic symptom of CTS is dysesthesia in the first three fingers of the hand, which is commonly exacerbated at night. Nocturnal exacerbation is so common in this condition that without it the diagnosis should be doubted. It is also true that there are many patients who complain of atypical symptoms, e.g., "sleeping hands," and pain radiating upward toward the forearm and shoulders. Many patients complain of numbness of the hands while driving a car. CTS is common in women and occurs most often in the 5th and 6th decades. Symptoms may appear during pregnancy and resolve after delivery. The most helpful diagnostic signs are Tinel's sign at the wrist and Phalen's sign (tingling sensation on the first three fingers after forceful wrist flexion for 1 min). Sensory loss, motor weakness, and wasting are seen in severe cases.

The causes of CTS are multiple, ranging from local trauma to systemic diseases. The systemic disorders that may produce CTS include diabetes mellitus, chronic renal failure, hypothyroidism, amyloidosis, rheumatoid arthritis, acromegaly, and mucopolysaccharidoses (57). Many patients develop the symptoms in the absence of other known causes, i.e., idiopathic CTS. It has been suggested that a nonspecific tendosynovitis is the most common cause of CTS (116), but this remains unproved.

The nerve conduction study (NCS) is the most definite diagnostic test for CTS, being positive in 91–98% of patients with clinically diagnosed CTS on the basis of their signs and symptoms (Table 21.7). The NCS shows *focal demyelination. The most sensitive diagnostic test is the sensory nerve conduction study*. However, it should be stressed that the extent of motor and/or sensory conduction abnormalities is *not proportional* to the duration or severity of symptoms (117).

Abnormalities in the sensory NCS in the finger-wrist segments have been reported in 63–97.8% of patients. With surface electrodes and without the signal averager, the absence of CNAP in the finger-wrist segment is the most common abnormality, and a slow sensory NCV or prolonged sensory latency is the next. Diminished amplitude is

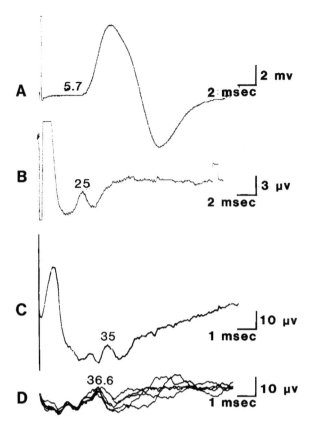

Figure 21.12.   Motor and sensory nerve conduction in carpal tunnel syndrome. **A**, Prolonged terminal latency (5.7 msec). **B**, Low amplitude of the CNAP (3 μv) and slow sensory NCV over the finger-wrist segment (25 msec). **C**, Dispersion (two peaks) and smaller amplitude (9 μv) of the sensory CNAP and slow sensory NCV (35.0 msec) over the palm-wrist segment. **D**, Dispersion (two peaks and 3.3 msec duration) of the sensory CNAP and slow sensory NCV (36.6 msec) over the finger-wrist segment.

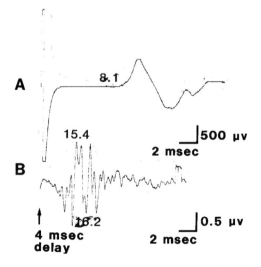

Figure 21.13.   Motor and sensory nerve conduction in carpal tunnel syndrome. **A**, Prolonged terminal latency (8.1 msec) and low amplitude of the CMAP (1500 μv). **B**, Sensory CNAP recorded with needle electrodes: the maximum NCV is 16.2 m/sec; the negative peak NCV is 15.4 m/sec; the dispersion phenomenon is obvious. Surface electrode was not able to record any sensory CNAP.

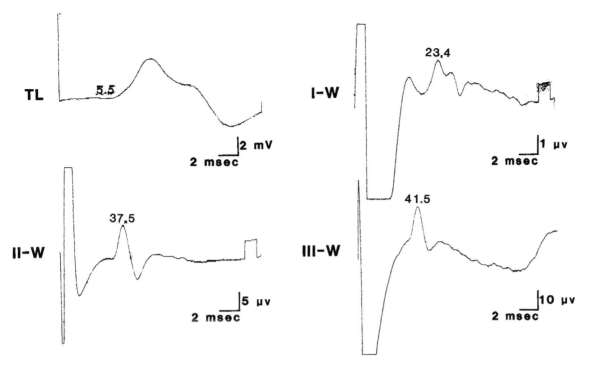

Figure 21.14. Carpal tunnel syndrome involving the motor and sensory branches to the thumb. (*TL*) Terminal latency 5.5 msec. *Roman numerals* indicate the digit number. (*W*) Wrist. Note normal III-W sensory nerve conduction: NCV is 41.5 m/sec. The II-W sensory NCV is slightly slow (37.5 m/sec). Note the marked abnormalities in I-W CNAP: dispersion; low amplitude; markedly slow NCV (23.4 m/sec).

Table 21.7.
Diagnostic Sensitivity (%) of Various Nerve Conduction Tests in Carpal Tunnel Syndrome

Test	Buchthal(120) (N=118)	Duensing(357) (N=138)	Kaeser(127) (N=298)	Kimura(11) (N=172)	Sedal(125) (N=234)	Ludin(358) (N=169)	Thomas(141) (N=476)	Kimura(359) (N=639)	Steven(360) (N=885)
Sensory nerve conduction	**86**[a]	**97.8**[a]	**96**	**63**[b]	**88**	**88**	**85**	**92**[b]	**88**[b]
Slow sensory NCV in finger-wrist segment	86	93.6	41	55	88	88	35[c]	68[c]	
Absent CNAP	0	4.2	55	13			50	24	64
Diminished amplitude	73		3		76.5	58			88
Abnormal temporal dispersion	67					77			
Slow sensory NCV in forearm segment	3								9
Slow sensory NCV in palm-wrist segment	100[d]			86					
			87						
Motor nerve conduction	87	90.7	70	61	65	71	64.4	56.3	39.5
Prolonged terminal latency	82	90.7	63	58	65	71	60	54.3	37.5
Absent CMAP	5		7	3			4.4	2	2
Slow motor NCV in forearm segment	20				35.4		17		11
Normal motor and sensory nerve conduction	5		3	8					

[a]Surface electrodes used unless stated. Near-nerve technique with averager.
[b]Antidromic sensory NCV.
[c]Prolonged latency.
[d]Palm-wrist NCV was performed in 40 cases.

not a basis for electrophysiological diagnosis of CTS with the surface electrode technique. However, with the near-nerve needle technique and the aid of the signal averager, the incidence of an absent CNAP can be drastically reduced to 4.2–0.0%. A slow sensory NCS in the finger-wrist segment was present in 85–97.8%, and diminished amplitude of the largest components of CNAP and abnormal temporal dispersion were observed in about two-thirds of patients (13).

The motor nerve conduction is less sensitive in the diagnosis of CTS, being positive in 64–82% of patients. The CMAP is absent in 3–7% of the cases. In some patients the dispersion phenomenon may be observed.

In recent years palm-wrist sensory nerve conduction methods have been devised and have successfully increased the diagnostic capability in CTS. Using the antidromic sensory nerve conduction method, Kimura (11) was able to confirm CTS in 63% of patients by the conventional sensory NCS over the finger-wrist segment, and additionally in 23% of patients by palmar stimulation. Buchthal and Rosenfalck (13) showed a significant decrease in sensory NCV in the palm-wrist segment in six of eight patients in whom the motor latency was normal and sensory conduction in the finger-wrist segment was near-normal. They also reported that slow sensory NCV in the palm-wrist segment was seen in all tested cases among 40 CTS patients. Mills also reported slow sensory NCV of the palm-wrist segment in 67% of 72 patients with a tentative diagnosis of CTS, in contrast to 53% of cases when the conventional criteria were used (118). Thus, the palm-wrist sensory NCS is the procedure of choice when motor latency and sensory NCS over the finger-wrist segment are normal. *In many laboratories, including our own, the palm-wrist sensory nerve conduction study has become a standard test in the workup of CTS.* Moreover, the faster velocity from digit to palm compared with that from palm to wrist helps to distinguish entrapment at the wrist from a distal neuropathy (119).

It is worthwhile to remember that the various branches of the median nerve are not impaired to the same degree in CTS. Although it is rare, the terminal latency may be abnormal when the sensory NCS is normal. This phenomenon was observed in four of 19 patients in whom sensory potentials were normal (120) and can be explained by the various courses taken, in particular, by the motor thenar branch of the median nerve (121). In 10% of patients in whom sensory NCV from digit to wrist was slow, slowing was observed in half the fingers tested. This fact may be due to the variability of compression on the fascicles of the median nerve, resulting in greater slowing in some digital nerves than others. This emphasizes the need for testing the sensory nerve conduction from each digit in suspected cases of CTS.

To make the diagnosis of CTS, one or more of the following criteria have been used traditionally:

1. *Abnormal sensory nerve conduction in the finger-wrist segment;*
2. *Abnormal sensory nerve conduction in palm-wrist segment;* and
3. *Prolonged terminal latency.*

With increasing awareness of the reliability of this test in the diagnosis of CTS, many patients who do not have CTS are referred to the EMG laboratory with the request to rule out this disorder. Among these "suspected CTS patients," for obvious reasons, the diagnostic sensitivities of the conventional motor and sensory nerve conduction test are lower, being 49% (122) to 78% (123). To increase the diagnostic yield in these patients in whom the conventional tests are normal, various "comparison methods" of analysis have been proposed (Table 21.8).

These methods depend on the inherently flawed assumption that the nerve, with which the comparison is made, is normal. In practice, *this is not always the case.* In 32% of CTS patients, an asymptomatic CTS was detected by the nerve conduction in the opposite hand (124). Asymptomatic ulnar neuropathy was detected in 15% (101) to 39% (125) of CTS patients. Another problem with these comparison methods is that certain proposed criteria for CTS are abnormal in an unacceptably high percentage of "normal" subjects (126). Redmond and Rivner found that a 0.4 msec difference

Table 21.8.
Other Suggested Diagnostic Tests in Carpal Tunnel Syndrome

Suggested Tests	Comments
Comparison of the terminal latency and sensory latency between two median nerves (141)	In 32% of cases, asymptomatic CTS was present in the unaffected side (141)
Comparison of the terminal latency and sensory nerve conduction between the median and ulnar nerves on the affected side (128, 356)	In 15–39% of cases, asymptomatic ulnar neuropathy was found on the unaffected side (120, 125)
Comparison of the sensory nerve conduction between the median and radial nerves on the affected side (123, 122)	Rate of asymptomatic radial neuropathy is not determined. Some prefer this comparison, claiming that radial entrapment neuropathy is rare
Comparison of the sensory nerve conduction between the palmar cutaneous nerve and the conventional methods (133)	
Phalen's maneuver (139)	Dunnan and Waylonis did not confirm this (140)

between median and ulnar palmar sensory latencies was observed in 8% of 50 normal subjects, a reduced median and ulnar sensory amplitude ratio of less than 1.1 was found in 30%, and a residual latency greater than 2.6 msec was noted in 14% (126). Thus, it must be understood that these comparison methods have their own limitations, clearly compromising their usefulness.

The first comparison test proposed was that of the terminal latency and sensory nerve conduction between the symptomatic and asymptomatic median nerves (124, 127). This technique proved to be almost useless for the reason described above. Comparison between the terminal latencies in the median and ulnar nerves in the affected limb was the next comparative test proposed (128). Because of the low diagnostic sensitivity of the motor conduction test in CTS, this is no longer recommended.

The most popular comparative test has been between the sensory nerve conduction in the median and ulnar nerves in the affected hand (122, 123, 129–131). Jackson and Clifford reported an abnormal median/ulnar sensory latency difference by the antidromic technique in 40% of 40 patients referred to rule out CTS in whom the conventional test was normal (129). Pease et al. also observed such abnormalities by the antidromic technique in 88% of 333 "CTS referred patients," whereas the conventional test was diagnostic in only 78% of cases. A clever method is to record the median and ulnar CNAPs simultaneously on the median nerve at the wrist with stimulation of the ring finger because this finger is innervated by the medial and ulnar nerves (130, 131). Using this technique, Uncini et al. recorded a double-peaked response which allowed immediate diagnosis in 78% of 42 patients with electrophysiologically confirmed CTS: the two peaks representing the volume-conducted sensory CNAP from ulnar- and median-nerve stimulation, respectively (Fig. 21.15). Even when the double peaks were not recognized, these authors considered a median and ulnar latency difference greater than 0.5 msec to be suggestive of CTS. Thus, of all methods using median/ulnar differences, the "ring finger technique" was the most sensitive for detection of CTS. Using the same technique, Vallis and Llanas also found double peaks in 87% of 70 patients with clinical evidence of CTS (131). The conventional median nerve conduction study was diagnostic in 81% of cases in their series. Buchthal et al. did not find any advantage in this technique (120).

The most recent comparative test has been between the sensory nerve conduction in the median and radial nerves (122, 123, 129). This method is popular because entrapment neuropathy of the superficial radial nerve is rare. Using this comparison by the antidromic technique, Pease et al. reported an 87% diagnostic sensitivity in 333 patients suspected of having CTS in contrast to 78% by the conventional method (123). They used 0.5 msec as the normal limit. By using 0.4 msec as the upper normal limit with the orthodromic technique, Carrol found an increased diagnostic sensitivity of from 49% by the median sensory nerve conduction to 60% in 161 patients referred for confirmation of CTS (122). Jackson and Clifford reported abnormality in 40% of 40 patients in whom

Figure 21.15. Double-peak potentials recorded over the median nerve after D4 stimulation in seven different patients with CTS. (From Uncini A, Lange DJ, Solomon M, Soliven B, Meer J, Lovelace RE. Ring finger testing in carpal tunnel syndrome: a comparative study of diagnostic utility. Muscle Nerve 1989;12:739.)

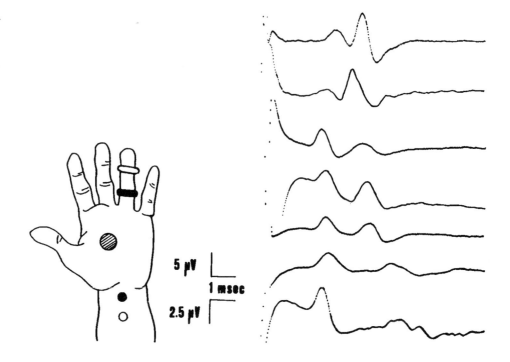

the conventional tests were normal (129). They recorded the median and radial CNAPs from the thumb. As yet there has not been any study reporting an asymptomatic radial nerve abnormality in CTS patients. Harrison found no significant difference in the CNAP amplitude of the radial nerve between controls and CTS patients (132).

From this review, it appears that the best comparative technique available for CTS is between the sensory nerve conduction latency of the median nerve and that of the radial nerve; this method increases the diagnostic sensitivity by 9–11% (122, 123). If a 0.5 msec difference is used as the upper normal limit of the sensory latency between the median and ulnar or radial nerves, it seems to be a safe practice as long as the distance is kept equal for the tested nerves (123, 126, 130).

Chang and Lien compared the difference in the latency and sensory NCV between the palmar cutaneous branch and first digital branch of the median nerve and were able to make the diagnosis of CTS in 84% of 50 "suspected" CTS patients (133). In contrast, the conventional sensory nerve conduction study in the digit-wrist segment was successful in diagnosing CTS in 75% of the cases.

Recently, two formulas have been proposed to increase the diagnostic sensitivity of the median motor nerve terminal latency. They are the Terminal Latency Index (TLI) and the Residual Index (RI) (134, 135). These formulas are:

$$TLI = \frac{\text{Terminal distance (mm)}}{\text{Conduction velocity (m/sec)} \times \text{terminal latency (msec)}}$$

$$RL = TL - \frac{\text{Distal distance (mm)}}{\text{Proximal NCV (m/sec)}}$$

The lower normal limit of the TLI is reported to be 0.34 for the median and ulnar nerves (135). In patients with CTS the median TLI fell below the normal range. In some patients this may have been the earliest electrophysiological abnormality. The residual latency in the normal median nerve ranged from 1.3–2.6 msec, with a mean of 1.97 ± 0.27 msec (134). Kraft and Halvorson reported three patients with CTS who had a prolonged residual latency as their only abnormality. The value of residual latency in CTS has not been proved because it has not been tested in a sufficiently large number of patients (134). Evans and Daube compared the conventional tests with the TLI and RL in 140 patients referred to confirm CTS, finding abnormal conventional tests in

80% of cases, a low TLI in 39%, and a prolonged RL in 56% (136). These complex formulas do not increase the diagnostic sensitivity for CTS.

It has been well known that wrist flexion for 30–60 sec produces paresthesia in 80% of CTS cases, and this has been labeled "Phalen's sign" (137). With this in mind, Schwartz et al. studied the change in the motor and sensory latency of the median nerve after full wrist flexion to approximately 80° for 2 min in 10 controls and 20 patients suspected of having CTS (138). The distal motor and sensory latencies were never increased by more than 0.1 msec in the control subjects. In CTS patients motor or sensory latencies were increased by 0.2 msec or more in 16 of the 40 hands studied. Phalen's test produced paresthesia in only six of these 16 hands. The diagnosis of CTS could be made only after wrist flexion in two hands. Marin et al. also found that extreme flexion and extension of the wrist increased the motor and sensory latencies in controls and, with extreme extension and especially flexion for 5 min, the latency was increased to above normal in three, thus raising the diagnostic sensitivity from 75% to 100% in 12 patients with CTS (139). Dunnan and Waylonis, on the other hand, did not find any significant difference between 87 controls and 19 CTS patients in latency prolongation after 5 min of wrist flexion to establish the value of adding wrist flexion to the conventional screening methods (140). Thus, the diagnostic value of this "stress test" has not been confirmed as yet.

The motor NCV in the wrist-elbow segment of the median nerve is normal in a majority of patients suspected of having CTS. However, mild slowing of motor NCV has been reported in 11–35% of patients. Thomas (124) found reduced velocities in the upper arm in 50% of patients studied, but even in the most severely affected patients, proximal velocity was found to be less than 30% below the lower limit of the normal range. Thomas et al. also determined the reduced NCV to be most marked in patients with prolonged terminal latencies (124, 141). This is due to a retrograde change in the proximal motor axon, similar to that which is known to occur after nerve section. This change has been well documented in human subjects (7).

The sensory nerve conduction velocity over the wrist-elbow segment, though within the normal range, tended to be slower, in proportion to the slowing in the proximal motor conduction. In 3–9% of cases the sensory NCV was below the 95% confidence limit (120). Kimura (11) reported a significant reduction in sensory NCV in patients with CTS. We have observed a similar reduction in mixed NCV in the forearm segment. These observations suggest that the large afferent fibers from muscle behave like motor fibers when separated from their end-organs (7).

In addition to their purely physiological interest, these findings are *of practical value*. A mildly decreased motor, mixed, or sensory NCV on the forearm segment *does not*, therefore, exclude the diagnosis of CTS.

Slow conduction distal to the compression is also common in CTS. Buchthal and Rosenfalck (13) reported slow sensory NCV in the digit-palm segment in 73%, and Casey and LeQuesne (142) found slow digital NCV in 56% of their patients. According to Gilliatt (7), this distal slowing is the result of wallerian degeneration followed by regeneration of nerve fibers.

Brown and Yates (143) studied the motor nerve conduction during surgery in 23 median nerves. They obtained CMAP from the thenar muscle after stimulation of the exposed median nerve at 1–2 cm proximal to the origin of the flexor retinaculum and, in most instances, distal as far as the origin of the recurrent thenar motor branch. By measuring the amplitude of CMAP, the latency, and the negative potential area, they were able to localize the most frequent sites of the abnormalities, as observed in 15 median nerves, to the first 1–2 cm distal to the beginning of the carpal tunnel. The maximum conduction abnormalities were located proximal to the flexor retinaculum, and in four median nerves, 2 cm distal. This is in sharp contrast to Kimura's study, which localized the most abnormal conduction to the 2–4 cm distal to the origin of the transverse carpal ligament in 52% of 91 affected nerves (11). Kimura used the antidromic sensory NCS after stimulation of the nonexposed nerve along the carpal tunnel in 1-cm increments. By using Kimura's technique, but in 2-cm increments, Brown et al. (10) found the worst conduction delays in patients with carpal tunnel syndrome toward the distal end of the flexor retinaculum, in agreement with Kimura's observation (11).

With regard to the prediction of the postoperative prognosis by the nerve conduction study, Thomas stated that the extent of motor and/or sensory conduction abnormalities does not provide any clue (124). However, Harris et al. found that those patients with motor nerve conduction abnormalities appeared to have more favorable results than did those with only sensory abnormalities (144); seven of 10 patients with poor postoperative results had purely sensory nerve conduction abnormalities.

Serial nerve conduction changes after decompression of the flexor retinaculum in CTS have been well studied by four groups (142, 145–147). All these studies demonstrated definite electrophysiological improvement after decompression surgery, as indicated below:

1. Electrophysiological parameters that improve most after surgery are the sensory and motor latencies in the finger-wrist segment and the amplitude of the sensory CNAP at the wrist. The sensory and motor latencies showed a highly significant decrease, while the sensory CNAP amplitude at the wrist showed a correspondingly significant increase in relation to the elapsed time after decompression (147, 148).

2. Electrophysiological improvement can occur rapidly within 30 min after decompression. This is well documented in Hongell and Mattsson's study (146), in which the sensory NCS was performed during seven operations. All seven patients showed a slight but definite improvement of the sensory conduction within 30 min (Fig. 21.16). Microelectrode recordings of the sensory CNAP showed similar findings. In 1980, Gilliatt (7) concluded that the removal of ischemia of the compressed nerve fibers is responsible for the rapid nerve conduction change.

3. This electrophysiological improvement was curvilinear, with rapid initial improvement within 6–8 weeks followed by slower improvement over a 12– to 18–month period. This pattern may be due to faster initial segmental remyelination of the affected nerve fibers, which becomes progressively slower as the fibers return toward normal (145, 147).

Evermann and Ritsick (149) studied terminal latency across the carpal tunnel before and after release of the deep transverse ligament using the intraoperative nerve conduction test. They reported a dramatic improvement in the terminal latency in 44 of 51 hands within 15 min after release of the ligament, and further improvement in five of the remaining seven hands after internal neurolysis of the median nerve. They suggested that this immediate improvement was due to an immediately reversible mechanical or metabolic block.

4. Regardless of the severity of CTS, all patients showed postoperative electrophysiological improvement which paralleled the clinical improvement (145–147), although the electrophysiological changes lagged behind the clinical improvement.

5. Patients with more marked electrophysiological abnormalities showed a faster initial rate of electrophysiological improvement in proportion to the clinical improvement when compared with patients with less severe involvement (145).

6. There was evidence that some electrophysiological measurements did not return to normal mean values for a considerable time after clinical improvement had commenced. This was attributed to a reduction of some nerve fiber diameters that failed to be regenerated to their previous size after clinical improvement from CTS. There is disagreement over the percentage of patients with normal nerve conduction over the years after the surgery. Garland et al. (150) reported that all 27 patients operated on were completely relieved of symptoms for at least 1 year, and in all cases, motor and sensory nerve conduction in the distal segment of the median nerve returned to normal.

Goodman and Gilliatt (145) reported that serial examinations of motor conduction in 24 patients for up to 2 postsurgical years showed satisfactory recovery in all cases and the return to normal motor latency occurred within 18 months after the surgery. However, their data showed that sensory NCV remained abnormal in two of six patients tested. On the other hand, Melvin et al. (151) reported normal motor and sensory nerve conductions in only 23% of 30 patients 1 year after surgery. Sixty percent of patients had an abnormal sensory latency and 27% had a prolonged terminal latency in the later study. We have also observed many patients with abnormal sensory NCV many years after their operations, even though they were symptom-free.

Splinting of the wrist is one conservative mode of therapy for mild CTS that induced partial symptomatic improvement in two-thirds of patients (145). Goodman and Gilliatt

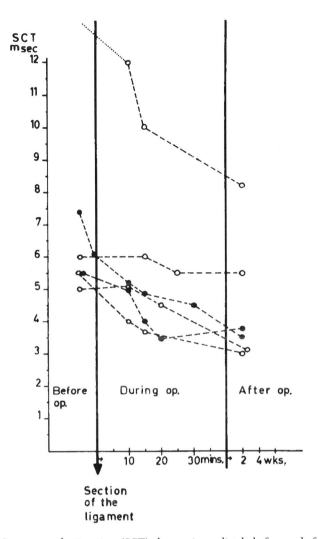

Figure 21.16. Sensory conduction time (SCT) changes immediately before and after sectioning of the volar carpal ligament in six patients with carpal tunnel syndrome. Sensory CNAP is recorded with a bipolar electrode consisting of a pair of silver hooks placed around the exposed nerve at the same level as in the pre- and postoperative studies. Improvement of the SCT is apparent within 30 min after section of the ligament. (From Hongell A, Mattsson HS. Neurographic studies before, after, and during operation for median nerve compression in carpal tunnel syndrome. Scand J Plast Surg 1971;5:108.)

(145) studied the motor latency serially before and during splinting in 23 patients for periods of 9–105 weeks. Their results were not uniform, some of the patients showing improvement in latency, some deteriorating, and others showing no change. Kruger et al. reported symptomatic relief in 67% of 105 patients with CTS who were treated with a Jobst JU 1000 splint and who had a follow-up nerve conduction study within 17 months of treatment (152). Significant improvement was observed in the sensory latency but not in the motor latency. Their study suggests that optimal results are obtained if the splint is applied within the first 3 months after onset of symptoms, and that patients with no structural damage may have a more favorable response.

Local steroid injection has been used as a conservative mode of treatment in mild CTS. Goodman and Foster (153) measured the motor latency during the follow-up period in patients treated with injections of 10 mg prednisolone butyl-acetate repeated three times, 1 week apart. All showed clinical improvement, particularly those with mild (latency 5–7 msec) or moderately severe (latency 7–10 msec) CTS. In some patients, the authors were able to demonstrate improvement in the distal latency as much as 1 year after treatment. In an 18-month follow-up prospective study, Gelberman et al. reported complete relief of symptoms in 22% of 50 CTS patients who were treated with local triamcinolone injections and night splinting for a 3-week period (154). The most favorable response was observed among patients with mild CTS (duration less than 1 year, pure sensory symptoms, absence of weakness or atrophy, no fibrillations, and only a 1- or 2-msec prolongation in the motor or sensory latencies). Giannini et al. (155) reported complete symptomatic relief in 35% and partial symptomatic relief in 58% of 22 patients with mild CTS who were treated with a single 40-mg injection of triamcinolone and were followed for 6 months. Significant electrophysiological improvement in the motor latency and sensory NCV over the finger-wrist segment was observed during the follow-up period.

The needle EMG is helpful in defining the severity of a lesion by indicating the presence of axonal degeneration as fibrillation potentials and the severity of the MUP abnormality (57). It was the least sensitive test, however. Buchthal et al. found reduced recruitment and prolonged duration in 50% of muscles tested, polyphasic MUPs in 60%, and abnormal spontaneous activity in 50%. Fasciculation was observed in 18% of muscles (120). In Stevens's series, of 603 APB muscles examined, 59% were normal and 41% showed decreased recruitment or MUP abnormalities (156). Fibrillation with or without positive sharp waves was present in 18%. Studying a more severely affected series of patients, Thomas et al. found fibrillation potentials in 44% (141). The presence of fibrillation potentials by the needle examination suggests that surgical intervention is necessary.

Ulnar Nerve

The ulnar nerve is derived from the C8 and T1 spinal nerves and passes through the lower trunk and medial cord of the brachial plexus (see Fig. 5.7). At the proximal axilla, the ulnar nerve arises from the brachial plexus, lies against the lateral wall of the axilla and on the medial aspect of the upper arm. It courses down to the elbow close to the brachial artery and median nerve. At the elbow, it passes through the ulnar (condylar) groove behind the medial epicondyle. As it emerges from this groove, it passes under the aponeurotic arch (cubital tunnel) between the two heads of the FCU muscle. The nerve courses down through the remainder of the forearm between the flexor digitorum profundus and FCU muscles. At the wrist, the ulnar nerve passes through Guyon's canal between the pisiform bone and the hook of the hamate. As it emerges from Guyon's canal, it divides into a sensory branch and a motor branch. Sensory fibers innervate sensation on the last 1.5 digits of the hand. The motor branch innervates the hypothenar muscles by the superficial terminal branch and many other ulnar-innervated hand intrinsic muscles through the deep branch. The ulnar nerve does not have any branch to the upper arm. In the forearm, it innervates the FCU and the flexor digitorum profundus muscles (digits 4 and 5). The palmar cutaneous branch arises from the ulnar nerve at the midforearm and innervates sensation on the hypothenar area. The dorsal ulnar cutaneous nerve arises about 5 cm above the wrist and winds around the ulnar nerve to innervate the ulnar side of the dorsum of the hand.

Proximal Ulnar Neuropathy

Two patients with demyelinating proximal ulnar neuropathy have been reported (Fig. 21.17) (157, 158). Both developed ulnar neuropathy as a variant of acute brachial plexopathy and had conduction block between the axilla and Erb's point in the motor nerve conduction study. Both patients improved within 8 weeks. Krarup and Sethi's case showed a sensory NCV across the brachial plexus of 36 m/sec (158). The needle EMG in Katirji and Katirji's series revealed a marked decrease in recruitment in all ulnar-innervated muscles (157); Krarup and Sethi found fibrillations and positive sharp waves in the ADQ and APB muscles (158).

Ulnar Neuropathy at the Elbow

Ulnar nerve compression (Fig. 21.17) occurs most commonly at the elbow because of the superficial location of the ulnar nerve at the elbow sulcus. Acute compression of the

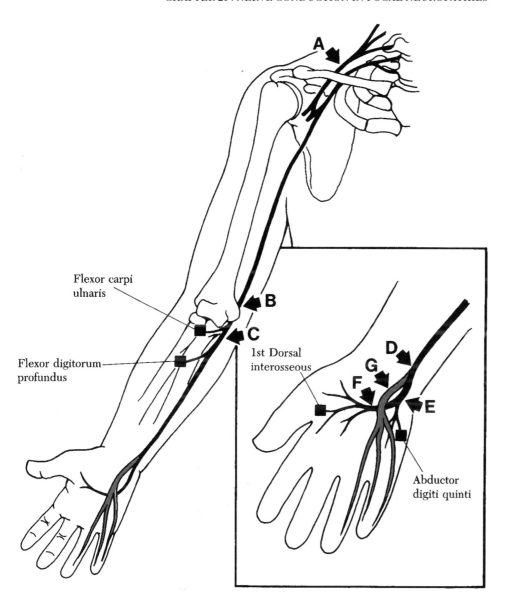

Figure 21.17. Entrapment sites in the ulnar nerve. **A**, Thoracic outlet syndrome. **B**, Tardy ulnar nerve palsy at the sulcus of the ulnar nerve. **C**, Cubital tunnel syndrome. **D**, Proximal portion of Guyon's canal (Type I). **E**, Distal portion of Guyon's canal (Type II). **F**, Within the palm (Type III). **G**, In the palmaris brevis muscle (Type IV).

ulnar nerve may occur after prolonged pressure on the nerve during surgery. This is a rare but well-known complication of operations under general anesthesia. Chronic ulnar nerve compression can be divided into two syndromes: tardy ulnar nerve palsy and cubital tunnel syndrome. Tardy ulnar nerve palsy refers to chronic neuropathy at the elbow sulcus resulting from several mechanisms, including habitual elbowing, recurrent subluxation of the nerve, joint deformity after arthritis, trauma, or fracture. Cubital tunnel syndrome refers to ulnar nerve compression at the cubital tunnel, which is formed by the FCU aponeurotic bands covering the sulcus. This compression is caused by thickening of the fibromuscular bands. Eisen and Danon (159) stated that cubital tunnel syndrome is the most common cause of an ulnar nerve lesion at the elbow. However, Brown and Yates (160) found from their experience that this syndrome is not very common.

Ulnar neuropathy at the elbow is characterized clinically by sensory loss on the palm and dorsum of the ulnar aspect of the hand, weakness of the FCU, the flexor digitorum profundus of the ring and little fingers, and the intrinsic hand muscles. In advanced cases a "claw hand" is typically noted. Although Miller (12) suggested that clinical differentiation between cubital tunnel syndrome and tardy ulnar nerve palsy is possible, our experience suggests the contrary.

The precise location of the lesion in ulnar neuropathy at the elbow can be determined by the NCV test in 95% of cases. The study shows focal demyelination across the elbow. The most common abnormality is seen in the sensory or mixed nerve conduction because sensory fibers are more likely to be damaged than motor fibers (Table 21.9).

Unlike the situation in CTS, the electrophysiological abnormalities are *relatively well* correlated with the clinical severity in these disorders (Figs. 21.18 and 21.19) (8, 161–163). Payan (164) found that the velocity in the fastest conduction fibers across the sulcus indicate the severity.

The sensory and/or mixed nerve conduction study produced a higher diagnostic yield than the motor conduction study, being positive in 73–91% of patients. When utilizing surface electrodes without signal averaging, the most helpful localizing findings are the combined abnormalities in sensory nerve conduction over the finger-wrist segment and in mixed nerve conduction over the wrist-elbow segment in the presence of normal mixed nerve conduction above the elbow. To document the latter, it is important to stimulate the ulnar nerve 4 cm above the sulcus to avoid stimulating the compressed area of the nerve. These CNAP abnormalities were observed in 73% of the cases in our series (163) and in 100% in Gilliatt's series (124). More precise localization of the lesion

Table 21.9.
Diagnostic Sensitivity of Nerve Conduction Tests in Ulnar Compression Neuropathy at the Elbow

Investigator	Diagnostic Rate (%): Motor Nerve Conduction				Diagnostic Rate (%): Sensory Nerve Conduction				Electrophysiological Localization by All Tests (%)
	Slow NCV at Elbow	Disproportionate Slowing at Elbow	Above Elbow, Prolonged Latency to — FCU	ADQ	Slow NCV at Elbow	Disproportionate Slowing at Elbow	Change in Amplitude Across Elbow	Abnormal Conduction Below Elbow	
Kaeser (162) (N = 29))	86								86
Payan (164) (N = 50)	85	50	41		91	60	8	94	96
Eisen (161) (N = 90)		32	73					50	91
Nishihira and Oh (163) (N = 40)	68	68	⌞————⌟		93[a]	58[a]		73[b]	96
Blatt-Lyon (165) (N = 66)	98		79		91	75	16		98
Miller (12) (N = 15)		87						93[c]	93
Bhala (361) (N = 78)	51							45[d]	
Pickett (362) (N = 61)	51							57[d]	
Tackmann et al. (363)									
Pure sensory (N = 40)	33		30		40		33		82
Motor and sensory (N = 63)	65		70		70		59		95

[a]Mixed nerve conduction.
[b]Sensory nerve conduction at wrist and mixed nerve conduction at elbow.
[c]Absent sensory CNAP at wrist.
[d]Absent or reduced CNAP amplitude.

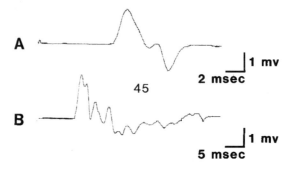

Figure 21.18. Motor nerve conduction in ulnar compression neuropathy at the elbow. **A**, CMAP with stimulation below the elbow. **B**, CMAP with stimulation above the elbow. The motor NCV is normal (45 m/sec). No conduction block is noted. Dispersion in (**B**) is indicative of focal demyelination across the elbow. Note the calibration change in (**B**).

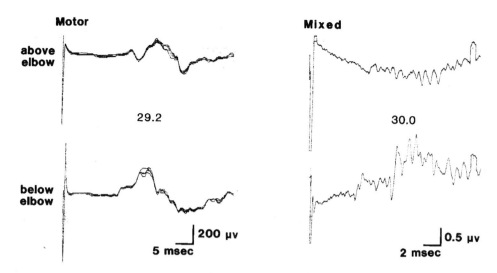

Figure 21.19.   Motor and mixed nerve conduction in ulnar compression neuropathy at the elbow. Motor nerve conduction: low amplitude (400 μV) and slow motor NCV (29.2 m/sec) across the elbow. The mixed CNAP with needle electrodes with wrist stimulation: dispersion phenomenon and slow mixed NCV across the elbow (30.0m/sec); a conduction block is also obvious across the elbow. Stimulation at the finger did not produce any sensory potentials at sites below or above the elbow.

can be achieved with the near-nerve needle technique used together with signal averaging, as confirmed by Payan (164).

With Payan's technique (164), slowing of the sensory NCV at the elbow was observed in 91% of cases (164, 165). However, to achieve maximum localization value, Payan (164) recommended the following criteria: (*a*) disproportionate slowing of sensory NCV at the elbow compared with the forearm; and (*b*) change in amplitude, duration, or shape of the sensory potential from below to above the elbow. For the second criterion, Blatt-Lyon (165) required a drop in amplitude of sensory CNAP of more than 50% above as compared to below the sulcus. Following these strict criteria, Payan (164) was able to localize the lesion at the elbow unequivocally in 68% and Blatt-Lyon (165) in 91% of patients studied, confirming the superiority of this technique. Tackmann et al. also addressed this question (166). Their technique was able to localize the lesion at the elbow in 60% of patients with pure sensory symptoms and signs and in 81% of patients with mixed motor and sensory symptoms and signs. It is our experience that the sensory CNAP, obtained by stimulating the 5th finger, was not recordable below and above the elbow in many severe cases. In these cases, mixed nerve conduction across the elbow can be substituted for the sensory nerve conduction with similar results (163).

To localize the lesion at the elbow by the motor nerve conduction study, the minimal requirement is stimulating the nerve below and above the elbow. There are two important details one must observe to obtain a technically satisfactory NCV: the position of the elbow and the distance below and above the elbow. These two variables must be strictly adhered to according to the method with which normal values were collected. Depending on the angle of flexion of the elbow, the distance varies. The distance becomes longer, and consequently the NCV faster, in the flexed position of the elbow. Although Checkles et al. (167) recommended a 70° flexed position, many laboratories— including our own—test the nerve conduction with the elbow extended and the forearm supinated because of greater convenience. With regard to the distance, Payan (164) and Eisen (161) used a 10-cm distance below and above the elbow, and Kaiser used 6–10 cm. We use 9–10 cm because we were able to localize the lesion at the elbow with our method in a few patients in whom the NCV was normal with a 10-cm distance.

The most sensitive motor conduction abnormality is slow NCV at the elbow. However, to localize the lesion better at the elbow, Payan (164) used as the diagnostic criterion the disproportionate slowing at elbow compared with the distal segment. This abnormality was observed in 50–87% of patients. Eisen (161) considered a decrease in motor NCV of at least 10 m/sec across the elbow in relation to the conduction above and below this region significant for localization, but was able to localize the lesion in only 32% of the patients. We believe that Eisen's criteria are too rigid to be of practical value.

Conduction block is another motor conduction abnormality frequently observed in this disorder. The amplitude and area are normal with stimulation at the wrist and below the elbow, but it is reduced by more than 50% with stimulation just above the elbow and proximally. Conduction block was observed in 60% of Miller's patients (12). Conduction block is often associated with abnormal temporal dispersion and focal slowing. In some cases this is the only abnormality indicative of the lesion at the elbow, as was the case in 7% of Miller's patients.

Prolonged latency to the FCU when stimulating the ulnar nerve above the elbow is also helpful in localizing the lesion. This abnormality was observed in 41% of Payan's patients and had localizing value in 20% of his patients when all other motor conductions were normal (164). This finding was also observed in 30% of Tackmann et al.'s patients with pure sensory symptoms and signs and in 70% of those with mixed motor and sensory symptoms and signs (166).

Prolonged latency to the ADQ when stimulating the ulnar nerve above the elbow is the most frequently observed abnormality in Eisen's study, being found in 91% of patients compared with focal slowing in only 53% (161). Unfortunately, however, this simple examination does not have any localizing value.

Nerve conduction abnormalities in other segments of the ulnar nerve are not uncommon in patients with this compression neuropathy. In sensory and mixed nerves, the most prominent abnormalities are noted in the finger-wrist-elbow segments, as discussed above. In the above elbow-axilla segment, we observed minimal mixed nerve conduction slowing (less than 19% of normal) in 40% of 13 tested cases (163); and Payan (164) reported minimal sensory nerve conduction slowing in 50% of 10 tested cases. For motor nerve conduction, prolonged terminal latency was reported in 10–40% of cases. The slow motor NCV (less than 23% of normal) was observed in 17–75% of cases in the forearm. In the above elbow-axilla segment, much less slowing (less than 14% of normal) was observed in 13–30% of cases. These distal and proximal nerve conduction abnormalities are caused by wallerian and retrograde degeneration of nerve fibers after prolonged focal compression (124). These findings have practical importance for the interpretation of nerve conduction abnormalities, suggesting that minor abnormalities in other segments of the ulnar nerve *do not* rule out ulnar neuropathy at the elbow and that *disproportionate slowing* at the elbow is important in localization of the lesion to the elbow.

Routinely, most ulnar nerve lesions at the elbow can be localized by the motor conduction study and the recording of sensory CNAPs at the wrist and mixed CNAPs at the elbow. These procedures localized the lesion in 78% of our patients. For the remaining cases, the use of Payan's techniques is recommended. According to Odusote and Eisen (168), the dispersion or extent of desynchronization of the above-sulcus sensory CNAP proved to be the most useful characteristic in 28.5% of nerves in which the authors were not able to localize the lesion by routine studies. The combination of these techniques increases the diagnostic sensitivity to 96–98%.

In summary, the following criteria are used to localize the lesion at the elbow:

1. Motor nerve conduction
   a. *Disproportionate slowing of motor NCV at the elbow* compared with the forearm or upper arm segment
   b. *Conduction block with dispersion phenomenon at the elbow*
   c. Prolonged terminal latency to the FCU
2. Sensory and mixed nerve conduction
   a. *Abnormal sensory nerve conduction in the finger-wrist segment and abnormal mixed nerve conduction in the wrist-elbow segment* by the routine surface electrode technique

b. With the near-nerve technique: *(a) disproportionate slowing of sensory or mixed NCV at the elbow; and (b) more than 50% reduction in amplitude and/or dispersion phenomenon* in the sensory or mixed CNAP above compared with below the elbow.

The "short-segment stimulation (SSS) technique" (or "inching technique") of the motor conduction has become a standard method of testing for ulnar neuropathy at the elbow. Campbell et al. used 1-cm segments (169), and others have used 2-cm segments (12, 170). This technique can pinpoint a lesion to the exact site of compression and can distinguish cubital tunnel syndrome from tardy ulnar nerve palsy (retrocondylar compression). *If the lesion is localized to more than 2 cm distal to the medial epicondyle, the diagnosis of cubital tunnel syndrome can be made* (169) (Fig. 21.20). On the other hand, if the lesion is localized to the medial epicondyle or proximal to it, retrocondylar compression syndrome can be diagnosed (Fig. 21.21). This distinction is important in determining therapeutic strategy: in cubital tunnel syndrome decompression of the cubital tunnel is required, whereas for retrocondylar compression syndrome anterior transposition of the ulnar nerve is recommended.

Using this technique, Campbell et al. (169) were able to localize the lesion at the cubital tunnel in six of 19 cases and to the rectrocondylar sulcus in eight cases. In one case, the cubital tunnel and retrocondylar sulcus were equally involved. In four cases, the test was nonlocalizing. By using this technique during surgery, they were able to pinpoint the lesion better in six cases, including four patients with no localizing lesion.

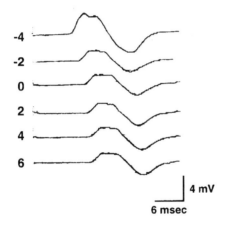

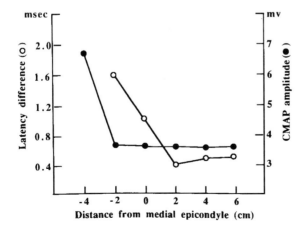

Figure 21.20. Cubital tunnel syndrome identified by the "inching" technique of motor nerve conduction across the elbow. Serial CMAPs at various sites along the ulnar groove. Conduction block (47% decrease in the CMAP) and prolonged latency (1.6 msec) between 4 cm and 2 cm distal to the medial epicondyle. −, distal to the medial epicondyle.

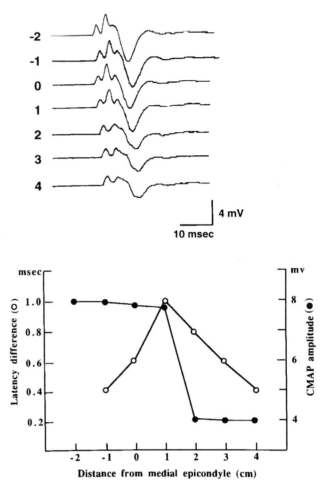

Figure 21.21. Tardy ulnar nerve palsy identified by the "inching" technique of motor nerve conduction across the elbow. Serial CMAPs at the various sites along the ulnar groove. Conduction block (48% decrease in the CMAP) between 1 and 2 cm proximal to medial epicondyle and the prolonged latency (1.0 msec) between 0 and 1 cm proximal to the medial epicondyle.

In 11 patients with ulnar compression neuropathy at the elbow, Kanakamedala et al. (170) localized the lesion by the 2 cm-SSS technique to the cubital tunnel in three cases and to the medial epicondyle in nine. These studies clearly showed that there are two distinct compression syndromes involving the ulnar nerve at the elbow: (*a*) cubital tunnel syndrome, and (*b*) sulcal (retrocondylar) compression syndrome, and that sulcal compression syndrome is more common.

The needle EMG in ulnar compression neuropathy at the elbow should theoretically show denervation in all the ulnar-innervated muscles because an innervating branch to the FCU arises at or below the elbow most of the time (171). However, repeated studies have shown that the FDI and ADQ are commonly involved, whereas the FCU and FDP are less frequently involved both clinically and electrophysiologically (172). This finding has a practical implication in that *"sparing of the FCU and FDP muscle"* in the *needle EMG study does not necessarily localize the lesion to the wrist.*

There are a few studies (159, 173) reporting spontaneous recovery from ulnar neuropathy at the elbow. DeJesus and Steiner (173) reported clinical improvement in 85% of the 13 unoperated cases with excellent recovery in 62% for a mean follow-up period of 20 months. In 30 patients with mild cubital tunnel syndrome, which was diagnosed by subjective symptoms in the ulnar nerve territory alone, Eisen and Danon (159) reported clinical improvement in 90% of cases over a mean follow-up period of 22 months. An improvement in the motor NCV at the elbow, in the mean latency of

CMAP from above the elbow, and in the mean latency of the sensory nerve conduction in the finger-wrist segment was documented in the follow-up study of improved cases. Eisen and Danon further suggested that a motor NCV across the elbow of 41 m/sec may be a criterion for surgery. However, the considerable overlap in their data between the motor NCV at the elbow of their patients and normal controls and the fact that 41 m/sec is still within two standard deviations from the normal mean raised serious questions on the validity of their criterion. Assmus et al. (174) reported clinical and electrophysiological improvement (motor NCV across the elbow) in 36 patients with uncomplicated pressure palsies during a 2-year follow-up period. These data suggest that surgery should be considered after an adequate trial of conservative management of ulnar nerve palsy at the elbow, especially in uncomplicated cases.

Intraoperative nerve conduction was studied by three groups (12, 143, 169). Brown et al. (143) studied 14 ulnar nerves intraoperatively by utilizing the motor nerve conduction and localized the most abnormal conduction to 1 cm proximal and distal to the medial epicondyle. None of their cases showed the most abnormal conduction at the cubital tunnel. Miller (12), on the other hand, studied motor nerve conduction during surgery in seven patients with cubital tunnel syndrome and confirmed the localization of the abnormal conduction to the cubital tunnel. It was difficult to reconcile these conflicting observations, but a recent study by Campbell et al. (169) resolved this issue, confirming clearly that there are two subgroups in ulnar neuropathy at the elbow: sulcal compression syndrome and cubital tunnel syndrome. By intraoperative motor nerve conduction study in 19 patients, they showed cubital tunnel syndrome in six cases, retrocondylar compression syndrome in eight cases, and compression at both sites in two cases.

Postoperative nerve conduction changes have been studied by various groups. All four studies (174, 175–177) on the anterior transposition of the ulnar nerve documented electrophysiological improvement. Payan (176) reported electrophysiological improvement in both sensory and motor conduction (by 5–10 m/sec) across the elbow in 10 and in motor conduction only in one of 12 patients. The earliest electrophysiological improvement was seen in motor fibers at 3 months and in sensory fibers at 5 months. An increase in conduction velocity across the elbow was the first sign of recovery in both sensory and motor fibers. The amplitude of sensory CNAP was low even after transposition regardless of whether velocity increased. Restoration of the sensory CNAP at the wrist occurred late, and only then was there significant clinical improvement.

Assmus et al. (174) observed a significant increase in the motor NCV across the elbow during first postoperative year in 39 patients. In 36 nonsurgical cases there was no improvement in the NCV in a group where the elbow joint abnormalities were verified by x-ray. In a group where no abnormalities were documented, there was minimal improvement in the NCV. Lunnegard et al. (175) also reported a significant increase (roughly 10 m/sec) in the motor NCV across the elbow postoperatively in 10 of 11 patients. There was no improvement in the motor NCV in other segments. The mixed CNAP was recorded in the wrist-below elbow-axilla segment postoperatively in two cases where no measurable potential could be recorded preoperatively.

After simple decompression of the cubital tunnel, Miller and Hummel (178) observed clinical and electrophysiological improvement in 11 of 12 patients. Electrophysiological improvement was characterized by increased motor NCV across the elbow in nine, a tendency of the amplitude of the CMAP toward normal in seven, and an increase in amplitude of the sensory CNAP at the wrist in four. They noted the best result in patients with mild weakness, recent onset of symptoms, and mild abnormality of the sensory CNAP preoperatively.

Friedman and Cochran observed clinical improvement in 70% of 23 patients and a highly significant improvement in the motor NCV after a mean follow-up period of 33 months after anterior transposition of the ulnar nerve (177). The motor NCV improved regardless of the clinical outcome. Nielsen et al. (179) investigated nine patients with moderate to severe ulnar palsy after interfascicular neurolysis and reported no electrophysiological or clinical improvement within the first postoperative year. On the contrary, there were changes suggesting deterioration in some patients. Thus, they concluded that interfascicular neurolysis of the ulnar nerve should be abandoned.

Acute Ulnar Compression Neuropathy at the Elbow

Acute ulnar compression neuropathy may occur during operations involving general anesthesia and is an example of acute compression neuropathies in man. The initial symptom is usually numbness in the ulnar nerve territory in the affected hand, immediately on awaking from general anesthesia or within 24–48 hr after surgery (180). There are classic sensory and motor deficits of ulnar neuropathy at the elbow. Miller observed a motor NCV below 42 m/sec in all but one of 14 patients, localizing the lesion at the elbow (181). Though the CMAP amplitude was abnormal in 12 patients, a conduction block across the elbow was seen in three patients. Precise localization of the cubital tunnel by demonstration of the conduction block with the inching technique was possible in only one patient. Sensory nerve conduction in the finger-wrist segment was abnormal in all of eight tested cases, absent in six, and reduction of amplitude in two. Miller believes, on the basis of intraoperative observations, that compression in this neuropathy occurs at the cubital tunnel (180).

Ulnar Neuropathy at the Forearm

A few cases of compression ulnar neuropathy at the forearm have been reported. Holtzman et al. described a patient with a spontaneous ulnar neuropathy and complete conduction block 5 cm proximal to the ulnar styloid, caused by two fibrovascular bands crossing from the ulnar artery to the distal belly of the FCU muscle (182). After resection of the bands, there was nearly complete clinical and electrophysiological recovery within 6 months. Harrelson et al. also reported a case of ulnar neuropathy due to "hypertrophy of the FCU muscle" in the distal part of the forearm (183), which was identified by prolonged terminal latency from a point proximal to the hypertrophied muscle. Campbell reported a distal forearm ulnar neuropathy due to a dense fibrovascular band from the ulnar artery to the abnormal FCU muscle (184). A distal forearm lesion was localized to 7 cm proximal to the ulnar styloid by the demonstration of a conduction block with the percutaneous "short-segment stimulation technique" (SSS). Campbell et al. described a proximal forearm ulnar compression neuropathy at its exit from the FCU muscle (185). Using the SSS method, they were able to identify the entrapment site by demonstrating a conduction block 6 cm distal to the epicondyle.

Ulnar Nerve Lesions at the Wrist and Hand

The ulnar nerve (Fig. 21.15) can be compressed at various critical locations along its pathway at the wrist and hand. Proximally at the wrist the entire ulnar nerve, containing both motor and sensory branches, passes through Guyon's canal. At the distal portion of the canal, the ulnar nerve divides into the superficial sensory and deep motor branches. The superficial sensory branch passes through a fat pad down to the palmaris brevis muscles before continuing subcutaneously to provide sensation to the ulnar 1.5 fingers of the palmar aspect of the hand. The deep motor branch, innervating the hypothenar muscles, takes an abrupt turn around the hook of the hamate to follow along the deep palmar arch, innervating the interossei, the medial two lumbricalis, the abductor pollicis, and the deep head of the flexor pollicis brevis muscles.

Thus, ulnar compression neuropathy at the wrist and hand can be divided into four groups according to the site of the lesion. Because of the distinct combination of signs, the diagnosis of ulnar nerve compression syndromes of the wrist and hand and the precise localization of the lesion are usually apparent clinically. Although Shea and McClain (186) classified these lesions into three types, we prefer four types depending on the four possible combinations of clinical findings (Table 21.10). Among a total of 136 cases, 30% were type I (type I according to Shea and McClain's classification)

Table 21.10.
Types of Ulnar Nerve Lesions at the Wrist and Hand

Parameter	Type I	Type II	Type III	Type IV
Site of lesion	Proximal portion of Guyon's canal	Distal portion of Guyon's canal	Within the palm	In the palmaris brevis muscle
Branch of nerve involved	Superficial and entire deep	Entire deep	Palmar deep	Superficial
Signs and symptoms	Sensory and motor deficits involving hypothenar and intrinsic muscles	Motor deficits involving hypothenar and intrinsic muscles	Motor deficit involving intrinsic muscles	Sensory deficits
Electrophysiological abnormalities				
Sensory nerve conduction	Abnormal	Normal	Normal	Abnormal
Terminal latency to				
Abductor digiti quinti	Prolonged	Prolonged	Normal	Normal
First dorsal interosseous	Prolonged	Prolonged	Prolonged	Normal
Shea and McClain's classification (186)	Type I	Type II		Type III

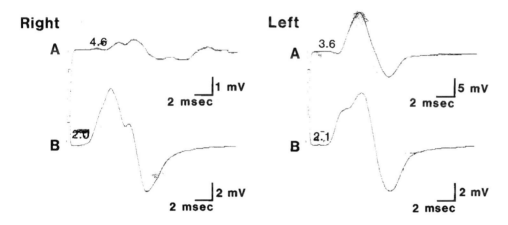

Figure 21.22. Motor nerve conduction in a lesion in the deep palmar branch of the right ulnar nerve. The patient had a schwannoma. **A**, CMAP from the right first dorsal interossei: low amplitude (1 mV) and dispersion phenomenon. The terminal latency is within normal limit (4.6 msec). These are compared with the normal CMAP from the left first dorsal interosseous. **B**, The CMAPs from the right and left ADQ are comparable.

(186), 52% were types II and III (Shea and McClain's type II), and 18% were type IV (Shea and McClain's type III). The most common lesion in Ebeling et al.'s series was type III, followed by type II (187). Shea and McClain listed 19 different causes for this disorder, the most frequent being ganglionic compression (28.7% of reported cases) and then occupational neuritis (23.5%), laceration (10.3%), ulnar artery disease (8.1%), and others.

The nerve conduction study is essential for precisely localizing the lesion as well as for ascertaining the extent of the conduction defect (Fig. 21.22). The nerve conduction study should include sensory nerve conduction and terminal latency to the ADQ and the first dorsal interosseus muscles (148). These studies localize the lesion precisely according to Table 21.11.

The most extensive electrophysiological data are available in the classic paper by Ebeling et al. (187). In two patients with type I lesions, the prolonged terminal latencies to the ADQ and first dorsal interossei were prominent together with the absence of sensory nerve potential in one tested case. In seven patients with type III lesions, the marked prolongation of terminal latency to the first dorsal interossei and the dispersion phenomenon in CMAP (up to 29 msec) were the cardinal findings in the presence of normal terminal latency to the ADQ muscle and normal sensory nerve conduction. Similar findings were also observed in Bhala and Goodgold's case (188). In one patient with type II (189), the terminal latencies to the ADQ and first dorsal interossei were prolonged, whereas sensory nerve conduction was normal. We were not able to find any type IV case with well-documented electrophysiological findings in the literature.

Table 21.11.
Ulnar Nerve Conduction Abnormalities in Thoracic Outlet Syndrome

	Nerve Conduction/ Thoracic Outlet (%)		Distal Sensory Conduction (%)			
	Slow Motor NCV	Low Mixed Amp	Low Amp	Slow NCV	Prolonged F-wave (%)	Low CMAP (%)
Nonneurogenic TOS						
Urschel et al. (364)						
(N = 17)	94					
Kremer and Ahlquist (204)						
(N = 5)	0					
Shahani et al. (206) (N = 8)	0					
Oh (N = 7)a	0	0[b]	0	0		
Ryding et al. (207) (N = 37)	11[c]		8		22	
Aminoff et al. (67) (N = 10)			0		0	0 (ADQ/APB)
Neurogenic TOS						
Krogness (202) (N = 5)	60[d]					
Wilbourne et al. (211)						
(N = 11)	0		100		80	45 (ADQ)
						73 (APB)
Oh (N = 3)	0	67	67	100		33 (ADQ)
Gillatt et al. (209) (N = 14)			71			
Wulff and Gilliatt (214)						
(N = 5)					100	
Smith and Trojaborg (212)						
(N = 10)	0		80 (Ulnar)			30 (ADQ)
			33 (Med)			50 (APB)
Aminoff et al. (67) (N = 5)			80 (Ulnar)		50 (Med)	80 (APB)
					40 (Ulnar)	60 (ADQ)

[a]Unpublished data.
[b]Mixed NCV is normal.
[c]Latency from the Erb's point is prolonged.
[d]Proximal stimulation was applied closer to the 7th transverse process.

Distal ulnar sensory and motor neuropathy caused by the wearing of tight handcuffs has been reported in two cases, mimicking type I lesion (190), both of which demonstrated a prolonged terminal latency and absent sensory CNAP over the finger-wrist segment in the ulnar nerve. In one case, both ulnar nerves were involved. In the other case, a distal median motor and sensory neuropathy was also present.

In this disorder, Ebeling et al. (187) reported a normal NCV over the wrist-elbow segment in motor nerve fibers to the ADQ, whereas motor nerve fibers to the interossei showed slightly slower conduction in seven of nine tested cases. This is caused by the selective retrograde degeneration of motor fibers to the interossei proximal to the compression.

Spontaneous improvement of motor terminal latency was the usual rule in five patients who showed spontaneous clinical improvement. In two cases motor nerve conduction was found to be markedly improved, although clinical recovery at that stage was slight. Thus Ebeling et al. stressed the value of serial measurements of conduction time for detecting early recovery (187).

Thoracic Outlet Syndrome

Thoracic outlet syndrome (TOS) refers to the compression syndrome of the neurovascular bundles at the point between the neck and axilla (50). The causes of TOS include congenital abnormalities (cervical ribs, abnormal first rib with fibrous band, the scalenus muscle band) and trauma (fractures of the clavicle and first rib, pseudoarthrosis of the clavicle, and crushing injury to the upper thorax) (191). TOS can be conveniently divided into two major categories: (a) neurogenic TOS, or cases with neurological deficits; and (b) nonneurogenic TOS, or cases without neurological deficits.

Neurogenic TOS is extremely rare and has distinct clinical features: (*a*) pain and sensory loss in the C8 and T1 dermatomes; and (*b*) selective weakness and wasting of the thenar muscles (192). In severe cases, weakness and wasting of all the intrinsic hand muscles are observed.

A majority of nonneurogenic TOS patients have an ill-defined pain complex, best described by the term "droopy shoulder syndrome" (193). Most of these are women who have low-set, droopy shoulders, and a long, swan-like neck. This results in traction of the brachial plexus, producing pain in the neck, shoulders, chest, arms, or hands. Symptoms are aggravated by pulling down on the shoulder and are relieved by passive posture elevation. There may be a Tinel's sign over the brachial plexus, and lateral cervical spine films may show that the second thoracic vertebra is visible above the shoulders. The most valuable diagnostic test for nonneurogenic TOS is the duplication of the patient's symptoms with or without pulse change during one of three tests: Adson's test, the exaggerated military maneuver, and the hyperabduction/external rotation test (194–196). The specificity of such tests in TOS has been questioned since positive studies are also often found in normal individuals (197–199).

In 1971 Urschel et al. (200) and Caldwell et al. (201) claimed that the motor NCV of the ulnar nerve across the thoracic outlet was helpful in the diagnosis of TOS (Table 21.11). Their results can be summarized as follows: (*a*) slow segmental motor NCV in 94% of 17 cases (200); the average NCV was 57.8 m/sec in TOS versus 72.2 m/sec in normal controls; (*b*) the majority of patients having a segmental NCV below 60 m/sec required operative decompression; and (*c*) an average improvement of 18 m/sec in motor NCV postoperatively. In 1973 Krogness (202) observed the slowing of motor NCV across the thoracic outlet in three of five patients with neurogenic TOS in whom cervical rib and scalenus anticus syndrome were confirmed by surgery and postoperative improvement in nerve conduction. He stimulated the ulnar nerve trunk above the clavicle corresponding to the 7th cervical transverse process instead of Erb's point. However, these findings were not confirmed by subsequent studies (203–206), which showed normal motor NCV across the thoracic outlet.

Among 37 patients with nonneurogenic TOS, Ryding et al. found low sensory CNAP amplitude in three, plexus latency prolongation in four, and prolongation of F-wave latency in eight cases in the ulnar nerve study, together with denervation in the C8-innervated muscle in 13 patients, and concluded that the nerve conduction test was able to identify brachial plexus compression in only two (5%) of cases (207). Assessing the motor conduction from C8 to the supraclavicular fossa by stimulating the C8 root with a needle electrode, Pavot and Gargour found significant prolongation of the mean conduction time in 50 nonneurogenic TOS patients (208). They did not say how many TOS patients showed such a prolongation.

In neurogenic TOS (patients with neurological deficits), *the reduction of amplitude in the ulnar sensory CNAP and a prolonged F-wave latency* were the most consistent nerve conduction abnormalities (Figs. 21.23 and 21.24). Gilliatt et al. (209) observed reduced amplitude of the sensory CNAP in the ulnar nerve in 10 of 14 patients with wasting of the hand due to a cervical rib and band, and concluded that this abnormality is due to wallerian degeneration of the afferent sensory fibers of the ulnar nerve distal to the cervical rib or band. They also observed a significant reduction in mean motor NCV over the forearm segment in the median nerve, which was ascribed to loss of the fast conducting fibers in some severely affected patients. Lascelles et al. (210) also reported a reduced sensory CNAP amplitude in the ulnar nerve in five patients with cervical rib syndrome. Among 11 patients with neurogenic true TOS, Wilbourn et al. (211) reported a relatively low amplitude of ulnar sensory CNAP in all (less than 50% of contralateral amplitude but never below 5 μv), a relatively low or a low amplitude of the CMAP in the ulnar nerve in five cases, and an invariably low amplitude of the CMAP in the median nerve (often less than 2 mv), and a normal median sensory amplitude. NCVs and distal latencies were unaffected, except when axon loss was marked; proximal ulnar motor conduction (Erb's point stimulation) was normal. Of 10 patients with neurogenic TOS caused by a cervical rib, Smith and Trojaborg found normal

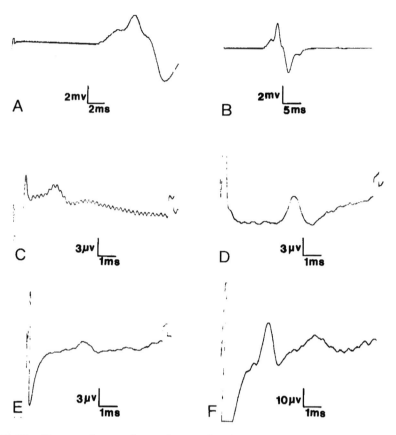

Figure 21.23. Nerve conduction abnormalities in the ulnar nerve in a patient with thoracic outlet syndrome. *A*, CMAP with stimulation at the axilla. *B*, CMAP with stimulation at Erb's point. *C*, Low-amplitude sensory CNAP over the finger-wrist segment. *D*, Low-amplitude mixed CNAP over the wrist-elbow segment. *E*, Low-amplitude CNAP over the axilla-Erb's point segment. *F*, Normal mixed CNAP over the axilla-Erb's point segment on the normal side for comparison.

motor ulnar and median NCV in all cases, low CNAP amplitude of the ulnar nerve in eight and of the median nerve in three, low CMAP of the ADQ in three and of the APB in five, enabling them to localize the lesion to the thoracic outlet in all patients (212). The needle EMG in nonneurogenic TOS was normal (208). However, in neurogenic TOS, chronic denervation was seen in the ADQ and APB muscles in all tested cases (212). Fibrillation and positive sharp waves were rare in these muscles.

We observed similar findings: A low amplitude of the CNAP in ulnar sensory nerve conduction and mixed nerve conduction over the Erb's point-wrist segment in two of three cases of neurogenic TOS (Figs. 21.23 and 21.24). Low-amplitude CMAPs were observed in one case. The proximal motor NCV across the thoracic outlet was normal in all three patients with neurogenic TOS. All motor, sensory, and mixed nerve conduction parameters were normal in all seven cases of nonneurogenic TOS.

F-wave latency was studied by several investigators. Weber and Piero (213) found that there was a significant prolongation of the F-wave latency in 16 patients with TOS. Wulff and Gilliatt (214) found the F-wave latency to be consistently increased in the affected hands of the patients, compared with results from their unaffected hands and from the hands of normal controls. Each of these five patients had unilateral wasting of the hand muscles as a result of cervical rib and band. This increase persisted after removal of the cervical band in four patients and was thought to be caused mainly by degeneration of the fast-conducting fibers. In the 5th patient, F-wave latency decreased after surgery. Wilbourn et al. (211) found prolonged F-wave latency in four of five tested patients with neurogenic TOS.

Recently, two articles reported brachial plexus injuries sustained during TOS

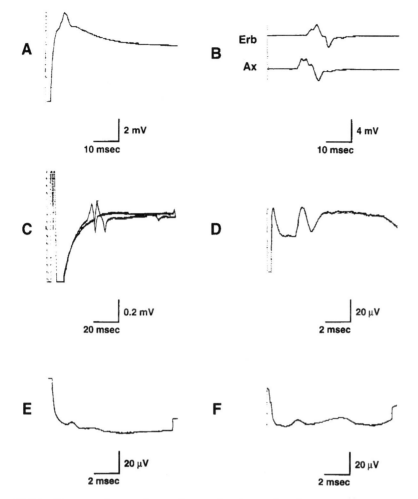

Figure 21.24.   Nerve conduction abnormalities in the ulnar and median nerves in a patient with thoracic outlet syndrome due to a hypertrophied anticus sclenius muscle. **A**, Low CMAP in the median nerve. **B**, Normal CMAP in the ulnar nerve with stimulation at the Erb's point (**Erb**) and axilla (**Ax**). **C**, Prolonged F-wave latency in the ulnar nerve. **D**, Normal sensory CNAP in the median nerve. **E**, Low sensory CNAP amplitude in the ulnar nerve. **F**, Low mixed CNAP amplitude in the axilla-Erb's point segment in the ulnar nerve.

surgery, warning of potentially serious neurological deficits in nonneurogenic TOS (215, 216). Cherington reported five patients who sustained serious injuries during TOS surgery (215). Four of these had neurological complaints, predominantly hand weakness and/or causalgic pain, consistent with a brachial plexus injury. Wilbourn reported eight patients with severe brachial plexopathy during TOS surgery: lower trunk/medial cord brachial plexus lesions in five, diffuse plexus lesions with lower trunk accentuation in two, and diffuse but patchy plexus involvement in one (216).

Based on our review, we conclude with the following points:

1. At this time, there is no single nerve conduction test sensitive and typical enough to be diagnostic of nonneurogenic TOS. In the nonneurogenic group, the motor, sensory and mixed nerve conductions in the distal as well as the thoracic outlet segments in the ulnar nerve are normal.

2. In a majority of patients with neurogenic TOS, *a distinct electrophysiological pattern exists: (a) a low CNAP amplitude in the distal as well as the thoracic outlet segment of the ulnar nerve; (b) prolonged ulnar F-wave latency; and (c) low CMAP more often in the median nerve than in the ulnar nerve* (Fig. 21.24).

3. At this time, *nerve conduction studies are more valuable in ruling out the common distal entrapment neuropathies in nonneurogenic TOS* (e.g., carpal tunnel syndrome or ulnar entrapment neuropathy). The diagnostic value of the SEP test in TOS is discussed in Chapter 19.

Medial Antebrachial Cutaneous Nerve

The medial antebrachial cutaneous (MABC) nerve arises from the medial cord of the brachial plexus, follows the medial side of the brachial artery in the arm, pierces the deep fascia in the middle arm, then becomes superficial and divides into anterior and posterior branches (see Fig. 11.33). The larger anterior branch innervates the medial aspect of the elbow and forearm and terminates at the wrist (Fig. 21.25). Because of its superficial location and proximity to the brachial artery, the MABC nerve is vulnerable to injury. Three cases of MABC neuropathy were reported (217, 218). In one case, the CNAP amplitude was low and in the other, the CNAP was absent, confirming MABC neuropathy by the nerve conduction technique (Fig. 21.26) (218).

Digital Neuropathy of the Median and Ulnar Nerves

Digital neuropathy of the median and ulnar nerves has been described. A median sensory CNAP with a notched configuration was recorded in two patients with old unsuspected lesions of the digital branch of the median nerve. The notch was caused by the

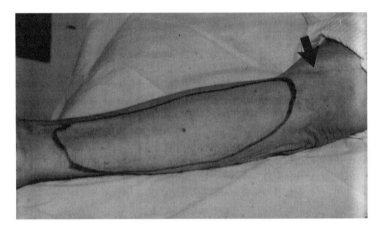

Figure 21.25. *Encircled area* represents decreased sensation to pin-prick corresponding to the medial antebrachial cutaneous nerve. Scar is indicated by *arrow*. (From Chang CW, Oh SJ. Medial antebrachial cutaneous neuropathy: case report. EMG Clin Neurophysiol 1988;28:4.)

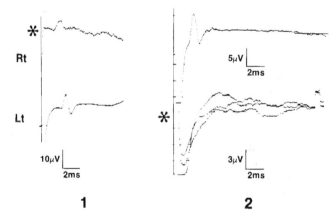

Figure 21.26. Nerve conduction abnormalities in two cases (**1** and **2**) of medial antebrachial cutaneous neuropathy. Symptomatic side is indicated by *asterisk*. Low sensory CNAP (6 μV) in case 1. In case 2, no consistent CNAP is obtained even with three averagings. (From Chang CW, Oh SJ. Medial antebrachial cutaneous neuropathy: case report. EMG Clin Neurophysiol 1988;28:4.)

presence in the injured nerves of two groups of fibers with different mean NCVs (219). Digital neuropathy can be diagnosed by sensory nerve conduction testing of the affected digital nerve. This could be achieved by stimulating the affected digital nerve with metal electrodes instead of ring electrodes.

Double Crush Syndrome of the Median and Ulnar Nerves

In 1973 Upton and McComes (220) found cervical root lesions in 70% of 115 patients with carpal tunnel syndrome or lesions of the ulnar nerve at the elbow. They thought that this association was not fortuitous but, rather, the result of serial constraints of axoplasmic flow in nerve fibers. They termed this combination "double crush syndrome." Unfortunately, the evidence for a cervical root lesion was not entirely based on objective findings, e.g., the EMG finding of denervation. This explains the high frequency (70%) of cervical root lesions in carpal tunnel syndrome. Yu et al. (221) found 20% of 525 patients with carpal tunnel syndrome had other neurological disorders. The associated disorders consisted primarily of involvement of the cervical roots (53%), the ulnar nerve at the elbow (28%), or both (9%). In his review on entrapment neuropathy, Nakano (222) stated that ulnar nerve entrapment may occur concomitantly with lower cervical spine disease or with the thoracic outlet syndrome, but no firm data were presented. Nakano further stated that the patient responds only if treatment is directed toward both processes, and that the EMG and x-ray studies should be performed in patients with entrapment neuropathy with symptoms referable to the neck.

Radial Nerve

The radial nerve is a major continuation of the posterior cord of the brachial plexus, which is formed from the C5–T1 spinal roots. On emerging from the posterior cord, the radial nerve courses down the lateral wall of the axilla, then gains the upper arm where it winds obliquely around the humerus in the spiral groove, and proceeds downward to the radial aspect of the bend of the elbow. Before it reaches the spiral groove, it gives off branches to the triceps muscles (see Fig. 11.53). At the distal portion of the spiral groove, the posterior antebrachial cutaneous nerve branches off from the main nerve. As the radial nerve emerges from the spiral groove, it gives off a first branch to the brachioradialis muscle and then to the extensor carpi radialis muscle. At the elbow, the radial nerve divides into two major terminal branches: (*a*) the superficial branch—the superficial radial sensory nerve; and (*b*) the deep branch—the posterior interosseous nerve.

Saturday Night Palsy

The radial nerve (Fig. 21.27) is vulnerable to compression near its emergence from the intermuscular septum in the spiral groove in the upper arm. Radial nerve palsy is frequently seen in patients who have been in an alcoholic stupor after a Saturday night binge. Hence this disorder is often called "Saturday night palsy."

Clinically, the condition produces weakness or paralysis of the wrist and finger extensor muscles. The triceps muscle is spared, but the brachioradialis muscle is invariably involved. Sensory impairment is rare.

Even though radial nerve compression is not unusual, there is only one article reporting nerve conduction findings obtained with special attention to technical accuracy. This fact is most likely due to the difficulty of performing reliable motor and sensory conduction across the spiral groove.

Trojaborg's study (223) showed an acute compression block at the spiral groove in 29 patients with this disorder (Fig. 21.28), including:

1. Normal amplitude of the CMAP and latencies to the forearm muscles when stimulating at the elbow;

2. Normal distal motor latency and sensory conduction velocity between the wrist and elbow in all but 7% of patients in whom conduction was absent in both motor and sensory fibers above the elbow;

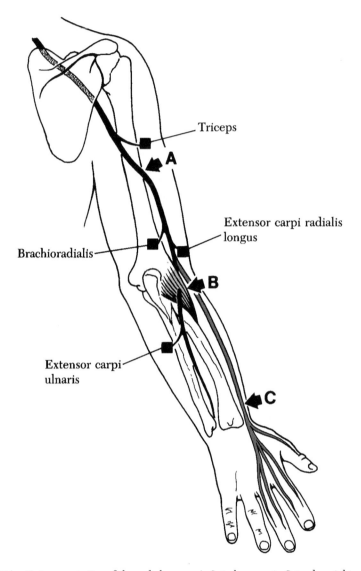

Triceps

Extensor carpi radialis
longus

Brachioradialis

Extensor carpi
ulnaris

Figure 21.27.   Entrapment sites of the radial nerve. **A**, Spiral groove in Saturday night palsy. **B**, The arcade of Frohse in posterior interosseous neuropathy. **C**, At the wrist in superficial radial sensory neuropathy.

3. Considerable variation in the amplitude of sensory CNAP at the elbow among patients studied;

4. Severe reduction in the amplitude of the CMAP and sensory CNAP (with dispersion) proximal to the spiral groove and *marked slowing (less than 50% of normal) in motor and sensory NCVs between axilla and elbow;* and

5. Electrophysiological and clinical improvement within 6–8 weeks.

The EMG shows acute denervation in all radial-innervated muscles except the triceps and anconeus muscles.

Posterior Interosseous Syndrome

The posterior interosseous nerve is the major terminal motor branch that passes through the supinator muscle (sometimes called the "radial tunnel" or "supinator channel"), entering through the arcade of Frohse, and innervating the supinator, all the forearm and finger extensors except the extensor carpi radialis and abductor pollicis longus muscles (Fig. 21.27). In contrast to the wrist drop seen in radial nerve palsy, this neuropathy produces "finger drop": an inability to extend the fingers at the metapha-

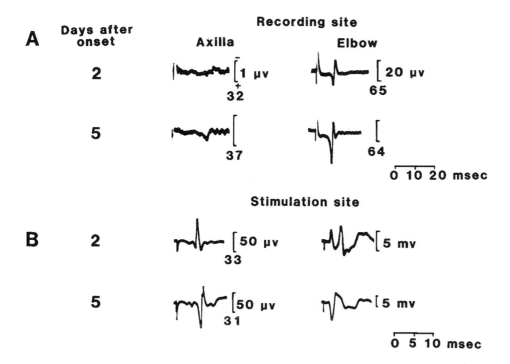

Figure 21.28. Nerve conduction abnormalities in Saturday night palsy. *A*, Sensory nerve conduction across the spiral groove. CNAP at the elbow and axilla. The number under each record denotes the conduction velocity. *B*, Motor nerve conduction across the spiral groove. CMAP from brachioradialis muscle. The number under each record denotes the conduction velocity between the axilla and the elbow. (Modified from Trojaborg W. Rate of recovery in motor and sensory fibers of the radial nerve: clinical and electrophysiological aspects. J Neurol Neurosurg Psychiatry 1970;33:628–629.)

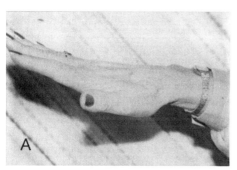
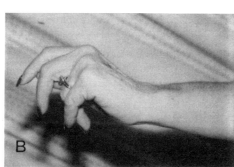

Figure 21.29. Fingerdrop in posterior interosseous syndrome (*B*) compared with normal finger extension (*A*).

langeal joint (Fig. 21.29). Various causes of posterior interosseous neuropathy have been described, the most common being trauma (224).

In the radial nerve conduction test with a needle in the extensor indicis proprius muscle and stimulation above the elbow, Carfi and Ma (224) found normal response in three of eight patients and prolonged latency or absent response in five. In a study of 15 patients, Kaplan observed significant prolongation in the distal motor latency to the extensor digitorum communis muscle with elbow stimulation compared with the normal side and normalization of this latency with conservative treatment during a 5-year follow-up period (225). Falck and Hurme described a motor and mixed nerve conduction technique for the posterior interosseous branch of the radial nerve (226). In two cases of posterior interosseous syndrome, the NCV across the arcade of Frohse was slow but normalized after surgery. The superficial radial sensory nerve conduction is classically normal in posterior interosseous neuropathy.

The needle EMG classically shows denervation in all the radial nerve-innervated forearm muscles except the extensor carpi radialis and brachioradialis muscles. In two-thirds of 12 patients with this neuropathy, Carfi and Ma found denervation in the supinator muscle and proposed that supinator syndrome is a special case of posterior interosseous syndrome (224).

Radial Tunnel Syndrome

In recent years, there have been many orthopaedic surgeons who claimed that resistant tennis elbow is caused by entrapment of the posterior interosseous nerve at the arcade of Frohse (radial tunnel) and thus labeled this disorder "radial tunnel syndrome" (227, 228). Their claim is based on two studies (227, 229). Roles et al. (227) found some needle EMG abnormality in 16 of 18 patients with resistant tennis elbow: fibrillations in the extensor digitorum in two and "EMG confirmation of radial tunnel syndrome" in the others. Narakas found needle EMG abnormalities in nine of 12 patients (229), none of whom had a nerve conduction study.

Four groups performed the posterior interosseous nerve conduction test in patients for whom pain was the main symptom and arrived at opposing conclusions. In electrophysiological studies of 25 of 90 patients who had surgery, Werner found a slow radial motor NCV across the supinator in 13 and a slight increase in the MUPs in the EDC muscle in eight cases (230). None of these cases showed any abnormal spontaneous potentials. Rosen and Werner studied the radial motor nerve conduction across the supinator in 28 patients at rest and during forceful supination of the muscle (231). The standard posterior interosseous nerve conduction was normal, but there was a significant delay in latency when the test was repeated during forceful supination of the forearm. EMG studies of the EDC were mildly abnormal. These authors claimed that their study supports the possibility of an entrapment etiology of the posterior interosseous nerve in patients with refractory tennis elbow. In contrast, Rossum et al. found no abnormality in the needle EMG or the radial motor nerve conduction in 10 patients with tennis elbow (232). In another study by Verhaar and Spaans in 16 patients with radial tunnel syndrome, only one patient had a major increase in latency of the radial nerve conduction across the radial tunnel (233). Thus, the diagnosis of radial tunnel syndrome is based solely on the clinical features: pain in the proximal radial part of the forearm which is aggravated by work and intense tenderness over the posterior interosseous nerve, especially where it passes under the proximal edge of the superficial supinator muscle, approximately 5 cm distal to the lateral epicondyle (230). There is *no solid evidence* as yet to suggest that refractory tennis elbow or radial tunnel syndrome is due to entrapment of the posterior interosseous nerve.

Superficial Radial Sensory Nerve

The superficial radial sensory nerve is a long nerve, originating from the main radial nerve just above the elbow, and dividing into terminal digital branches that supply the dorsolateral aspect of the hand and the first three digits. This neuropathy produces sensory impairment over the territory of the nerve, which is usually compressed at the wrist where it lies close to the distal end of the radius. This produces cheiralgia paresthetica, or "handcuff neuropathy." In this neuropathy, the sensory CNAP was either absent or low in amplitude or the sensory NCV was slow (234, 235). Sometimes, handcuff neuropathy may involve the median or ulnar nerve in addition to the superficial radial sensory nerve (236).

Entrapment of the superficial radial sensory nerve at the forearm where it exits from the deep fascia beneath the tendon of the brachioradialis muscle has been described (237). Tinel's sign is usually present at the entrapment site and symptoms are aggravated by hyperpronation of the forearm with ulnar flexion at the wrist (237). In 16 of 19 patients, the sensory nerve conduction of this nerve at the wrist was abnormal: absent CNAP in three cases, slow NCV in eight, and decreased amplitude in five. Spindler and Dellon found slow NCV in the superficial radial sensory nerve conduction in the forearm in one of three patients and normal NCV in the other two (238), which, however, showed relative slowing compared with lateral antebrachial cutaneous nerve.

Posterior Antebrachial Cutaneous Nerve

The posterior antebrachial cutaneous nerve branches off from the radial nerve at the distal portion of the spiral groove and continues down along the lateral side of the elbow and the dorsal side of the forearm to the wrist, innervating sensation over the dorsolateral aspect of the forearm (see Fig. 11.53).

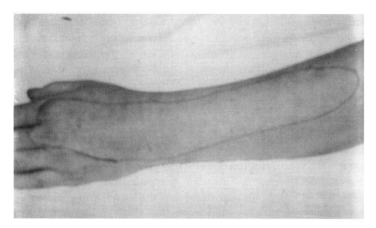

Figure 21.30. *Encircled area* of decreased sensation to pin-prick corresponding to the territory of the left posterior antebrachial cutaneous nerve. (From Chang CW, Cho HK, Oh SJ. Posterior antebrachial cutaneous neuropathy: case report. EMG Clin Neurophysiol 1989;29:109.)

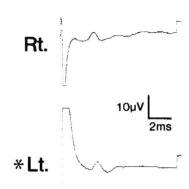

Figure 21.31. Nerve conduction abnormality in posterior antebrachial cutaneous neuropathy. *Asterisk* indicates the symptomatic side. Slow sensory NCV (47.6 m/sec) in the symptomatic side in contrast to normal sensory NCV (61.3 m/sec) in the normal side.

A nerve conduction technique for this nerve has been described (239). Three cases of posterior antebrachial cutaneous neuropathy were reported (Fig. 21.30) (240, 241): one case was caused by an intramuscular injection and the others by trauma. Sensory nerve conduction in this nerve was abnormal in all three cases: slow NCV, low CNAP amplitude, or absent CNAP (Fig. 21.31).

Thoracic Spinal Nerve

The thoracic spinal nerve forms the intercostal nerves at the T2–T6 level and the intercostoabdominal nerve at the T7–T12 level. These nerves divide into the lateral cutaneous branches about halfway around the chest and form the medial cutaneous branch at the end. The lateral cutaneous branch of the thoracic spinal nerve innervates the intercostal and abdominal muscles.

Thoracic spinal neuropathy is accompanied by pain and sensory impairment on the affected segment. Muscle weakness is rarely demonstrable. However, bulging of the abdomen has been reported as a sign of diabetic thoracic radiculoneuropathy (242).

Techniques for the intercostal nerve conduction have been described, but no cases of thoracic spinal neuropathy have been studied with these techniques.

Three disorders can be affected by the disease process in the thoracic spinal nerves: (*a*) diabetic thoracic radiculopathy; (*b*) herpes zoster; and (*c*) abdominal cutaneous nerve entrapment. Among these, diabetic thoracic radiculopathy is the most common. This neuropathy occurs most commonly in adult-onset diabetics and is often the first manifestation of diabetic amyotrophy. This entity is diagnosed only by the demonstration of denervation process in the paraspinal muscles with the needle EMG. This is discussed further in Chapter 22.

Herpes zoster typically involves the dorsal root ganglia, producing "shingles" and pain in the affected spinal nerve. Segmental zoster paralysis has been reported in 5% of patients with herpes zoster because of the concomitant involvement of motor nerve fibers (243). The needle EMG in patients with segmental zoster paralysis showed fibrillations universally in the affected muscles (243, 244). In 71% of 17 cases of acute herpes zoster, fibrillations were observed in the paraspinal muscles corresponding to the cutaneous lesions, indicating that segmental motor involvement is more common than was previously thought (245).

Notalgia paresthetica is a sensory neuropathy involving the posterior rami of several thoracic spinal nerves, causing pruritis, burning, and dysesthesia, with an objective hypesthesia of the posterior thorax (246). Needle EMG was not performed in these cases.

Entrapment of the anterior cutaneous nerves of the abdomen has been found to occur where this nerve pierces the rectus abdominalis muscle and sheath (247). Sharp pain in the anterior abdominal wall, tenderness at the entrapment site, and sensory abnormalities were usually present. The needle EMG of the rectus abdominalis muscle showed chronic denervation (long-duration and high amplitude MUPs) in two cases (247).

Lumbosacral Plexus Nerve

The lumbosacral plexus is formed from the spinal L1–L5 and S1–S4 roots (see Fig. 5.12). The major nerves arising from the lumbar plexus are the femoral and obturator nerves: the femoral nerve from the posterior division and the obturator nerve from the anterior division. The major nerve arising from the lumbosacral plexus is the sciatic nerve, which is formed by two main nerves: the common peroneal and posterior tibial nerves. *The motor branch to the iliopsoas muscle originates from the lumbar plexus, and the superior and inferior gluteal nerves originate from the lumbosacral plexus.*

Lumbosacral plexopathy is characterized clinically by neurological deficits that extend beyond a single root or peripheral nerve. A thorough examination of the girdle (iliopsoas and gluteus) muscles can localize the lesion to the plexus, since these muscles are innervated by branches from the lumbosacral plexus. To evaluate for lumbosacral plexopathy, sensory examination of the saddle and perineal areas, the anal sphincter tone and reflex, and the bulbocavernosus reflex are essential.

There is no nerve conduction test of the lumbosacral plexus. There are, however, two essential tests to help localize a lesion to the plexus: (*a*) the needle EMG of the paraspinal muscles (denervation process in the paraspinal muscles is indicative of a root disorder but not of plexopathy); and (*b*) the sensory nerve conduction (abnormal in plexopathies but not in root disease). The most important electrophysiological test for lumbosacral plexopathy is the needle EMG study, which *must* include testing of the paraspinal and girdle muscles innervated by the branches from the lumbosacral plexus: *the iliopsoas muscle* for the lumbar plexus and *the gluteal* muscles for the lumbosacral plexus. Needle EMG evidence of denervation process in the girdle muscles in the absence of such findings in the paraspinal muscles is indicative of a lumbosacral plexopathy.

Tumor-Induced Plexopathy

Malignant invasion is one of the most frequent causes of lumbosacral plexopathy. The lumbosacral plexus can easily be invaded by malignant tumors arising from the pelvic, abdominal, and retroperitoneal areas. The insidious onset of pelvic or radicular leg pain followed weeks or months later by sensory symptoms and weakness is a typical history. The quintet of leg pain, weakness, edema, rectal mass, and hydronephrosis suggests plexopathy due to cancer (248). The CT scan is the test of choice, revealing the pelvic tumor in 96% of cases. The needle EMG showed active and chronic denervation in the clinically involved muscles in more than 95% of cases (248, 249). The needle EMG study successfully identified bilateral involvement in 24% of cases with clinically unilateral involvement (248). The paraspinal EMG was helpful in identifying the epidural extension of malignancy (248, 249).

Radiation-Induced Plexopathy

Radiation-induced lumbosacral plexopathy is a well-known entity. It may develop 1–31 years (median 5 years) after radiation therapy (249). In general, higher doses of radiation are more likely to produce this disorder. *Painless* leg weakness was a classic feature in radiation-induced plexopathy, whereas pain marks the presence of a tumor (249). In the nerve conduction study, NCVs in the peroneal and posterior tibial nerves were slow in 15% of cases, but CMAPs were normal in some patients with normal NCV (249). The sural nerve conduction was abnormal in 50% of cases: absent in seven and of low amplitude in three. The needle EMG study showed fibrillations and chronic denervation in all cases, with paraspinal EMG abnormalities in 50% of cases. The most striking

EMG abnormality, which distinguishes this disorder from tumor-induced plexopathy, is myokymia (249, 250). *Myokymia* was observed in 60% of cases in one series, whereas in tumor-induced plexopathy it was not found (249). Fasciculations are also helpful in diagnosis of this disorder because they were observed in one-third of patients with radiation-induced plexopathy but in only one of 30 cases of tumor induced plexopathy (249, 251).

Hematoma-Induced Plexopathy

Retroperitoneal hematoma, which may occur as a complication of hemophilia or anticoagulant therapy, is a well-known cause of lumbosacral plexopathy and can produce three distinct syndromes: (*a*) femoral neuropathy with an iliacus hematoma; (*b*) lumbar plexopathy with a psoas hematoma; and (*c*) lumbosacral plexopathy with an extensive retroperitoneal hematoma (252, 253). The needle EMG showed active denervation in the involved muscles. The femoral nerve was inexcitable at the groin in one case of lumbar plexopathy caused by a psoas hematoma (252). The CT scan is diagnostic of this disorder.

Acute Lumbosacral Plexopathy

As a counterpart to the well-known acute brachial plexus neuropathy, acute lumbosacral plexus neuropathy can present with a sudden onset of severe pain followed by insidious weakness of the muscles innervated by the lumbosacral plexus. Only one leg is involved in a majority of patients. The proximal muscles are more frequently affected than the distal leg muscles. Usually the prognosis is good with a slow recovery.

The needle EMG shows evidence of a patchy pattern of denervation in the distribution of part or all of the lumbosacral plexus but not in the paraspinal muscles (254, 255). Peroneal nerve conduction was normal in six tested cases. Sural nerve conduction was also normal in four cases. Femoral nerve conduction, F-wave latency, and H-reflex latency were not studied in the reported cases. The paraspinal EMG showed denervation in one case (256).

Bradley et al. described six patients with a syndrome of acute or subacute painful lumbosacral plexopathy, elevated sedimentation rate, and perivascular mononuclear cells in the sural nerve biopsy (257). One autopsy case showed perivascular collections of mononuclear cells in the epineurium of the cauda equina, brachial plexus, sympathetic ganglia, and sciatic, femoral and recurrent laryngeal nerves. Four of five patients treated with immunosuppressive drugs improved. Three patients were diabetic. There were no features of a necrotizing vasculitis. Initial electrophysiological findings were consistent with multiple mononeuropathies in all patients. The paraspinal EMG was normal in all but one patient, indicating that the spinal roots were usually not involved.

Subacute lumbosacral plexopathy with recovery within a few weeks was reported in addicts using intravenous heroin, sometimes in association with rhabdomyolysis (258–260). The needle EMG study usually confirmed acute denervation in the involved muscles with sparing of paraspinal muscles (258, 260).

Diabetic Lumbosacral Radiculopathy

Clinical and EMG evidence of unilateral lower lumbosacral radiculopathy has been described in a few diabetic patients. This radiculopathy is different from classic diabetic amyotrophy in that the femoral nerve territory is not predominantly involved (see Chapter 22). Electrophysiologically, multiple lumbosacral radiculopathies and diffuse peripheral neuropathy were present. No evidence of disc disease was noted on an imaging study. This entity follows the usual course of diabetic amyotrophy.

Lateral Femoral Cutaneous Nerve

The lateral femoral cutaneous nerve originates from the L2 and L3 spinal nerves. Meralgia paresthetica is a clinically benign entrapment neuropathy of the lateral femoral

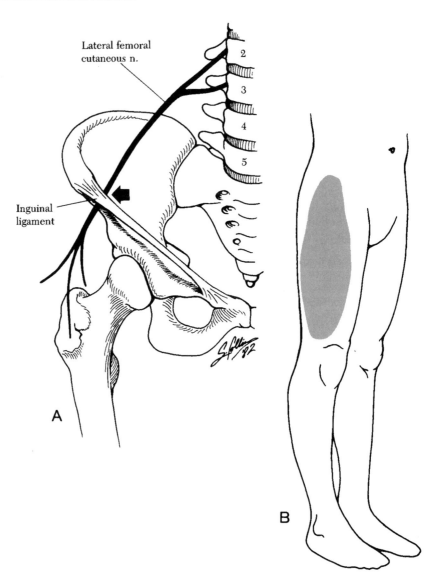

Figure 21.32. Entrapment site of the lateral femoral cutaneous nerve in meralgia paresthetica (*arrow* is at the anterior superior iliac spine). Typical territory of lateral femoral cutaneous nerve is the blackened area.

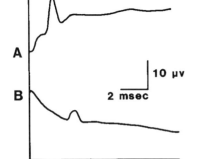

Figure 21.33. Nerve conduction abnormality in meralgia paresthetica. *A*, Normal sensory CNAP. Sensory NCV is 66.7 m/sec. *B*, Sensory CNAP in a patient. Sensory NCV is 34.8 m/sec. (From Sarala PK, Nishihara T, Oh SJ. Meralgia paresthetica: electrophysiologic study. Arch Phys Med Rehabil 1979;60:30).

Table 21.12.
Nerve Conduction Abnormalities in Meralgia Paresthetica

Investigator	No. of Patients	No. with Sensory Nerve Conduction			
		Normal	Low Amplitude	Slow NCV	Absent
Stevens and Roselle (261)		2	1		1
Butler et al. (262)	1				1
Sarala et al. (263)	9			3	6
Lysens et al. (264)	5				5
Lagueny et al. (265)	9	6	4	2	9

cutaneous nerve of the thigh. The site of entrapment is the point at which the nerve pierces the inguinal ligament or the fascia lata upon entering the thigh at or near the level of the anterior superior iliac spine (Fig. 21.32). The diagnosis is usually based on the presence of dysesthesia over the usual territory of the lateral femoral cutaneous nerve.

A conduction study of the lateral femoral cutaneous nerve can be used as an objective diagnostic aid in this disorder. The most prominent abnormality is an absence of sensory CNAP, as observed in 58% of the reported cases (261–265) (Table 21.12). The sensory NCV was slow in 17% (Fig. 21.33). The somatosensory evoked potential test has also been used to detect this disorder.

Synek found a prolonged latency of the first negative cortical potential in the lateral femoral cutaneous cortical SEP in five of six patients with meralgia paresthesica (266, 267). Lagueny et al. (268) reported normal absolute latency in 17 of 19 cases, a prolonged latency of the first positive cortical potential in two, an abnormal side-to-side latency difference in four, and an abnormal side-to-side amplitude difference (>50%) in six. Thus, 11 (58%) of 19 cases showed a normal SEP by any standard. According to Lagueny, no electrophysiological parameter has shown any predictive value in the outcome of this disorder (268).

Iliohypogastric, Ilioinguinal, and Genitofemoral Nerves

These nerves arise from the upper lumbar plexus and innervate the inguinal region, the upper anterior and medial thigh, and a small part of the genitalia. Neuropathy involving these nerves is usually due to surgical incision and postoperative adhesions in the lower abdomen and inguinal area (57). Diagnosis of these disorders is based purely on the demonstration of sensory abnormalities confined to the sensory territory of each nerve. There is no electrophysiological test confirming these disorders.

Obturator Nerve

The obturator nerve is formed within the psoas muscle from the ventral divisions of the L2, L3, and L4 spinal nerves and descends through the psoas muscle. It passes through the obturator foramen, where it divides into anterior and posterior branches that innervate the hip adductors magnus, longus, and brevis, and the obturator externus muscles. Sensory fibers supply a small area of skin on the medial aspect of the middle and lower thirds of the thigh. Patients with obturator neuropathy have hip adductor weakness and sensory loss in a small area on the medial thigh.

No nerve conduction technique has been described for the obturator nerve. The electrophysiological diagnosis of this neuropathy is best confirmed by the presence of denervation process confined to the hip adductors on the needle EMG. Pellegrino et al. reported active denervation process in the adductor longus muscles in a patient who developed bilateral obturator neuropathy, most likely compressing the nerve at the bony obturator foramen, during prolonged dorsal lithotomy positioning (269). Obturator neuropathy after hip replacement has also been reported (270, 271). This nerve is also frequently damaged during labor (272).

Femoral Nerve

The femoral nerve is formed within the psoas muscle from the posterior divisions of the L2, L3, and L4 spinal nerves and emerges beneath the inguinal ligament lateral to the femoral artery and vein. In the thigh, it divides into motor branches to the quadriceps muscles and a sensory branch to the anterior thigh (Fig. 21.34). The saphenous nerve is the terminal branch of the femoral nerve that descends through the subsartorial (Hunter's) canal and emerges from it just above the knee, innervating the medial aspect of the lower leg and the arch of the foot.

Various causes, including trauma and iliacus hematoma, are known to be responsible for femoral neuropathy (57). *The most common cause of femoral neuropathy, however, is often said to be diabetes* (273). Though the femoral nerve is predominantly involved in diabetic amyotrophy, there is a more widespread denervation process involving the roots and lumbosacral plexus.

Femoral neuropathy is clinically characterized by the presence of one or more of three findings: (*a*) weakness of the quadriceps; (*b*) reduced or absent knee reflex; and

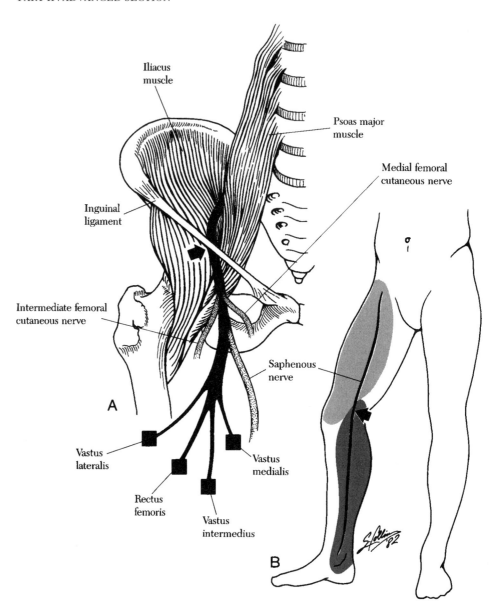

Figure 21.34. Entrapment sites of the femoral nerve. **A**, Entrapment at the inguinal ligament produces motor and sensory impairment. **B**, Entrapment of the saphenous nerve at the knee. Lightly shaded area represents the sensory territory of the intermediate and medial femoral cutaneous nerves.

(*c*) sensory impairment over the anteromedial aspect of the thigh and the medial aspect of the lower leg. Weakness of the iliopsoas muscle indicates that either the upper lumbar plexus or the L2 or L3 roots are involved. Weakness of the hip adductors also indicates that the patient has either a lumbar plexopathy or an L2, L3, L4 radiculopathy.

A femoral nerve conduction technique is available. The needle EMG study shows denervation process in the quadriceps muscles. The femoral and saphenous nerve conduction studies distinguish femoral neuropathy from lumbar radiculopathy. Even in patients with diabetic amyotrophy, a prolonged terminal latency in the femoral nerve was noted in 64–67% of cases (274, 275). This is in addition to widespread evidence of polyradiculopathy and peripheral neuropathy (Oh, unpublished data). In a few patients with traumatic injury of the femoral nerve at the inguinal area, prolonged latency of the femoral nerve and absence of the saphenous CNAP were consistent findings (276–280).

Anterior femoral cutaneous neuropathy producing sensory loss over its territory with sparing of the femoral and saphenous nerves following femoral artery reconstructive surgery was reported (281). No nerve conduction technique is available for this nerve.

Saphenous Nerve

The saphenous nerve is the terminal sensory branch of the femoral nerve that supplies the cutaneous branches to the medial aspect of the knee and lower leg (Fig. 21.32). Saphenous neuropathy is clinically characterized by sensory impairment on the medial aspect of the knee and lower leg. In spite of its long and superficial course, this nerve is infrequently injured except by lacerations (57). The most common cause of saphenous neuropathy is a complication of the removal of the adjacent saphenous vein during coronary bypass surgery, occurring in 12 of 421 patients in one prospective study (282). A rare entrapment of the saphenous nerve at the exit from Hunter's canal was reported (283). This nerve is also vulnerable during operations on varicose veins (284).

Nerve conduction techniques for this nerve are available. The saphenous nerve conduction was abnormal in a few patients with this disorder, revealing either a slow NCV or absent CNAPs (Oh, unpublished data).

Goyalgia paresthetica is an isolated neuropathy of the infrapatellar branch of the saphenous nerve characterized by hypesthesia and hypalgesia on a small affected area outside the knee (285). This disorder is well known to the orthopaedic surgeon because it is a relatively frequent postoperative complication that develops after medial knee incisions. House and Ahmed reported a case of spontaneous entrapment of this nerve behind the sartorius tendon against the prominent edge of the medial femoral condyle (286).

Sciatic Nerve

The sciatic nerve is the major nerve originating from the L4–S3 spinal nerves (see Fig. 5.12). The lumbar roots form the lumbosacral trunk, which is joined by the sacral rami, eventually becoming the sciatic nerve. Four nerves originate from the lumbosacral plexus: the superior gluteal nerve (L4, L5, S1), the inferior gluteal nerve (L5, S1, S2), the posterior femoral cutaneous nerve (S1, S2, S3), and pudendal nerve (S2, S3, S4). The sciatic nerve leaves the pelvis through the greater sciatic foramen (the sciatic notch) below the piriformis muscle. The inferior gluteal nerve and the posterior femoral cutaneous nerve also pass through the sciatic notch below the piriformis muscle. *The only nerve that passes above the piriformis is the superior gluteal nerve.* Thus, the sciatic nerve may be entrapped by the piriformis muscle as it leaves the pelvis through the greater sciatic notch and crosses its sharp edge (287). Other nerves (the inferior gluteal and posterior femoral cutaneous nerves) are usually also involved.

The sciatic nerve consists of two distinct nerve trunks, the medial trunk (the posterior tibial nerve) and the lateral trunk (the common peroneal nerve). The medial trunk arises from the posterior divisions and the lateral trunk from the anterior divisions of the L4–S2 spinal nerves.

The sciatic nerve innervates the hamstring muscles. The short head of the biceps femoris is *the only muscle innervated by the lateral trunk*, all other hamstring muscles being innervated by the medial trunk. *No sensory branch arises from the sciatic nerve itself.* Proximal sciatic neuropathy should be differentiated clinically from common peroneal nerve palsy because the peroneal branch is always more involved in sciatic neuropathy (288, 289). The greater vulnerability of the lateral trunk is most likely due to a combination of factors: (*a*) it is more firmly fixed and angulated at the sciatic notch; and (*b*) it contains larger and fewer fascicles and less connective tissue than the medial trunk, and so has less tensible strength (290).

The most common cause of proximal sciatic neuropathy is trauma because of the proximity of the sciatic nerve to the hip joint (272). Hip surgery and the insertion of prostheses can also cause sciatic nerve injuries. In one study, sciatic neuropathy developed after total hip arthroplasty in about 1% of patients (271). Sciatic neuropathy is the most common neurological complication from intramuscular gluteal injections, accounting for 96% of cases (291). An experimental study showed that the intrafascicular injection of drugs causes injury and that benzylpenicillin and diazepam produce the most severe damage (292). Sciatic neuropathy usually develops immediately after the injection, mostly without pain, but a few patients develop neuropathy later, presumably due to scar formation (291). Endometriosis in the pelvis or near the proximal sciatic nerve is also known to produce a rare sciatic neuropathy (293, 294).

Compression of the proximal sciatic nerve occurs infrequently, accounting for 25% of cases of sciatic neuropathy (293). Crisci et al. reported a case of trochanteric sciatic neuropathy caused by the combination of an underlying prominent lesser trochanter and sitting on hard benches (295). The needle EMG study localized the lesion to the proximal scitaic nerve. The nerve conduction study showed no response in the peroneal and posterior tibial nerves and absent CNAP in the sural and superficial peroneal nerves. Wilbourn and Mitsumoto reported four cases of proximal sciatic neuropathy caused by prolonged sitting (296). All patients had footdrop. The needle EMG showed denervation process in the sciatic-innervated muscles, typically including the hamstrings. Nerve conduction studies showed absent CNAPs in the sural and superficial peroneal nerves and low CMAP amplitude in the peroneal and posterior tibial nerves.

Piriformis syndrome is a pure pain syndrome characterized by hip pain radiating down the back of the thigh and dyspareunia in a female patient (297, 298). Pain and "weakness" with resisted abduction-external rotation of the thigh and a positive straight-leg raise are the usual findings. This syndrome is confirmed by tenderness and reproduction of the patient's complaint when digital pressure is applied over the belly of the piriformis muscle, either through vaginal or rectal examination or through external examination in the sciatic notch. Diagnostic injection of local anesthetics in the piriformis muscle relieves the pain. Classic piriformis syndrome should not be associated with any neurological abnormality (297).

Sciatic neuropathy is less common in the thigh and is most frequently caused by missile wounds (272). Other causes include schwannomas, myositis ossificans, trauma, and hematomas. A Baker's cyst in the popliteal fossa occasionally entraps the lower sciatic nerve (299). The peroneal, posterior tibial, sural, or all three nerves may be involved.

A sciatic nerve conduction test is available. We have not found any study of proximal sciatic nerve conduction in proximal sciatic neuropathy. We had one case of sciatic neuropathy in a thin alcoholic patient in whom the sciatic motor nerve conduction was slow.

Superior Gluteal Nerve

The superior gluteal nerve is the *only nerve* that passes through the sciatic notch above the piriformis muscle. Thus, it may be damaged while other nerves of the sciatic notch are spared. This nerve innervates the gluteus medius and minimus and tensor fascia latae muscles. One case of entrapment of this nerve in the suprapiriformis foramen was reported (300). Two cases of injection-induced superior gluteal neuropathy were also reported in which the needle EMG showed denervation process in the gluteus medius and minimus muscles (301).

Inferior Gluteal Nerve

The inferior gluteal nerve is one of four nerves that pass through the sciatic notch below the piriformis muscle. The others are the sciatic, posterior femoral, and pudendal nerves. Thus, the inferior gluteal nerve is almost never damaged without associated lesions of the other three nerves.

This nerve innervates the gluteus maximus muscle alone. A syndrome of buttock pain, cutaneous anesthesia in the distribution of the posterior femoral cutaneous nerve, and EMG evidence of marked denervation of the gluteus maximus has been described in five patients with recurrence of colorectal carcinoma (302). The authors suggested that malignant tissue compressed the inferior gluteal and posterior cutaneous nerves of the thigh as they passed below the piriformis muscle. Two cases of infrapiriformis foramen syndrome resulting from infragluteal injection with involvement of the inferior gluteal, posterior femoral cutaneous, pudendal, and sciatic nerves (291) have been reported. The most prominent needle EMG findings in these two cases were denervation in the gluteus maximus muscles with less involvement of the sciatic-innervated muscles.

Posterior Femoral Cutaneous Nerve

Posterior femoral cutaneous neuropathy produces paresthesias over the lower buttock and/or the posterior aspect of the thigh and is caused by injections, pressure from prolonged bicycle riding, and tumors in the presacral region that presumably compress the nerve in its intrapelvic course (272).

A nerve conduction method for the posterior femoral cutaneous nerve has been described (303). Iyer and Shields confirmed a case of injection-induced posterior femoral cutaneous neuropathy in which the sensory CNAP was absent in the involved posterior femoral cutaneous nerve but obtained in the normal side (304). Dumitru and Marquis reported an attenuation of amplitude in the posterior femoral cutaneous cortical SEP compared with the opposite side in a case of posterior femoral cutaneous neuropathy (305).

Pudendal Nerve

The pudendal nerve is the main nerve innervating the sensory and motor functions in the perineal area. Pudendal nerve injury is extremely rare because the nerve is deeply located and well protected. This nerve is occasionally damaged together with other nerves by injection and pelvic fracture (272, 301). On the basis of a prolonged anal reflex latency and SFEMG evidence of denervation of the anal sphincter, Swash et al. (306) suggested that idiopathic fecal incontinence is caused by a stretch injury of the pudendal nerve as a result of the descent of the pelvic floor during childbirth or repeated straining during defecation. A nerve conduction technique for the dorsal nerve of the penis is available. Abnormal nerve conduction of this nerve was reported in diabetic patients with erectile dysfunction. The pudendal SEP and bulbocavernosus reflex tests have been used to evaluate the pudendal nerve as a portion of the pathway (see Chapters 17 and 19).

Common Peroneal Nerve

The common peroneal nerve is the continuation of the lateral trunk of the sciatic nerve, formed from the anterior divisions of the L4–S2 spinal nerves and separating from the sciatic nerve in the upper popliteal fossa, descending downward and laterally through the popliteal fossa, and passing behind and around the fibular head (Fig. 5.13). The sural nerve and lateral cutaneous sensory nerve of the calf branch out from the common peroneal nerve before it reaches the fibular head. As it pierces the fibular tunnel, it divides into its two major branches: the superficial and deep peroneal nerves.

Common peroneal neuropathy is clinically characterized by weakness of the anterior tibialis and peroneus muscles and sensory impairment in the territory of the superficial peroneal nerve (lower lateral aspect of the calf). More weakness is usually noted in the muscles innervated by the deep peroneal nerve than in those innervated by the superficial peroneal nerve (289, 307). Thus, the sensory symptoms and findings are usually minimal. If the lesion is above the fibular head, *sensory loss over the lateral aspect of the calf* is an added clinical feature which differentiates it from a lesion at the fibular head. Peroneal neuropathy can also be differentiated from L5 radiculopathy by *preservation of foot inversion,* which is controlled by the posterior tibial muscle innervated by the posterior tibial nerve and the L5 root.

Crossed-Leg Palsy

The peroneal nerve is susceptible to compression at the point where it passes through the osteomuscular channel in the fibular head (Fig. 21.35). Acute compression neu-

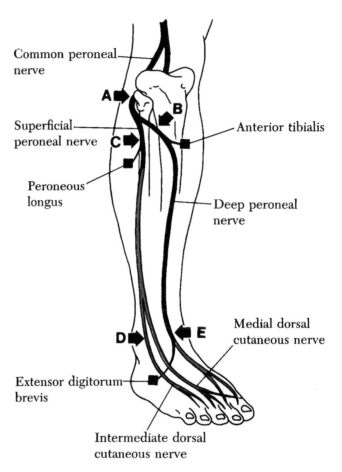

Figure 21.35.   Entrapment sites of the peroneal nerve. **A**, Fibular head compression in crossed-leg palsy. **B**, Deep peroneal nerve palsy. **C**, Superficial nerve palsy. **D**, Superficial peroneal neuropathy at the ankle. **E**, Anterior tarsal tunnel syndrome.

Table 21.13.
Nerve Conduction Findings in Peroneal Neuropathy at the Fibular Head

| Investigator | Motor Conduction (%) | | | | Sensory Conduction (%)[*] | | |
	SNCV	CB	NP	Diagnostic Sensitivity (%)	SNCV	Low amplitude	Diagnostic Sensitivity (%)
Singh et al. (308) (N = 47)	36	13[a]	36	36	82	77	82
	62 (AT)	19		62			
Redford (312) (N = 10)	90 (AT)	100		100			
Smith and Trojaborg (309) (N = 14)	64	50[b]	21	79	71	86	86
Pickett (310) (N = 3)	74[c]	53[c]	13	74			
Sourkes and Stewart (307) (N = 22)	45	45		64[°°]			
Katirji and Wilbourn (311) (N = 116)	4	45[d]	39 (EDB)	45[°°°]			
			13 (AT)				

[a]75% decrease in the proximal CMAP with the needle stimulation.
[b]CB >30% decrease in the proximal CMAP amplitude.
[c]SNCV, slowing in NCV >6m/sec; CB >20% decrease in the proximal CMAP amplitude.
[d]>50% decrease in the proximal CMAP amplitude. Test was performed by recording from the anterior tibialis muscle.
[*]The near-nerve sensory nerve conduction.
[°°]Axonal loss in 64% of cases.
[°°°]Pure axonal loss <50% amplitude in 55%.
Abbreviations: SNCV, slow NCV. CB, conduction block. NP, no potential. AT, anterior tibialis. EDB, extensor digitorum brevis.

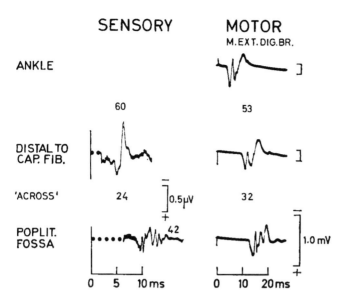

Figure 21.36. Sensory and motor conduction along the peroneal nerve in crossed leg palsy. Slowing in conduction across fibular head is most severe along sensory fibers (24 m/sec); conduction is normal along the segment of the nerve distal to the fibular head (sensory NCV 60 m/sec; motor NCV 53 m/sec). Sensory NCV from the superior retinaculum to the popliteal fossa is 42 m/sec. (From Singh N, Behse F, Buchthal F. Electrophysiological study of peroneal palsy. J Neurol Neurosurg Psychiatry 1974;37:1209.)

ropathy commonly occurs after prolonged crossing of the legs, squatting, or incorrect positioning of the legs. Clinically, this palsy is characterized by acute onset of footdrop occasionally associated with sensory impairment in the territory of the superficial peroneal nerve.

The most sensitive electrophysiological test is the sensory conduction study with the near-nerve needle technique, which should include the segments distal and proximal to the fibular head (Table 21.13) (308, 309). The diagnostic sensitivity is more than 80%. Comparison of the slow sensory NCV across the fibular head with the distal NCV is the best method (Fig. 21.36) (308, 309). The amplitude was a poor indicator of the site of the lesion (only 15%). Although the CNAPs in the popliteal fossa were dispersed to more than six components in 80% of patients with crossed-leg palsy, compared with 10% in normal nerves, this phenomenon was also unsatisfactory in localizing the lesion because it was also observed in peroneal paresis due to causes other than acute compression.

The motor conduction velocity was effective in localizing the lesion in 36–79% of patients (Table 21.13). Motor nerve conduction criteria commonly used to localize the lesion across the fibular head are:

1. NCV across the fibular head below the normal range, and NCV below the fibular head within the normal range;

2. *NCV across the fibular head slower than the distal NCV by more than 6–10 m/sec,* although both values are within the normal range, or the distal NCV is slightly slow (Fig. 21.36) (308, 310); and

3. *Conduction block or abnormal temporal dispersion across the fibular head* (Fig. 21.37).

This test is severely limited by the frequent difficulty of obtaining the CMAP in the extensor digitorum brevis in these patients. *An alternative method under this circumstance is the recording of the CMAP in the anterior tibialis or peroneus longus muscle* (308, 311, 312). Slowing across the fibular head in this method was noted in 62% of patients, a substantial increase from 36% by the conventional method (308). The disadvantage of this latter technique, however, is that the NCV across the fibular head cannot be compared with the distal NCV, but by comparing the amplitude difference

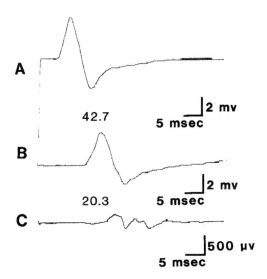

Figure 21.37. Motor nerve conduction in peroneal compression neuropathy at the fibular head. *A*, CMAP with stimulation at the ankle. *B*, CMAP with stimulation below the fibular head. Motor NCV of the over ankle-below fibular head segment is 42.7 m/sec *C*, CMAP with stimulation at the popliteal fossa 10 cm from the point in (*B*). The motor NCV across the fibular head is 20.3 m/sec. Conduction block is also obvious.

below and above the fibular head, the conduction block can be recognized in addition to the slow NCV. Using this technique, Redford (312) reported slow NCV in nine and conduction block in all 10 patients studied with peroneal palsy. One unusual finding in this neuropathy is the high frequency of axonal loss (low CMAP without any evidence of focal demyelination): 55–64% of cases (307, 311).

Mixed nerve conduction was studied in four patients by Gilliatt et al. (313). In every case, diminution in the mixed CNAP with slowing of the NCV was found on the affected side compared with the unaffected leg.

By using an "inching" technique at an interval of 2 cm for motor conduction, Brown and Yates (10) were able to localize the major abnormalities at or adjacent to the fibular head. Using the short-segment stimulation technique, Kanakamedala and Hong found that a majority of the lesions were located just proximal to the fibular head (314). Brown et al. (143) also performed the intraoperative motor nerve conduction in two patients with this disorder and found the most abnormal conduction to be proximal or distal to the entry of the common peroneal nerve into the peroneus longus muscle. These abnormalities were characterized by conduction block and delayed latency. In patients with common peroneal nerve palsy due to multiple causes, including 14 cases of spontaneous or compression palsy, it was found that those in whom motor NCV in the fibular head-ankle segment was greater than 30 m/sec made good recovery, but that patients with a motor NCV of less than 30 m/sec (or where the motor NCV could not be recorded) had a worse prognosis (315).

The needle EMG found active denervation in some muscles innervated by the peroneal nerve in all cases (307, 311). However, Sourkes et al. found that muscles innervated by the deep peroneal nerve were more frequently and severely denervated than those innervated by the superficial peroneal nerve (307).

One study compared the electrophysiological findings in six patients with complete recovery and eight patients with incomplete recovery (309). The authors concluded that normal sensory conduction distal to the fibular head is compatible with a good prognosis, whereas slowing along this segment, reduced or absent sensory CNAPs, slowing along the distal motor fibers to the EDB, or absent motor conduction suggest a poorer prognosis.

The lateral half of the extensor digitorum brevis muscle may be innervated by a branch of the superficial peroneal nerve (accessory deep peroneal nerve) (see Chapter

14). Gutmann (316) described two patients with complete deep peroneal nerve palsy caused by a fibular chondroma and a ganglion cyst who showed relatively normal motor conduction of the accessory deep peroneal nerve. This finding led him initially to conclude that the deep peroneal neuropathy was only partial in one case. An awareness of the anatomical variation in the innervation of the extensor digitorum brevis muscle is important for correct clinical and electrophysiological evaluations of deep peroneal nerve lesions but is of limited practical value in the diagnosis of crossed leg palsy since most lesions are found proximal to or at the neck of the fibula and thus above the origin of the accessory branch of the nerve.

Deep Peroneal Nerve

The deep peroneal nerve is the main branch of the common peroneal nerve running along the anterior compartment of the leg between the anterior tibialis and extensor hallucis muscles and tendons. It innervates the anterior tibialis, extensor hallucis, digitorum longus, and peroneus tertius muscles. At the ankle it passes under the extensor retinaculum and divides into two terminal branches: the lateral branch to the extensor digitorum brevis muscle and the medial branch to the small sensory territory in the web space between the first and second toes.

Deep peroneal neuropathy is characterized by footdrop with sparing of the peroneus muscles and is a rare entity. This nerve can be compressed in anterior tibial compartment syndrome (317) as well as by a ganglion or mass (316).

Superficial Peroneal Nerve

The superficial peroneal nerve is a branch of the common peroneal nerve innervating the peroneus longus and brevis muscles and then becoming a pure sensory nerve with two terminal branches (medial and intermediate). Thus, it supplies the sensory function in the lateral portion of the lower leg and almost all the dorsum of the foot except for the adjoining web of the first and second toes, which is supplied by the deep peroneal nerve.

Superficial peroneal neuropathy can occur in rare peroneal compartment syndrome, which is similar to anterior compartment syndrome in that muscle swelling and necrosis are confined to the peroneal muscles (318). There may be concomitant involvement of the deep peroneal nerve because this nerve passes through the most proximal portion of the peroneal compartment (319). The needle EMG shows denervation process in the peroneus longus and brevis muscles. Electrical stimulation on the exposed superficial peroneal nerve during surgery did not produce twitching in one case (318). This nerve can also be compressed where it passes through the deep fascia and becomes the superficial sensory branch. Patients with this neuropathy complain of paresthesia, pain, and sensory impairment in the distribution of the nerve (320–323). This neuropathy can easily be confirmed by the sensory nerve conduction technique of the superficial sensory nerve. In fact, the sensory nerve conduction test confirmed this neuropathy by showing an absent CNAP in one case and a prolonged latency in the other (323).

The terminal branches of this nerve can be compressed or injured at the ankle, usually as a result of local trauma or tight shoes.

Peroneal Nerve at the Ankle

Sensory Neuropathy of the Deep Peroneal Nerve

The sensory branch is the terminal branch of the deep peroneal nerve innervating the sensory fibers of the first dorsal web space. Sensory impairment in this small area is observed in this neuropathy. Compression of this nerve may be due to local trauma or tight shoes. A nerve conduction technique for this sensory nerve has been described. One patient with the entrapment of sensory branch of the deep peroneal nerve showed a low CNAP amplitude (0.6 μV) and prolonged latency (4.6 msec), confirming this neuropathy (324).

Anterior Tarsal Tunnel Syndrome

Compression neuropathy of the deep peroneal nerve at the ankle (Fig. 21.21) (anterior tarsal tunnel syndrome) may produce motor impairment of the extensor digitorum brevis and impaired sensation between the first and second toes. This compression neuropathy is most commonly caused by a tight rim or strap of a shoe, especially those with high heels, according to Marinacci (325).

Compression neuropathy of the superficial peroneal nerve at the ankle may also produce sensory impairment over the medial and intermediate dorsal cutaneous nerve territory. This is also often caused by a tight rim or strap of a shoe. The diagnosis of this disorder can be confirmed electrophysiologically by testing sensory nerve conduction of the superficial peroneal nerve for the toe-ankle segment.

Sural Nerve

The sural nerve has been infrequently reported to be the site of an isolated compression or traumatic neuropathy. Gross et al. (326) reported two cases of sural neuropathy in which sural nerve conduction was abnormal: a slow NCV in a patient with compression neuropathy and a low sensory CNAP amplitude in a patient with an iatrogenic stretch injury. Schuchmann et al. (327) also reported two cases of this disorder: one caused by compression of the nerve by a combat boot and the other due to chronic traumatic or irritative neuritis. In both cases, the sural CNAPs were absent. Gradual electrophysiological improvement was documented in Schuchmann et al.'s cases.

Posterior Tibial Nerve

Posterior Tibial Neuropathy

The posterior tibial nerve is a continuation of the medial trunk of the sciatic nerve. It passes through the popliteal fossa and then deep between the two heads of the gastrocnemius muscle (see Fig. 5.15). In the calf, it innervates the gastrocnemius, soleus, posterior tibialis, flexor digitorum longus, and hallucis longus muscles. At the ankle, it passes through the tarsal tunnel. Within the tarsal tunnel it is divided into three branches: the medial and lateral plantar nerves and the calcaneal branch.

Since the posterior tibial nerve is deeply located in the popliteal fossa and calf, this nerve is rarely compressed externally. This neuropathy is characterized by clinical weakness of the plantar flexor and inverter muscles and the intrinsic muscles of the foot. Sensory loss is confined to the sole of the foot and sometimes the sural nerve territory. A Baker's cyst high in the calf was responsible for this neuropathy in one case (328). As expected, no response was observed with posterior tibial stimulation at the ankle. Fibrillation was detected in the flexor hallucis longus, abductor hallucis, and abductor digiti minimi muscles.

Tarsal Tunnel Syndrome

The tarsal tunnel syndrome (TTS) is a compression neuropathy of the posterior tibial nerve and its branches within the fibroosseous tunnel that lies beneath the flexor retinaculum on the medial side of the ankle (Fig. 21.38). Typical symptoms include burning pain and paresthesia on the toes and along the sole of the foot. Classically, the symptoms are increased by activity, are diminished by rest, and often become worse at night. The most helpful diagnostic criteria are a positive Tinel's sign at the ankle and objective sensory loss in the territory of any of the terminal branches of the posterior tibial nerve. Weakness of toe flexion and atrophy of the abductor hallucis muscle are rare. The needle EMG study shows denervation process in the involved intrinsic muscles of the foot.

The nerve conduction study is the test of choice for confirming the diagnosis of TTS in more than 90% of cases (329, 330) (Table 21.14) (Figs. 21.39 and 21.40). Until 1979, prolonged terminal latency of the medial and lateral plantar nerves was used as an objective diagnostic criterion for TTS. However, the diagnostic sensitivity of the termi-

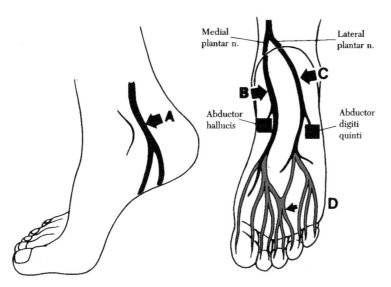

Figure 21.38. Entrapment sites of the posterior tibial nerve. **A**, Tarsal tunnel syndrome. **B**, Medial plantar neuropathy. **C**, Lateral plantar neuropathy. **D**, Morton's neuroma.

Table 21.14.
Nerve Conduction Findings in Tarsal Tunnel Syndrome

Recording Electrodes:	Surface Electrode (329) (N = 21)	Near-nerve Needle Electrode (330) (N = 25)
Terminal latency		
Prolonged latency	11 (54.4%)	4 (17%)
Medial plantar nerve	10	1
Lateral plantar nerve	7	3
Low CMAP amplitude		
Medial plantar nerve	7	1
Lateral plantar nerve	7	0
Sensory nerve conduction	19 (90.5%)	24 (96%)
Medial plantar nerve	(N = 21)	
Absent CNAP	11	2
Slow NCV	5	16
Low CNAP amplitude	6	10
Dispersion phenomenon		14
Lateral plantar nerve	(N = 18)	
Absent	10	6
Slow NCV	2	4
Low CNAP amplitude	3	5
Dispersion phenomenon		5

nal latency is low, prolongation having been observed in 17–52% of cases (329, 330). Overall diagnostic sensitivity of the terminal latency in the literature is 47%. In contrast, sensory nerve conduction studies using a surface electrode and signal averaging have been found to be far superior in confirming the diagnosis of TTS, being abnormal in 90.5% of cases (331) (Table 21.14). Sensory nerve conduction was abnormal in all nerves in which the terminal latency was prolonged. Both plantar nerves should be tested because in some cases only one is affected. Abnormality of sensory nerve conduction may be expressed either by absent CNAP or slow NCV. Since the CNAP of plantar nerves cannot be obtained in some older normal individuals, we used the near-nerve needle technique for the sensory nerve conduction of the plantar nerve for diagnosis of TTS (330). This technique improved the diagnostic sensitivity from 90.5% to 96% and, further, was able to elucidate the basic pathological process of TTS as a focal segmental demyelination.

Saeed and Gatens described a technique for recording mixed nerve conduction in

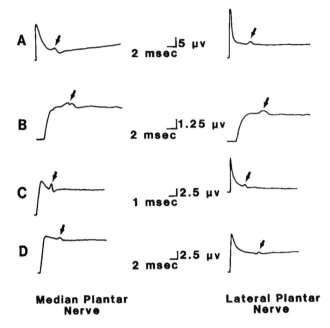

**Median Plantar
Nerve**

**Lateral Plantar
Nerve**

Figure 21.39. Sensory nerve conduction abnormalities in tarsal tunnel syndrome. CNAPs were obtained with surface electrodes. **A**, CNAP in a normal control: NCVs in the medial and lateral plantar nerves are 36.96 and 34.44 m/sec, respectively. **B**, CNAP in a patient, showing slow sensory NCV in the medial plantar nerve; NCVs in right medial and lateral plantar nerves are 24.66 and 24.36 m/sec, respectively. **C**, CNAP in a normal control: slow sensory NCVs in the medial and lateral plantar nerves are 41.25 and 34.80 m/sec, respectively. **D**, CNAP in a patient, showing slow sensory NCVs in the medial and lateral plantar nerves: NCVs in medial and lateral plantar nerves are 26.10 and 17.78 m/sec, respectively. The *arrow* in each case indicates the sensory CNAP. (From Oh SJ, Sarala PK, Kuba T, Elmore RS. Tarsal tunnel syndrome: electrophysiological study. Ann Neurol 1979;5:328.)

Figure 21.40. Sensory nerve conduction abnormalities in tarsal tunnel syndrome. The CNAPs are obtained with the near-nerve technique. The Roman numeral indicates the stimulating digit; the arabic number under each CNAP denotes the maximum sensory NCV in m/sec. No CNAP is obtained with V digit stimulation.

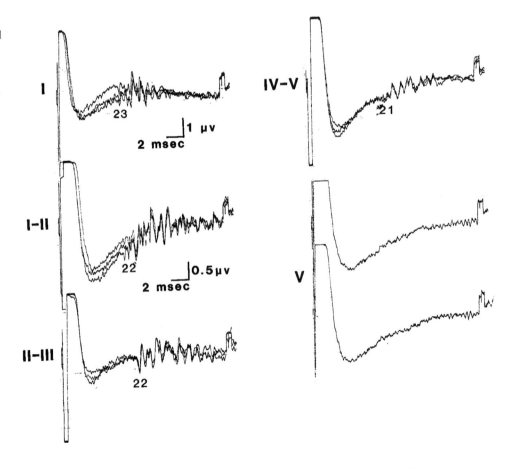

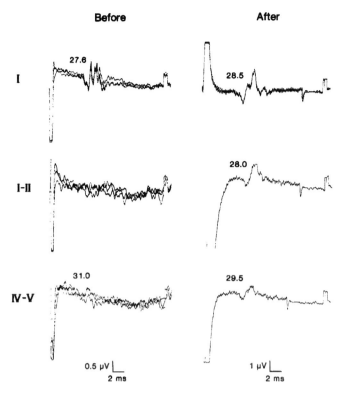

Figure 21.41.   Sensory nerve conduction in a patient with TTS before and after the decompression surgery. In the I–II interdigital nerve, the CNAP was absent before the surgery but recorded after the surgery. Numbers above the potentials represent the maximal NCV in m/sec. Notice the difference in the amplitude calibration before and after the surgery. (From Oh SJ, Arnold TW, Park KH, Kim DE. Electrophysiological improvement following decompression surgery in tarsal tunnel syndrome. Muscle Nerve 1991;14:409.)

the medial and lateral plantar nerves (332). This technique has the advantage of not depending on the signal averager. As yet, there has been no report dealing with a large number of TTS patients using this technique. We have had some difficulty in consistently obtaining the CNAP from the lateral plantar nerve with this technique. Saeed and Gatens reported absent CNAP in the medial and lateral plantar nerves in one case of TTS (332). Delisa and Saeed reported one case of TTS in which CNAP was absent in the lateral plantar nerve (333).

The needle EMG study shows a denervation process in the involved intrinsic muscles of the feet. However, this study does not provide any additional diagnostic information. In some cases where the differential diagnosis from lumbosacral radiculopathy or distal peripheral neuropathy is clinically difficult, the appropriate electrophysiological tests are needed to examine for these possibilities (329, 330).

Electrophysiological improvement was recently documented in three patients with TTS who had clinical improvement after surgical decompression (Fig. 21.41) (334). The near-nerve sensory nerve conduction of the plantar nerve 14 months–3.5 years after surgery showed improvements in motor and sensory nerve conduction. However, minor abnormalities still existed in the sensory nerve conduction in all three cases.

Medial Plantar Neuropathy

The medial plantar nerve can be compressed in isolation along its pathway distal to the tarsal tunnel, thereby producing medial plantar neuropathy (MPN). MPN has been reported with malignant schwannoma, leprosy, tenosynovial cysts, entrapment at the abductor tunnel, and reversible "jogger's foot" (335). The common site of compression in MPN is at the abductor tunnel (the fibromuscular tunnel behind the navicular tuberosity). Clinically, these patients have burning pain/tingling numbness over the

Figure 21.42. The CNAPs of the interdigital nerves in a patient with medial plantar neuropathy. The Roman numerals indicate the stimulated digits. The Arabic numbers under and above each CNAP denote the maximum sensory NCV and the negative NCV, respectively, in m/sec. The Arabic number between two arrows indicates the duration of CNAPs in msec. (From Oh SJ, Lee KW. Medial plantar neuropathy. Neurology 1987;37:1410.)

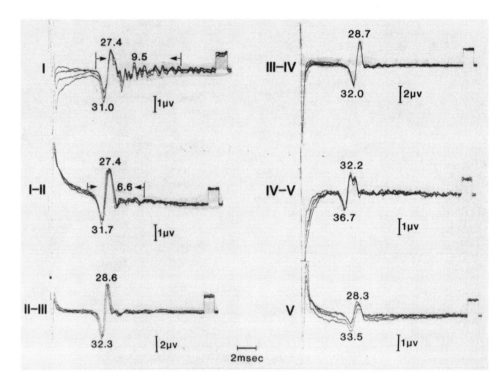

medial two-thirds of the sole of the foot and Tinel's sign and tenderness over the medial plantar nerve at the entrance of the abductor tunnel.

The sensory nerve conduction study of the plantar nerves can confirm the diagnosis of MPN, being selectively abnormal in the medial plantar nerve and normal in the lateral plantar nerve (Fig. 21.42) (335). Absent sensory CNAPs or slow NCV with low CNAP amplitude were observed in the medial plantar nerve in four cases. The needle EMG in the abductor hallucis brevis and flexor digitorum brevis (I–III) muscles may show denervation in this disorder.

Lateral Plantar Neuropathy

The lateral plantar nerve can also be compressed or injured in isolation along its pathway distal to the tarsal tunnel, producing lateral plantar neuropathy. Sensory loss is confined to the lateral one-third of the sole of the foot. We were able to confirm this neuropathy in three cases by the plantar nerve conduction study, showing abnormal sensory nerve conduction confined to the lateral plantar nerve. Terminal latency to the ADQ muscle was normal in all three cases. Denervation by the needle EMG should be confined to the ADQ muscle.

Interdigital Neuropathy (Morton's Neuroma)

Morton's neuroma refers to digits 3–4 interdigital neuropathy and is not uncommon. Typically, the patient complains of pain on the plantar aspect precisely localized between the 3rd to 4th metatarsal heads, often with radiation to the toes. Walking or standing precipitates the pain, and rest gives relief. Nearly all patients have tenderness on the interdigital nerve between the metatarsal heads. Sensory impairments are often detectable in the affected clefts and toes. Repeated trauma on the interdigital nerve is the most commonly accepted cause of this disorder. Pathologists have consistently found a proliferation of fibrous connective tissue within the plantar digital nerve and its supporting stroma in Morton's neuroma. Thus, Morton's "neuroma" is really a misnomer and should be more accurately described as a fibroma. Recently Oh et al. (336) devised a method for recording CNAPs from the various interdigital nerves on the foot and reported the electrophysiological abnormalities in five cases of interdigital neuropa-

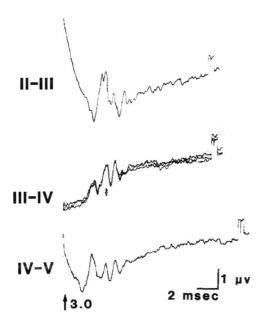

Figure 21.43. Sensory nerve conduction abnormalities in a patient with Morton's neuroma. The shape of the III–IV interdigital CNAP is abnormal, and a dip phenomenon is obvious. (Modified from Oh SJ, Kim HS, Ahmad BK. Electrophysiological diagnosis of the interdigital neuropathy of the foot. Muscle Nerve 1984;7:224.)

thy. They were characterized by a selective decrease in the amplitude of the CNAP in the involved interdigital nerve *("abnormal dip phenomenon")*, a relatively normal NCV, and normal duration of CNAP (Fig. 21.43). "Dip phenomenon" (a selective decrease in the amplitude of the CNAP in one interdigital nerve between neighboring interdigital nerves with normal amplitude) was present in 18% of normal controls (337). However, the amplitude of CNAPs in the interdigital nerve with "dip" was always greater than 50% of the CNAP amplitude in the preceding interdigital nerve. In patients with interdigital neuropathy, the amplitude of the CNAP in the involved nerve was less than 50% of that in the preceding interdigital nerve. This is called "abnormal dip phenomenon." Diagnosis of interdigital neuropathy was confirmed electrophysiologically by the abnormal dip phenomenon in four cases and by the abnormal shape and prolonged duration of the CNAP in one case.

On the other hand, Falck et al. used a different technique to measure the sensory nerve conduction in the interdigital plantar nerves of the foot (see Chapter 11) (338). In the diagnosis of Morton's neuroma, these authors suggested comparing the NCVs of the four interdigital nerves with each other, rather than comparing individual interdigital nerves with the normal mean. In patients with Morton's neuroma, the NCV of the affected nerve was abnormally slow in six cases. The amplitude of CNAP was not affected. This finding is in contrast to that of Oh et al., who reported that the amplitude was selectively decreased in the affected nerve (dip phenomenon) in Morton's neuroma (337). This discrepancy was apparently due to the difference in techniques.

Medial Plantar Digital Proper Nerve Syndrome (Joplin's Neuroma)

Joplin described a pain syndrome due to traumatic perineurial fibrosis of the proper digital nerve, which is sometimes called "Joplin's neuroma" (339, 340). This syndrome is usually characterized by pain in the medial aspect of the foot involving the great toe and an enlarged (cord-like) nerve immediately proximal to the interphalangeal joint, which is painful to palpation. Hypesthesia or hyperesthesia to pin-prick over the medial aspect of the great toe was found in some cases (341). This syndrome can be diagnosed by selective stimulation of the first digital nerve. However, there has not been any report of such a study. Excision of the "neuroma" usually relieves the symptoms.

Hereditary Compression Neuropathy

Hereditary compression neuropathy is a rare disorder characterized by susceptibility to pressure palsies (342, 343). The characteristic features are: (*a*) susceptibility to pressure palsies following relatively minor episodes of compression or ischemia; (*b*) improvement of symptoms within weeks or months; (*c*) frequent recurrence of pressure palsies; and (*d*) autosomal dominant inheritance (344). The disorder may present along with recurrent brachial plexus neuropathy (345–347). Tomacula, ballooned internodal "sausages" caused by the formation of extra myelin lamellae and segmental demyelination, are pathognomonic of this disorder (Fig. 21.44) (347, 348).

Electrophysiological abnormalities in this disorder are *those of mild segmental demyelination:*

1. Unequivocal abnormalities in sensory or mixed nerve conduction are noted in clinically affected and unaffected nerves. Mayer and Garcia-Mullin (349) observed absent or low-amplitude sensory and mixed CNAPs with surface electrodes in all nerves tested, and Behse et al. (348) found a 20–70% slowing in sensory conduction along the distal segments of clinically affected and unaffected nerves in six patients using the needle technique. The amplitude of the sensory potentials was moderately diminished, and the potentials were more "split up" than usual.

2. Motor conduction was slowed to a lesser degree and not as consistently as the sensory conduction (20, 348, 349).

3. The slow velocities were especially prominent in segments of nerves at sites of chronic compression (350). Thus, in clinically affected nerves the dysfunction can be localized to sites of chronic compression by electrophysiological studies. Two studies in this disorder showed conduction block at the entrapment site (351, 352). Sellman and Mayer reported conduction block in five of 23 nerves studied in four affected patients from two families with this disorder (351). Magistris and Roth detected 29 conduction blocks in 12 patients with this disorder (352).

4. Slowing of the NCV was more pronounced in distal than in proximal segments of the nerves. NCV was sometimes normal in proximal segments, whereas distal segments were clearly abnormal.

Of three patients with recurrent brachial plexus neuropathy (347), two showed electrophysiological evidence of proximal and distal neuropathy, and one was normal. There was a considerable increase in the distal latency in severely affected shoulder girdle muscles in two patients: diffuse neuropathy in one and evidence of entrapment of the median nerve at the wrist and of the ulnar nerve at the elbow in the other.

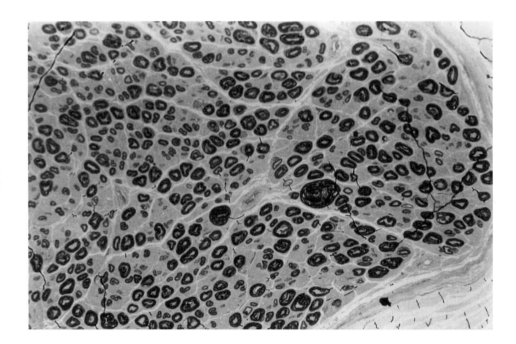

Figure 21.44. Tomaculous formation in a case of hereditary compression neuropathy. Two tomaculous formations with thick myelin layers are noted in the center. Diameter of larger tomaculous formation is twice that of the larger diameter normal fibers. Otherwise, there are relatively normal findings. Streaky lines are artifacts. Semithin section, Toludine blue, ×200. (From Oh SJ. Diagnostic usefulness and limitations of the sural nerve biopsy. Yonsei Med J 1990;31:21.)

REFERENCES

1. Ochoa J, Fowler TJ, Gilliatt RW. Changes produced by a pneumatic tourniquet. In: Desmedt JE, ed. New developments in EMG and clinical neurophysiology. Basel: Karger, 1973;2:174–180.
2. Trojaborg W. Prolonged conduction block with axonal degeneration: an electrophysiological study. J Neurol Neurosurg Psychiatry 1977;40:50–57.
3. Bolton CF, McFarlane RM. Human pneumatic tourniquet paralysis. Neurology 1978;28:787–793.
4. Rudge P. Tourniquet paralysis with prolonged conduction block: an electrophysiological study. J Bone Joint Surg (Br) 1974;56b:716.
5. Fowler TJ, Danta G, Gilliatt RW. Recovery of nerve conduction after a pneumatic tourniquet: observations on the hind limb of the baboon. J Neurol Neurosurg Psychiatry 1972;35:638–647.
6. Aguayo AJ. Neuropathy due to compression and entrapment. In: Dyck P, Thomas PK, Lambert EH, eds. Peripheral neuropathy. Philadelphia: WB Saunders, 1975:688–713.
7. Gilliatt RW. Chronic nerve compression and entrapment. In: Sumner AJ, ed. The physiology of peripheral nerve disease. Philadelphia: WB Saunders, 1980:316–339.
8. Kaeser HE. Nerve conduction velocity measurements. In: Vinken PJ, Bruyn GW, eds. Handbook of clinical neurology. Amsterdam: North Holland, 1970;7:116–196.
9. Simpson JA. Electrical signs in the diagnosis of carpal tunnel and related syndromes. J Neurol Neurosurg Psychiatry 1956;19:275–280.
10. Brown WF, Yates SK. Percutaneous localization of conduction abnormalities in human entrapment neuropathies. Can J Neurol Sci 1982;9:391–400.
11. Kimura J. The carpal tunnel syndrome. Brain 1979;102:619–635.
12. Miller RG. The cubital tunnel syndrome: diagnosis and precise localization. Ann Neurol 1979;6:56–59.
13. Buchthal F, Rosenfalck A. Sensory conduction from digit to palm and from palm to wrist in the carpal tunnel syndrome. J Neurol Neurosurg Psychiatry 1971;34:243–252.
14. Kimura J, Rodnitzky R, Van Allen M. Electrodiagnostic study of trigeminal nerve. Neurology 1970;20:574–583.
15. Ongerboer de Visser B, Goor C. Electromyographic and reflex study in idiopathic and symptomatic trigeminal neuralgias: latency of the jaw and blink reflexes. J Neurol Neurosurg Psychiatry 1974;37:1225–1230.
16. Lecky B, Hughes R, Murray N. Trigeminal sensory neuropathy. Brain 1987;110:1465–1485.
17. Ashmore B, Tait G. Trigeminal neuropathy in connective tissue disease. Neurology 1971;21:609–614.
18. Hess K, Kern S, Schiller H. Blink reflex in trigeminal sensory neuropathy. EMG Clin Neurophysiol 1984;24:185–190.
19. Zander Olsen P. Prediction of recovery in Bell's palsy. Acta Neurol Scand 1975;52 (Suppl 61):1–121.
20. Adour KK. Diagnosis and management of facial paralysis. NEJM 1982;307:348–351.
21. Fisch U. Surgery for Bell's palsy. Arch Otolaryngol 1981;107:1–11.
22. May M. Facial paralysis: differential diagnosis and indications for surgical therapy. Clin Plast Surg 1979;6:275–291.
23. Devi S, Challenor Y, Duarte N, Lovelace RE. Prognostic value of minimal excitability of facial nerve in Bell's palsy. J Neurol Neurosurg Psychiatry 1978;41:649–652.
24. Campbell EDR, Hickey RP, Nixon KH. Value of nerve excitability measurements in prognosis of facial palsy. Brit Med J 1962;2:7–10.
25. Alford BR, Weber SC, Session RB. 1970 Neurodiagnostic studies in facial paralysis. Ann Otol Rhinol Laryngol 1970;79:227–234.
26. Laumans EPJ. Nerve excitability in facial paralysis. Arch Otolaryngol 1965;81:478–485.
27. LeClaire R, Tremblay L, Dupuis M. Prognostic value of nerve excitability test in Bell's palsy. Can J Otolaryngol 1975;4:352–357.
28. Saade B, Karam F. Simple electrodiagnostic test for Bell's palsy. JAMA 1966;195:824–826.
29. May M, Harvey JE, Marovitz WF, Stroud M. The prognostic accuracy of the maximal stimulation test compared with that of the nerve excitability test in Bell's palsy. Laryngoscopy 1971;81:931–938.
30. Yanagihara N, Kishimoto M. Electrodiagnosis in facial palsy. Arch Otolaryngol 1979;95:376–382.
31. Adour KK, Wingerd J, Bell DN, Manning J, Hurley JP. Prednisone treatment for idiopathic facial paralysis. NEJM 1972;287:1268–1272.
32. Gilliatt RW, Taylor JC. Electrical changes following section of the facial nerve. Proc R Soc Med 1959;52:1080–1083.
33. Langworth EP, Taverner D. The prognosis in facial palsy. Brain 1963;86:465–480.
34. Brown E, Arno S, Twedt DC. Bell's palsy: Nerve conduction and recovery time. Phys Ther 1970;50:799–806.
35. Esselen E. Quantification of nerve fiber degeneration and time course of regeneration in Bell's palsy. EEG Clin Neurophys 1973;34:810.
36. Redhead J, Mugliston T. Facial electroneuronography: action potential amplitude and latency studies in 50 normal subjects. J Laryngol Otol 1985;99:369–372.
37. Cantar RJ, Nedzelski JM, McLean JA. Evoked electromyography in Bell's palsy: a clinically useful test? J Otolaryngol 1986;15:344–347.
38. Schenck E, Manz F. The blink reflex in Bell's palsy. In: Desmedt JE, ed. New developments in electromyography and clinical neurophysiology. Basel: Karger, 1973;3:678–681.
39. Kimura J, Giron LT, Young SM. Electrophysiological study of Bell's palsy. Arch Otolaryngol 1976;102:140–143.
40. Granger C. Prognosis in Bell's palsy. Arch Phys Med Rehabil 1976;57:33–35.

41. Granger C. Toward an earlier forecast of recovery in Bell's palsy. Arch Phys Med Rehabil 1967;48:273–278.
42. Blom S, Ekstrand T. Electromyography and sialometry in the prognosis of Bell's palsy. Acta Otolaryngol 1981;91:289–295.
43. May M, Blumenthal FS, Klein SR. Acute Bell's palsy: prognostic value of evoked electromyography, maximal stimulation, and other electrical tests. Amer J Otol 1983;5:1–7.
44. Tarvener D. Bell's palsy. A clinical and electromyographic study. Brain 1955;78:209–228.
45. Alford B. Electrodiagnostic studies in facial paralysis. Arch Otolaryngol 1967;85:259–264.
46. Steidel L. Prognosis and course of Bell's palsy. Arch Psychiat Nervenkr 1972;216:311–322.
47. Krogness K. Early EMG studies in Bell's palsy. EMG Clin Neurophysiol 1974;14:227–233.
48. Berry H, MacDonald EA, Mrazek AC. Accessory nerve palsy: a review of 23 cases. Can J Neurol Sci 1991;18:337–341.
49. Eisen A, Bertrand G. Isolated accessory nerve palsy of spontaneous origin. Arch Neurol 1970;27:496–502.
50. Cherington M. Accessory nerve conduction studies. Arch Neurol 1968;18:708–709.
51. Fahrer H, Ludin HP, Mumenthaler M, Neiger M. The innervation of the trapezius muscle: an electrophysiological study. J Neurol 1974;207:183–188.
52. Krogness K. Serial conduction studies of the spinal accessory nerve used as a prognostic tool in a lesion caused by lymph node biopsy. Acta Chir Scand 1974;140:7–11.
53. Logigian El, McInnes JM, Berger AR, Busis NA, Lehrich JR, Shahani BT. Stretch-induced spinal accessory nerve palsy. Muscle Nerve 11:146–150, 1988.
54. Petrera JE, Trojaborg W. Conduction studies along the accessory nerve and follow-up of patients with trapezius palsy. J Neurol Neurosurg Psychiatry 1984;47:630–636.
55. Barkhaus PE, Means ED, Sawaya R. Ligature injury to the accessory nerve. J Neurol Neurosurg Psychiatry 1987;50:1382–1386.
56. Palliyath SK. A technique for studying the greater auricular nerve conduction velocity. Muscle Nerve 1984;7:232–234.
57. Stewart JD. Focal peripheral neuropathies. New York: Elsevier, 1987.
58. Riley EA. Idiopathic diaphragmatic paralysis. Am J Med 1962;32:404–416.
59. Wolfe E, Shochina M, Fidel Y, et al. Phrenic neuropathy in patients with diabetes mellitus. EMG Clin Neurophysiol 1983;23:523–530.
60. Dourie-Devi M, Ganapathy GR. Phrenic nerve conduction time in Guillain-Barré syndrome. J Neurol Neurosurg Psychiatry 1985;48:245–249.
61. Tsarris P, Dyck PJ, Mulder DW. Natural history of brachial plexus neuropathy. Arch Neurol 1972;27:109–117.
62. England JD, Sumner AJ. Neuralgic amyotrophy: an increasingly diverse entity. Muscle Nerve 1967;10:60–68.
63. Weikers NJ, Mattson RH. Acute paralytic brachial neuritis: a clinical and electrodiagnostic study. Neurology 1969;19:1153–1158.
64. Flaggman P, Kelly JJ. Brachial plexus neuropathy: An electrophysiological evaluation. Arch Neurol 1980;37:160–164.
65. Martin WA, Kraft GH. Shoulder girdle neuritis: a clinical and electrophysiological evaluation. Milit Med 1974;139:21–25.
66. Gassell MM. A test of nerve conduction to muscles of the shoulder girdle as an aid in the diagnosis of proximal neurogenic and muscular disease. J Neurol Neurosurg Psychiatry 1964;27:200–205.
67. Aminoff MJ, Olney RK, Parry GJ, Raskin NH. Relative utility of different electrophysiologic techniques in the evaluation of brachial plexopathies. Neurology 1988;38:546–550.
68. Kori SH, Foley KM, Posner JB. Brachial plexus lesions in patients with cancer: 100 cases. Neurology 1981;31:45–50.
69. Lederman RJ, Wibourn AJ. Brachial plexopathy: recurrent cancer or radiation? Neurology 1984;34:1331–1335.
70. Stoll BA, Andrews JT. Radiation-induced peripheral neuropathy. Br Med J 1966;1:834–837.
71. Albers JW, Allen AA, Bastron JA, Daube JR. Limb myokymia. Muscle Nerve 1981;4:494–504.
72. Stohr M. Special types of spontaneous electrical activity in radiogenic nerve injuries. Muscle Nerve 1982;5:S78–S83.
73. Bufalini C, Pescatori G. Posterior cervical electromyography in the diagnosis and prognosis of brachial plexus injuries. J Bone Joint Surg 1969;51B:627–631.
74. Warren J, Gutmann L, Figueroa AF, et al. Electromyographic changes of brachial plexus root avulsion. J Neurosurg 1969;31:1237–1240.
75. Bonney G. Prognosis in traction lesions of the brachial plexus. J Bone Joint Surg 1959;41B:4–35.
76. Lederman RJ, Breuer AC, Hanson MR, et al. Peripheral nervous system complications of coronary artery bypass graft surgery. Ann Neurol 1982;12:297–301.
77. Graham JG, Pye IF, McQueen INF. Brachial plexus injury after median sternotomy. J Neurol Neurosurg Psychiatry 1981;44:621–625.
78. Hanson M, Wibourn A, Breuer A, Lederman R, Furlan A. EMG findings in a characteristic type of brachial plexopathy seen in open heart surgery. Muscle Nerve 1981;4:439.
79. Petrera JE, Trojaborg W. Conduction studies of the long thoracic nerve in serratus anterior palsy of different etiology. Neurology 1984;34:1033–1037.
80. Kaplan PE. Electrodiagnostic confirmation of long thoracic nerve palsy. J Neurol Neurosurg Psychiatry 1980;43:50–52.
81. Saeed MA, Singh S. Winging of the scapula. Am Fam Phys 1981;24:139–143.

82. Aiello I, Serra G, Triana CC, Tugnoli V. Entrapment of the suprascapular nerve at the sphinoglenoid notch. Ann Neurol 1982;12:314–316.

83. Garcia G, McQueen D. Bilateral suprascapular nerve entrapment syndrome. J Bone Joint Surg (Am) 1981;63a:491–492.

84. Hirayama T, Takemitsu Y. Compression of the suprascapular nerve by a ganglion at the suprascapular notch. Clin Orthop 1981;155:95–96.

85. Post M, Mayer J. Suprascapular nerve entrapment: diagnosis and treatment. Clin Orthop 1987;223:126–136.

86. Marrero JL, Godfine LJ. Isolated lateral pectoral nerve injury: trauma from a seat belt. Arch Phys Med Rehabil 1989;70:239–240.

87. Berry H, Bril V. Axillary nerve palsy following blunt trauma to the shoulder region: a clinical and electrophysiological review. J Neurol Neurosurg Psychiatry 1982;45:1027–1032.

88. Kirby JF, Kraft GH. Entrapment neuropathy of anterior branch of axillary nerve: report of case. Arch Phys Med Rehabil 1972;53:338–340.

89. Liveson JA. Nerve lesions associated with shoulder dislocation; an electrodiagnostic study of 11 cases. J Neurol Neurosurg Psychiatry 1984;47:742–744.

90. Kim SM, Goodrich A. Isolated proximal musculocutaneous nerve palsy: case report. Arch Phys Med Rehabil 1984;65:735–736.

91. Braddom RL, Wolfe C. Musculocutaneous nerve injury after heavy exercise. Arch Phys Med Rehabil 1978;59:290–293.

92. Dundore DE, DeLisa JA. Musculocutaneous nerve palsy; an isolated complication of surgery. Arch Phys Med Rehabil 1979;60:130–133.

93. Trojaborg W. Motor and sensory conduction in the musculocutaneous nerve. J Neurol Neurosurg Psychiatry 1976;39:890–899.

94. Felsenthal G, Mondell DL, Reischer MA, Mack RH. Forearm pain secondary to compression syndrome of the lateral cutaneous nerve of the forearm. Arch Phys Med Rehabil 1984;65:139–141.

95. Roth G, Ludy JP, Egloff-Baer S. Isolated proximal and median neuropathy. Muscle Nerve 1982;5:247–249.

96. Suranyi L. Median nerve compression by Struther's ligament. J Neurol Neurosurg Psychiatry 1983;46:1047–1049.

97. Hart CR, Linscheid RL, Reed Gramse RR, Daube JR. The pronator teres syndrome: compressive neuropathy of the median nerve. J Bone Joint Surg 1981;63A:885–890.

98. Mysiew WJ, Colachis SC. The pronator syndrome. Am J Phys Med Rehabil 1991;70:274–277.

99. Morris HJ, Peters BH. Pronator syndrome: clinical and electrophysiological features in seven cases. J Neurol Neurosurg Psychiatry 1976;39:461–464.

100. Werner CO, Rosen I, Thorngreen KG. Clinical and neurophysiologic characteristics of the pronator syndrome. Clin Orthop Relat Res 1985;197:231–236.

101. Buchthal F, Rosenfalck A, Trojaborg W. Electrophysiological findings in the entrapment of the median nerve at wrist and elbow. J Neurol Neurosurg Psychiatry 1974;37:340–360.

102. Gessini L, Jandolo B, Pietrangeli A. Entrapment neuropathies of the median nerve at and above the elbow. Surg Neurol 1983;19:112–116.

103. Martinelli P, Gambellini A, Poppi M, Gallassi R, Pozzati E. Pronator syndrome due to thickened bicipital aponeurosis. J Neurol Neurosurg Psychiatry 1982;45:181–182.

104. Aiken BM, Moritz MJ. Atypical electromyographic findings in pronator teres syndrome. Arch Phys Med Rehabil 1987;68:173–175.

105. Gross PT, Jones HR. Proximal median neuropathies: Electromyographic and clinical correlation. Muscle Nerve 1992;15:390–395.

106. Rennels GD, Ochoa J. Neuralgic amyotrophy manifesting as anterior interosseous nerve palsy. Muscle Nerve 1980;3:160–164.

107. Nakano KK, Lundergon MM, Okihiro M. Anterior interosseous nerve syndrome. Diagnostic methods and alternative treatment. Arch Neurol 1977;34:477–480.

108. O'Brien MD, Upton ARM. Anterior interosseous nerve syndrome: a case report with neurophysiological investigation. J Neurol Neurosurg Psychiatry 1972;35:531–536.

109. Gardner-Thorpe C. Anterior interosseous nerve palsy. Spontaneous recovery in two patients. J Neurol Neurosurg Psychiatry 1974;37:1146–1150.

110. Rosenberg JN. Anterior interosseous/median nerve latency ratio. Arch Phys Med Rehabil 1990;71:228–230.

111. Stern MB. The anterior interosseous nerve syndrome. Clin Orthop 1984;187:223–227.

112. Bolton CF, Driedger AA, Lindsay RM. Ischemic neuropathy in uraemic patients caused by bovine arterovenous shunt. J Neurol Neurosurg Psychiatry 1970;42:810–814.

113. Wilbourn AJ, Furlan AJ, Hulley W, Ruschhaupt W. Ischemic monomelic neuropathy. Neurology 1983;33:447–451.

114. Knezevic W, Mastaglia FL. Neuropathy associated with Brescia-Cimino arteriovenous fistulas. Arch Neurol 1984;41:1184–1186.

115. Bennett JB, Crouch CC. Compression syndrome of the recurrent motor branch of the median nerve. J Hand Surg 1982;7:407–409.

116. Dawson DM, Hallett M, Millender LH. Entrapment neuropathy. 2nd ed. Boston: Little, Brown & Co., 1990.

117. Goodwill CJ. The carpal tunnel syndrome: long-term follow-up showing relation of latency measurements to response to treatment. Ann Phys Med 1965;3:12–27.
118. Mills KR. Orthodromic sensory action potentials from palmar stimulation in the diagnosis of carpal tunnel syndrome. J Neurol Neurosurg Psychiatry 1984;48:250–255.
119. Casey EB, LeQuesne PM. Digital nerve action potentials in healthy subjects, and in carpal tunnel syndrome and diabetic patients. J Neurol Neurosurg Psychiatry 1972;35:612–623.
120. Buchthal F, Rosenfalck A, Trojaborg W. Electrophysiological findings in entrapment of the median nerve at wrist and elbow. J Neurol Neurosurg Psychiatry 1974;37:340–360.
121. Benini A. Die anatomischen Varianten des Ramus thenaris nervi mediani und ihre klinischchirurgische Bedeutung. Neurochirurgia (Stuttg) 1975;18:51–57.
122. Carrol GJ. Comparison of median and radial nerve sensory latencies in the electrophysiological diagnosis of carpal tunnel syndrome. EEG Clin Neurophysiology 1987;68:101–106.
123. Pease WS, Cannell CD, Johnson EW. Median to radial latency difference test in mild carpal tunnel syndrome. Muscle Nerve 1989;12:905–909.
124. Thomas PK. Motor nerve conduction in the carpal tunnel syndrome. Neurology 1960;10:1045–1050.
125. Sedal L, McLeod JG, Walsh JC. Ulnar nerve lesions associated with the carpal tunnel syndrome. J Neurol Neurosurg Psychiatry 1973;36:118–123.
126. Redmond MD, Rivner MH. False positive electrodiagnostic tests in carpal tunnel syndrome. Muscle Nerve 1988;11:511–517.
127. Kaeser HE. Diagnostische Probleme beim Karpaltunnelsyndrom. Dtsch Z Nervenheilk 1963;185:453–470.
128. Downie AJ. Studies in nerve conduction. In: Walton JD, ed. Disorders of voluntary muscle. London: Churchill, 1969:800.
129. Jackson DA, Clifford JC. Electrodiagnosis of mild carpal tunnel syndrome. Arch Phys Med Rehabil 1989;70:199–204.
130. Uncini A, Lange DJ, Solomon M, Soliven B, Meer J, Lovelace R. Ring finger testing in carpal tunnel syndrome: a comparative study of diagnostic utility. Muscle Nerve 1989;12:735–741.
131. Vallis J, Llanas J. Orthodromic study of the sensory fibers innervating the fourth finger. Muscle Nerve 1988;11:546–552.
132. Harrison MJG. Lack of evidence of generalized sensory neuropathy in patients with carpal tunnel syndrome. J Neurol Neurosurg Psychiatry 1978;41:957–959.
133. Chang CW, Lien IN. Comparison of sensory nerve conduction in the palmar cutaneous branch and first digital branch of the median nerve: a new diagnostic method for carpal tunnel syndrome. Muscle Nerve 1991;14:1173–1176.
134. Kraft GH, Halvorson GA. Median nerve residual latency: normal value and use in diagnosis of carpal tunnel syndrome. Arch Phys Med Rehabil 1983;64:221–226.
135. Shahani BT, Young RR, Potts F, Maccabee P. Terminal latency index (TLI) and late response studies in motor neuron disease, peripheral neuropathies, and entrapment syndrome (abstract). Acta Neurol Scand (Suppl) 1979;73:118.
136. Evans BA, Daube JR. A comparison of three electrodiagnostic methods of diagnosing carpal tunnel syndrome. Muscle Nerve 1984;7:565.
137. Phalen GS. The carpal tunnel syndrome: clinical evaluation of 588 hands. Clin Orthop 1972;83:29–40.
138. Schwartz MS, Gordon JA, Swash M. Slowed nerve conduction with wrist flexion in carpal tunnel syndrome. Ann Neurology 1980;8:69–70.
139. Marin EL, Vernick S, Freidmann LW. Carpal tunnel syndrome: median nerve stress test. Arch Phys Med Rehabil 1983;64:206–208.
140. Dunnan JB, Waylonis GW. Wrist flexion as an adjunct to the diagnosis of carpal tunnel syndrome. Arch Phys Med Rehabil 1991;72:211–213.
141. Thomas JE, Lambert EH, Dseuz KA. Electrodiagnostic aspects of the carpal tunnel syndrome. Arch Neurol 1967;16:635–641.
142. LeQuesne PM, Casey EB. Recovery of conduction velocity distal to a compressive lesion. J Neurol Neurosurg Psychiatry 1974;37:1346–1351.
143. Brown WF, Ferguson GG, Jones MW, Yates SK. The location of conduction abnormalities in human entrapment neuropathies. Can Neurol Sci 1976;3:111–122.
144. Harris CM, Tanner E, Goldstein MN, Pettee DS. The surgical treatment of the carpal tunnel syndrome correlated with preoperative nerve-conduction studies. J Bone Joint Surg 1979;61A:93–98.
145. Goodman HV, Gilliatt RW. The effect of treatment on median nerve conduction in patients with the carpal tunnel syndrome. Ann Phys Med 1961;6:137–155.
146. Hongell A, Mattsson HS. Neurographic studies before, after, and during operation for median nerve compression in the carpal tunnel syndrome. Scand J Plast Surg 1971;5:103–109.
147. Kemble F. Clinical and electrophysiological improvement from the carpal tunnel syndrome. EMG Clin Neurophysiol 1968;8:27–38.
148. Carpendale MT. The localization of ulnar nerve compression in the hand and arm: an improved method of electroneuromyography. Arch Phys Med Rehabil 1966;47:325–330.
149. Evermann WW, Ritsick JA. Intraoperative changes in motor nerve conduction latency in carpal tunnel syndrome. J Hand Surg 1978;3:77–81.
150. Garland H, Langworth EP, Taverner D, Clark JMP. Surgical treatment for the carpal tunnel syndrome. Lancet 1964;1:1129–1130.

151. Melvin JL, Johnson EW, Duran R. Electrodiagnosis after surgery for the carpal tunnel syndrome. Arch Phys Med Rehabil 1968;49:502–507.
152. Kruger VL, Kraft GH, Deitz JC, Ameis A. Carpal tunnel syndrome: objective measures and splint use. Arch Phys Med Rehabil 1991;72:517–520.
153. Goodman HV, Foster JB. Effect of local corticosteroid injection on median nerve conduction in carpal tunnel syndrome. Ann Phys Med 1962;6:287–294.
154. Gelberman RH, Aronson D, Weisman MH. Carpal tunnel syndrome: results of a prospective trial of steroid injection and splinting. J Bone Joint Surg 1980;62A:1181–1184.
155. Giannini F, Passero S, Cioni R, et al. Electrophysiological evaluation of local steroid injection in carpal tunnel syndrome. Arch Phys Med Rehabil 1991;72:738–742.
156. Stevens JC. AAEM Minimonograph # 26: The electrodiagnosis of carpal tunnel syndrome. Muscle Nerve 1987;10:99–113.
157. Katirji MB, Katirji PM. Proximal ulnar mononeuropathy caused by conduction block at Erb's point. Arch Neurol 1988;45:460–461.
158. Krarup C, Sethi RK. Idiopathic brachial plexus lesion with conduction block of the ulnar nerve. EEG Clin Neurophysiol 1989;72:259–267.
159. Eisen A, Danon J. The mild cubital tunnel syndrome. Neurology 1974;4:608–613.
160. Brown WF, Yates SK. Cubital tunnel syndrome and ulnar neuropathy. Ann Neurol 1980;7:289–290.
161. Eisen A. Early diagnosis of ulnar nerve palsy. Neurology 1974;24:256–262.
162. Kaeser HE. Erregungsleitungsstoerungen bei Ulnarisparesen Deutsch Zeit Nerveheik 1963;185:231–243.
163. Nishihira T, Oh SJ. Ulnar neuropathy: an improved method of diagnosis. Arch Phys Med Rehabil 1976;57:602.
164. Payan J. Electrophysiological localization of ulnar nerve lesions. J Neurol Neurosurg Psychiatry 1969;32:208–220.
165. Blatt-Lyon B. Sensory and motor conduction across and distal to the cubital sulcus in cubital tunnel syndrome. EEG Clin Neurophysiol 1973;34:798.
166. Tackmann W, Vogel P, Kaeser HE, Ettlin T. Sensitivity and localizing significance of motor and sensory electroneurographic parameters in the diagnosis of ulnar nerve lesions at the elbow: a reappraisal. J Neurol 1984;231:204–211.
167. Checkles NS, Russaken AD, Piero DL. Ulnar nerve conduction velocity of elbow position on measurement. Arch Phys Med Rehabil 1971;52:362–365.
168. Odusote K, Eisen A. An electrophysiological quantitation of the cubital tunnel syndrome. Can J Neurol Sci 1979;6:403–410.
169. Campbell WW, Sahni SK, Pridgeon RM, Riaz G, Leshner RT. Intraoperative electroneurography: management of ulnar neuropathy at the elbow. Muscle Nerve 11:75–81, 1988.
170. Kanakamedala RV, Simons DG, Porter RW, Zucker RS. Ulnar nerve entrapment at the elbow localized by short segment stimulation. Arch Phys Med Rehabil 1988;69:959–963.
171. Campbell WW, Pridgeon RM, Riaz G, Astruc J, Learhy M, Crostic EG. Sparing of the flexor carpi ulnaris in ulnar neuropathy at the elbow. Muscle Nerve 1989;12:965–967.
172. Stewart JD. The variable clinical manifestations of ulnar neuropathies at the elbow. J Neurol Neurosurg Psychiatry 1987;50:252–258.
173. DeJesus PV, Steiner JC. Spontaneous recovery of ulnar neuropathy at the elbow. EMG Clin Neurophysiol 1976;16:239–248.
174. Assmus H, Klug N, Kontopoulos B, Penzholz H. Das Suleus ulnaris Syndrom. J Neurol 1974;208:109–122.
175. Lunnegard H, Walheim G, Wennberg A. Operative treatment of ulnar nerve neuropathy in the elbow region. Acta Orthop Scand 1977;48:168–176.
176. Payan J. Anterior transposition of the ulnar nerve: an electrophysiological study. J Neurol Neurosurg Psychiatry 1970;33:157–165.
177. Friedman RJ, Cochran TP. A clinical and electrophysiological investigation of anterior transposition for ulnar neuropathy at the elbow. Arch Orthop Trauma Surg 1987;106:375–380.
178. Miller RG, Hummel EE. The cubital tunnel syndrome: treatment with simple decompression. Ann Neurol 1980;7:567–569.
179. Nielsen VK, Osgaard O, Trojaborg W. Interfascicular neurolysis in chronic ulnar nerve lesions at the elbow; an electrophysiological study. J Neurol Neurosurg Psychiatry 1980;43:272–280.
180. Miller RG, Camp PE. Postoperative ulnar neuropathy. JAMA 1979:242:1636–1639.
181. Miller RG. Ulnar nerve lesions. In: Brown WF, Bolton CF, eds. Clinical electromyography. Boston: Butterworths, 1987:97–117.
182. Holtzman RNN, Mark MH, Patel MR. Wiener LM. Ulnar nerve entrapment neuropathy in the forearm. J Hand Surg 1984;9A:576–578.
183. Harrelson JM, Newman M. Hypertrophy of the flexor carpi ulnaris as a cause of ulnar-nerve compression in the distal part of the forearm. J Bone Joint Surg 1975;57A:554–555.
184. Campbell WW. Ulnar neuropathy in the distal forearm. Muscle Nerve 1989;12:347–352.
185. Campbell WW, Pridgeon RM, Sahni SK. Entrapment neuropathy of the ulnar nerve at its point of exit from the flexor carpi ulnaris muscle. Muscle Nerve 1988;11:467–470.
186. Shea JD, McClain EJ. Ulnar nerve compression syndrome at and below the wrist. J Bone Joint Surg (Am) 1969;51a:1095–1103.
187. Ebeling P, Gilliatt RW, Thomas PK. A clinical and electrical study of ulnar nerve lesions in the hand. J Neurol Neurosurg Psychiatry 1960;23:1–9.

188. Bhala RP, Goodgold J. Motor conduction in the deep palmar branch of the ulnar nerve. Arch Phys Med Rehabil 1968;49:460–466.
189. Eckman PB. Ulnar neuropathy in bicycle riders. Arch Neurol 1975;32:130–131.
190. Scott TF, Yager JG, Gross JA. Handcuff neuropathy revisited. Muscle Nerve 1989;12:219–220.
191. Cuetter AC, Bartoszek DM. The thoracic outlet syndrome: controversies, overdiagnosis, overtreatment, and recommendations for management. Muscle Nerve 1989;12:410–419.
192. Gilliatt RW, LeQuesne PM, Logue V, Sumner AJ. Wasting of the hand associated with cervical rib or band. J Neurol Neurosurg Psychiatry 1970;33:615–624.
193. Swift TTR, Nichols FT. The droopy shoulder syndrome. Neurology 1984;34:212–215.
194. Conn J. Thoracic outlet syndromes. Surg Clin North Am 1974;54:155–164.
195. Kelly TR. Thoracic outlet syndrome. Current concepts of treatment. Ann Surg 1979;190:657–662.
196. Roos DB. Thoracic outlet syndromes: symptoms, diagnosis, anatomy and surgical treatment. Medical Problems in the Performing Arts 1986:1:90–93.
197. Costigan DA, Wilbourn AJ. The elevated arm stress test: specificity in the diagnosis of the thoracic outlet syndrome. Neurology 1985;35 (suppl 1):74–75.
198. Wright IS. The neurovascular syndrome produced by hyperabduction of the arms: the immediate changes produced in 150 normal controls and the effects on some persons of prolonged hyperabduction of the arms, as in sleeping, and in certain occupations. Am Heart J 1945;29:1–19.
199. Gergoudis R, Barnesw RW. Thoracic outlet arterial compression: prevalence in normal persons. Angiography 1980;31:538–541.
200. Urschel HC, Razzuk MA, Wood RE, Parekh M, Paulson DL. Objective diagnosis (ulnar nerve conduction velocity) and current therapy of the thoracic outlet syndrome. Ann Thorac Surg 1971;12:608–616.
201. Caldwell JW, Crane CR, Krusen EM. Nerve conduction studies: an aid in the diagnosis of thoracic outlet syndrome. South Med J 1971;64:211–212.
202. Krogness K. Ulnar trunk conduction studies in the diagnosis of the thoracic outlet syndrome. Acta Chir Scand 1973;139:597–603.
203. Daube JR. Nerve conduction studies in the thoracic outlet syndrome. Neurology 1975;25:347.
204. Kremer RM, Ahlquist RE. Thoracic outlet compression syndrome. Am J Surg 1975;130:612–616.
205. Sanders RJ, Monsour JW, Gerber WF, Adams WR, Thompson N. Scalenectomy versus first rib resection for treatment of the thoracic outlet syndrome. Surgery 1979;85:109–121.
206. Shahani BT, Potts F, Juguilon A, Young RR. Electrophysiological studies in "thoracic outlet syndrome." EEG Clin Neurophysiol 1980;50:172.
207. Ryding E, Ribbe E, Roséen I, Norgren L. A neurophysiologic investigation of thoracic outlet syndrome. Acta Chir Scand 1985;151:327–331.
208. Pavot AP, Gargour GW. Assessment of conduction from C_8 nerve root exit to supraclavicular fossa—its value in the diagnosis of thoracic outlet syndrome. EMG Clin Neurophysiol 1989;29:445–451.
209. Gilliatt RW, LeQuesne PM, Logue V, Sumner AJ. Wasting of the hand associated with a cervical rib or band. J Neurol Neurosurg Psychiatry 1970;33:615–624.
210. Lascelles RG, Mohr PD, Neary D, Bloor K. The thoracic outlet syndrome. Brain 1977;100:601–612.
211. Wilbourn A, Hansen M, Hardy R. Neurogenic true thoracic outlet syndrome: electrodiagnostic features in 11 patients. Muscle Nerve 1982;5:558.
212. Smith T, Trojaborg W. Diagnosis of thoracic outlet syndrome. Value of sensory and motor conduction studies and quantitative electromyography. Arch Neurol 1987;44:1161–1163.
213. Weber RJ, Piero DL. F-wave evaluation of thoracic outlet syndrome: a multiple regression derived F-wave latency predicting technique. Arch Phys Med Rehabil 1978;9:464–469.
214. Wulff CH, Gilliatt RW. F-waves in patients with hand wasting caused by a cervical rib and band. Muscle Nerve 1979;2:452–457.
215. Cherington M, Happer I, Machanic B, Parry L. Surgery for the thoracic outlet syndrome may be hazardous to your health. Muscle Nerve 1986;9:632–634.
216. Wilbourn AJ. Thoracic outlet syndrome surgery causing severe brachial plexopathy. Muscle Nerve 1988;11:66–74.
217. Pribyl R, You SB, Jantra P. Sensory nerve conduction velocity of medial antebrachial cutaneous nerve. EMG Clin Neurophysiol 1979;19:41–46.
218. Chang CW, Oh SJ. Medial antebrachial cutaneous neuropathy: case report. EMG Clin Neurophysiol 1988;28:3–5.
219. Jablecki C, Nazemi R. Unsuspected digital nerve lesions responsible for abnormal median sensory responses. Arch Phys Med Rehabil 1982;63:135–138.
220. Upton ARM, McComas AJ. The double crush in nerve entrapment syndromes. Lancet 1973;359–362.
221. Yu J, Bendler EM, Mentari A. Neurological disorders associated with carpal tunnel syndrome. EMG Clin Neurophysiol 1979;19:27–32.
222. Nakano KK. The entrapment neuropathies. Muscle Nerve 1978;1:264–279.
223. Trojaborg W. Rate of recovery in motor and sensory fibers of the radial nerve: clinical and electrophysiological aspects. J Neurol Neurosurg Psychiatry 1970;33:625–638.
224. Carfi J, Ma DM. Posterior interosseous syndrome revisited. Muscle Nerve 1985;8:499–502.
225. Kaplan PE. Posterior interosseous neuropathies: natural history. Arch Phys Med Rehabil 1984;65:399–400.
226. Falck B, Hurme M. Conduction velocity of the posterior interosseous nerve across the arcade of Frohse. Electromyograph Clin Neurophysiol 23:567–576, 1983.

227. Roles NC, Maudsley RH, Berkshire A. Radial tunnel syndrome. J Bone Joint Surg 1972;54B:499–508.
228. Hagart CG, Lundborg G, Hansen T. Entrapment of the posterior interosseous nerve. Scand J Plast Reconstr Surg 1977;11:205–212.
229. Narakas A. Epicondylite et syndrome compressif du nerf radial. Méd Hyg (Genève). 1974;32:2067–2070.
230. Werner C. Lateral elbow pain and posterior interosseous nerve entrapment. Acta Orthopaedica Scandinavica (Suppl.) 1979;174;1–62.
231. Rosen I, Werner C. Neurophysiological investigation of posterior interosseous nerve entrapment causing lateral elbow pain. EEG Clin Neurophysiol 1980;50:125–133.
232. Rossum JV, Buruma OJS, Kamphuisen HAC, Onvlee GJ. Tennis elbow—a radial tunnel syndrome? J Bone Joint Surg 1978;60B;197–198.
233. Verhaar J, Spaans F. Radial tunnel syndrome. J Bone Joint Surg 1991:73A:539–544.
234. Massey EW, Pleet AB. Handcuffs and cheiralgia paresthetica. Neurology 1978;28:1312–1313.
235. Dorfman LJ, Jayaram AR. Handcuff neuropathy. JAMA 1978;239:957.
236. Levin RA, Felsenthal G. Handcuff neuropathy: two unusual cases. Arch Phys Med Rehabil 1984;65:41–43.
237. Dellon AL, Mackinnon SE. Radial sensory nerve entrapment. Arch Neurol 1986;43:833–835.
238. Spindler HA, Dellon AL. Nerve conduction studies in the superficial radial nerve entrapment. Muscle Nerve 1990;13:1–5.
239. Ma DM, Liveson JA. Nerve conduction handbook. Philadelphia: FA Davis, 1983:79–81.
240. Chang CW, Oh SJ. Posterior antebrachial cutaneous neuropathy: a case report. EMG Clin Neurophysiol 1989;29:109–111.
241. Chang WC, Oh SJ. Posterior antebrachial cutaneous neuropathy. Case report. EMG Clin Neurophysiol 1990;30:3–5.
242. Boulton AMJ, Angus E, Ayyar DR, et al. Diabetic polyradiculopathy presenting as abdominal swelling. Br Med J 1984;289:798–799.
243. Thomas JE, Howard FM. Segmental zoster paresis—a disease profile. Neurology 1972;22:459–466.
244. Gardner-Thorpe C, Foster JB, Barwick DD. Unusual manifestations of herpes zoster: a clinical and electrophysiological study. J Neurol Sci 1976;28:427–447.
245. Greenverg MK, McVey AL, Hayes T. Segmental motor involvement in herpes zoster: an EMG study. Neurology 1992;42:1122–1123.
246. Fleet AB, Massey EW. Notalgia paresthetica. Neurology 1978;28:1310–1312.
247. Komar J, Vargass B. Syndrome of the rectus abdominis muscle: a peripheral neurological condition causing abdominal diagnostic problems. J Neurol 1975;210:121–125.
248. Jaeckle KA, Young DF, Foley KM. The natural history of lumbosacral plexopathy in cancer. Neurology 1985;35:8–15.
249. Thomas JE, Cascino TL, Earle JD. Differential diagnosis between radiation and tumor plexopathy of the pelvis. Neurology 1985;34:1–7.
250. Aho K, Sanio K. Late irradiation induced lesions of the lumbosacral plexus. Neurology 1983;33:953–955.
251. Ashenburst EM, Quartey GRC, Starreveld A. Lumbo-sacral radiculopathy induced by radiation. Can J Neurol Sci 1977;4:259–263.
252. Emery S, Ochoa J. Lumbar plexus neuropathy resulting from retroperitoneal hemorrhage. Muscle Nerve 1978;1:330–334.
253. Rajashekhar TP, Herbison GJ. Lumbosacral plexopathy caused by retroperitoneal hemorrhage: report of two cases. Arch Phys Med Rehabil 1974;55:91–93.
254. Evans BA, Stevens C, Dyck PJ. Lumbo-sacral plexus neuropathy. Neurology 1981;31:1327–1330.
255. Sanders JE, Sharp FR. Lumbosacral plexus neuropathy. Neurology 1981;31:470–473.
256. Torras MV, Tejedor ED, Tella PB. Lumbosacral plexus neuropathy and paraspinal muscle denervation. Neurology 1985;35:448–449.
257. Bradley WG, Chad D, Verghese JP, Liu HC, Good P, Gabbai AA, Adelman LS. Painful lumbosacral plexopathy with elevated erythrocyte sedimentation rate: a treatable inflammatory syndrome. Ann Neurol 1974;15:457–464.
258. Jacome DE. Neurogenic bladder, lumbosacral plexus neuropathy and drug-associated rhabdomyolysis. J Urol 1982;127:994–995.
259. Greenwood RJ. Lumbar plexitis and rhabdomyolysis following abuse of heroin. Postgrad Med J 1974;50:772–773.
260. Challenor YB, Richter RW, Bruun B, Pearson J. Nontraumatic plexitis and heroin addiction. JAMA 1973;225:958–961.
261. Stevens A, Roselle N. Sensory nerve conduction velocity of n. cutaneous femoris lateralis. Electromyography 1970;10:397–398.
262. Butler ET, Johnson EW, Kaye AZ. Normal conduction velocity in lateral femoral cutaneous nerve. Arch Phys Med Rehabil 1974;55:31–32.
263. Sarala PK, Nishihira T, Oh SJ. Meralgia paresthesica: electrophysiological study. Arch Phys Med Rehabil 1979;60:30–31.
264. Lysens R, Vandendriessche G, VanMol Y, Rosselle N. The sensory conduction velocity in the cutaneous femoris lateralis nerve in normal adult subjects and in patients with complaints suggesting meralgia paresthesica. EMG Clin Neurophysiol 1981;21:505–510.
265. Lagueny A. Deliac MM, Deliac P, Durandeau A. Diagnostic and prognostic value of electrophysiologic tests in meralgia paresthetica. Muscle Nerve 1991;14:51–56.

266. Synek VM. Assessing sensory involvement in lower limb nerve lesions using somatosensory evoked potential techniques. Muscle Nerve 1985;8:511–515.

267. Synek VM, Synek BJL. Intractable meralgia paresthetica after repeated abdominal surgery. EMG Clin Neurophysiol 1986;26:103–106.

268. Lagueny A, Deliac MM, Deliac P, Durandeau A. Diagnostic and prognostic value of electrophysiological tests in meralgia paresthetica. Muscle Nerve 1991;14:51–56.

269. Pellegrino MJ, Johnson EW. Bilateral obturator nerve injuries during urologic surgery. Arch Phys Med Rehabil 1988;69:46–47.

270. Melamed NB, Satya-Murti S. Obturator neuropathy after total hip replacement. Ann Neurol 1983;1:578–579.

271. Weber ER, Daube JR, Coventry MB. Peripheral neuropathies associated with total hip arthroplasty. J Bone Joint Surg 1976;58A:66–69.

272. Stewart JD. Focal peripheral neuropathies. New York: Elsevier, 1987.

273. Calverley JR, Mulder DW. Femoral neuropathy. Neurology 1960;10:963–967.

274. Chokroverty S, Reyes MG, Rubino FA, Tonaki H. The syndrome of diabetic amyotrophy. Ann Neurol 1977;1:181–194.

275. Subramony SH, Wilborn AJ. Diabetic proximal neuropathy: clinical and electrodiagnostic features. J Neurol Sci 1982;53:293–304.

276. Rottenberg MF, DeLisa JA. Severe femoral neuropathy with "hanging leg" syndrome. Arch Phys Med Rehabil 1981;62:404–406.

277. Young MR, Norris JW. Femoral neuropathy during anticoagulant therapy. Neurology 1976;26:1173–1175.

278. Cranberg L. Femoral neuropathy from iliac hematoma: report of a case. Neurology 1979;29:1071–1072.

279. Reinstein L, Alevizatos AC, Twardzik FG, et al. Femoral nerve dysfunction after retroperitoneal hemorrhage: pathophysiology revealed by computed tomography. Arch Phys Med Rehabil 1984;65:37–40.

280. Synek VM, Cowan JC. Saphenous nerve evoked potentials in the assessment of the intraabdominal lesions of the femoral nerve. Muscle Nerve 1983;6:453–456.

281. Belsch JM. Anterior femoral cutaneous nerve injury following femoral artery reconstructive surgery. Arch Neurol 1991;48:230–232.

282. Lederman RJ, Breuer AC, Hanson MR, et al. Peripheral nervous system complications of coronary artery bypass graft surgery. Ann Neurol 1982;12:297–301.

283. Mozes M, Ouaknine G, Nathan H. Saphenous nerve entrapment simulating vascular disorders. Surgery 1975;77:299–303.

284. Garnjobst W. Injuries to the saphenous nerve following operations for varicose veins. Surg Gynecol Obstet 1964;119:359–361.

285. Massey EW. Gonyalgia paresthetica. Muscle Nerve 1981;4:80–81.

286. House JH, Ahmed K. Entrapment neuropathy of the infrapatellar branch of the saphenous nerve. Am J Sports Med 1977;5:217–224.

287. Kopec HP, Thompson WAL. Peripheral entrapment neuropathies. Baltimore: Williams & Wilkins, 1963.

288. Stookey B. Gunshot wounds of peripheral nerves. Surg Gynecol Obstet 1916;23:639–656.

289. Van Langenhove M, Pollefliet A, Vanderstraeten G. A retrospective electrodiagnostic evaluation of footdrop in 303 patients. EMG Clin Neurophysiol 1989;29:145–152.

290. Sunderland S. The relative susceptibility of injury of the medial and lateral popliteal divisions of the sciatic nerve. Br J Surg 1953;41:2–4.

291. Obach J, Aragones JM, Ruano D. The infrapiriformis foramen syndrome resulting from intragluteal injection. J Neurol Sci 1983;58:135–142.

292. Gentili F, Hudson AR, Hunter D. Clinical and experimental aspects of injection injuries of peripheral nerves. Can J Neurol Sci 1980;7:143–151.

293. Stewart JD, Angus E, Gendron D. Sciatic neuropathies. Br Med J 1983;287:1108–1109.

294. Baker GS, Parson WR, Welch JS. Endometriosis within the sheath of the sciatic nerve: report of two patients with progressive paralysis. J Neurosurg 1966;25:652–655.

295. Crisci C, Baker MK, Wood MB, Litchy WJ, Dyck PJ. Trochanteric sciatic neuropathy. Neurology 1989;39:1539–1541.

296. Wilbourn A, Mitsumoto H. Proximal sciatic neuropathies caused by prolonged sitting. Neurology 1988;38 (Suppl):400.

297. Pace JB, Nagle D. Piriform syndrome. West J Med 1976;124:435–439.

298. Solheim LF, Siewers P, Paus B. The piriformis muscle syndrome. Acta Orthop Scand 1981;52:73–75.

299. Nakano KK. Entrapment neuropathy from Baker's cyst. JAMA 1978;1:264–279.

300. Rask MR. Superior gluteal nerve entrapment syndrome. Muscle Nerve 1980;3:304–307.

301. Obach J, Aragones JM, Ruano D. The infrapiriformis foramen syndrome resulting from intragluteal injection. J Neurol Sci 1983;58:135–142.

302. LaBan MM, Meerschaert JR, Taylor RS. Electromyographic evidence of inferior nerve compromise: an early representation of recurrent colorectal carcinoma. Arch Phys Med Rehabil 1982;63:138–141.

303. Dumitru D, Nelson M. Posterior femoral cutaneous nerve conduction. Arch Phys Med Rehabil 1990;979–982.

304. Iyer VG, Shields CB. Isolated injection injury to the posterior femoral cutaneous nerve. Neurosurgery 1989;25:835–838.

305. Dumitru D, Marquis S. Posterior femoral cutaneous nerve neuropathy and somatosensory evoked potentials. Arch Phys Med Rehabil 1988;69:44–45.

306. Swash M, Snooks SJ, Henry MM. A unifying concept of pelvic floor disorders and incontinence. J R Soc Med 1985;78:906–911.
307. Sourkes M, Stewart JD. Common peroneal neuropathy: a study of selective motor and sensory involvement. Neurology 1991;41:1029–1033.
308. Singh N, Behse F, Buchthal F. Electrophysiological study of peroneal palsy. J Neurol Neurosurg Psychiatry 1974;37:1202–1213.
309. Smith T, Trojaborg W. Clinical and electrophysiological recovery from peroneal palsy. Acta Neurol Scand 1986;74:328–335.
310. Pickett JB. Localizing peroneal nerve lesions to the knee by motor conduction studies. Arch Neurol 1984;41:192–199.
311. Katirji MB, Wilbourn AJ. Common peroneal mononeuropathy. Neurology 1988;38:1723–1728.
312. Redford JB. Nerve conduction in motor fibers to the anterior tibial muscle in peroneal palsy. Arch Phys Med Rehabil 1964;45:500–504.
313. Gilliatt RW, Goodman HV, Willison RG. The recording of lateral popliteal nerve action potentials in man. J Neurol Neurosurg Psychiatry 1961;24:305–318.
314. Kanakamedala RV, Hong CZ. Peroneal nerve entrapment at the knee localized by short segment stimulation. Am J Phys Med Rehabil 1989;68:116–122.
315. Berry H, Richardson PM. Common peroneal palsy: a clinical and electrophysiological review. J Neurol Neurosurg Psychiatry 1976;39:1162–1171.
316. Gutmann L. Atypical deep peroneal neuropathy in presence of accessory deep peroneal nerve. J Neurol Neurosurg Psychiatry 1970;33:453–456.
317. Rorabeck CH, Macnab J, Waddell JP. Anterior tibial compartment syndrome; a clinical and experimental review. Can J Surg 1972;15:249–256.
318. Davies JAK. Peroneal compartment syndrome secondary to rupture of the peroneus longus: a case report. J Bone Joint Surg 1979;61A:783–784.
319. Lipscomb AB, Ibrahim AA. Acute peroneal compartment syndrome in a well conditioned athlete: report of a case. Am J Sports Med 1977;5:154–157.
320. Low IMR. Superficial peroneal nerve entrapment. J Bone Joint Surg 1985;67B;58–59.
321. Kernohan J, Levack B, Wilson JN. Entrapment of the superficial peroneal nerve. J Bone Joint Surg 1985;67B;60–61.
322. McAuliffe TB, Fiddian NJ, Browett JP. Entrapment neuropathy of the superficial peroneal nerve. J Bone Joint Surg 1985;67B;62–63.
323. Sridhara CR, Izzo KL. Terminal sensory branches of the superficial peroneal nerve: an entrapment syndrome. Arch Phys Med Rehabil 1985;66:789–791.
324. Posas HN, Rivner MH. Nerve conduction studies of the medial branch of the deep peroneal nerve. Muscle Nerve 1990;13:862.
325. Marinacci AA. The neuropathies of the nerves of the foot. In: Applied electromyography. Philadelphia: Lea & Febiger, 1968:191–197.
326. Gross JA, Hamilton WJ, Swift TR. Isolated mechanical lesions of the sural nerve. Muscle Nerve 1980;3:248–249.
327. Schuchmann JA. Isolated sural neuropathy: report of two cases. Arch Phys Med Rehabil 1980;61:329–331.
328. Kashani SR, Moon AH, Gaunt WD. Tibial nerve entrapment by a Baker cyst: case report. Arch Phys Med Rehabil 1985;66:49–51.
329. Oh SJ, Sarala PK, Kuba T, Elmore R. Tarsal tunnel syndrome: electrophysiological study. Ann Neurol 1979;5:327–330.
330. Oh SJ, Kim HS, Ahmad B. The near-nerve sensory nerve conduction in tarsal tunnel syndrome. J Neurol Neurosurgery Psychiatry 1985;45:999–1003.
331. Fowler CP, Harrison MJ, Snaith ML. Familial carpal and tarsal tunnel syndrome. J Neurol Neurosurg Psychiatry 1986;49:717–718.
332. Saeed MA, Gatens PF. Compound nerve action potentials of the medial and lateral plantar nerves through the tarsal tunnel. Arch Phys Med Rehabil 1982;63:304–307.
333. Delisa JA, Saeed M. The tarsal tunnel syndrome. Muscle Nerve 1983;6:664–670.
334. Oh SJ, Arnold TW, Park KH, Kim DE. Electrophysiological improvement following decompression surgery in tarsal tunnel syndrome. Muscle Nerve 1991;14:407–410.
335. Oh SJ, Lee KW. Medial plantar neuropathy. Neurology 1987;37:1408–1410.
336. Oh SJ, Kim HS, Ahmad BK. Electrophysiological diagnosis of the interdigital nerves of the foot. Muscle Nerve 1982;5:566–567.
337. Oh SJ, Kim HS, Ahmad BK. Electrophysiological diagnosis of the interdigital neuropathy of the foot. Muscle Nerve 1984;7:218–225.
338. Falck B, Hurme M, Hakkarainen S, Aarnio P. Sensory conduction velocity of plantar digital nerves in Morton's metatarsalgia. Neurology 1984;34:698–701.
339. Joplin RJ. The proper digital nerve, vitallkium stem arthroplasty, and some thoughts about foot surgery in general. Clin Orthop 1971;76:199–212.
340. Merritt GN, Subotnick SI. Medial plantar digital proper nerve syndrome (Joplin's neuroma)—typical presentation. J Foot Surg 1982;21:166–169.
341. Ginnestras NJ. Foot disorders, medical and surgical management. Philadelphia: Lea & Febiger, 1973:440–442.
342. Earl CJ, Fullerton PM, Wakefield GS, Schutta HS. Hereditary neuropathy with liability to pressure palsies. Q J Med 1964;33:481–498.

343. Staal A, DeWeerdt CJ, Went LN. Hereditary compression syndrome of peripheral nerves. Neurology 1965;15:1008–1017.
344. Meier C, Moll C. Hereditary neuropathy with liability to pressure palsies. Report of two families and review of the literature. J Neurol 1982;228:73–79.
345. Arts WFM, Busch HFM, Van Den Brand HJ, et al. Hereditary neuralgic amyotrophy: clinical, genetic, electrophysiological and histopathological studies. J Neurol Sci 1983;62:261–679.
346. Dunn HG, Daube JR, Gomez MR. Heredofamilial brachial plexus neuropathy (hereditary neuralgic amyotrophy with brachial predilection) in childhood. Dev Med Child Neurol 1978;20:28–46.
347. Bradley WG, Madrid R, Thrush DC, Campbell MJ. Recurrent brachial plexus neuropathy. Brain 1975;98:381–398.
348. Behse F, Buchthal F, Carlsen F, Knappeis GG. Hereditary neuropathy with liability to pressure palsies: electrophysiological and histopathological aspects. Brain 1972;95:777–794.
349. Mayer RF, Garcia-Mullin R. Hereditary neuropathy manifested by pressure palsies: a Schwann cell disorder? Trans Am Neurol Assoc 1968;93:238–240.
350. Bosch EP, Chui HC, Martin MA, Cancilla PA. Brachial plexus involvement in familial pressure-sensitive neuropathy: electrophysiological and morphological findings. Ann Neurol 1980;8:620–624.
351. Sellman MS, Mayer RF. Conduction block in hereditary neuropathy with susceptibility to pressure palsies. Muscle Nerve 1987;10:621–625.
352. Magistris MR, Roth G. Long-lasting conduction block in hereditary neuropathy with liability to pressure palsies. Neurology 1985;35:1639–1641.
353. Logigian EL, McInnes JM, Berger AR, Busis NA, Lehrich JR, Shahani BT. Stretch-induced spinal accessory nerve palsy. Muscle Nerve 1988;11:146–150.
354. Petrera JE, Trojaborg W. Conduction studies along the accessory nerve and follow-up of patients with trapezius palsy. J Neurol Neurosurg Psychiatry 1984;47:630–636.
355. Barkhaus PE, Means ED, Sawaya R. Ligature injury to the accessory nerve. J Neurol Neurosurg Psychiatry 1987;50:1382–1386.
356. Loong SC, Seanj OS. Comparison of median and ulnar sensory nerve action potentials in the diagnosis of the carpal tunnel syndrome. J Neurol Neurosurg Psychiatry 1971;34:750–754.
357. Duensing F, Lowitzsch K, Thorwirth V, Vogel P. Neurophysiologische Befunde beim Karpaltunnelsyndrom. Z Neurol 1974;206:267–284.
358. Ludin H, Parkmann W. Sensory neurography. New York: Thieme-Stratton, 1980.
359. Kimura I, Ayyar DR. The carpal tunnel syndrome: electrophysiological aspects of 639 symptomatic extremities. EMG Clin Neurophysiol 1985;25:151–164.
360. Stevens JC. AAEM Minimonograph #26: The electrodiagnosis of carpal tunnel syndrome. Muscle Nerve 1987;10:99–113.
361. Bhala RP. Electrodiagnosis of ulnar nerve lesion at the elbow. Arch Phys Med Rehabil 1976;57:206–212.
362. Pickett JB, Coleman L. Localizing ulnar nerve lesions to the elbow by motor nerve conduction studies. EMG Clin Neurophysiol 1984;24:343–360.
363. Tackmann W, Vogel P, Kaeser HE, Ettlin TH. Sensitivity and localizing significance of motor and sensory electroneurographic parameters in the diagnosis of ulnar nerve lesions at the elbow. J Neurol 1984;231:204–211.
364. Urschel HC, Paulson DL, McNamara JJ. Thoracic outlet syndrome. Ann Thorac Surg 1968;6:1–9.

22

Nerve Conduction in Polyneuropathies

Peripheral Neuropathies

Peripheral neuropathy refers to the clinical syndrome produced by widespread involvement of the peripheral nerves with resultant motor weakness, impairment of sensation, loss of muscle stretch reflexes, and wasting.

There are two major components in peripheral nerves—axon and myelin—and it is logical to classify a peripheral neuropathy according to the predominant pathological involvement: axonal degeneration and segmental demyelination (Figs. 22.1–22.3). The pathophysiological differences between axonal degeneration and segmental demyelination are given in Table 22.1. The majority of peripheral neuropathies can be classified into these categories (Table 22.2).

The major clinical manifestations of neuropathy are: (a) weakness and atrophy of muscle; (b) sensory loss in all modalities; (c) diminished or absent reflexes; and (d) trophic changes in the skin. Among these, sensory impairment is the most important sign indicative of peripheral neuropathy because it is not observed in myopathy or anterior horn cell diseases.

The next step in the diagnosis of peripheral neuropathy is to decide what kind of neuropathy the patient has: polyneuropathy, mononeuropathy multiplex, or mononeuropathy. This distinction is important because it suggests the etiological diagnosis.

Polyneuropathy. The common clinical syndrome of mixed sensorimotor polyneuropathy is characterized by ascending and symmetrical paresthesia and distal impairment of sensation (stocking glove dysesthesia), flaccid weakness often including footdrop, loss of muscle stretch reflexes, and wasting. Pure sensory and motor polyneuropathies are also possible.

Mixed sensorimotor polyneuropathies include the nutritional neuropathies (alcoholism, beriberi, pellagra, vitamin B deficiency, pernicious anemia), and the metabolic neuropathies (diabetes mellitus and uremia). Sensory polyneuropathies include arsenic or carcinomatous polyneuropathy. Motor polyneuropathies include the Guillain-Barré syndrome, porphyria, and chronic inflammatory demyelinating polyneuropathy.

Mononeuropathy Multiplex. Two or more nerves in more than one extremity are involved, e.g., the ulnar nerve in one arm and the peroneal nerve in one leg. This is

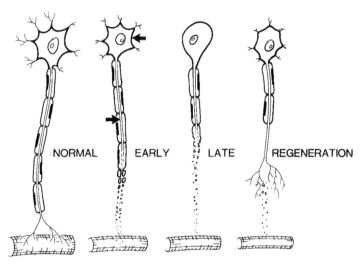

Figure 22.1. Mechanism of axonal degeneration and regeneration. Axonal degeneration is induced either by a metabolic derangement in the neuron (neuronopathy) or throughout the axon (dying-back axonal degeneration) (early; *arrows*). Damage to the neurons and disruption of proximal axonal integrity result in rapid degeneration of the entire distal portion of the axon, producing breakdown of the myelin sheath (late). Regeneration occurs with axonal sprouting. (From Oh SJ. Diagnostic usefulness and limitations of the sural nerve biopsy. Yonsei Medical Journal 1990;31:2.)

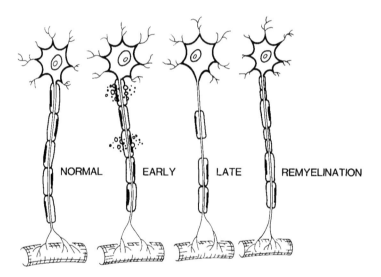

Figure 22.2. Mechanism of segmental demyelination and remyelination. Segmental demyelination is induced by metabolic damage of Schwann cells or peeling and engulfment by activated inflammatory cells (early). This process affects the myelin sheath producing primary segmental demyelination and leaving the axon intact (late). Remyelination occurs with myelination over the demyelinated segment. (From Oh SJ. Diagnostic usefulness and limitations of the sural nerve biopsy. Yonsei Medical Journal 1990;31:2.)

seen classically in patients with periarteritis nodosa and collagen vascular diseases. Three other important causes of mononeuropathy multiplex are leprosy, diabetes mellitus, and multifocal demyelinating neuropathy (1).

Mononeuropathy. Certain mononeuropathies are common to certain diseases: femoral neuropathy and oculomotor nerve palsy with sparing of pupillary function in diabetes mellitus, recurrent or bilateral facial nerve palsy in sarcoidosis, bilateral radial nerve palsy in lead neuropathy.

Despite extensive and costly examinations, the cause of peripheral neuropathy remains unknown in 24% of all cases (2). The most common cause of peripheral neuropathy in the United States is diabetes mellitus, followed by chronic alcoholism.

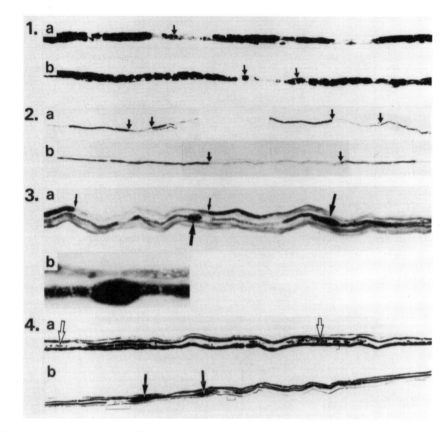

Figure 22.3. Teased nerve fibers. 1. Axonal degeneration: *arrows* indicate row of myelin ovoids. 2. Demyelination: *arrows* indicate demyelinated segments. 3. Tomaculous change: **a**, *Thin arrows* indicate a demyelinated segment. *Thick arrows* indicate "tomaculous change"; **b**, Enlarged tomaculous change. 4. Giant axons: **a**, *white arrows* indicate rows of myelin ovoids; **b**, *arrows* indicate giant axons. (From Oh SJ. Diagnostic usefulness and limitations of the sural nerve biopsy. Yonsei Medical Journal 1990;31:16.)

Table 22.1.
Pathophysiology of Two Types of Peripheral Neuropathy[a]

Parameter	Axonal Degeneration	Segmental Demyelination
Primary lesion	Axon	Myelin
Pathology	Clumping of myelin	Segmental demyelination (at Ranvier node)
Regeneration mechanism	Axonal sprouting	Remyelination
Regeneration speed	Slow	Rapid
NCV	Mildly slow or normal	Markedly slow
Peripheral neuropathies: examples	Alcoholic or nutritional neuropathy	Guillain-Barré syndrome Diphtheric neuropathy

[a]From Oh (692) with permission.

Nerve Conduction Abnormalities in Peripheral Neuropathy

The nerve conduction study is an essential part of the workup in patients with a peripheral neuropathy (3). This study helps in: (*a*) confirming peripheral neuropathy; (*b*) determining the type of neuropathy; and (*c*) following the course of the disease.

The nerve conduction study identifies neuropathy in 76–80% of patients with diabetic neuropathy and in 81–100% of patients with the Guillain-Barré syndrome (Table 22.3). To obtain a greater diagnostic yield in the nerve conduction investigation of patients with peripheral neuropathy, it is important to follow two important guidelines. First, the tests should be performed on several nerves. McLeod et al. (4) recommended

Table 22.2.
Classification of Peripheral Neuropathies

Axonal Degeneration	Segmental Demyelination
Metabolic Neuropathies	
Uremia	Uremia (secondary)
Diabetes mellitus	Diabetes mellitus
Alcoholism	Acromegaly
Hypothyroidism	Tetrodotoxin
Vitamin deficiency including vitamin B12	Saxitoxin
Pyridoxin toxicity	
Acute porphyria	
Critical illness polyneuropathy	
Autoimmune Neuropathies	
Fisher's syndrome	GBS
Chronic ataxic neuropathy	CIDP
Neuropathy with serum autoantibody to sulfatide	Multifocal demyelinating neuropathy
Neuropathy with anti-Hu antibody	Chronic sensory demyelinating neuropathy
Sarcoid neuropathy	Anti-GM1 autoantibody neuropathy
Vasculitic neuropathies	
Neuropathies with Infectious Diseases	
AIDS (late)	AIDS (early)
Lyme disease	Diphtheric neuropathy
Neuropathy associated with tetanus	Leprosy
Paraneoplastic Neuropathies	
Carcinoma	Lymphoma
Toxic Neuropathies	
Lead (human)	Lead (animal)
Almost all drugs except:	Perhexiline
	Amidarone
Almost all solvents including n-Hexane	
Arsenic	
Thallium	
Gold	
Cisplatinum	
Spanish toxic oil neuropathy	
Dysproteinemic Neuropathies	
Multiple myeloma	Multiple myeloma
Amyloidosis	MUGUS neuropathy
Cryoglobulinemia	Osteosclerotic myeloma
	Waldenström's macroglobulinemia
	Angiofollicular lymph node hyperplasia
Hereditary Neuropathies	
Neuronatal HMSN Type II	Hypertrophic CMT (HMSN Type I)
Hereditary ataxias including Freidreich's ataxia	Dejerine-Sottas Disease (HMSN Type III)
Giant axonal sensory neuropathy	Refsum's disease (HMSN Type IV)
Hereditary sensory autonomic neuropathy	Roussy-Levy syndrome
Fabry's disease	Metachromatic leukodystrophy
Infantile neuroaxonal dystrophy	Krabbe's disease
Cerebral lipofuchsinosis	Hereditary compression neuropathy
Mucopolysaccharidoses	Cockayne's syndrome
Pelizaeus-Merzbacher disease	Adrenomyeloneuropathy
	Cerebroxanthomatosis

Table 22.3.
Incidence of Nerve Conduction Abnormalities in Major Peripheral Neuropathies[a]

Neuropathy	Conduction Abnormalities (%)
Guillain-Barré syndrome	81–100
Alcoholic	88
Uremic	97
Diabetic	76–80
Childhood	94.8

[a]Data from Evans (693).

several nerves in both upper and lower limbs. We recommend several nerves in one upper and both lower limbs (5). Second, the test should include both sensory and mixed nerve conduction studies. Abnormalities in sensory conduction are a more sensitive indicator of impairment than the motor response (6–10). Motor conduction was normal in about half of 25 patients with slight but definite changes in the sensory nerve conduction distally (digit to wrist) in Buchthal's series (11).

Types of peripheral neuropathy can be determined by the criteria outlined in Chapter 20. Changes in nerve conduction in response to the changing clinical status are discussed under the headings of the separate diseases.

Metabolic Neuropathies

Diabetic Neuropathy

Neuropathy is the most common of the so-called "late complications of diabetes." Whereas symptomatic distal symmetrical polyneuropathy is present in roughly 25% of patients with diabetes mellitus (12), recent studies have revealed that electrophysiological evidence of abnormal peripheral nerve function can be found in 75–85% of all diabetic subjects (13, 14).

The various types of diabetic neuropathy are listed in Table 22.4. Several hypotheses suggest the causes of diabetic neuropathy. At one time it was believed that vascular infarction or ischemia might play a role (15). At present, only diabetic ophthalmoplegia and the acute form of mononeuropathy multiplex are believed to be related to sudden ischemia (16–18). Other forms of diabetic neuropathy are thought to be due to metabolic abnormalities (19).

Though an earlier study found segmental demyelination to be the salient feature in diabetic neuropathy (20), others have maintained that diabetic neuropathy represents a primary degeneration of the lower motor and first sensory neurons (21), or a combination of segmental demyelination and axonal degeneration (22). Though *teased nerve fiber studies clearly show that the predominant change in diabetic neuropathy is segmental demyelination* (23–25), Thomas and Eliasson concluded in a 1984 review that *axonal loss of the peripheral nerve trunk is clearly present and that widespread segmental demyelination may be a feature in diabetic neuropathy* (26). Behse et al. believed demyelination and axonal loss to be independent processes (24). Dyck emphasized "ischemia" as an important factor in axonal loss in diabetic neuropathy (27).

One study correlated nerve biopsy and nerve conduction studies in diabetic neuropathy (24). This study showed that a grossly diminished conduction velocity of the sural nerve was caused by loss of the large fibers, but that slowing of 20–30% was due to causes other than fiber loss. These causes should include mild demyelination in relatively intact myelin and metabolic defects.

Though the basis of nerve conduction abnormalities in diabetic neuropathy is segmental demyelination according to the teased nerve fiber data, a recent study showed that conduction block, an electrophysiological hallmark of segmental demyelination, is

Table 22.4.
Types of Diabetic Neuropathy[a]

Polyneuropathy
  Symmetrical
  Asymmetrical
Diabetic amyotrophy (proximal neuropathy)
Diabetic radiculopathy
Autonomic neuropathy
Mononeuropathy multiplex
Mononeuropathy
Diabetic ophthalmoplegia

[a]Compression neuropathies are more common in diabetics.

uncommon in diabetic neuropathy (28). Abu-shakra et al. observed conduction block in only six of 76 tested nerve segments in six of 24 patients with diabetic neuropathy (28). This is in contrast to findings in many acquired demyelinating neuropathies that show the characteristic pattern of nonuniform demyelinating neuropathy. *This electrophysiological and histopathological discrepancy may be explained by a metabolic factor: the effect of hyperglycemia on nerve conduction slowing, as discussed later.* Asbury et al. proposed that the hyperosmolarity of tissue interstitial fluid caused by hyperglycemia produces axon shrinkage that is responsible for "metabolic slowing of nerve conduction" (29). It is well known that subclinical neuropathy is not uncommon in diabetes. Subclinical neuropathy is best detected by the sensory nerve conduction study (Table 22.5). The motor nerve conduction test is able to detect subclinical neuropathy in only 16–17% of diabetics, whereas the sensory nerve conduction is abnormal in 46–50% of diabetic patients.

In diabetics with subclinical neuropathy, the mean motor nerve conduction studies showed statistically significant slowing in all tested nerves (30–32). The average slowing ranged from 5 to 12% below normal mean values. In sensory and mixed nerve conduction studies, Downie and Newell (33) were unable to record the compound nerve action potentials (CNAP) of the median and ulnar nerves in 25% of patients, and Mayer (31) found no recordable CNAP in the peroneal nerve in 50% of his patients. Slowing of sensory and mixed NCV was also significant statistically. The average slowing ranged from 7 to 14% below normal values. The H-reflex conduction velocity was also slow in this group.

In diabetics with clinical neuropathy, motor nerve conduction abnormalities are observed in 76–80% of patients, and sensory nerve conduction abnormalities in 80% (Table 22.6). Statistically significant slowing in motor, mixed, and sensory NCVs has been consistently reported (31–36). The average slowing of motor nerve conduction

Table 22.5.
Subclinical Neuropathy in Diabetics

Investigator	Test Performed	Abnormality	Incidence of Abnormalities (%)
Lawrence and Locke (30)	Motor NC; peroneal	Slowing	16 (N = 50)[a,b]
Skillman et al. (32)	Motor NC; peroneal	Slowing	17 (N = 30)
Downie and Newell (33)	Sensory and mixed NC with surface electrode; median/ulnar	Absent potential / Slowing	25 (N = 16)[a] / 25
Noel (14)	Sensory NC with needle; median	Slow NCV / Desynchronization	42 (N = 26) / 4

[a]The present author's analysis.
[b]N, No. of patients.

Table 22.6.
Electrophysiological Abnormalities in Patients with Diabetic Neuropathy

Investigator	Test Performed	Abnormality	Incidence of Abnormalities (%)
Skillman et al. (32)	Motor NC; peroneal	Slowing	77 (N = 23)[a]
Lawrence and Locke (30)	Motor; peroneal	Slowing	76 (N = 50)
Downie and Newell (33)	Sensory and mixed; median, ulnar with surface electrode	Absent / Slowing	59 (N = 23) / 21
Lamontagne and Buchthal (34)	Sensory with needle; median / Peroneal motor	Abnormalities / Slowing	80 (N = 30) / 80

[a]N, No. of patients.

was 18–28% in the peroneal nerve (31, 34), and 14–17% in the median nerve (31). In sensory and mixed nerve conduction, Downie and Newell were not able to obtain any CNAP in the median or ulnar nerves in 59% of patients (33), and Mayer in 25–35% of patients in the peroneal and posterior tibial nerves (31). The average slowing in sensory and mixed NCV was 22–28% below normal values. The H-reflex was not obtainable in 60% of the patients and was usually small in amplitude (31). *Thus, the nerve conduction abnormalities in diabetic neuropathy fall into a "gray zone" where they can be equally attributted to mild segmental demyelination or to axonal degeneration.*

Among the various electrophysiological parameters, the sensory potentials have been shown to be the most sensitive indicator for neuropathy in diabetic patients (34). Median sensory conduction abnormalities were observed in 80% of patients, whereas the motor distal latency was abnormally delayed in 40%. This finding indicates that sensory nerve fibers may be affected before the motor fibers. Nerve conduction abnormalities in diabetic neuropathy are more pronounced distally and in the lower extremities. This observation is consistent with the more pronounced clinical involvement of the legs in diabetic neuropathy.

The relationship between the nerve conduction changes and the clinical status of the patient has been studied by various workers and can be summarized as follows:

1. The nerve conduction abnormalities are correlated with the clinical severity of the neuropathy. According to Lamontagne and Buchthal (34), the slowing in the peroneal nerve was the electrophysiological parameter most closely related to the severity of the neuropathy. Noel (14) found that sensory nerve conduction abnormalities in the median nerve also correlated well with the clinical severity of the disease.

2. The nerve conduction abnormalities are proportional to the duration of the disease. Gregersen (37) studied the peroneal motor conduction and found that the mean NCV decreased with the increasing time since the onset of diabetes, but the change was statistically significant in young patients only. Kraft et al. (38) longitudinally reviewed peroneal conduction values over a period of 1–8 years in diabetics and found a mean drop of 8.8 m/sec.

3. The nerve conduction abnormalities are worse in patients with poorly controlled diabetes than in well-controlled patients (39). Gregerson (39) demonstrated that peroneal motor NCV in a group of "badly controlled" diabetic patients (fasting hyperglycemia greater than 140 mg/dl and urine sugar greater than 1%) was much slower than that of "well-controlled diabetic patients."

4. The nerve conduction changes reflect the type of neuropathy. Gilliatt and Willison (40) found that in patients with symmetrical sensory neuropathy, the most consistent abnormality was the loss of the peroneal CNAP, which depends largely on conduction in the sensory fibers. When a mixed motor and sensory neuropathy coexist, motor conduction velocity is greatly reduced. Finally, in patients with isolated peripheral nerve lesions, the changes tend to be restricted to the clinically affected nerves. This fact has a practical value in diagnosing a mononeuropathy, e.g., carpal tunnel syndrome, in diabetic patients. In diabetic amyotrophy, a prolongation of distal latency in the femoral nerve is common (see the section entitled *Diabetic Amyotrophy*).

5. The nerve conduction abnormalities can occur early in the course of diabetes. The mean NCV in the ulnar and peroneal motor fibers was already slow at the time of diagnosis in 10 newly diagnosed patients who had had symptoms less than 12 weeks (41). Similar observations were also made by other researchers (34, 39, 42), and are consistent with the view that neuropathy can present as the initial manifestation of diabetes (43).

The F-wave was studied by Kimura et al. (44) and Conrad et al. (45). Both showed that F-wave latencies were prolonged in diabetic neuropathy, suggesting that motor conduction abnormalities in diabetic polyneuropathy are diffuse over the total length of the nerve. Kimura et al. (44) measured the latency ratio of the proximal to the distal segment (F-ratio) and found that the F-ratio was slightly but significantly smaller in patients than controls, indicating more intense impairment in the distal than in the proximal segment.

Johnson and Waylonis (46) studied the conduction latency of the facial nerve in 59 patients with diabetes and found a significant delay (mean 6.0 msec) compared with the mean value of 3.4 msec in normal controls. The delay paralleled a slowed motor NCV in the peroneal nerve.

There is mounting electrophysiological evidence to suggest that symmetrical diabetic polyneuropathy is due to metabolic changes and that some nerve conduction abnormalities are at least partly dependent on a metabolic abnormality (47). A recent study (13) has shown that fasting plasma glucose levels in diabetic subjects were inversely related to the motor NCV of the median, peroneal, and posterior tibial nerves, but not to the sensory NCV of median and sural nerves in 20 untreated adult-onset diabetic patients. The H-reflex latency was similarly correlated with fasting plasma glucose. Levels of glycosylated hemoglobin, an index of long-term glycemia, were correlated with slowing of peroneal motor NCV in diabetic patients. Graf et al. (13) added that these associations could not be explained by the patients' age or the duration of their diabetes. They further documented that there was a direct linear relationship between changes in fasting plasma glucose and NCV improvement in the median and peroneal nerves during the 3rd month of treatment. This relationship was maintained in the median nerve for up to 12 months of treatment.

These findings support the hypothesis that some abnormalities of nerve function in adult-onset diabetic subjects are related to their level of hyperglycemia. However, Ward and associates (42) did not find a relation between the motor NCV and 1- to 3-hr postprandial blood glucose levels in their patients.

The metabolic basis of diabetic neuropathy is further supported by the favorable changes in NCV during treatment (Table 22.7). All five studies of this subject showed clear improvement in the motor nerve conduction with a satisfactory fall in the blood sugar level. A single study with sensory nerve conduction did not show any improvement (48). This discrepancy is not well explained.

When the NCV was measured within a few days after treatment, early improvement was clearly documented in a given nerve. It seemed to Gregersen (39) that a reliable increase in motor NCV is first seen after 2–3 days of treatment in recently diagnosed untreated patients. Fraser et al. (41) observed significant improvement in peroneal motor NCV after 6 days of treatment in newly diagnosed patients, and Campbell et al. (49) in the peroneal distal latency within the same period of time. This early improvement of nerve conduction seems to persist throughout the period of observation (1.5–12 months). After 1 month of treatment, Graf et al. (48) noticed significant improvement in median motor NCV in known diabetics. Ward et al. (42) reported a significant mean change in the median motor NCV after 6 weeks of treatment. By 3 months after initiation of treatment, a significant improvement was also seen in peroneal and ulnar nerves (48, 49). A majority of tested nerves had improved NCVs after 6 months of treatment (48). All of these investigations show that *treatment of hyper-*

Table 22.7.
Nerve Conduction Changes with Conventional Insulin Treatment in Diabetics

Investigator	Patients Tested	Duration of Observation; Tests Performed[a]	Findings
Ward et al. (42) (N = 39)[b]	Newly diagnosed	6 weeks, 6 months Motor: M,P	6 weeks: Significant improvement in median NCV.
Gregersen (37) (N = 14)	Recently diagnosed, untreated	8–35 days Motor: P	6 months: Significant improvement; increase in the NCV during treatment in most cases.
Campbell et al. (49) (N = 5)	Known diabetics with ketoacidosis	2,6 days; 1,2,3 months Motor: U,P	Peroneal TL improved in 6 days; ulnar and peroneal NCV improved by 2–3 months.
Fraser et al. (41) (N = 20)	Newly diagnosed	1,6 days; 3,6 months Motor: M,U,P	Peroneal NCV improved by 6 days; peroneal TL improved by 3 months.
Graf et al. (13) (N = 18)	Known diabetics	1,3,6,12 months Motor: M,P,T Sensory: M,S	Median NCV improved at 1 month; peroneal NCV improved at 3 months; posterior tibial NCV improved at 6 months.

[a]Nerves: M = median. U = ulnar. P = peroneal. T = posterior tibial. S = sural.
[b]N, No. of patients.

glycemia is accompanied by improved nerve conduction in diabetic patients, indicating that treatment for diabetes is beneficial to nerve function. We propose that metabolic improvement is responsible for the early improvement of NCV, and that remyelination of the damaged nerves causes continuing late improvement. Hence, prevention of sustained hyperglycemia may theoretically result in prevention of diabetic neuropathy.

After development of the portable insulin infusion pump, it was used in several studies to monitor the nerve conduction change. Service et al. (50) recorded 25 conduction measurements, including motor, sensory, and F-wave latency during a 3-day study. Except for the sensory NCV in the ulnar nerve, there was no significant improvement. They concluded that any significant effect on nerve function resulting from correction of hyperglycemia probably required more than 3 days to be manifested. Tolaymat et al. (51) reported convincing improvement in the motor and sensory NCV in one patient during 4 weeks of observation. Pietri et al. (52) reported a significant increase in motor NCV in the median and peroneal nerves after 6 weeks of continuous insulin infusion. They did not find any significant change in median nerve sensory latency and amplitude. In our study, two patients who had satisfactory control of hyperglycemia according to a 24-hr glucose profile showed definite improvement in median motor and sensory NCV on the 9th day of treatment (unpublished). These studies again show the early response of NCV to adequate treatment for diabetes.

The improvement of the nerve conduction by long-term continuous subcutaneous insulin infusion (CSII) has also been consistently reported (53–55). In a prospective study of 45 type I diabetics who were randomized to treatment with CSII, multiple insulin injections (five or six daily), or conventional twice-daily insulin injections, the motor NCV deteriorated in patients given conventional treatment, whereas in those given CSII it was unchanged during the 1st year but had improved significantly in all nerves tested after 2 years (55). Two studies showed a significant improvement in the NCVs after 1 year with CSII treatment compared with the conventional treatments (53, 54). Warmolts et al. reported that the mean motor and sensory NCVs had increased 6.4% in the CSII group versus 1.3% in the split-mixed injection group, even though glucose regulation was equally and significantly improved in both groups (53). Ehle et al. reported an average increase of the motor NCV of 2.5 m/sec in the CSII group but no change in the conventional treatment group (54). No significant change was noted in the median sensory CNAP amplitude or latency.

Along with the control of diabetes, other modes of therapy have been tried for diabetic neuropathy. There were two therapeutic trials with myoinositol (56, 57) and one trial with aldose reductase inhibitors (58). These therapeutic trials were based on the sorbitol pathway hypothesis of diabetic neuropathy. Many recent animal studies have provided evidence that the polyol pathway is normally present and active in mammalian peripheral nerves and that its activity is influenced by the ambient glucose concentration (19). Increased polyol pathway activity resulting from hyperglycemia produces increased sorbitol, fructose, and water concentrations and decreased free myoinositol concentrations in the peripheral nerves. These alterations are associated with a decrease in NCV, which can be prevented by correction of the hyperglycemia through careful insulin administration and reversed by the restoration of nerve myoinositol concentrations to normal through dietary myoinositol supplementation.

Two studies reported improvement in nerve conduction after dietary myoinositol supplementation in patients with diabetic peripheral neuropathy. Salway et al. (57) found a significant increase in the amplitude of the CNAP in the median and sural nerves and of the compound muscle action potential (CMAP) in the peroneal nerve in seven diabetic patients following myoinositol supplementation (500 mg twice a day for 2 weeks). Improvement was not observed in the placebo group. No significant change in NCV was found irrespective of whether the patient was taking myoinositol or placebo. Clements et al. (56) tried a high-myoinositol diet (1.6 g/day) in 20 patients with diabetic neuropathy for a period of 16 weeks and found a significant improvement in the sensory NCV in the median and sural nerves but no improvement in the motor NCV in the median and peroneal nerves. Gregersen et al. (59) observed no significant changes in the mean motor NCV when dietary myoinositol supplementation (3.0 g/day) was provided in 60 treated diabetic human subjects. Thus, increased dietary myoinositol intake appears to have a salutary effect upon sensory nerve conduction in diabetics.

Faguns and Jameson (58) assessed the efficacy of treatment with aldose reductase inhibitor on peripheral nerve function in diabetic polyneuropathy using a double-blind placebo trial. Aldose reductase inhibitor inhibits the conversion of D-glucose to sorbitol, resulting in a decrease in sorbitol content in the peripheral nerves. Significant differences favoring aldose reductase inhibitor over the placebo group (no change) were found in ulnar motor NCV and F-wave latency. Judzewitsch et al. reported NCV improvement in the peroneal and median motor and the median sensory nerve conduction during 9 weeks of treatment with Sorbinil (250 mg per day) in a randomized, double-blind crossover study. The NCV for all three nerves declined significantly within 3 weeks after cessation of the drug (60). Jaspan et al. also reported the relief of pain in eight of 11 patients and improvement of median motor and sensory NCVs in four of seven tested cases after 1 week of Sorbinil treatment (61). In each case the improvement was reversed after withdrawal of therapy. These studies thus provide support for the sorbitol pathway hypothesis.

Bassi et al. (62) studied the effect of cerebral gangliosides in patients with diabetic neuropathy. Cerebral gangliosides (50 mg/day intramuscularly) were given for 40 days to 15 diabetic patients. A significant increase was found in the CMAP in all tested nerves and in a number of patients in whom the sural CNAP was obtained. This improvement was proposed to be due to an improvement in the excitability of nerve fibers and a subsequent facilitation of reinnervation in the denervated muscle by cerebral gangliosides.

In recent years, pancreatic transplantation has become a mode of treatment for diabetes. Some investigators maintain that this is the most effective method of replacing islet cells and restoring lasting euglycemia (63). Kennedy et al. found *significant improvement* in the mean motor and sensory NCVs (about 2 m/sec in the upper extremities and 1.5 m/sec in the lower extremities) 12 months after transplantation in 61 type I diabetics (63). They also observed a slight increase of the mean CMAP and CNAP amplitudes in the upper but not in the lower extremities. This was in contrast to the control group in which the NCV did not change but there was significant deterioration in the CMAP and CNAP amplitude after 12 months. They attributed the change in the course of diabetic neuropathy to the transplanted pancreas and concluded that the progression of diabetic polyneuropathy may be halted through the restoration of a euglycemic state by successful pancreatic transplantation. Solders et al. studied the effect of combined pancreatic and renal transplantation on diabetic neuropathy in 13 patients and found a small but significant improvement in NCV during a 24-month follow-up period (64). Similar improvement was also observed in 15 diabetics with renal transplantation only. In view of the latter observation, they attributed the improvement of nerve conduction more to the elimination of uremia.

Diabetic Amyotrophy

Diabetic amyotrophy is a syndrome consisting of unilateral or bilateral, but often asymmetrical, marked weakness and atrophy primarily affecting the pelvifemoral muscles and accompanied by pain in the back and thighs (65). The patellar reflex is frequently decreased or absent but sensation is little affected. This disorder is usually subacute in onset and occurs in middle-aged or elderly male patients with poorly controlled or previously unrecognized diabetes mellitus. Severe weight loss is a common concomitant. Prognosis is favorable in that most patients improve within 6–18 months.

Generalized peripheral neuropathy was documented by the nerve conduction study in 63% (66) to 100% (67) of patients. In all three patients studied by Williams and Mayer (68), the sensory and mixed nerve conductions were abnormal (either slow NCV or absent CNAP). In the series of Chokroverty et al. (69), a motor nerve conduction study was performed on 12 patients with conduction velocities reduced in the peroneal and posterior tibial nerves in all 12 patients and in the median and ulnar nerves in four. The most extensive nerve conduction study was performed on 27 patients by Subramony and Wilborn (66). Among the sensory nerve conductions, the most common abnormality was absence of a sural CNAP (61%), followed by abnormality in the median nerve (52%) and the ulnar nerve (37%). The motor NCV was slow in the ulnar nerve in 63% of patients and in the posterior tibial nerve in 52%. These authors found generalized peripheral neuropathy clinically in 41% of patients and electromyographically in 63%. This discrepancy seems to indicate that diabetic amyotrophy is commonly accompanied by subclinical generalized peripheral neuropathy (70) and is a strong argument for the metabolic cause for diabetic amyotrophy.

The femoral nerve conduction study is extremely useful in recognizing this condition. The prolonged distal latency of the femoral nerve (> 6 msec) was noted in 64% (66) to 67% (69) of patients. Saphenous nerve conduction was abnormal in all the cases we have studied (unpublished data). The common nerve conduction abnormalities in the femoral and saphenous nerves are most helpful in differentiating this disorder from lumbar radiculopathy of other etiologies, in which the femoral nerve latency and saphenous nerve conduction are normal.

The F-wave in the peroneal nerve at the knee was studied by Chokroverty et al. (69) in 11 patients with diabetic amyotrophy; F-wave latencies and the F-wave ratio were longer and F-wave conduction and distal motor NCVs were slower than in control subjects. The F-wave ratio data indicate a more severe disorder in the proximal peroneal segments of the sciatic nerves. This finding contrasts with Kimura et al.'s (44) observation that conduction abnormalities in diabetic neuropathy are more severe distally. The needle EMG is *invariably abnormal* in diabetic amyotrophy. Fibrillations and positive sharp waves are often detectable in the lumbar paraspinal muscles as well as in the quadriceps, iliopsoas, and adductors of the thigh muscles. In one series, fibrillations were present in the lumbar paraspinal muscles in over half the patients (66) and often only in a single area of the paraspinal muscles. If more extensive paraspinal muscle searches are performed, as recommended by Bastron and Thomas (71), most of these patients are likely to show evidence of active denervation in the paraspinal muscles, typically in the multiple roots beyond the clinically suspected level. The MUPs in the limb muscles in diabetic amyotrophy are typical of acute or chronic denervation, depending upon the duration of the lesion. When the reinnervation is active, small polyphasic MUPs are present mimicking myopathy (34, 72). Usually, these polyphasic MUPs caused by reinnervation have normal duration.

In many patients with diabetic amyotrophy the needle EMG abnormalities are strictly unilateral, found only in the thigh muscles and often in the ipsilateral lumbar paraspinal muscles. However, in some patients, the EMG test shows abnormalities on the contralateral side and extension of the lesion caudally to the L5–S1 roots in the symptomatic limbs.

Diabetic Polyradiculopathy

Diabetic polyradiculopathy is a not uncommon complication of diabetes mellitus and is now a well-recognized form of diabetic peripheral neuropathy (71). Most patients are elderly male type II diabetics who have experienced weight loss. Onset is usually subacute, reaching maximal intensity in weeks. Though presenting symptoms are sensory—pain, paresthesias, or dysesthesias—in over 90% of patients, motor weakness ultimately develops in most patients, unilaterally in almost one-third of cases. Muscle stretch reflexes are decreased or absent in the affected area. An increased CSF protein is an almost universal finding, suggesting root involvement and correlating well with the presence of widespread fibrillation and positive sharp wave potentials in the paraspinal muscles. *The best diagnostic test for this entity is the needle EMG study.*

Though any part of the spinal roots may be involved, the most commonly involved area is the thoracic roots. On rare occasions diffuse diabetic polyradiculopathy occurs together with diabetic polyneuropathy, producing diabetic neuropathic cachexia (73).

Diabetic Thoracic Radiculopathy

Of the forms of diabetic polyradiculopathy, diabetic thoracic radiculopathy is the most common. Though it has been well recognized for years that thoracic or abdominal pain can be a manifestation of diabetic neuropathy, this entity has been relatively well delineated only in the past few years (74). It can affect any part of the thoracic segments, but it has a striking tendency to involve the lower thoracic roots, especially the T8–T12 roots, and to involve two or more contiguous roots (74). Involvement is almost always unilateral and asymmetrical. The most prominent symptom is pain over the thorax or abdomen, often distressingly dysesthetic and with nocturnal exacerbation. In only a few cases does the pain radiate around the trunk in a "radicular" fashion. Loss of sensation in the body parts afflicted by sensory symptoms is usually inconspicuous (75). When present, various combinations of sensory loss involving the branches of the spinal nerves have been described (76). There is usually no obvious motor involvement (75), but abdominal swelling caused by weakness of the abdominal muscles is rarely reported (77). Prognosis for recovery is good, as this is often a self-limiting entity. Since diabetic thoracic radiculopathy can mimic a number of intraabdominal and intrathoracic diseases, numerous diagnostic workups are often performed before a definite diagnosis is made by the needle EMG study.

Although intercostal nerve conduction tests are available (78, 79), so far these tests have not been used for diagnosis of diabetic thoracic radiculopathy. Because of the undue risk of pneumothorax associated with testing (80), the intercostal nerve conduction test with the needle recording electrode is not practical. Thus far, *the needle EMG test is essentially the sole means of identifying diabetic thoracic radiculopathy.*

Fibrillation and positive sharp waves are typically found in the involved thoracic paraspinal muscles, usually in multiple contiguous segments (71, 75, 76, 81–83), and sometimes corresponding almost exactly to the area of maximal pain (82). Bastron and Thomas reported fibrillations on both sides of the spine in most patients (71). Because of the inherent difficulty of relaxation of the thoracic paraspinal muscles, Streib et al. recommended the needle EMG in the abdominal muscles in patients suspected of having diabetic thoracic radiculopathy (81, 84): in three cases in which the thoracic needle EMG was impossible because of poor relaxation, the needle EMG in the abdominal muscles showed abnormalities, identifying diabetic thoracic radiculopathy (84). The needle EMG for the intercostal muscles is not recommended because of the possible risk of pneumothorax.

Concomitant polyneuropathy has been reported in 33% (82), 47% (81), and 75% (71) of patients with diabetic thoracic radiculopathy. Extensive nerve conduction studies of this disorder are few. Sun and Streib (81) tested motor nerve conduction in the median and peroneal nerves and sensory nerve conduction in the median, ulnar, and sural nerves in five patients, and observed abnormalities in two of these. Massey (83) tested one sural sensory latency and one peroneal motor conduction velocity as a minimal study in 15 patients and found some abnormality of nerve conduction in 11 (73%). The abnormalities in the sural sensory nerve conduction and low amplitudes of CMAP in the peroneal nerve were the two most common findings. According to our experience, almost all patients with this disorder demonstrate some degree of peripheral neuropathy when the nerve conduction study includes many nerves in one arm and both legs (unpublished data).

Diabetic Cervical and L5–S1 Radiculopathy

Diabetic cervical radiculopathy as an extension of diabetic amyotrophy is rare and has been reported in passing in a few studies of diabetic amyotrophy (74). Typically, this disorder appears bilaterally, sometimes asymmetrically, and involves the shoulder girdle muscles (74). Recently, the clinical and EMG findings in four such patients were described, all of whom also had diabetic amyotrophy (85).

Diabetic L5–S1 radiculopathy is known to occur as an occasional extension of diabetic amyotrophy. When it occurs in isolation, it is difficult to attribute the radiculopathy to diabetes. Child and Yates reported a diabetic patient with pain in the distribution of both sciatic nerves, who showed denervation bilaterally in the L5-innervated muscles with definite fibrillations in the L5 paraspinal muscles, and attributed to diabetes the bilateral L5 radiculopathy following a normal myelogram (86).

Unless cervical or L5–S1 radiculopathy occurs together with diabetic thoracic radiculopathy or diabetic amyotrophy, it is difficult to make a diagnosis of diabetic cervical or L5–S1 radiculopathy. However, even when it occurs in isolation, such a diagnosis is reasonable if the imaging study is negative, the needle EMG documents polyradiculopathy, and peripheral neuropathy is present in a diabetic patient.

Uremic Neuropathy

Uremic polyneuropathy is a well-known and frequent complication of chronic renal failure, being present in 22–26% of patients with that disorder (87–91) and for some reason seeming not to occur in those with acute renal failure. The exact cause is unknown. However, the improvement that can be produced by adequate hemodialysis or, more effectively, renal transplantation suggests that *a retained dialysable metabolite* is responsible for uremic polyneuropathy. Clinically this neuropathy is dominated by an initial distal sensory impairment, followed by later motor weakness involving the lower limbs more than the upper. Clinical signs of cranial or autonomic neuropathy are usually absent.

In uremic neuropathy, the pathological process is characterized by *primary axonal degeneration and secondary segmental demyelination.* Thomas et al. (92) found that the predominant finding was axonal loss, particularly of the larger myelinated nerve fibers, together with some demyelination. Dyck et al. (93) observed that the main type of fiber degeneration is axonal degeneration with secondary segmental demyelination.

The basis of nerve conduction abnormalities in uremic neuropathy is predominantly axonal degeneration and secondary segmental demyelination. It has been well known that subclinical neuropathy is common in chronic renal failure. The nerve conduction study is the most sensitive aid in the detection of subclinical neuropathy. Subclinical neuropathy was detected in 48–70% of patients with chronic renal failure, only 22–29% of whom had clinical neuropathy (Table 22.8). Slow nerve conduction was detected in a higher rate of patients when multiple nerves were tested. The highest incidence (70%) was reported by Nielsen (94), who employed median and peroneal motor and median sensory nerve conductions. Among 29 patients with clinical neuropathy, nerve conduction abnormalities in one or more segments were observed in 97% of cases.

In uremic patients without clinical neuropathy, the mean motor NCVs in the median nerve were slower than normal means by 10% and in peroneal nerves by 13–17% than the normal mean values (20, 94). Sensory and mixed nerve conductions in the median nerve were slower than the normal mean by 11–12% (95).

Table 22.8.
Frequency of Clinical Neuropathy and Nerve Conduction Abnormalities in Uremic Patients

Investigator	No. of Patients	Frequency (%)	
		Clinical Neuropathy	Slow NCV[a]
Tenckhoff et al. (90)	35	26	49
			(motor: U,M,P,T)
Ackil et al. (100)	27	29	59
			(sensory: S; F-wave, H reflex)
Thomas et al. (92)	54	22	48
			(motor: P)
Nielsen (694)	27[b]		70
			(motor: M,P; sensory: M)

[a]Nerves: U = ulnar. M = median. P = peroneal. T = posterior tibial. S = sural.
[b]Patients without any clinical neuropathy.

Nerve conduction abnormalities in one or more segments were observed in 97% of 29 patients with uremic neuropathy (94). The nerve conduction abnormalities are more prominent in this group than in the subclinical group. The average slowing of the motor NCV was 22–39% below normal in peroneal nerves and 15% in median nerves. In sensory nerve conduction, the average slowing was 16–19% in median nerves. For sensory nerve conduction, the average slowing was 16–19% in median nerves. The amplitude of the sensory CNAP was reduced, primarily because of increased temporal dispersion and an increased incidence of irregularities in the potential shapes. On more proximal recording, there was considerable dispersion of sensory CNAPs recorded orthodromically with needle electrodes, suggesting a disproportionate slowing of conduction along some fibers due to *segmental demyelination*. On the other hand, Bolton (96) observed that the most marked electrophysiological abnormality in uremic neuropathy was decreased CMAP and sensory CNAP amplitudes, suggesting that *axonal degeneration* is the predominant change in this neuropathy. Thus, the nerve conduction abnormalities in uremic neuropathy are characterized by a *combination of axonal and segmental degeneration.*

The H-reflex latency was significantly prolonged by 10–13% of normal in uremic patients (97–99). Halar et al. (98) observed a prolonged H-reflex latency in 40% of patients in contrast to an NCV abnormality in 30%. In the posterior tibial nerve, the F-wave latency from the gastrocnemius and soleus muscles was prolonged by 11% of normal in 32 patients with chronic renal failure (99). The F-wave latency in the peroneal nerve from the extensor digitorum brevis was prolonged by 38% of normal in nine patients with chronic renal failure (69). Because of the predominant clinical involvement of the legs, these are not unexpected. Ackil et al. (100) studied the late response and sural nerve conduction in addition to conventional motor and sensory conduction in 30 patients with chronic renal failure. Abnormalities of sural nerve conduction and/or late responses were present in 100% of cases. In contrast, abnormalities of motor conduction were present in 83% of cases, and of sensory conduction, in 87%. Although it seems that these late responses are more sensitive for detecting neuropathy, their practical value is limited because of their nonspecificity for neuropathies.

Mitz et al. (101) studied facial nerve latency in 84 patients with chronic renal failure. Electrophysiological evidence of motor neuropathy was found in 72 patients. Of the four motor nerves studied, the facial nerve was the most sensitive indicator of uremic neuropathy: prolonged terminal latency in 82% of the patients; abnormal nerve conduction in the peroneal nerve in 68%, in the median nerve in 35%, and in the ulnar nerve in 36%. This is contrary to what is observed clinically.

In contrast to other peripheral neuropathies, in uremic neuropathy studies have shown that the motor and sensory NCVs are affected with equal frequency (94) and to approximately the same degree (102) in uremic neuropathy. Although some studies (94, 103) found that nerve conduction abnormalities are observed with equal frequency in the lower and upper extremities, another study (104) clearly showed a higher incidence of nerve conduction abnormalities in peroneal and posterior tibial nerves. All studies showed that nerve conduction abnormalities are more pronounced in the lower extremities. These findings are consistent with the clinical findings.

Nielsen (94) found that distal and proximal segments of nerves are equally affected in this disorder. On the other hand, Miyoshi and Oh (105) found more marked involvement of the motor and mixed nerve conduction distally. Although Bolton (96) claimed that the peroneal nerve motor NCV is usually the first electrophysiological sign to become abnormal and that it most accurately reflects the severity of the neuropathy, others (103, 106) expressed the view that slowing of conduction is detected as early in the median as in the peroneal nerve. The needle EMG reveals fibrillation potentials and positive sharp waves in resting muscles as signs of denervation, most marked in distal limb muscles and particularly in those of the legs. With successful renal transplantation, these signs of denervation disappear. When motor unit potentials reappear, they are initially polyphasic, consistent with reinnervation (107).

The relationship between various renal functions and the NCVs has been well established in this disorder. Lindholm (108) showed that slowing of the ulnar motor NCV was significantly correlated with the nonprotein-nitrogen concentration in serum in patients with renal insufficiency. In 14 individual patients with chronic renal failure, Jebsen et al. (109) demonstrated that an increase in the serum creatinine concentration was accompanied by a reduction of the median motor NCV. Blaggs et al. (95) found that the correlation between the median motor, sensory, and mixed NCVs and the creatinine concentration was greater than that with blood urea. They inferred that this was probably because serum creatinine levels reflected renal function more accurately. They also observed that the mean NCVs became abnormal only when levels of serum creatinine become grossly abnormal (> 12 mg%).

Nielsen (110) found no significant correlation between peroneal motor NCV and the serum urea or creatinine but found a linear correlation of the sensory and motor NCVs in the median and peroneal nerves with endogenous creatinine clearance in a semilogarithmic system. A significant reduction of the NCV is expected in half the patients when kidney function is reduced to about 10% of normal (24-hr creatinine clearance below 10 ml/min/1.73 m^2); and only a few patients with terminal renal failure show conduction velocities within normal limits. Oh et al. (111) found that the median sensory NCV increased significantly as the serum creatinine, urea nitrogen, and plasma myoinositol fell in 12 patients following renal transplantation. The highest negative linear correlation coefficients were found to exist between the median sensory NCV and creatinine and myoinositol concentrations. A linear relationship between plasma urea nitrogen and plasma myoinositol levels was found in patients with chronic renal failure. Thus, all studies show *a good correlation between NCVs and renal function*. This finding indicates that the slowing of nerve conduction is dependent not only on structural changes but also on metabolic changes in uremic neuropathy (67).

Nerve conduction deteriorates slowly and gradually over a long follow-up period in conservatively treated patients with terminal renal failure. Nielsen (94) observed significant deterioration of the NCV in the median motor and sensory and the peroneal motor nerves. A mean decrease of 3.8 to 5.0 m/sec in the sensory NCVs and of 5.4 to 7.7 m/sec in the motor NCVs was observed in nine patients who were followed for 1–14 months (mean 5.1 months). In contrast, clinical neuropathy developed abruptly, the first indication being a sudden rise in vibratory perception threshold.

Compared with conservative treatment, *hemodialysis arrests deterioration or improves the NCV* (112). The effect of a single dialysis was studied by Jebsen et al. (109) and Stanley et al. (113). Jebsen et al. (109) studied nerve conduction changes in the median, ulnar, peroneal, and posterior tibial motor nerves and in the median and ulnar sensory nerves. There was a significant increase in the median sensory NCV: 2.4 m/sec after dialysis ($p < 0.01$). There was little change in NCVs of other nerves. Stanley et al. (113) also found a significant increase in the amplitude of the CMAP and mixed and sensory CNAPs in the median nerves after a single dialysis. They did not find any significant difference in motor and sensory NCVs before versus after dialysis. These studies show that even a single hemodialysis causes minor electrophysiological improvement, although this is only partial or transient. The effect of long-term hemodialysis on the nerve conduction and clinical neuropathy has been extensively studied. Nielsen (114) found no further slowing of nerve conduction in the median sensory and the median and peroneal motor nerves in nine patients during the 1st year of dialysis (mean observation period 5.6 months). Compared with the conservatively treated group, "no change" in the NCVs represents a substantial improvement in the hemodialyzed group. In a majority of patients, regular hemodialysis interrupted the progression of clinical neuropathy, and development of neuropathy during dialysis was not seen. Jebsen et al. (109) also did not find any significant increase in the NCVs of the median, ulnar, peroneal, and posterior tibial nerves in 10 patients on dialysis for 1 year or less. However, when dialysis was continued for more than 1 year (mean 47 months), all 10 patients showed an increase in mean motor NCVs, the mean increment being 16.4%, which is statistically significant. Some of Jebsen's patients have recovered from all clinical evidence of neuropathy with prolonged hemodialysis. Cadilhac et al. (104) reported that short-term hemodialysis over several months produced some deterioration in motor NCV followed by rapid recovery in almost half the patients, but long-term (1 year or more) hemodialysis produced no change or worsening in the nerve conduction in 36% of patients, improvement of NCV in 36%, and return of NCV to normal in 28%. Teschan et al. carried out a well-controlled multicenter trial on a total of 139 uremic patients (115). Patients were divided into four different groups according to the different methods of hemodialysis: low-BUN and long-dialysis time, high-BUN and short-dialysis time, low-BUN and long-dialysis time, or high-BUN and short-dialysis time. High-BUN values and short-dialysis time had the most deleterious effect on the NCV, latencies, and compound action potential amplitudes. Thus, the effect of hemodialysis on the nerve conduction can be summarized as follows:

1. Single dialysis produces little change in the majority of nerve conduction parameters but a minor transient improvement in a few parameters;

2. Short-term hemodialysis arrests the deterioration of nerve conduction, which is inevitable if conservatively treated; and

3. Long-term hemodialysis stabilizes the nerve conduction in most patients, with improvement or worsening occurring in only a few.

Continuous ambulatory peritoneal dialysis is a new and increasingly used form of maintenance dialysis therapy. Most studies showed that *it stabilized peripheral neuropathy,* as measured by the nerve conduction test, as did chronic hemodialysis, during follow-up periods ranging from 1 month to 3 years (116–119). However, one study in 15 nondiabetic patients during a mean 18-month follow-up period found that the motor NCV, vibratory sensation threshold, and clinical score deteriorated significantly, whereas the median sensory NCV was unchanged (120).

The remission of clinical neuropathy following renal transplantation is well documented (96, 121–123). In most uremic patients the remission of clinical neuropathy was completed within 1–6 months after a successful renal transplantation (122). *Nerve conduction improvement* has also been well documented repeatedly by several studies. Chaumont et al. (124) and Funk-Bretano et al. (125) showed that the increase in the motor NCV might continue for 1–2 years. Their data did not cover the initial phase after transplantation. Dobbelstein et al. (126) drew attention to an early rapid and a late slow phase in the remission of clinical neuropathy, and a similar pattern was seen in the recovery of the motor NCV. Nielsen (127) observed a *two-phase improvement* in the NCV of median motor and sensory nerves, an early rapid (within 6 weeks) and a late (after 6 months), slow improvement.

During the 1st year the greatest improvement was seen in the patients most severely affected before transplantation. Median sensory nerve function improved faster than motor nerve function. Nielsen (127) observed an earlier rise in sensory NCV within 6 weeks of transplantation. The amplitude of the sensory CNAP became normal after 6 months at the wrist and after 1 year at the elbow. Bolton (96) reported that major improvement in NCV was observed during the first 3 postoperative months in patients with mild neuropathy and that improvement was delayed 6 months in those with more severe neuropathy; relative stability occurred after 12 and 24 months, respectively. He did not observe any immediate effect of transplantation and concluded that the main reason for amelioration in neuropathy was segmental remyelination. Ibrahim et al. (21) observed a rapid rise in NCV within a few days of allografting in most of their patients and postulated that it was due to restoration of metabolic function in the kidney. Oh et al. (111) made frequent serial measurements of NCV in the first 3 weeks after renal transplantation and found a significant improvement in mean NCV on postoperative day 2 and 5 in the median sensory NCV in patients who had had subnormal NCVs preoperatively. A significant improvement in median sensory NCV was maintained throughout the test period. In patients who had had normal conduction velocities preoperatively, there was no statistically significant change. Furthermore, Oh et al. (111) found a close correlation between improvement in median sensory NCV and amelioration in renal function, indicating that metabolic phenomena are responsible for the rapid improvement in NCV following renal transplantation. The effects of transplantation on the NCV can be summarized as follows:

1. Motor and sensory NCV improve following successful renal transplantation in patients with chronic renal failure;

2. Two-phase improvement in the NCV—an early rapid (within a few days up to 6 weeks), and a late slow recovery (up to 12 months)—followed by a relatively stable course afterward (after 12 months) is noted following successful transplantation;

3. Sensory NCV improves more rapidly and to a greater degree than the motor NCV (21, 96, 111);

4. There is a close correlation between improvement of sensory nerve conduction and the amelioration in renal function (111); and

5. The aggravation of NCV occurs in the presence of a nonfunctioning transplanted kidney and rejection phenomena during the postoperative period.

These dramatic changes of NCV after successful transplantation are strongly indicative of the metabolic basis in the pathogenesis of uremic neuropathy and demonstrate the superiority of a successful renal transplantation compared with regular hemodialysis treatment in patients with chronic renal failure. The initial rapid improvement is most likely due to improvement of overall kidney function. This is followed by segmental remyelination and axonal regeneration.

There are two distinct focal neuropathies in uremic neuropathy: *carpal tunnel syndrome (CTS) and ischemic neuropathy* due to an arteriovenous shunt.

CTS is known to be common in patients with chronic renal failure on chronic hemodialysis. CTS is now also recognized commonly to arise distal to an arteriovenous fistula implanted into the forearm for access during hemodialysis (128). Distal ischemia in the region of the carpal tunnel due to a vascular steal mechanism related to the fistula is the presumed mechanism. Surgical decompression, closure of the fistula, or both, improve symptoms and signs of CTS.

Bovine shunts inserted between the brachial artery and cephalic vein in the upper arm for access during chronic hemodialysis may rarely induce excessive arteriovenous shunting and a severe ischemic neuropathy involving the median, ulnar, and radial nerves in the forearm and/or hand (129, 130). This develops immediately or within a few hours of fistula creation. Nerve conduction and needle EMG tests can identify the involved nerves (see Chapter 21). Ischemic neuropathy involving median and ulnar nerves in the hand and forearm has also been reported following a bovine shunt inserted between the radial artery and cephalic vein in the forearm (131). Banding of the graft may improve the symptoms and signs of ischemic neuropathy, despite an incomplete recovery (129).

Alcoholic Neuropathy

Alcoholic neuropathy is one of the most common forms of peripheral neuropathy. It is a mixed sensory and motor disorder, involving predominantly the distal segments and the legs (132). Sensory neuropathy is typical in mild cases, with complaints of burning feet or painful paresthesia. In advanced cases, motor weakness is present together with sensory impairment. The neuropathy develops slowly, and recovery is slow. The predominant pathological process in this disorder is *axonal degeneration* of the heavily myelinated fibers (133, 134).

The basis of nerve conduction abnormalities in alcoholic neuropathy is thus axonal degeneration (135). Two studies correlate nerve biopsy and nerve conduction in alcoholic neuropathy. Behse and Buchthal (133) found a linear correlation between the maximum sural sensory NCV and the fiber diameter of the intact large nerve fibers in 33 of 37 studied nerves. This finding, together with a marked reduction in amplitude of the sural sensory CNAPs, is consistent with axonal degeneration, which was found in teased preparations and electron microscopic studies. Tackmann et al. (136), on the other hand, found a linear correlation between the sensory NCV and the nerve fiber diameter in only 17 of 27 sural nerves studied. They concluded that in some cases the predominant pathological process is segmental demyelination.

About 20% of alcoholic patients are known to have peripheral neuropathy (137). Subclinical neuropathy is best detected by sensory nerve conduction study. The motor nerve conduction is able to detect subclinical neuropathy in only 16% of alcoholics (137), whereas the sensory nerve conduction is abnormal in 31% (138).

In alcoholics without clinical neuropathy, subclinical neuropathy is well documented by the nerve conduction studies. Blackstock et al. (137) found no significant abnormalities in the median and peroneal motor nerve conductions, but did find a marked reduction of the mean sensory NCV and prolonged H-reflex latency among 24 cases. On the other hand, a significant slowing in the motor and sensory NCVs and prolongation of the H-reflex latency were reported by Mawsley and Mayer (139). The slowing of mean motor NCVs ranged from 9.7% of normal in the median nerve to 14% in the peroneal nerve. The mean NCVs were slowed 18% below normal in the median sensory nerve and 7.6% in the median mixed nerve. The H-reflex latency was prolonged by 17%.

In alcoholics with peripheral neuropathy, nerve conduction abnormalities are observed in 88% of cases in at least two out of four nerves in sensory nerve conduction tests and two out of three nerves in motor nerve conduction tests (133). Sensory nerve conduction abnormalities are seen in 52–78% of cases (137, 140), and motor conduction abnormalities in 33–69% (133, 137), indicating that sensory fibers are more often affected in alcoholic neuropathy and that sensory conduction tests are superior in the detection of this disorder.

Several studies of maximal motor NCV showed a slight reduction: 9.7–14% reduction from normal in the median nerve (134, 139) and 17–18% reduction in the peroneal nerve. The CMAP amplitude was low in 50–60% of cases, and a low CMAP amplitude was the only abnormality in one-quarter of the tested motor conductions (133). In sensory nerve conduction, a marked reduction of amplitude of the sensory CNAP is typical of this disorder (134, 136–138, 141), the average being a 50–90% reduction from normal (134, 137). The sensory NCV was slowed by 20–26% of normal in the median nerve (137). Mixed nerve conduction was studied by Mawsley and Mayer (139) and Walsh and McLeod (134). The latter authors (134) found a 60% reduction in amplitude from normal, and the latency was prolonged by only 25% in the median nerve. They were not able to record any mixed nerve potential in peroneal nerve in 10 of 11 cases. Mawsley and Mayer (139) found a 10–13% reduction of mean NCV of mixed nerve in median and ulnar nerves. The H-reflex latency was prolonged by 23–27% of normal (137, 139) and the ankle jerk latency by 38% of normal (137). The minimal motor NCV was studied in eight patients with no clinical neuropathy, and pathological changes were found in the smaller motor fibers in 5 (63% versus 0% in maximum NCV) (137).

Tackmann et al. (136) examined the slow components of the sensory CNAP in the sural nerves of nine patients; the NCV of these components were slowed in seven. Four of the seven showed normal maximum NCV and normal potential amplitude of the main components of the CNAP. The nerve conduction abnormalities were worse (137, 139) and more frequent in severe form of neuropathy (133). Consistent with the clinical findings, the legs show more frequent and severe involvement electrophysiologically than the arms (133, 134, 139).

Comprehensive needle EMG studies by Behse and Buchthal showed some evidence of denervation and reinnervation in virtually all muscles in patients with alcoholic polyneuropathy (133). The abnormalities were most marked distally in the lower limbs and in those patients with more severe signs of neuropathy.

In alcoholic neuropathy, the nerve conduction abnormalities are *typical of axonal neuropathy:*

1. The amplitude of the CMAP and sensory CNAP is markedly reduced, whereas the motor and sensory NCVs are only mildly slow and the H-reflex and F-wave latencies are mildly prolonged; and

2. The nerve conduction abnormalities are more frequent and severe distally and in the legs.

Neuropathies Due to Nutritional Disturbances

Beriberi Neuropathy

Vitamin B_1 deficiency produces beriberi, which is characterized by edema, cardiomyopathy, and predominantly sensory neuropathy. Beriberi neuropathy has been cited as the best example of a nutritional neuropathy, but has been rare in recent years. Administration of thiamine results in clinical recovery. Sural nerve biopsies from Japanese patients, who developed beriberi neuropathy from eating milled rice without supplementary B_1, showed that axonal degeneration is the predominant change involving primarily the large-diameter fibers (142, 143). Nerve conduction studies in seven cases showed no response in the peroneal nerve in five of six tested cases, normal NCV in the median nerve, and low normal or absent sensory CNAP amplitudes with normal latencies in the sural nerve (143). Needle EMG showed fibrillations and reduced interference pattern in the affected muscles in the legs. Thus, the electrophysiological findings were *typical of axonal neuropathy.*

Neuropathy Due to Folate Deficiency

Neuropathy caused by folate deficiency is rare. Botez et al. (144) reported five patients with this neuropathy, two of whom had signs of subacute combined degeneration of the spinal cord and three of whom had signs of polyneuropathy only. Clinically the patients had sensorimotor neuropathy with mainly sensory deficits. All had reduced folic acid levels, long-standing gastrointestinal diseases, and deficient folate intake. Both motor and sensory NCVs were normal, but the CNAPs were either absent or reduced. The needle EMG did not show any evidence of denervation. Mild improvement in nerve conduction occurred after folate therapy. Fehling et al. showed similar clinical and electrophysiological findings and response to treatment in a single case (145). Initial nerve conduction studies in this case showed mild slowing in motor and sensory NCVs with reduced CMAP amplitude and no sensory CNAPs in the median nerve. These findings were typical of a mild *axonal neuropathy.*

Neuropathy Due to Niacin Deficiency

Pellagra, a disease caused by niacin deficiency, is characterized by the triad of dermatological, gastrointestinal (diarrhea), and neurological (dementia) manifestations. In underdeveloped countries this disorder is still a problem, but in developing countries niacin deficiency is most likely to occur in chronic alcoholics. Ischii and Nishihara found neuropathologic evidence of pellagra in 20 of 74 patients who died of chronic alcoholism (146). Seven of 20 patients had sensory-motor polyneuropathy with severe paresthesias and burning pains in the extremities. In pellagric neuropathy, Taher et al. (147) studied motor NCVs in eight Egyptian pellagrins showing clinical neuropathy. Values of 32–40 m/sec were reported in the ulnar and peroneal nerves. There was no good correlation between the severity of the clinical picture and the slowing of conduction. All patients responded clinically to antipellagra treatment within 4–6 weeks, although no significant change in the conduction velocity was reported.

Neuropathy Due to Pyridoxin Deficiency

This neuropathy develops in man as a side effect of isoniazid and hydralzine, which inhibit the phosphorylation of pyridoxine and cause a decrease in the tissue levels of pyridoxal phosphate. This neuropathy is clinically characterized by sensory-motor neuropathy with predominant sensory symptoms and responds favorably to discontinuation of the drugs and to the administration of pyridoxine (148). Sural nerve biopsy in this neuropathy showed all the changes of axonal degeneration (148, 149). Motor NCV was mildly slow in the peroneal nerve in four of five tested cases and in the ulner nerve in all five cases (148). These findings are compatible with *axonal neuropathy.* A report of detailed nerve conduction studies is lacking in this neuropathy.

Neuropathy Due to Pyridoxin Toxicity

Toxic peripheral neuropathy may be produced by a high daily dose of pyridoxin. In 1983, Schaumburg et al. described seven patients who developed sensory ataxic neuropathy after daily megadose (2–6 g) pyridoxin consumption (150). Parry and Bredesen reported such a neuropathy following pyridoxin abuse with a much lower (0.1–2 g) dose (151). All these patients improved after withdrawal of pyridoxin. Sural nerve biopsy in two cases showed widespread axonal degeneration (150, 151). The classic nerve conduction pattern of *sensory neuronopathy pattern* was observed in this neuropathy: absent sensory CNAP or severely reduced sensory CNAP amplitude and normal motor nerve conduction (150, 151). The sensory NCV was mildly slow in the peroneal nerve in two of Schaumburg et al.'s seven cases and in three of Parry and Bredesen's 16 cases. The needle EMG was normal in all cases (151). In fact, experimentally selective degeneration of sensory neurons of the dorsal root and gasserian ganglia was reported in this condition (152).

Neuropathy Due to Vitamin B$_{12}$ Deficiency

Vitamin B$_{12}$ deficiency usually occurs in individuals with pernicious anemia but rarely in those with blind loop syndrome, ileal resection, or fish tapeworm, or in strict vegetarians. Peripheral neuropathy, posterior column signs, and pyramidal tract signs are the classic triad of this disorder. Megaloblastic anemia and dementia are usually present.

Mayer (153) reported the nerve conduction findings in 53 patients with this disorder. In group 1, which consisted of 16 patients who never had symptoms or signs of neurological disorder, the motor, sensory, and mixed NCVs and the H-reflex latency were all normal. In group 2, which consisted of five patients who previously had neurological symptoms that were abolished by specific therapy, the NCVs were also normal. In group 3, which consisted of patients with neurological dysfunction, reduced mean sensory NCVs in the median and ulnar nerves were the sole abnormality. In no case were the sensory or mixed CNAPs absent in median or ulnar nerves. Lockner et al. observed a reduced median sensory CNAP amplitude in 33% of 34 patients, 7% of whom had subjective symptoms (154). Eleven patients were followed with repeated examinations during treatment, but the amplitude did not change. Hahn et al. reported a mildly reduced motor NCV and absent sensory CNAPs in a patient with a predominantly distal sensory neuropathy (155). The needle EMG was normal. In three patients, McCombe and McLeod observed mildly slow motor NCV in two cases and abnormal sensory conduction in two cases (156). Thus, the nerve conduction abnormalities in pernicious anemia are *typical of axonal neuropathy* and are consistent with axonal degeneration observed in this disorder (153, 156, 157). With vitamin B$_{12}$ treatment, the sensory NCVs returned to normal within a year (153).

Neuropathy Due to Vitamin E Deficiency

Vitamin E deficiency has been reported in chronic fat malabsorption, in association with long-standing cholestatic liver disease, and in a-β-lipoproteinemia (158–160). Harding et al.'s patients had dysarthria, cerebellar ataxia, and the peripheral nerve signs of loss of proprioception and reduced deep tendon reflexes (159). Werlin et al.'s patients showed severe hyporeflexia and decreased vibratory sensation (160). Nerve conduction abnormalities were typical of *a sensory neuronopathy pattern*: normal motor nerve conduction (159, 160) and absent sensory CNAP or markedly reduced sensory CNAP amplitude (159). The needle EMG showed a myopathic pattern in Harding et al.'s two cases (159) and normal findings in Werlin et al.'s cases (160). Two patients reported by Harding et al. showed a central delay in the somatosensory evoked potential studies consistent with dysfunction of the posterior columns (159). Clinical and electrophysiological improvement were observed in one case after oral therapy with vitamin E (159).

Neuropathy Due to Hypophosphatemia

Hypophosphatemia occurs as a complication of diabetic ketoacidosis, chronic alcoholism, hyperalimentation, and during recovery from burns. Peripheral neuropathy due to hypophosphatemia has been reported (161, 162). In a patient with an areflexic paralysis necessitating respiratory assistance associated with a low serum phosphorus level during intravenous hyperalimentation, nerve conduction studies showed a slow motor NCV, a low and dispersed CMAP, and absent sensory CNAP and F-response (162). The needle EMG showed profuse fibrillations and positive sharp waves with occasional MUPs on voluntary contraction. With correction of the serum phosphorus level, the patient gradually improved.

Neuropathy Due to Tropical Sprue

Peripheral neuropathy and proximal myopathy may occur as complications of tropical sprue (163). Tropical sprue is a malabsorption syndrome of as yet unknown cause confined to residents of tropical climates. Among 24 cases of tropical sprue in southern India, 15 patients had myopathy and one had sensory neuropathy. Among 15 myopathy patients, the needle EMG showed a myopathic pattern in 10 cases and pseudomyotonia in six. Nerve conduction studies showed mildly slow motor and sensory NCV with a reduced sensory CNAP is eight cases. There was no correlation with serum folate levels, but five of eight patients with peripheral neuropathy had a megaloblastic bone marrow, and four had a low serum B_{12} level.

Postgastrectomy Neuropathy

Neuropathy develops in a few patients following gastrectomy (164). One cause is vitamin B_{12} deficiency, which invariably occurs after total gastrectomy. In six patients who developed a sensory motor polyneuropathy 1–15 years after surgery for peptic ulcer, a moderately slow motor and sensory NCV and severe reduction of the sensory CNAP amplitude were observed (133). The needle EMG showed signs of denervation and reinnervation in all muscles. Sural nerve biopsy revealed substantial fiber loss, and teased fiber preparations suggested a combination of segmental and paranodal demyelination.

Neuropathy after Gastric Restriction Surgery for Morbid Obesity

Various neurological complications occur 3–30 months after gastric restriction surgery for morbid obesity (165). These include Wernicke's encephalopathy, peripheral neuropathy, and optic atrophy. Among these, peripheral neuropathy is the most common, accounting for 52% of the cases of neurological complications. Chronic or subacute sensory polyneuropathy is the most common presentation, whereas acute polyneuropathy or burning feet syndrome is rarely seen. Nerve conduction tests showed normal motor NCV in two patients with burning feet syndrome and mildly slow motor NCV in 12 patients with chronic or subacute sensory polyneuropathy and in one patient with acute sensory neuropathy. No other nerve conduction data were available. A therapeutic trial with IM multivitamins and increased protein and calorie intake resulted in improvement in patients with acute sensory neuropathy and burning feet syndrome but not in those with subacute or chronic neuropathy.

Acromegalic Neuropathy

The carpal tunnel syndrome is a well-recognized complication of acromegaly. In a study of 11 patients with this disorder, Low et al. (166) found clinical and electrophysiological evidence of peripheral neuropathy in eight patients and of carpal tunnel syndrome in nine. There was a significant reduction in the mean motor NCV and in the mean amplitude of sensory CNAPs and mixed CNAPs. The sural nerve biopsy showed segmental demyelination with onion-bulb formation (166, 167). Oh et al. (168) also observed a case of tarsal tunnel syndrome in a patient with acromegaly.

Thyrotoxic Neuropathy

Thyrotoxic neuropathy (Basedow's paraplegia) is a rare but possible manifestation of severe hyperthyroidism. Feibel and Campa (169) reported a case of motor-sensory neuropathy in hyperthyroidism. Motor NCVs were mild to moderately slow. Sural CNAP was absent, and the sural sensory NCV was slow.

Hypothyroid Neuropathy

Two types of neuropathy occur in patients with hypothyroidism. The most common type is carpal tunnel syndrome (31, 170, 171). Typical nerve conduction abnormalities seen in carpal tunnel syndrome are also seen here. The disorder can be successfully treated with thyroid replacement. Kaeser (172) observed a case of bilateral carpal and tarsal tunnel syndromes. In nine patients with myxedema and carpal tunnel syndrome, Schwartz et al. found four cases of tarsal tunnel syndrome on the basis of prolonged terminal latency in the posterior tibial nerve, three of whom were only mildly symptomatic, suggesting that tarsal tunnel syndrome is frequently encountered in myxedema (173).

The second type is diffuse sensory neuropathy. Recent studies have showed that *axonal degeneration* is the basic pathology of this neuropathy (174, 175), although previously it was thought to be segmental demyelination (170, 176). Nerve conduction data are more typical of axonal neuropathy and superimposed carpal tunnel syndrome (174, 175). Fincham and Cape (171) studied nerve conduction in 16 patients with myxedema, of whom 14 had had sensory neuropathy. The motor NCVs were normal for the most part. In the median nerve, carpal tunnel syndrome was present in six. Mild slowing of the NCV in the ulnar and peroneal nerves was noted in six and three patients, respectively. The amplitude of sensory CNAPs is reduced or the sensory NCVs are slow in almost all patients. Similar nerve conduction abnormalities have also been reported by others (174, 175). These findings can be reversed with good thyroid treatment.

Acute Porphyric Neuropathy

Porphyric neuropathy is an acute or subacute, symmetrical or asymmetrical, predominantly motor neuropathy, occurring in three dominantly inherited hepatic porphyrias—acute intermittent porphyria, hepatic coproporphyria, and variegate porphyria. Acute neurological crises occur in patients with acute intermittent porphyria. They take the form of severe episodes of abdominal pain, psychiatric disorders, and peripheral neuropathies. Attacks of acute intermittent porphyria occur either spontaneously or are precipitated by drugs. Excessive intake of alcohol, barbiturates, or sulfonamides is particularly responsible. Diagnosis is confirmed by an increased porphobilinogen level in the urine. Pathological changes are predominantly those of *axonal degeneration* (177, 178).

Motor NCVs are either normal (9, 179, 180) or mildly decreased in both upper and lower extremities with a reduction in amplitude of the CMAP (181, 182). Distal motor latencies are normal or only slightly prolonged. The sensory NCV is borderline, but the amplitude of the CNAP in the sural and superficial peroneal nerve is markedly diminished (183). In Albers et al.'s series, sensory conduction was normal in four of six patients in whom this was examined. In the other two individuals, sensory potentials were either absent or of reduced amplitude but with normal latencies (181). Thus, nerve conduction abnormalities are characteristic of an *axonal neuropathy with relative preservation of sensory fibers.* Needle EMG showed prominent fibrillation potentials, first in the proximal muscles and later in the distal muscles (181). Recruitment of MUPs was reduced. In the earlier stages the MUPs were of normal appearance; later they tended to be polyphasic and of increased amplitude and duration.

Hepatic Neuropathy

Clinical peripheral neuropathy has been reported in 9% of patients with chronic liver disease (184). Nerve conduction abnormalities have been reported in 14–68% of patients with chronic liver diseases (184, 185). Sural nerve biopsy showed segmental demyelination (184, 186). Nerve conduction abnormalities consisted of slowing of the motor NCV (which can be quite marked in some patients), reduction in the CMAPs, prolonged terminal latencies, reduced sensory CNAPs, and slowing of the sensory NCV (187). Among 14 cases of neuropathy, Knill-Jones et al. found six cases of diabetes mellitus and five of alcoholic cirrhosis. Thus, 79% of their patients had other causes for peripheral neuropathy. Considering this, it is not clear if hepatic neuropathy is a separate entity. There is a distinct painful sensory neuropathy associated with biliary cirrhosis (188, 189). Patients with this disorder demonstrate biliary cirrhosis, xanthomatosis, and xanthoma in the sural nerve biopsy (188, 190). Nerve conduction studies in these cases showed typical sensory neuropathy: normal motor nerve conduction with absent sensory CNAPs or reduced CNAP amplitude (188, 189).

Hypoglycemic Neuropathy

Danta reviewed the subject of hypoglycemic neuropathy in 1969 (191). He reviewed 24 cases of spontaneous hypoglycemia that showed evidence of peripheral neuropathy. In seven patients the neuropathy was entirely motor; in only four was it predominantly sensory. Peripheral neurological symptoms usually appeared in the course of hypoglycemic attacks or sometimes after a severe attack. The motor NCV was mildly slow (191). Because most of these patients have adenoma of the pancreas, it has been suggested that this may be a paraneoplastic carcinomatous neuropathy (192).

Critical Illness Polyneuropathy

Critical illness polyneuropathy was first described in five patients in 1984 (193). Since then the clinical, electrophysiological, and pathological features have been delineated (194–196). Sepsis and critical illness occur as complications of disease, injury, or surgery in approximately 5% of patients in the critical care unit (194, 195). Critical illness polyneuropathy occurs in at least 50% of such patients and may be mild or severe. Its causes are not clearly known (193, 194) but are most likely multifactorial. Patients have usually been septic and in critical condition for more than 2 weeks. Difficulty in weaning from the ventilator as the critical illness subsides and the development of flaccid and areflexic limbs are early clinical signs (193). Thus, this neuropathy is a significant cause of respiratory insufficiency in the critical care unit. The spinal fluid examination in one study was usually normal: three of 11 patients had mildly elevated protein; one had 12 mononuclear cells/cm^3 (195). The polyneuropathy is a predominantly distal axonal degeneration of motor and sensory fibers with minimal evidence of segmental demyelination (193, 195). The electrophysiological study is the key diagnostic test in the recognition of this entity (196). The nerve conduction study (195) showed the *classical pattern of axonal neuropathy:* normal or mildly slow motor and sensory NCV with a severely reduced CMAP and CNAP amplitude. The phrenic nerve latency was normal. The needle EMG revealed fibrillation potentials, positive sharp waves, and MUPs that were reduced in number, somewhat polyphasic, but not increased in size, predominantly in the distal muscles. In comparison with the Guillain-Barré syndrome (GBS), there was no significant difference in the various nerve conduction parameters (196). However, Bolton et al. stated that, in eight of 16 GBS patients, there was conduction block in the proximal segments, which was not observed in the patients with critical illness polyneuropathy (196). CSF protein and the presence of abundant fibrillation and positive sharp waves in the needle EMG further differentiate this neuropathy from GBS. No defect in neuromuscular transmission was demonstrated despite the use of aminoglycoside antibiotics in some patients. In those who survived the critical illness, clinical and electrophysiological improvement occurred.

Paraneoplastic Neuropathies

Paraneoplastic neuropathies have been better delineated in recent years. Among 692 patients presenting over a 1-year period with clinically and electrophysiologically confirmed polyneuropathy, paraneoplastic neuropathy was found in 1.7% (197). When patients with known malignancy were screened, the frequency of clinically detectable polyneuropathy varied from 1.7 to 5.5% in retrospective studies (198, 199) to about 50% in prospective studies when electrophysiological or morphological techniques were used (200–202). These latter subclinical patients usually had mild axonal neuropathies with known and advanced malignancies.

Various forms of polyneuropathy are observed as paraneoplastic neuropathy (Table 20.9). Among these, *subacute sensory neuronopathy* is most distinctive as a paraneoplastic neuropathy (203, 204). In 86% of 14 cases, the anti-Hu antibody was found (205), and the immunological basis of this neuropathy is now well established. Patients typically present with this neuropathy before discovery of a malignancy. In men, the association is mainly with oat cell carcinoma of the lung, and in women with breast carcinoma. This neuropathy is usually subacute and characterized by sensory ataxia because of severe sensory impairments, particularly in proprioception. Motor strength is surprisingly unaffected. The nerve conduction in this disorder is *characterized by the pattern of sensory neuronopathy: absence of sensory CNAPs and normal or near-normal motor nerve conduction* (206). This characteristic pattern is caused by inflammation and degeneration of the dorsal root ganglia and degeneration of the posterior roots and posterior columns of the spinal cord (206). The needle EMG generally shows normal MUPs or increased polyphasic MUPs but no definite evidence of fibrillation or fasciculation (206). In rare cases fibrillation or positive sharp waves were observed in muscles (206).

Among patients with paraneoplastic neuropathy, axonal neuropathy is the most common. Since this neuropathy occurs as a complication of known malignancies, parallels progressive malnutrition and weight loss, and develops with administration of universal chemotherapies, the causes of this neuropathy are most likely multiple. The pathology in this neuropathy is most likely a distal "dying back" axonopathy (207). Nerve conduction studies reveal a typical axonal mixed neuropathy pattern: little or no slowing of motor and sensory NCVs with reduction of amplitude of the distal CMAPs or sensory CNAPs (198, 200, 202, 208–210). The needle EMG shows mild distal signs of an acute or a chronic mixed denervation-reinnervation pattern.

Acute or chronic inflammatory demyelinating polyneuropathy (AIDP or CIDP) may also herald the presence of an underlying malignancy. However, these neuropathies are extremely rare (211) and more commonly associated with lymphomas than with carcinoma (198, 202, 212–217). Clinical and electrophysiological features are not different from AIDP or CIDP (218). CIDP commonly occurs in the early stages of acquired immunodeficiency syndrome (AIDS) (see below).

Paraneoplastic vasculitis is an extremely rare form of paraneoplastic neuropathy. The

Table 22.9.
Paraneoplastic Polyneuropathies

Neuropathy	Clinical Features	CSF Protein	Pathology	Nerve Conduction Pattern	Common Malignancies
Axonal neuropathy	Distal mixed	Usually normal	Axonal degeneration	Axonal mixed	Lung cancers
Demyelinating neuropathy (AIDP or CIDP)	Relatively motor	Usually high	Segmental demyelination	Nonuniform demyelination	Lymphoma, leukemia, malignant dysproteinemia
Paraneoplastic vasculitis	Subacute distal	Usually high	Microvasculitis	Axonal mixed	Lung cancers, lymphoma
Paraneoplastic LMND[a]	Subacute pure motor	Normal	Anterior horn cell degeneration	Pure motor axonal	Lymphoma, lung cancers
Sensory neuronopathy	Subacute sensory ataxic	Usually high; some cells	Dorsal root ganglion degeneration	Pure sensory	Lung cancers in man; breast cancer in women

[a]Abbreviations: LMND, lower motor neuron disease; AIDP, acute inflammatory demyelinating polyneuropathy; CIDP, chronic inflammatory demyelinating polyneuropathy.

hallmark of this neuropathy is vasculitis or microvasculitis in the nerve (219–222). This neuropathy is commonly associated with lung cancer and lymphoma and is clinically characterized by a subacute symmetrical or asymmetrical polyneuropathy and a high sedimentation rate and spinal fluid protein (222). The nerve conduction studies showed a typical axonal mixed neuropathy pattern (219, 221, 222). The needle EMG revealed active and chronic denervation process (222).

Paraneoplastic motor neuron disease is another extremely rare form of paraneoplastic neuropathy. This neuropathy is characterized by subacute progression of motor weakness without any sensory impairment, thus mimicking motor neuron disease, and is reported in association with lung cancer, lymphoma, and renal cell carcinoma (223–225). The motor NCV was normal or mildly slow (223, 224), whereas the sensory and mixed nerve conduction were essentially normal (223). The needle EMG showed widespread denervation process (223, 224, 226–229). Two of Younger's patients had multifocal conduction block in the nerve conduction study, and these cases should have been reclassified as multifocal demyelinating neuropathy (225).

Lymphomatous Peripheral Neuropathy

Lymphomatous infiltration of the nerves is a *sine qua non* in this disease. A recent review found 39 previously reported patients with this disorder (230). Diagnosis was confirmed either by autopsy in 25 cases or by nerve biopsy in 15. The majority of patients had non-Hodgkin's lymphoma. Systemic lymphoma was confirmed in only 48% of cases. Thus, peripheral neuropathy can be the sole manifestation of this disease. The most common presentation was subacute progressive neuropathy, seen in 72% of cases. Acute neuropathy resembling GBS was observed in six cases, and others showed a focal neuropathy. Spinal fluid showed elevated protein and cells in half the cases. Various nerve conduction abnormalities were reported: axonal mixed neuropathy (231–233), as well as demyelinating neuropathy (234, 235), motor axonal neuropathy (230), and sciatic neuropathy (236, 237).

Toxic Neuropathies

Heavy Metal Neuropathies

Arsenic Neuropathy

Arsenic neuropathy is a mixed motor-sensory polyneuropathy with predominant sensory symptoms that follows the hyperkeratosis and acute gastrointestinal symptoms seen at the time of exposure to arsenic. Often encephalopathy is also present. Mees' lines (transverse white line on the nails) appear within 6 weeks of exposure. Arsenic is often used with homicidal intent.

There are distinct nerve conduction abnormalities in arsenic neuropathy: a marked abnormality in sensory nerve conduction in the presence of moderate abnormalities in motor nerve conduction. According to Oh (238), the most prominent abnormality in the motor nerve conduction was abnormal CMAP: either absent or low amplitude in almost all cases. In this study, the mean terminal latencies were prolonged by 29–44% from the normal mean, and the mean NCV was reduced minimally by 22–35% of the normal mean. Thus, the motor nerve conduction abnormalities were *typical of axonal degeneration.* On the other hand, *sensory and mixed CNAPs were absent* in almost all cases. Similar findings were also observed by others (239–243). These nerve conduction abnormalities are caused predominantly by axonal degeneration of the peripheral nerve (238) (Fig. 22.4). It should be noted that transient conduction block has been reported in a few cases during the worsening period of neuropathy (238, 240). This, together with elevated spinal fluid protein in some patients with arsenic neuropathy, may lead clinicians to the diagnosis of GBS in an otherwise classic case of arsenic neuropathy.

The motor NCV changes showed two distinct phases: During the first 3 months the velocity was progressively reduced, reaching its nadir some 90 days after exposure, fol-

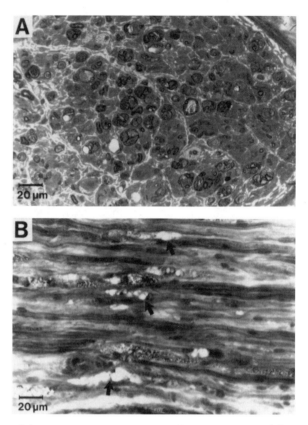

Figure 22.4.   Axonal degeneration in arsenic neuropathy. **A**, Active axonal degeneration producing bizarre myelin ovoids (Semithin section). **B**, Axonal degeneration producing myelin digestion chambers (modified trichrome stain on frozen section).

lowed by a gradual increase in velocity thereafter (242). During recovery, motor conduction improved, but sensory nerve conduction remained abnormal (241, 243, 244). The needle EMG showed active denervation process characterized by prominent fibrillations and positive sharp waves, increased polyphasic MUPs, and reduced interference pattern in all cases (238).

Lead Neuropathy

Lead neuropathy is predominantly a motor polyneuropathy accompanied by wristdrop and occasional footdrop. It can thus mimic motor neuron disease (245, 246). Anemia and basophilic stippling are noted in the peripheral blood. Nephropathy and encephalopathy may be present. Lead encephalopathy is common in children, while lead neuropathy is more frequent in adults. This disorder is commonly seen in those who work with lead, acetylene torches, and batteries, as well as in wine makers and in alcoholics who drink lead-contaminated "moonshine."

   Since Gombault's (247) classic description of segmental demyelination in guinea pigs with chronic lead intoxication, lead neuropathy has been referred to as a classic example of segmental demyelination. In human lead neuropathy, there is more evidence to suggest that axonal degeneration is a leading process (183, 246, 248). Also, nerve conduction abnormalities are more consistent with *axonal degeneration* than segmental demyelination. Motor NCVs were either normal or minimally slow (245, 246, 249–251). Terminal latency was prolonged, and there was a striking reduction in the amplitude of the CMAP (246). Sensory and mixed nerve conduction were abnormal, with absent CNAPs or slow NCV (245, 246). This has been best documented in Oh's case in which the primary findings were fibrillation potentials in distal and proximal muscles, low amplitudes of the CMAP, normal or mildly slowed motor NCV, disproportionate involvement of the radial nerve, and abnormal sensory and mixed nerve conduction, either with absent CNAPs or slow NCV. Biopsy of the sural nerve revealed evidence of axonal degeneration (246).

Lead neuropathy mimicking motor neuron disease was studied electrophysiologically in a battery worker who had clinical signs of weakness of all the hand muscles with fingerdrop, atrophy of the hypothenar muscle with a few fasciculations, and brisk reflexes (245). The needle EMG showed high-amplitude MUPs with reduced recruitment and increased polyphasic MUPs in the hand muscles. Motor NCVs in median and ulnar nerves were normal. Borderline slowing of sensory NCVs was present in median and ulnar nerves. The patient improved clinically after treatment with penicillamine.

The nerve conduction study in 20 workers exposed to a combination of organic and inorganic lead showed that the mean motor NCV of the median and posterior tibial nerves was lower and the terminal latencies were prolonged compared with the nonexposed group, whereas median sensory and sural nerve conduction showed no significant differences between the two groups (252).

In lead workers who have no neurological symptoms or signs, the mean values of the motor NCV were significantly reduced from control values (249, 253, 254). In children with known plumbism, Feldman et al. (255) reported mild slowing of the motor NCV. Although Feldman et al. (255) suggested that measurement of the motor NCV may be used as a screening test for subclinical lead toxicity, Fiaschi et al. (256) suggested that sensory conduction studies are most sensitive in detecting subclinical chronic lead toxicity.

Lead toxicity is treated with chelating agents. Oh (246) and Feldman et al. (249) documented an improvement in nerve conduction in patients with lead neuropathy after treatment with chelating agents.

Thallium Neuropathy

Thallium neuropathy is a predominantly sensory neuropathy. It may mimic arsenic neuropathy in that they both produce hyperkeratosis and Mees' lines. The hallmark of thallitoxicosis is alopecia, which rarely occurs, however, until 2–4 weeks after the patient is poisoned with thallium. Thallium produces a clear-cut polyneuropathy of *axonal degeneration* in human subjects (257–259) as well as in animals (260). Thallium poisoning is caused by the intentional or nonintentional ingestion of rodenticides.

Nerve conduction data for this disorder are limited. Bank et al. (261) reported normal motor and sensory NCVs in one case and mild slowing in motor and sensory NCVs in another. Roby et al. (262) stated that the electrodiagnostic study showed an axonal sensorimotor neuropathy that was greatest in the legs. No detailed information has been published. In Davis et al.'s patient, no CMAP was obtained in the legs or distally in the arms (259). Limos et al. elicited no CMAP in the peroneal or posterior tibial nerves and no CNAP in the sural nerve (258).

Mercury Neuropathy

Generally, the mercury toxicity is industrially related. Encephalopathy associated with tremor, irritability, emotional lability, and rigidity are the most prominent symptoms. Sensory changes clinically resemble those of peripheral neuropathy (263). A helpful clue is the high frequency of gum abnormalities and loose teeth in suspected patients (264). Mercury neuropathy is said to be predominantly sensory. However, LeQuesne et al. (265) conducted an extensive electrophysiological evaluation in 19 patients with organic mercury poisoning and found normal motor, sensory, and mixed nerve conductions. They concluded that the sensory disturbances are predominantly or entirely due to damage to the central nervous system. Thus, there is some question about the existence of mercury neuropathy due to organic mercury compounds. However, there are recent reports of clinical neuropathy following accidental (266, 267) or occupational exposure (268–270) to mercury vapors. Vroom and Greer (264) observed normal motor and sensory NCV in nine patients with inorganic mercury poisoning. However, statistical analysis showed borderline abnormalities in motor and sensory nerve conductions. The needle EMG showed denervation in eight patients. In one case, Goldstein et al. reported a normal motor NCV but "mildly abnormal sensory nerve conduction" (271).

Iyer et al. found absent CNAPs in the superficial peroneal nerve and a low CNAP amplitude in the sural nerve in the presence of normal motor nerve conduction in a dentist with chronic elemental mercury poisoning and sensory neuropathy (269). Following treatment with penicillamine, sensory conductions returned to normal. Albers et al. found mild clinical neuropathy in 13% of 138 chlor-alkali workers, who showed significantly prolonged distal latencies with reduced CNAP amplitudes and increased likelihood of denervation in the needle EMG (270). These findings are consistent with *mild axonal neuropathy*. Adams et al. reported a patient with mercury poisoning who was initially suspected of having ALS because of clinical and electrophysiological fasciculations (267). Positive sharp waves and an increased MUP amplitude and duration in affected muscles and normal motor and sensory NCVs were also reported.

Gold Neuropathy

Gold salts are sometimes used in the treatment of rheumatoid arthritis. Gold neuropathy is an infrequent complication of gold therapy (272, 273). It is predominantly sensory and usually occurs during or a few days after a full course of gold therapy. Axonal degeneration is the predominant pathological finding in gold neuropathy (272, 274).

Nerve conduction data were available in four cases (272, 274). Normal or mild to moderate slowing of motor NCVs and increased terminal latency were noted, together with mild slowing of sensory NCVs or absent sensory CNAPs. Mixed CNAPs were also absent in one case (272). These nerve conduction findings are typical of *axonal neuropathy*. The needle EMG showed active denervation in the involved muscles (274).

Generalized myokymia syndrome has been reported with gold therapy (274–276). Because of brisk reflexes and myokymia mimicking continuous fasciculations, these patients were often thought to have motor neuron disease. Motor and sensory nerve conductions were normal. The needle EMG showed typical *myokymic discharges,* consisting of doublets, triplets, or quadruplets of MUPs (274, 275). These myokymic discharges are thought to be generated from the distal nerve segments because myokymia was noted to persist with a local nerve block but was stopped by succinylcholine (276) or reduced by regional curare administration (274). The myokymia responded well to carbamazepine (274, 275).

Platinum Neuropathy

Platinum in the form of cis-diamminedichloroplatinum(cisplatin) is used in the chemotherapeutic treatment of cancer. Sensory neuropathy is a common complication of cisplatin therapy. Roelofs et al. (278) detected sensory neuropathy in 92% of patients. Some developed this neuropathy 3–8 weeks after the last dose of the drug (277). The neuropathy is dose-dependent, with most patients becoming symptomatic after receiving a total cumulative dose of 300–600 mg/m^2 (277). Nerve conduction studies showed a *distinct sensory neuronopathy pattern:* either absent CNAP or reduced amplitude in the presence of normal motor nerve conduction (278–280). The needle EMG showed fibrillations and a mild increase in the MUP amplitude in 13% of cases (278). Sural nerve biopsy showed a combination of axonal degeneration and secondary segmental demyelination (278, 280).

Tetany has been described in several patients as a result of the nephrotoxic action of cisplatinum, causing impaired tubular reabsorption of magnesium and calcium (281, 282). One study showed EMG evidence of tetany in 75% of patients who developed hypomagnesemia during cisplatin therapy (282).

Drug-Induced Neuropathy

Table 22.10 shows the list of drugs responsible for neuropathy. Drug-induced neuropathy is characterized by: (*a*) symmetrical polyneuropathy; and (*b*) potential reversibility

(283). It is inconceivable that any drug will remain in clinical use long if it produces significant peripheral neuropathy. Clinoquinol and thalidomide are the best examples of drugs found to cause problems and later withdrawn from use; vincristine and cisplatinum-acromycin, on the other hand, are still used because they are effective anticancer medications.

Most drugs that induce neuropathy produce axonal neuropathy (283, 284) (Table 22.10). However, there are a few drugs that are an exception to this rule. *Amidarone (285–287) and perhexiline (288, 289) are known to induce a demyelinating neuropathy,* whereas pyridoxine and thalidomide produce a sensory neuronopathy. Thus, depending on the main pathological process, the clinical features and nerve conduction patterns are different. One should remember, however, that the *majority of drug-induced neuropathies are axonal neuropathy.*

Solvent Neuropathy

Peripheral neuropathies resulting from industrial toxins are usually caused by occupational exposures (284, 290) (Table 22.11). It is important to have detailed information about the occupation and potential for toxin exposure in the workplace. In the domestic

Table 22.10.
Drug-induced Neuropathies[a]

Drug	Clinical Features	Predominant Pathology[b]	Electrophysiological Features	Special Features
Amiodarone	Sensory-motor	Segmental demyelination	Demyelinating neuropathy	
Amitriptyline	Sensory-motor	Total loss of myelinated fibers	Axonal mixed neuropathy	Neuropathy with overdose
Chloramphenicol	Sensory	NA[c]	NA	Optic neuropathy more prominent
Chloroquine	Sensory-motor	Axonal degeneration/ segmental demyelination	Axonal neuropathy	Myopathy is also present.
Clioquinol	SMON	?	?	Subacute myelooptico-neuropathy
Colchicine	Sensory-motor	Axonal degeneration	Axonal mixed neuropathy	Vacuolar myopathy is present
Dapsone	Predominant motor	Axonal degeneration	Pure motor axonopathy	Sensory CNAP: normal
Diphenylhydantoin	Sensory-motor	Axonal atrophy	Axonal mixed neuropathy	
Disulfiram	Sensory-motor	Axonal degeneration with giant axon	Axonal mixed neuropathy	
Ethambutol	Sensory	NA	Axonal mixed neuropathy	Optic neuropathy more prominent
Glutehimide	Sensory	NA	Axonal neuropathy with absent sensory potentials	Cerebellar ataxia
Hydralazine	Sensory	NA	NA	Due to vitamin B6 deficiency
Isoniazide	Predominant sensory	Axonal degeneration	Axonal mixed neuropathy	Due to vitamin B6 deficiency
Lithium	Sensory-motor	Axonal degeneration	Axonal mixed neuropathy	
Metronidazole	Sensory	Axonal degeneration	Sensory neuropathy	
Misonidazole	Sensory	Axonal degeneration	Axonal mixed neuropathy	
Nitrofurantoin	Sensory-motor	NA	Axonal mixed neuropathy	
Nitrous oxide	Predominantly sensory	Axonal degeneration with giant axons	Axonal mixed neuropathy	Myelopathy is also present Vitamin B12 may be low
Perhexiline	Sensory-motor	Segmental demyelination	Demyelinating neuropathy	Facial diplegia may occur
Pyridoxine	Sensory neuronopathy	Axonal degeneration	Sensory neuronopathy	Dorsal root ganglia degeneration
Sodium cyanate	Sensory	Axonal degeneration	NA	Dorsal root ganglia degeneration
Taxol	Predominantly sensory	NA	Axonal mixed neuropathy	
Thalidomide	Sensory neuronopathy	Axonal degeneration	Sensory neuronopathy	Dorsal root ganglia degeneration
Triptophan	Sensory-motor	Axonal degeneration	Axonal mixed neuropathy	Demyelinating neuropathy is also reported
Vincristine	Predominantly motor	Axonal degeneration	Axonal mixed neuropathy	

[a]These data are based on a review of 57 articles. References are available on request.
[b]Pathological findings based on the human cases.
[c]NA, not available.

Table 22.11.
Solvent-Induced Neuropathies[a]

Toxic Agent	Clinical Features	Predominant Pathology[b]	Electrophysiological Features	Special Features
Acrylamide	Predominantly sensory	Axonal degeneration	Axonal mixed neuropathy	Exfoliative dermatitis
Carbon disulfide	Sensory-motor	Axonal degeneration	Axonal mixed neuropathy	
Chlorobiphenyl	Sensory	NA	Axonal mixed neuropathy	
DMAPN	Sacral plexopathy	Axonal degeneration	Axonal mixed neuropathy	
Ethylene oxide	Predominantly motor	Axonal degeneration	Axonal mixed neuropathy	
Hexacarbon	Sensory-motor	Giant axon neuropathy	Mild: axonal mixed neuropathy Severe: "demyelinating neuropathy"	Due to paranodal widening
Methylbromide	Sensory	NA	NA	
Organophosphate	Motor as delayed complication	Axonal degeneration	Axonal mixed neuropathy	Neuromuscular transmission defect may be present
Trichlorethylene	Cranial neuropathy	Axonal degeneration and demyelination	Prolonged facial nerve latency Prolonged R1 latency	Found in 28% of cases

[a]These data are based on a review of 22 articles. References provided on request.
[b]Pathological findings in human cases.

setting, such cases may occur through accidental exposure to chemicals, through addiction (glue sniffer's neuropathy or huffer's neuropathy), or as a result of attempted suicide or homicide (organophosphate poisoning).

These neuropathies are clinically characterized by symmetrical sensory or sensory motor polyneuropathy and the "coasting phenomenon": patients continue to worsen for up to 3–4 months after exposure is discontinued before improvement begins. Pathologically, all industrial agents that induce a peripheral neuropathy produce axonal neuropathy. However, *N-hexane and MBK are known to induce additional giant axonal swelling.* Thus N-hexane and MBK neuropathies are categorized under the generic term "giant axonal neuropathy" (291, 292). *In giant axonal neuropathy,* paranodal widening due to paranodal retraction of myelin occurs as the secondary change after axonal degeneration (293, 294). This creates a tremendous increase in nodal delay of conduction and thus results in *nerve conduction slowing to the degree of demyelination* (295).

N-Hexane Neuropathy (Glue Sniffer's Neuropathy)

N-hexane is an organic solvent widely used in printing, in the shoe industry, and in commercial glues (296, 297). This neuropathy is reported among "glue sniffers" (298, 293) and shoe factory workers. It is better known as glue sniffer's neuropathy (299). Clinically, an insidious and symmetrical sensorimotor neuropathy is the cardinal feature.

Motor NCVs are moderately slow, and terminal latencies are prolonged up to twice the normal values. Sensory NCVs are moderately slow, or sensory CNAPs are absent (297, 299, 300).

MBK Neuropathy (Huffer's Neuropathy)

MBK neuropathy was first observed as an industrial outbreak in a plant that produced plastic-coated and color-printed fabrics. In mild cases, sensory neuropathy was prominent, whereas in moderate to severe cases, motor and sensory neuropathies were present. Huffer's neuropathy is a toxic neuropathy occurring among "huffers" of the paint or lacquer thinner and characterized by giant axon in the nerve biopsy (294, 301) (Fig. 22.5). MBK is the agent possibly responsible for huffer's neuropathy (294). Motor NCVs are moderately slow, and terminal latencies are substantially prolonged. Either sensory CNAPs are absent or sensory NCVs are moderately slow. Mixed nerve conductions are mildly abnormal (294). In the cases of Allen et al. (302), the peroneal motor NCVs were higher than 35 m/sec in the mildly affected group and below 35 m/sec in the moderately severely affected group.

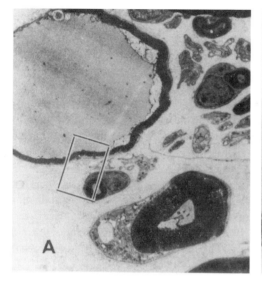
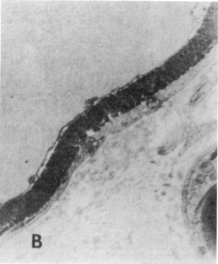

Figure 22.5. Giant axon in huffer's neuropathy. *A*, Transverse section, showing "swollen axon" surrounded by thin or no myelin sheath (× 1800). *B*, Axoplasm is filled with dense array of neurofilaments (× 95000). (From Oh SJ, Kim JM. Giant axonal swelling in "huffer's neuropathy." Arch Neurol 1976;33:585.)

Acrylamide Neuropathy

Acrylamide itself has little industrial use, but the polymer is extensively employed in tunneling operations to stabilize the soil, and as coating for paper. Acrylamide neuropathy is a sensory neuropathy and has been most extensively studied in animals as an example of axonal neuropathy that selectively destroys the large myelinated fibers.

In human acrylamide neuropathy, the motor NCV is either normal or just below normal in the nerves of affected limbs (303, 304). The sensory CNAP is reduced in amplitude or absent.

Clinical, pathological, and electrophysiological features of other industrial agent-induced neuropathies are summarized in Table 22.11.

Spanish Toxic Oil Syndrome

In 1981, an epidemic of toxic-allergic syndrome caused by ingestion of rapeseed oil denatured with aniline occurred in Spain (305). Myalgias, joint limitation, weight loss, cramps, progressive weakness and wasting, sensory disturbances, and scleroderma-like changes were the main clinical features. Electrophysiological studies showed that the neuromuscular impairments were caused by a slowly progressive mixed axonal neuropathy (306). Nerve biopsy confirmed neuropathy and showed perineuritis and perineurial fibrosis. Nerve conduction studies showed mild-to-moderate slowing of motor and sensory NCVs and severe reduction of sensory CNAPs. The needle EMG showed active denervation. Thus, nerve conduction findings were typical of axonal neuropathy.

Neuropathies Due to Biological Toxins

Tetrodotoxin Poisoning

It has been known for centuries that puff fish poisoning is usually fatal. This is caused by the ingestion of tetrodotoxin (TTX), which specifically blocks the sodium channels of excitable tissue (307). A fatal poisoning is characterized clinically by flaccid paralysis and respiratory failure, usually preceded by initial numbness of the lips and tongue. In one patient with tetrodotoxication, nerve conduction studies performed in the 36th hour after TTX ingestion showed an electrophysiologic pattern of *demyelination:* marked slowing (30 m/sec in the median nerve; 22 m/sec in the peroneal nerve) in the motor NCV, markedly prolonged F-wave latency (48 msec in the median nerve), and normal CMAP amplitude (308). Neither abnormal temporal dispersion nor focal conduction block was observed, indicating a uniform involvement of all fibers in a nerve trunk and resulting in a synchronous slowing of impulse conduction. There was a prolonged latency (5.2 msec) and a low CNAP amplitude in the sural nerve, which were checked at the 44th hour after TTX ingestion. Motor and sensory nerve conduction improved to completely normal at the 84th hour after TTX ingestion.

Saxitoxin Poisoning

Paralytic shellfish poisoning is an acute paralytic illness that follows ingestion of shellfish contaminated with saxitoxin and mimics botulism or the descending form of GBS. Saxitoxin, a diguanidinium compound similar to TTX, is produced by marine microorganisms that are eaten by shellfish such as clams and mussels. Nerve conduction studies in a patient at the time of respiratory failure showed marked prolongation of median motor (8.6 msec) and sensory (6.6 msec) latencies, a less dramatic decrease in median NCVs (34 m/sec), and moderately diminished CMAP and CNAP amplitudes (309). No conduction block or temporal dispersion was observed. The needle EMG did not show any abnormal spontaneous potentials. Nerve conduction became normal within 5 days, paralleling the patient's recovery. The nerve conduction data suggest that saxitoxin poisoning is based on physiological *demyelination* (309).

Ciguatera Poisoning

Ciguatera poisoning is the most common form of fish poisoning in man. It is characterized by the sudden onset of nausea, vomiting, diarrhea, and abdominal pain within 12 hours after ingestion of toxic fish, and by paresthesias, weakness, and myalgias in the extremities and perioral region. Nerve conduction studies in 15 cases of acute ciguatera poisoning showed a mild but significant slowing of sensory NCVs and prolongation of the absolute refractory, relative refractory, and supernormal periods (310). In nine cases of ciguatera poisoning, slow sensory NCVs without decrease in sensory CNAP amplitude were observed, documenting a *sensory neuropathy* (311). Mild slowing of motor NCVs was seen in all of three patients, one of whom died and who had both peripheral and central nervous system involvement (312). In one case in which the NCV was serially tested over a 6-week period, mildly slow motor NCV, prolonged distal motor (7.5 msec for the median nerve) and sensory latencies, reduced sensory CNAP amplitude, and prolonged F-wave latency were reported initially. These nerve conduction abnormalities improved during the 6-week observation period. Sural nerve biopsy showed edema in the adaxonal layer of the Schwann cell cytoplasm, with axonal compression and vesicular degeneration of the myelin. Cameron et al. (310) believed that Allsop's cases (312) were more representative of scaritoxin poisoning than ciguatera poisoning in view of the prominence of ataxia. These cases are most likely due to an abnormally prolonged sodium channel opening in the nerve membrane.

Tick Paralysis

Tick paralysis is a rare acute ascending flaccid paralysis caused by the bite of a tick. With removal of the offending tick, the patient usually recovers rapidly, although slow recovery has been reported (313). This disorder should be included in the differential diagnosis of the Guillain-Barré syndrome, and every patient with ascending paralysis should be carefully searched for the presence of a tick.

The mechanism of action of a toxin is unknown. Microelectrode studies have shown a temperature-dependent reduction in the number of acetylcholine quanta released by a nerve stimulus (314), suggesting a presynaptic abnormality. Hence, this disorder is discussed as a neuromuscular transmission disorder (315). However, the electrophysiological studies in a few human cases suggest that the basic defect is most likely *a physiological terminal axonal neuropathy*, as suggested by experimental results (316).

In recent years there have been several excellent reports on nerve conduction in this disorder (313, 317–321), and they can be summarized as follows:

1. CMAP amplitude is small, ranging from no response in peroneal nerves (313) to 3.5 mV in ulnar nerves (142). This is the most striking abnormality and is seen in all tested nerves in upper and lower extremities, the most severe reduction being in the lower extremities (313).

2. Distal latency is normal. An exception was noted in one case (320) in which terminal latency in the peroneal nerve was mildly prolonged.

3. Motor NCVs are normal or mildly slow. Half the tested motor nerves showed mild slowing. The other half showed normal NCV.

4. Sensory nerve conduction is normal. Exceptions were found in two cases: prolonged latency in sural nerves in Swift and Ignacio's case (321) and slow sensory NCV in median nerves in Donat and Donat's case (313). The amplitudes were all normal.

5. Repetitive nerve stimulation at 2–10/sec is normal. A normal response is noted at a high rate of stimulation (20–50/sec). Morris (322) reported a 20% decrement at 30/sec for 1.6 sec, and Donat and Donat (313) reported a 50% increment at 50/sec for 5 sec. These responses are not abnormal according to our data (323).

6. Rapid improvement has been documented in the nerve conductions. This corresponds to the rapid clinical improvement seen within hours or days after removal of the tick. Donat and Donat reported an exceptional case of slower clinical and electrophysiological recovery (313).

Hereditary Neuropathies

We have adopted Dyck's classification (324) for describing hereditary neuropathies. Their clinical and nerve conduction characteristics are listed in Tables 22.12 and 22.13.

Hereditary Motor and Sensory Neuropathies (HMSN)

Charcot-Marie-Tooth Disease (HMSN Type I and II)

Charcot-Marie-Tooth disease (CMT) is the most common hereditary neuropathy. It is inherited as an autosomal dominant trait and is characterized clinically by pes cavus (highly arched feet) and marked atrophy of the feet and lower legs resulting in a characteristic appearance sometimes described as "stork-leg" or "inverted champagne bottle leg." Weakness is seen predominantly in the peroneal muscle group, as a result of which the term peroneal muscular atrophy was coined for this disorder. This neuropathy is slowly progressive (325).

Table 22.12.
Nerve Conduction Abnormalities in Hereditary Motor and Sensory Neuropathies

Neuropathy	Clinical Findings	Electrophysiological Findings
Type I: Hypertrophic type of the Charcot-Marie-Tooth disease (CMT) including Roussy-Levy syndrome	Distinction between type I and II is not always possible. Earlier onset, weakness of intrinsic hand and neck flexor muscles, sensory impairment of hands and kyphosis are common in type I (329). Roussy-Levy syndrome has the combination of type I and essential tremor (478)	Marked slowing in motor NCV (below 20 m/sec) and sensory NCV. Frequent absence of CNAP. Dispersion phenomenon and marked diminution of the amplitude of CNAP (329).
Type II: Neuronal type of CMT		Normal or near-normal (NCVs are no more than 40% below normal) (40).
Type III: Hypertropic neuropathy of infancy (Dejerine Sottas disease)	Hypertrophic neuropathy from infancy. No pes cavus. Thickened nerves and high CSF protein.	Very marked slowing in motor NCV (2–10 m/sec). Frequent absence of CNAP.
Type IV: Refsum's disease	CMT-like findings, retinitis pigmentosa, neuronal hearing loss, ataxia, ichthyosis.	Very marked slowing of motor NCV (below 10 m/sec). Absence of CNAP (364).
Type V: Familial spastic paraplegia with neuronal type of CMT[a]	Combination of spastic paraplegia with CMT.	Normal motor NCV; low amplitude or absence of CNAP (324).

[a]Uncomplicated familial spastic paraplegia: normal motor and sensory NCV (695)

Table 22.13.
Nerve Conduction Abnormalities in Hereditary Sensory Autonomic Neuropathies

Neuropathy	Clinical Findings	Electrophysiological Findings
Type I: Hereditary sensory radicular neuropathy of Denny-Brown (371). Degeneration of the posterior root ganglion small neurons.	Onset after the first decade. Sensory dissociation in the legs. Lancinating pain. Ulceration of the foot.	Mildly slow (373) motor NCV. Sensory or mixed CNAP absent (373).
Type II: Congenital sensory neuropathy	Onset during early childhood. Painless blister and ulcers. Touch is more affected than pain and temperature. Position was absent.	Motor NCV just below normal. Sensory CNAP absent or reduced in amplitude (375, 696)
Type III: Familial dysautonomia (Riley-Day syndrome)	Mainly in Jewish children. Defective lacrimation, hyperhydrosis, episodic hypertension, hyperpyrexia and vomiting, seizures, areflexia, and hypotonia.	Normal or mild slowing (46–36 m/sec) of motor NCV. Normal sensory NCV but a reduced or absent sensory and mixed CNAP (380) (381). Mixed CNAP showed "double peak" in 7 of 9 cases (381)
Type IV: Congenital insensitivity to pain		Normal motor and sensory NCV.

Figure 22.6. Onion-bulb formation. Onion-bulb formations are recognized by many fine lines (proliferated Schwann cell processes) surrounding nerve fibers. Some fibers with onion-bulb formations have more than one Schwann cell. Many fibers have thin myelinated fibers. This example is from a patient with CIDP. (Semithin sections. Toluidine blue × 1000) (From Oh SJ. Diagnostic usefulness and limitations of the sural nerve biopsy. Yonsei Medical Journal 1990;31:12.)

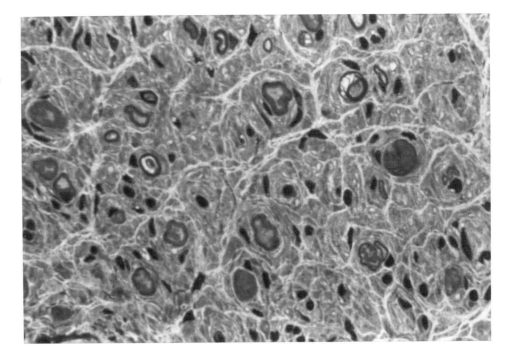

Dyck (324) concluded that CMT can be classified into two types: hypertrophic (onion-bulb formation) (Fig. 22.6) and neuronal. Although clinically it is not always possible to distinguish the type of neuropathy in the individual patient, the nerve conduction study has been a definite help in differentiating the type. Thomas and Calne (326) found evidence for genetic heterogeneity by measuring the motor NCV in 88 patients from 20 families with CMT. Their patients can be divided into two groups according to whether the values for the propositi are below or above 40 m/sec.

The nerve conduction abnormalities in CMT can be summarized as follows:

1. *Marked and uniform slowing in motor NCV* and marked abnormalities in sensory nerve conduction in the hypertrophic type (hereditary motor and sensory neuropathy [HMSN] Type 1)

(327, 328). The motor NCV is usually less than 60% of normal values (329). Dyck and Lambert (330) reported distal motor latencies averaging almost three times longer than normal, conduction velocities less than half normal, and the CMAP amplitudes less than half. Extreme slowing of the motor NCV was reported by Gilliatt and Thomas (331), who found a motor NCV of 11.2 m/sec. In sensory nerve conduction, either the CNAP was absent or there was marked slowing of the sensory NCV (172, 329). Buchthal and Behse (329) reported reduced amplitude of the sensory CNAP and a sensory NCV less than 60% of normal with the near-nerve needle technique. Studies of F-wave conduction velocities of the median and ulnar nerves showed that proximal nerve segments are affected but not so greatly as the more distal segments (332, 333). Marked slowing in NCVs is due to the segmental demyelination characterized by onion-bulb formation in the nerve in this disorder (Fig. 22.6) (334).

2. Normal or near-normal motor NCV and normal or mildly abnormal sensory nerve conduction in the neuronal type (HMSN Type 2) (324, 328, 329). Buchthal and Behse (329) reported normal motor and sensory conduction velocities (with the near-nerve technique) or velocities that are no more than 40% below normal. Dyck (324), using surface electrodes, reported absence of the sensory CNAP or normal sensory latency in this disorder.

3. The pattern of NCV changes seems to be constant within a family (326, 329, 331, 335, 336).

4. Slowing of the conduction velocity is found in members of families with this disorder showing only minimal or no abnormalities on clinical examination (330, 337).

5. A slowing of conduction precedes the onset of clinical symptoms and may even be present at birth (330, 337). Thus, conduction measurement is valuable as a screening test in preclinical stages of the disease. It should be mentioned that the NCV may be normal during early childhood and become abnormal at a later time (338). There has been some disagreement concerning the age at which the motor NCV may be considered abnormal in affected children. Berciano et al. reported marked slowing of motor NCV in a patient as young as 6 months (339), whereas the same group observed marked slowing of the motor NCV as early as 2.5 years of age in a prior study (340). In a study of two pairs of dizygotic twins, Gutmann et al. reported each born to a parent with HMSN Type 1, that maximal slowing of motor NCV evolves over the first 3–5 years of life. They further noted that prolonged terminal latency may be the earliest observable abnormality but that it evolves over a period of 10 or more years (341). These studies suggest that 3–5 *years of age* may be optimal for the study of potentially affected children. Thus, if the motor NCV is normal after 5 years of age, the diagnosis of HMSN Type 1 can safely be excluded in the tested child.

6. Conduction measurements are also helpful in detecting clinically *unaffected carriers* of the disease (330, 337, 342).

7. Longitudinal studies in patients aged 11–19 years showed that clinical deterioration was not associated with slowing in motor NCV but that a reduction in CMAP amplitude, reflecting progressive axonal loss, was correlated with clinical deterioration (343). The severity of the NCV abnormalities in young patients appeared to predict later neurological abnormalities (344).

Attempts have been made to distinguish HMSN Type 1 from chronic acquired demyelinating neuropathy. This distinction is important because some patients with acquired chronic demyelinating neuropathy may respond to steroid therapy or immunosuppressants. According to Lewis and Sumner's study (345), it is possible to make this distinction with the nerve conduction test. In HMSN Type 1, nerve conduction is *slowed uniformly* over all segments of nerves and conduction block is not observed (Fig. 22.7), whereas in chronic acquired demyelinating neuropathy multifocal slowing of nerve conduction and conduction block are typical. Although this rule is generally correct, it should not be regarded as always accurate because two studies showed exceptions in rare cases (Fig. 22.8) (346, 347). In fact, our study showed that conduction block was present in ulnar and median nerves in 28% of 30 cases (348).

Roussy-Levy syndrome resembles CMT in the following features: (*a*) its familial nature; (*b*) prevalence of clubfoot; (*c*) weakness and minimal atrophy of the distal extremity muscles; and (*d*) some distal sensory loss. It differs from CMT because there is a static tremor of the hands (337). Dyck and Lambert (337) classified this syndrome as Type 1 HMSN because they concluded that Roussy-Levy syndrome is nothing more than CMT plus an essential tremor. On the other hand, Oelschlager et al. (349) believed that the Roussy-Levy syndrome is a separate nosological entity. Nerve biopsy showed hypertrophic neuropathy (numerous onion bulb formations) (350). Marked

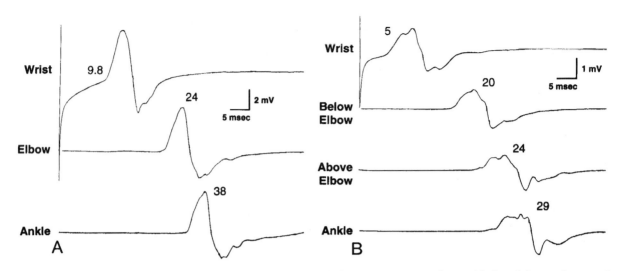

Figure 22.7. "Uniform slowing" typical of HMSN Type 1. Conduction block and abnormal temporal dispersion are absent. *A*, Median nerve: NCVs between the segments are "not uniformly slow." *B*, Ulnar nerve: NCVs between the segments are "uniformly slow." Numbers on the left represent the terminal latencies in msec. Numbers on the right represent the NCVs.

slowing of the motor NCV (349 351) has been reported in this condition. We found that sensory and mixed CNAPs were absent in most patients with this disorder.

Dejerine-Sottas Disease (HMSN Type 3)

Dejerine-Sottas disease, a recessively inherited disorder, usually begins during infancy and is associated with hypertrophic (onion bulb) neuropathy, thickened nerves, and a markedly increased cerebrospinal fluid (CSF) protein level (352). Marked slowing of the motor NCV has been a consistent finding in this disease (330, 353, 354). In fact, the slowest motor NCV among various peripheral neuropathies has been reported in this condition: Gilliatt and Sears (355) found values of 5–10 m/sec; Dyck and Gomez (352) measured motor NCVs of 3–4 m/sec; Joosten et al. (356) even found a value of only 2 m/sec. In sensory nerve conduction, the CNAP was not recordable (335, 354, 355).

Congenital Hypomyelination Neuropathy

Congenital hypomyelination neuropathy is most likely a variant of the HMSN Type 3 (Dejerine-Sottas disease). Except for its onset at birth, the clinical features are identical with those of Dejerine-Sottas disease (357, 358). The nerve biopsy shows a severe deficiency of myelin, an increase in collagen content, and onion bulb formation. There is no evidence of myelin breakdown. Thus, it is assumed that the Schwann cells are incapable of forming myelin. Motor nerve conduction was markedly abnormal: terminal latencies were markedly prolonged, and motor NCVs were markedly slow (357 360). Sensory CNAPs were absent (359). In fact, Kennedy et al. (357) recorded a terminal latency of 26 msec and a motor NCV of 1.8 m/sec in one patient.

Refsum's Disease (HMSN Type 4; Heredopathia Atactica Polyneuritiformis)

Refsum's disease is a hypertrophic neuropathy of autosomal recessive inheritance characterized by ataxia, retinitis pigmentosa, nerve deafness, ichthyosis, cardiomyopathy, and high CSF protein (361, 362). It is caused by an inborn error of metabolism in which the body accumulates exogenous phytanic acid. The disease is diagnosed by an elevated serum phytanic acid level.

Marked slowing of the motor NCV has been reported consistently in this disorder (363 366). Motor NCV below 10 m/sec was measured in the ulnar nerve. Oftedal (364) was unable to record sensory CNAPs in his patient. Clinical and nerve conduction

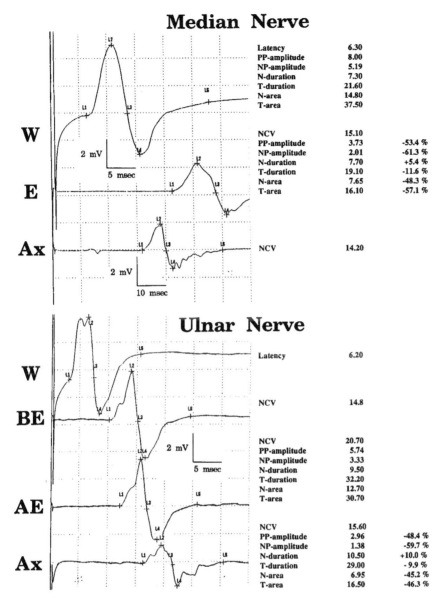

Figure 22.8. Nonuniform slowing in a case of HMSN Type 1. Conduction block in the wrist (*W*)-elbow (*E*) segment in the median and in the above elbow (*AE*)-axilla (*Ax*) segment in the ulnar nerve. Various electrophysiological data are listed to the right of figures. Latency, terminal latency in msec. PP-amplitude, peak-to-peak amplitude in mV. NP-amplitude, negative-peak amplitude in mV. N-duration, duration of negative wave in msec. T-duration, duration of total wave. N-area, area of the negative wave in mV/msec. T-area, area of the negative and positive areas. Percentage represents the difference between the proximal and distal CMAPs in the segment of conduction block in the various parameters. + represents an increase and −, a decrease. (From Oh SJ. Conduction block in hereditary motor sensory neuropathy, Type I; case report. Muscle Nerve 1992;15:522.)

improvement was documented consistently after a phytol- and phytanic acid-free diet treatment" (362, 363, 365, 367). A large-volume plasma exchange has also been found effective in improving the clinical condition (368, 369). Minimal nerve conduction improvement was documented with this procedure (368).

Infantile Refsum's disease was recently described (370). It is characterized by dysmorphic features, mental retardation, pigmentary retinopathy, severe sensorineural deafness, hepatomegaly, and sometimes peripheral neuropathy. Motor NCV was moderately slow and sensory CNAP was either absent or reduced in amplitude (370). The sural nerve biopsy showed demyelination.

Hereditary Sensory Autonomic Neuropathy (HSAN)

HSAN Type 1 (Hereditary Sensory Radicular Neuropathy of Denny-Brown; Dominant HSAN)

Hereditary sensory autonomic neuropathy (HSAN Type 1) is characterized by sensory dissociation (pain and temperature perceptions are markedly affected more than touch-pressure sensations), lancinating pain, and subsequent painless ulceration of the feet. The disease is insidious, with the first symptoms manifesting during the 2nd decade of life. The primary pathological change is degeneration of the small neurons of the dorsal root ganglia and of the small myelinated and unmyelinated fibers in the peripheral nerves (371, 372). Thus, the most prominent nerve conduction abnormality is absence of the sensory or mixed CNAP (373) in the presence of mildly slow motor NCV (373, 374). Buchthal and Rosenfalck (11) recorded a potential with an amplitude of only 1% of the normal value in the median nerve in one patient using the near-nerve needle technique and 1000 electronic averagings.

HSAN Type 2 (Congenital Sensory Autonomic Neuropathy; Recessively Inherited HSAN)

Symptoms of HSAN Type 2 appear during early childhood, taking the form of painless blisters and ulcers and sensory impairment. In contrast to Type 1, touch-pressure perception is more affected than pain and temperature. According to Ohta et al. (375), the nerve biopsy showed an almost total absence of myelinated fibers with a marked decrease in the number of unmyelinated fibers. The nerve conduction findings are characterized by absence of the sensory CNAP (342, 375, 376 379), whereas the motor NCV is at or just below the lower normal limit (375, 376, 378, 379). Ludin et al. (10) were not able to record a sensory CNAP from the median nerve in patients, even with the near-nerve needle technique.

HSAN Type 3 (Familial Dysautonomia; Riley-Day Syndrome)

HSAN Type 3, a rare familial disorder, occurs mainly in children of Jewish parentage. Involved children show early feeding difficulties, periodic vomiting, and fever. Characteristic symptoms are a lack of tears, hyperhidrosis, an absence of the fungiform papillae of the tongue, hypotonia, decreased or absent reflexes, and insensitivity to pain. Aguayo et al. (380) showed in the sural nerve biopsy the absence of myelinated fibers with a diameter of 12 μm or more and a greatly reduced number of unmyelinated fibers. The motor NCV was either normal or mildly slow (380, 381). Sensory and mixed NCVs were normal (380, 381), but sensory and mixed CNAPs were reduced in amplitude or absent (380). Brown and Johns (381) described "double peaks" in the mixed CNAPs in the ulnar nerve.

Nerve Conduction Abnormalities in Hereditary Ataxia

It is often difficult to categorize familial ataxia into a specific type on the basis of clinical findings alone. Nerve conduction has been of some help in this regard. Broadly speaking, there are two main groups of ataxia according to the nerve conduction abnormalities: hypertrophic neuropathy—Refsum's disease and Roussy-Levy syndrome; and the dorsal root ganglia degeneration group—Friedreich's ataxia, ataxia-telangiectasia, Bassen-Kornzweig's syndrome (Table 22.14).

Friedreich's Ataxia

Friedreich's ataxia, the most common form of spinocerebellar degeneration, is an autosomal recessive disorder with an onset almost always before the age of 20 years. Clinically it is characterized by ataxia, an absence of deep tendon reflexes, a loss of proprioceptive sensations in the extremities, extensor plantar responses, pes cavus, and kyphoscoliosis. Cardiomyopathy is also common. In the later stages of the disease, dis-

Table 22.14.
Nerve Conduction Abnormalities in Hereditary Ataxias

Pathology and Syndrome	Electrophysiological Findings

Degeneration of dorsal root ganglia
    Friedreich's ataxia
    Ataxia telangiectasia
    Bassen-Kornzweig syndrome
	Marked reduction in amplitude of sensory mixed CNAPs; normal or mild slowing of motor NCV.

Hypertrophic neuropathy
    Refsum's disease
    Roussy-Levy syndrome
	Marked slowing in motor NCV; marked slowing in sensory or mixed NCV or absent sensory or mixed CNAP.

tal amyotrophy in the limbs, because of the loss of anterior horn cells, may become apparent.

The characteristic nerve conduction abnormalities of sensory neuronopathy have been repeatedly reported: sensory or mixed nerve potentials are either absent or markedly reduced in amplitude, whereas the motor nerve conduction is normal or near normal (382 390). When the sensory or mixed CNAPs were recordable, the NCVs were either normal or only slightly reduced. Even when using the near-nerve needle technique and electronic averaging (383, 391), it was impossible to record the CNAP. These electrophysiological abnormalities are caused by *the selective degeneration of large cells of the dorsal root ganglia* without any segmental demyelination. Sural nerve biopsy showed loss of large myelinated fibers (387, 388).

These studies also showed that the characteristic sensory neuronopathy pattern in this disease is not related to the duration or severity of the disease (387) but is a constant finding even in mild cases (386) and as early as the age of 3 years (388). Thus, *the nerve conduction test has become the most important tool in the diagnosis of Friedreich's ataxia and is also an extremely useful test for early detection of this disorder.*

The needle EMG in the limb muscles showed increased polyphasic MUPs in three out of four cases in one series (387) and in one-third of the cases in another series (385). Reduced recruitment of MUPs was a constant finding, whereas fibrillation was extremely rare in both series (385, 387). In D'Angelo et al.'s series, fibrillation in the distal muscles was observed in 55% of cases and fasciculation in 28% (384). These needle EMG changes are due to mild anterior horn cell lesions in this disease.

Ataxia Telangiectasia (Louis-Barr Syndrome)

Ataxia telangiectasia is a heredofamilial syndrome transmitted by an autosomal recessive gene. The disease begins during infancy, and the main clinical features are progressive cerebellar ataxia, oculocutaneous telangiectasia, and frequent sinopulmonary infections. The nerve conduction abnormalities are identical with those found in Friedreich's ataxia (383, 392) and are related to loss of the larger myelinated fibers in the peripheral nerves. The needle EMG shows signs of denervation in the distal muscles.

Bassen-Kornzweig's Syndrome

Bassen-Kornzweig's syndrome is a rare disorder clinically manifested early in childhood with cerebellar ataxia, loss of proprioception, areflexia, retinitis pigmentosa, malabsorption, acanthocytosis, and a-β-lipoproteinemia. The nerve conduction abnormalities are identical with *those found in Friedreich's ataxia* (393 395). Two recent studies, each dealing with three cases, showed almost identical findings: absent sensory CNAPs, or a diminution in the sensory CNAP amplitude with a slight slowing in sensory NCV, in the presence of normal motor nerve conduction (396, 397). The needle EMG, however, showed subclinical signs of partial chronic denervation in both studies. The sural nerve biopsy consistently showed a decreased number of large fibers in three cases. In Wichman et al.'s three patients, the serum vitamin E level was extremely low (396). There is now good evidence for believing that the neurologic features associated with a-β-lipoproteinemia are related to vitamin E deficiency (398).

Olivopontocerebellar Atrophy (OPCA)

This is a chronic progressive cerebellar ataxia with onset in adult or late middle life characterized by progressive cerebellar ataxia of the trunk and limbs. It is variably associated with extrapyramidal features, disorders of eye movement, tremor of the head and trunk, and scanning speech. The reflexes are usually normal, but knee and ankle jerks may be lost and extensor responses may occur. In a study of 19 patients, McLeod and Evans reported normal motor and sensory nerve conduction studies in 10, mild slowing of motor NCV in one or more nerves and impaired sensory nerve conduction (predominantly reduced amplitude) in six cases, and impairment of sensory nerve conduction alone in three patients (399). Rossi et al. found a decrease in sensory CNAP amplitude and a slight slowing of sensory NCV in seven patients and slow motor NCV in four of nine cases of OPCA (400). The nerve biopsy showed a slight reduction of the large myelinated fibers in two cases. In eight OPCA patients with deficient glutamate dehydrogenase (GDH), Chokroverty et al. found reduced sensory CNAP amplitude or absent nerve potentials in the sural nerves, reduced CNAP sensory amplitude in the median and ulnar nerves, and low CMAP in the peroneal nerves (401). The above electrophysiological findings are best explained by the degeneration of dorsal root ganglia and anterior horn cells (402).

Peripheral Neuropathy in Progressive Central Nervous Disorders

There are many progressive central nervous system (CNS) diseases associated with peripheral neuropathy. It is often difficult to identify peripheral neuropathy on clinical grounds alone because of the superimposed CNS symptoms. Thus, nerve conduction has been used to identify peripheral neuropathy in patients suspected of these disorders. Often because of easy access to peripheral nerves, the sural nerve biopsy has been employed as a diagnostic aid in these disorders.

Metachromatic Leukodystrophy (Aryl-Sulfatase Deficiency)

Metachromatic leukodystrophy is a rare demyelinating disorder of the central nervous system (CNS) and peripheral nerves caused by deficiency of aryl-sulfatase. Pathologically, this disorder is diagnosed by the presence of metachromatic granules in the CNS white matter and peripheral nerves. Among five different types, the late infantile form of metachromatic leukodystrophy is the most common, occurring between the ages of 1 and 4 years. Severe mental regression, ataxia, hypertonia, flaccid paraplegia with pyramidal signs, peripheral neuropathy, and optic atrophy are characteristic clinical features. Nerve conduction abnormalities in this disorder are characterized by the *demyelinating neuropathy pattern: marked motor NCV slowing (below 25 m/sec) and absent sensory CNAPs* (403 407). The same nerve conduction findings have been reported in juvenile cases (408). The needle EMG usually showed chronic denervation.

Globoid Leukydystrophy (Krabbe's Disease; Galactosylceramidase Deficiency)

Globoid leukodystrophy or Krabbe's disease is another leukodystrophy involving the CNS and peripheral nerves. This disorder is of autosomal recessive inheritance and caused by a deficiency of galactosylceramidase. Pathologically, the CNS shows diffuse demyelination and the presence of large multinucleated "globoid" cells. Peripheral nerve pathology is typical of segmental demyelination (409, 410). Nerve conduction abnormalities are characteristic of *demyelinating neuropathy:* marked slowing in motor (below 25 m/sec) (410, 411–413) and sensory NCVs (below 25 m/sec) (411). Sensory CNAP was absent (410) or low in amplitude in this disorder (414). Slowing of nerve conduction may be detectable as early as 7 weeks postnatally (413). Cases with a later onset and a slower course also occur. Thomas et al. reported a patient with onset in early childhood and clinical features resembling a spinocerebellar degeneration accompanied by demyelinating neuropathy (410).

Adrenoleukodystrophy and Adrenomyeloneuropathy

This disorder occurs as a sex-linked recessive adrenal insufficiency and progressive myelopathy in young males. Associated symptoms may be peripheral neuropathy, cerebellar ataxia, and dementia. The disorder is associated with the accumulation of very long-chain fatty acids, particularly with a 25- and 26-carbon chain length. In five patients, a spectrum of nerve conduction abnormalities was observed: in three patients with asymptomatic neuropathy, normal or mildly slow motor and sensory NCVs were observed; in a patient with mild neuropathy, NCV was mildly slow; in one case with definite peripheral neuropathy, a moderately slow NCV was indicative of *demyelinating neuropathy* (415). Moderate slowing in motor NCV in peroneal and posterior tibial nerves was also found in four patients in another series (416).

Palizaeus-Merzbacher Disease

This disorder is a sex-linked recessive, slowly progressive, white-matter disease with onset in infancy. Pendular nystagmus, cerebellar ataxia, and spasticity are prominent clinical features. Mild slowing (39–32 m/sec) in motor NCV and low-amplitude or absent CNAPs were found in this disorder (417).

Infantile Axonal Dystrophy (Seitelberger Disease)

Infantile neuroaxonal dystrophy (INAD) is an autosomal recessive disorder characterized by infantile onset of slowly progressive upper and lower motor neuron dysfunction associated with visual and other sensory deficits. Mild slowing (36 m/sec) in motor NCV was found in one case (418).

Neuronal Ceroid Lipofuchscinosis (Batten-Spielmeyer-Vogt Disease)

This rare disease is characterized by a progressive myoclonic convulsions, blindness, and dementia due to neuronal ceroid lipofuchscinosis in the gray matter. Usually the onset occurs from late infancy to adulthood. Pyramidal, extrapyramidal and cerebellar dysfunction appear late. Slight decrease in sensory NCV (19% average) was reported in 75% of 23 cases (419).

Cockayne's Syndrome

This rare autosomal recessively inherited disorder is characterized by onset of disease after the 1st year of life, "bird face," progeria, cutaneous photosensitivity, growth and mental retardation, ataxia, pigmentary retinopathy, blindness, deafness, and basal ganglia calcification. Peripheral neuropathy has been documented in recent years (420, 421). The sural nerve biopsy showed demyelinating neuropathy (420, 421). Nerve conduction abnormalities are characterized by *demyelinating neuropathy with uniform slowing* (420). Markedly slow motor NCV (less than 25 m/sec) was reported (420, 421). Sural CNAP amplitude was reduced and latency was prolonged (420). Sensory NCV in the ulnar nerve was markedly slow in one case (421).

Cerebrotendinous Xanthomatosis

Cerebrotendinous xanthomatosis is a rare hereditary disease characterized by xanthomas of tendons, dementia, and a progressive spinocerebellar syndrome. Peripheral neuropathy is not clinically obvious but has been documented electrophysiologically. The sural nerve biopsy showed demyelinating neuropathy (422, 423). In three cases, nerve conduction studies showed *demyelinating neuropathy*: slow motor NCVs in the peroneal and posterior tibial nerves (12–34 m/sec) and in the median nerve (38–40 m/sec) (422). Sensory CNAPs were absent in the legs. In Katz et al.'s case, NCV was slow in the legs (31–34 m/sec) (423). Kuritzky et al. also found slow motor NCVs in the legs (26–39 m/sec) in four cases and absent sural CNAPs in two (424).

Xeroderma Pigmentosa

Xeroderma pigmentosa is an autosomal-recessive neurocutaneous disorder characterized by cutaneous photosensitivity and skin cancers. Neurological abnormalities include mental retardation, seizures, cerebellar ataxia, spasticity, choreoathetosis and peripheral neuropathy. Motor and sensory NCVs were normal or slightly slow and sensory CNAPs might be reduced (425–427). Denervation changes were present on needle EMG (425). This is caused by a selective loss of large myelinated fibers (426, 427).

Familial Amyloid Neuropathy

Peripheral neuropathy is a prominent feature in four types of inherited amyloidosis. All show an autosomal dominant inheritance pattern. Amyloid deposits in the endoneurium, perineurium, and epineurium, and around the vessels is pathognomonic of amyloid neuropathy. Axonal degeneration is the predominant feature (428) (same as 355). Nerve conduction findings are typical of *axonal degeneration.*

1. *Type 1 (Portuguese; Andurade type).* Onset is insidious, usually in the 3rd or 4th decade of life. Sensory neuropathy of the legs, preferentially affecting pain and temperature sensations, and autonomic neuropathy are the most prominent clinical features. The most prominent nerve conduction abnormality is the markedly abnormal sensory CNAP (either absent potential or reduced amplitude) in the presence of normal or mildly slow motor NCV (428–430). The most extensive electrophysiological findings were reported by Sales-Luis (430), who used the near-nerve needle technique to record the sensory CNAP. The motor nerve conduction was normal or mildly slow (above 37 m/sec in peroneal nerves and above 40 m/sec in median nerves), and the CMAP was decreased amplitude and polyphasic in shape. The most prominent abnormality was observed in the sensory nerve conduction: an absent CNAP in the distal sural nerve, an absent CNAP or reduced amplitude of CNAP in the proximal sural and median nerves, and a normal or slightly decreased sensory NCV when the CNAP was recordable. Sales-Luis (430) concluded that his findings were indicative of a peripheral neuropathy with predominantly axonal damage which first affects the distal segments of the sensory fibers and then the motor fibers.

2. *Type 2 (Indiana; Rukavian type).* This form begins in the 4th decade, frequently with carpal tunnel syndrome, and is relatively slow in progression. Sensory and autonomic neuropathy may follow. Carpal tunnel syndrome is confirmed electrophysiologically by the marked prolongation of terminal latency and abnormal sensory nerve potential (either absent or slow NCV) over the finger-wrist segment of the median nerve. A minimal decrease in motor NCV in the forearm segment of the median nerve was reported (431, 432). Sales Luis also provided evidence that suggested that nerve conduction abnormalities may be present before the disease becomes clinically overt. This early diagnosis may provide assistance in genetic counseling (433).

3. *Type 3 (Iowa; Van Allen type).* Onset is in the 3rd or 4th decade. Progressive painful distal sensorimotor polyneuropathy is most typical. Autonomic involvement is less obtrusive. No data for the nerve conduction are available, although findings typical of axonal degeneration are expected.

4. *Type 4 (Finnish; Meretoja type).* Cranial neuropathy associated with a corneal lattice dystrophy and cutaneous laxity are the cardinal features. There are only mild manifestations in other systems. Onset is usually in the 5th decade, and progression is slow. In one study, there was EMG evidence of denervation in the facial muscles and the tongue and increased latency in the facial nerve (434). In the limbs, the needle EMG showed mild signs of chronic denervation. Motor NCV in the extremities was normal except for two instances of a mild carpal tunnel syndrome. Sensory NCV was normal, but the amplitude of the sensory CNAP was reduced.

Other Hereditary Neuropathies

Tangier's Disease (High-Density Lipoprotein Deficiency)

Tangier's disease, a rare disorder, is characterized by tonsillar hypertrophy (bright yellow-orange), hepatosplenomegaly, high-density lipoprotein deficiency, and peripheral neuropathy (435, 436). Peripheral nerve involvement has been encountered in approximately one-half the patients diagnosed with Tangier's disease. Three variants of this neuropathy have been recognized (437): (*a*) relapsing multifocal neuropathy (438, 439); (*b*) the pseudosyringomyelic form (438 440); and (*c*) symmetrical polyneuropathy (441, 442). The pathology of the peripheral nerves is also different in each variant: demyelination in multifocal neuropathy, axonal degeneration of smaller fibers in the pseudosyringomyelic form and loss of larger myelinated fibers in symmetrical polyneuropathy. In relapsing multifocal neuropathy, normal or mildly slow motor and sensory NCVs were observed (438, 439). In the pseudosyringomyelic type, the sensory CNAP was usually absent and motor NCV was either absent or moderately slow (437–440). The absence of sensory CNAPs is important in distinguishing this form of Tangier's disease from true syringomyelia, in which CNAPs are well preserved. In symmetrical polyneuropathy, the motor NCVs were all found to be normal in one case (441), whereas in another case they were normal in the upper extremities but slow in the lower limbs (442).

Mucopolysaccharidosis II Peripheral Neuropathy (Hunter Syndrome)

Hunter syndrome, a sex-linked recessive trait, is characterized by short stature, coarse features, large head, deafness, skeletal deformities, cardiac abnormalities, protuberant abdomen with hepatosplenomegaly and umbilical hernia, intellectual impairment, skin lesions, and other features. Large amounts of acid mucopolysaccharides are stored in the tissues and excreted in the urine, due to deficiency of L-iduronosulfate sulfatase. In this disorder, multiple entrapment neuropathies are the classic neuropathic manifestations (443–445). Carpal tunnel syndrome is most commonly reported, followed by cubital tunnel syndrome. Electrophysiological findings are typical of carpal tunnel syndrome or cubital tunnel syndrome, respectively (443, 445). Sural nerve biopsy showed zebra bodies in the Schwann cell cytoplasm (443, 445).

Fabry's Disease (Angiokeratoma Corporis Diffusum)

Fabry's disease is a sex-linked recessive disorder characterized clinically by a painful sensory neuropathy, diminished sweating, a purplish maculopapular rash over the lower torso, corneal opacities, and eventual renal failure and hypertension. Ceramide accumulates in many tissues, including the peripheral nerves, because of a deficiency of ceramidetrihexosidase. *Motor and sensory nerve conductions are normal in this condition,* which is most likely due to the predominant loss of unmyelinated and small myelinated axons (446, 447). However, Sheth and Swick observed mild slowing in ulnar motor and peroneal motor NCVs in four patients affected with Fabry's disease (448).

Chediak-Higashi Syndrome

The Chediak-Higashi syndrome is an unusual inherited disease characterized by the presence of massive granulations in leukocytes of the peripheral blood and bone marrow, defective pigmentation of hair and skin, anemia, leukopenia, thrombocytopenia, marked susceptibility to infection, and a lymphoreticular malignancy. One case report of peripheral neuropathy was recorded (449). Motor NCVs in the involved nerves ranged from 30 to 32 m/sec. Conduction block was noted between the distal and proximal stimulation sites.

Niemann-Pick Disease

Niemann-Pick disease is an inborn error of lipid metabolism characterized by an accumulation of sphingomyelin in various organs caused by a deficiency of the enzyme sphingomyelinase. This disorder includes failure to thrive, hepatosplenomegaly, and intellectual deterioration in the first year of life. Peripheral neuropathy was reported in one patient (450), who also had striking hypotonia, areflexia, and marked slowing in motor NCVs (7.3–19.8 m/sec). Sural nerve biopsy showed the Schwann cells to be filled with numerous cytoplasmic bodies.

Giant Axonal Neuropathy

Giant axonal neuropathy, recently described, is a unique disorder characterized by giant axonal swellings in the nerve (451). Common clinical features include distal symmetrical progressive polyneuropathy with ataxia, onset at age 2–3 years, tightly curled hair, bilateral plantar responses, abnormal electroencephalogram (EEG), but with mental deterioration in some patients. It is probably of autosomal-recessive inheritance. This may be a general disorder of intermediate filaments (452).

Nerve conduction data are available for a few cases (452–456). The prominent finding is abnormal sensory nerve conduction: either an absent or reduced-amplitude CNAP. This sensory abnormality was reported in all cases. Mixed nerve conduction was normal in one case, motor NCVs were normal or mildly reduced, and in one case no response was obtained in peroneal and posterior tibial nerves (453). Needle EMG showed changes of chronic denervation.

Immunologically Mediated Neuropathies

Guillain-Barré Syndrome (Acute Postinfectious Neuropathy: Acute Inflammatory Demyelinating Neuropathy)

The Guillain-Barré syndrome (GBS) is an acutely evolving areflexic and usually symmetrical neuropathy that is commonly associated with antecedent infection and a high CSF protein, and which reaches its maximum severity within 4 weeks. The mandatory diagnostic criteria of GBS include a progressive motor weakness of more than one limb and areflexia; supportive diagnostic criteria include progressive motor weakness reaching the nadir by 4 weeks, elevated spinal fluid protein with 10 or fewer cells/mm^3, and nerve conduction evidence of demyelination (457). An antecedent event is evident within 1 month in 70% of cases, most commonly a respiratory tract infection or gastroenteritis. GBS has been associated with AIDS, Lyme disease, Hodgkin's disease, and non-Hodgkin's lymphoma (458). The pathological changes in peripheral nerves in GBS are those of primary demyelination and endoneurial inflammatory cells (Fig. 22.9) (459).

Electrophysiological studies have been found useful in diagnosing this disorder (Fig. 22.10). Nerve conduction abnormalities are observed in 81–100% of patients (Table

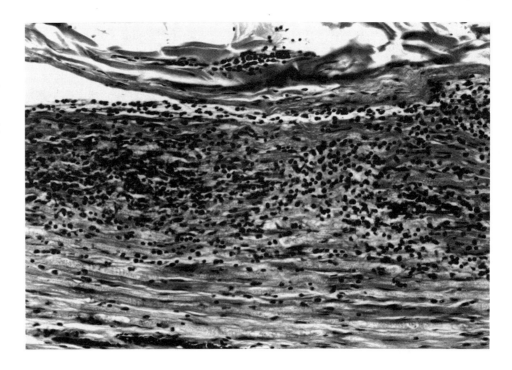

Figure 22.9. Endoneurial inflammatory cells in the Guillain-Barré syndrome. Mononuclear inflammatory cells are scattered in the epineurial space. At the top, minimal perivascular collections of inflammatory cells are noted in the perineurial space. Paraffin section, H & E, × 200. (From Oh SJ. Diagnostic usefulness and limitations of the sural nerve biopsy. Yonsei Medical Journal 1990;31:15.)

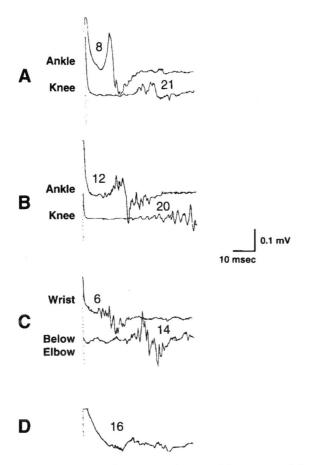

Figure 22.10. Conduction block. **A** and **B**, Abnormal temporal dispersion and slow NCVs typical of acquired demyelinating neuropathy in the GBS. Low CMAP amplitudes are also obvious. **A**, Peroneal nerve. **B**, Posterior tibial nerve. **C**, Ulnar nerve. **D**, Facial nerve. Numbers on the left represent the terminal latencies in msec. Numbers on the right represent the NCVs by m/sec.

Table 22.15.
Nerve Conduction Abnormalities in the Guillain-Barré Syndrome

			Percent of Cases	
Investigator	Tests Performed[a]	Normal	Mild Abnormality	Moderate/Marked Abnormality
Lambert and Mulder (465) (N = 49)[b]	Motor: M, U, P	15	25	61
McLeod et al. (467) (N = 242)	Motor: M, U, P	9	42	49
	Sensory: M, U	24	76	
Eisen and Humphreys (464) (N = 25)[c]	Motor: M, U, T	19	19	62
	Sensory: M, U	42	58	
Ramon and Taori (468) (N = 50)	Motor: M, U, T	18	14	68
	Sensory: M, R, S	32	68	
Cerra and Johnson (490) (N = 23)	Motor: U, M, P, T	0	100	
De Jesus (463) (N = 77)	Motor: M, P	0	18	82
	Sensory: M, P[d]	0	100	
Bradshaw and Jones (462) (N = 24)[e]	Motor: M, U, P, T	0	39	61
	Sensory:	30	70	
Roper et al. (461) (N = 113)	Motor: U, M, P, T	1	22	77
	Sensory: M, U	33	67	
Albers and Kelly (476) (N = 70)	Motor: U, M, P, T	0	13	87
	Sensory: M, S	35	65	

[a]Nerves: M, median. U, ulnar. P, peroneal. T, posterior tibial. S, sural.
[b]Number of patients.
[c]Subacute cases are included.
[d]Sensory NCV with needle.
[e]Children.

22.15). Recent studies showed nerve conduction abnormalities in 99–100% of patients (460–462). This may be due to the performance of more extensive nerve conduction studies, including the F-wave study. Because the primary pathological process is demyelination, it is expected that the typical electrophysiological patterns of *segmental demyelination* would be seen.

Compared with the mean values for control subjects, the patient with GBS has a statistically significant increase in distal motor latency and slowing of motor conduction as well as frequent abnormalities in sensory or mixed nerve potentials. However, the mean latencies and motor NCVs are not typical of demyelinating neuropathy according to the electrophysiological criteria; rather, there are a variety of patterns of nerve conduction abnormalities in GBS (460, 461, 463–468).

Diffuse slowing of conduction is the most common pattern encountered (465, 469) and is noted in the proximal and distal segments of the nerves, accompanied by a dispersion phenomenon and conduction block of some fibers.

Marked slowing of motor conduction velocity (35 m/sec in median and ulnar nerves or 30 m/sec in peroneal and posterior tibial nerves, or prolongation of distal motor latency in median and ulnar nerves beyond 6.0 msec and in peroneal and posterior tibial nerves beyond 10.0 msec) is characteristic of segmental demyelination and is found in 49–82% of patients (Table 22.15). On the other hand, normal nerve conduction is reported in up to 19% of patients, and mild nerve conduction abnormalities in 14–42% of patients. Thus, *a wide spectrum* of nerve conduction abnormalities is more characteristic of GBS, most likely reflecting the varying degree and location of the demyelination. Normal nerve conduction in the distal segment can be explained by the limited pathological involvement of the proximal segment, or the root, of the peripheral nerves. Mild nerve conduction abnormalities are seen in mild demyelination and will not differentiate between demyelinating neuropathy and axonal neuropathy unless the conduction block or dispersion phenomenon typical of demyelination is observed.

Even when the slowing of conduction is diffuse in GBS, the pattern of abnormalities is not homogeneous along the entire length of the nerves (470). Lambert and Mulder (465) stressed that the slowing was often most pronounced at common sites of nerve compression, and in some patients, interference with nerve conduction was predominantly at these sites. Miyoshi and Oh (469) compared median and ulnar motor and mixed nerve conduction between wrist-elbow and elbow-axilla segments and found more prominent and frequent slowing of NCV in the proximal segments, suggesting that the demyelination is more pronounced proximally.

Others have reported similar observations (471). Roper et al. also reported three common patterns of nerve conduction abnormalities: proximal conduction block (persistently absent or decreased F-wave in the presence of motor NCV > 80% of the normal lower limit) in 27% of cases, proximal block associated with a distal lesion in 22%, and generalized slowing in 22% (461). Thus, a *nonuniform demyelinating neuropathy* pattern is most typical in GBS, though this pattern is not observed in all cases.

Within the first 2 weeks, when the motor NCV is often within the normal range or only slightly reduced, conduction block and abnormal temporal dispersion are helpful in establishing the presence of demyelination. Brown and Feasby studied this issue in 25 patients with GBS (472). Motor NCV was within the normal range in the majority, even in the peroneal nerve, of these patients. In 13 of 19 nerves tested, there was evidence of generalized conduction block in at least one motor nerve; and in 15 of the 20 motor nerves in which such a block was demonstrable, the decline of the CMAP amplitude between the most proximal and distal sites of stimulation in the ulnar, median, and peroneal nerves exceeded 50%. On the basis of these observations, Brown and Feasby proposed that *acute paralysis in GBS is caused mainly by conduction block* (472).

Sensory nerve conduction abnormalities are less often seen in GBS, being observed in 56–76% of cases in contrast to the 80–100% of cases in which motor nerve conduction abnormalities are found (460–462, 464, 467). The most common sensory nerve conduction abnormality was a reduced or absent sensory CNAP (460, 467). The sensory NCV was less often abnormal (467). Normal distal sensory nerve conduction was observed in two-thirds of patients with an isolated proximal block in the motor conduction but was uncommon among those with generalized slowing (461). This finding indicates that the *motor neuropathy pattern of nerve conduction abnormalities is present in 15–35% of cases,* especially in the first 2 weeks of disease. According to Albers et al., a sensory nerve conduction abnormality was found in 32% of cases and a motor nerve conduction abnormality in 89% in the first 2 weeks (460). These figures are in contrast to sensory conduction abnormality in 83% and motor conduction abnormality in 89% in the later study.

Mixed nerve conduction abnormalities are more frequent than motor conduction abnormalities in the median and ulnar nerves, especially in the proximal segments (105). McLeod et al. found a significant reduction of mixed CNAP amplitudes but no significant prolongation of latencies in the peroneal nerves (467).

In recent years the F-wave has been used by several electromyographers as a means of measuring proximal motor conduction in GBS (473–475) (Table 22.15). Kimura and Butzer (473) used the F-wave conduction velocity as a measure of proximal conduction between the axilla and spinal cord in nine patients with mild GBS. In four of their nine patients, F-wave conduction velocity was slow despite normal or borderline distal motor nerve conduction velocities. King and Ashby (474), using techniques similar to Kimura's, also studied the F-wave in motor fibers of the ulnar nerve in 11 patients with GBS. They found that in two patients the conduction velocity in the proximal segment was disproportionately reduced, whereas in one of these the NCV in the distal segment was within normal limits. Lachman et al. (475) measured the F-wave latencies to the abductor pollicis brevis and the H-reflex latency to the soleus muscle in 11 patients with GBS. In two patients the F-wave latency was abnormal, although the distal motor NCV was within the normal range.

The F-wave study is therefore *of value* in establishing the diagnosis in some patients with GBS in whom the distal conduction velocities are normal, especially early in the course of disease (476). Furthermore, these studies support the hypothesis that the central segment of the peripheral nerves is predominantly involved in some patient.

In GBS, facial nerve involvement is common. This involvement is also confirmed by the electrophysiological study of the facial nerve. Facial nerve latency was abnormal (delayed or absent) in 77–79% of tested nerves (477, 478). Kimura observed that delayed conduction was associated with clinical facial weakness in a majority of cases (478). The blink-reflex showed abnormal responses (delay or absence of the early response) in 62–71% of tested patients, indicating that the blink reflex study does not have any advantage over the facial nerve latency test as a diagnostic test. Roper et al. observed abnormal blink reflex in 46% of 56 patients, all but one of whom had facial weakness (461). Autonomic testing showed absent sympathetic skin response in 17% of 23 cases and an abnormal R-R interval (461). No patients with abnormal autonomic testing had profound clinical dysautonomia.

To increase the electrodiagnostic sensitivity in GBS, it is important to remember the following facts:

1. The NCV abnormalities are often absent or far less marked during the first few days of the disease than they are 3–4 weeks later (467). Usually, the maximum nerve conduction abnormalities are observed at the time of a patient's maximum disability (479, 480). Albers et al. found the maximum abnormalities for the motor nerve conduction during the 3rd week and for the sensory nerve conduction during the 4th week (460). Serial nerve conduction studies are essential in some patients in whom an earlier study showed normal findings or only minor abnormalities.

2. Several different nerves should be studied. In McLeod et al.'s study (467), 34 of 114 patients (30%) had normal conduction in some nerves and abnormalities in others. The greater the number of nerves tested, the higher the percentage of abnormalities noted. In McLeod et al.'s study (467), abnormalities were present in 50% of patients when the test was done on one nerve, in 66.6% when performed on two nerves, and 92.3% when three nerves were tested.

3. The entire segment of a nerve should be tested, including the proximal segment (469). The F-wave study should be included in the workups of any suspected cases of GBS.

4. Mixed and sensory nerve conduction studies should be included in the study. Even though sensory impairment is less prominent in GBS, sensory and mixed nerve conduction abnormalities

are common (105, 460 462, 467, 477). Ludin and Tackmann (481) stated that the slowing of sensory conduction and abnormalities in potential configuration can also be found in patients with no sensory symptoms, and that such findings can be significant in the differential diagnosis between GBS and acute anterior poliomyelitis.

No apparent correlation exists between the degree of impairment of conduction and the severity of clinical symptoms in a group of patients with GBS (467, 469, 482). This finding reflects the variability of degree and distribution of demyelination in the peripheral nerve (459). Patients with demyelination in the roots and proximal segments of nerves may be severely paralyzed but have normal distal nerve conduction. Conduction may be mildly slowed in patients in whom demyelination is mild. In contrast, only minor clinical disability may be present in some patients who have severe nerve conduction slowing. Miyoshi and Oh (469) did not find any correlation between the degree of conduction abnormalities and the CSF protein level or the duration of the acute illness.

There are four views in regard to the prognostic value of the nerve conduction abnormalities. Eisen and Humphreys (464) found that patients with an acute progression of neurological deficit in the face of normal electrophysiological results throughout the illness recovered rapidly. The mean duration to complete recovery for this group was 5 weeks, compared with 25 weeks for the group of patients with conduction abnormalities. On the other hand, McQuillen (480) found the reverse to be true: There is a strong negative correlation between the degree of slowing and the length of the illness. The slowest conduction abnormalities were associated with the shortest clinical courses. McLeod et al. (467, 482) observed that there is no statistical correlation between the degree of impairment of conduction at the time of diagnosis and the period of disability or the clinical disability at follow-up examinations. The reason for this diversity of observations is not clear. Our findings are more concordant with those of McLeod (482).

Recent studies showed that *reduced distal CMAP amplitude is a predictor of poor outcome* even when motor conduction studies are performed early in the course of the disease (483–485). Cornblath et al. stated that a mean distal CMAP amplitude of 0–20% of the lower limit of normal is associated with a markedly increased probability of a poor outcome when the test was done during the first 30 days of illness (483). Miller et al. also observed that the most powerful predictor of a poor outcome was reduced CMAP amplitude (less than 10% of the lower limit of normal) and that the ideal time for the test may be 7 days after the nadir is reached (484). Winer et al. found a significant association between poor outcome and absent or small CMAP amplitude in the abductor pollicis brevis muscle (485). These findings, together with the needle EMG findings, support the general knowledge that segmental demyelination is correlated with relatively rapid recovery, whereas findings of severe axonal degeneration are correlated with slow recovery. Caution is expressed in this regard because the distal CMAP may be relatively spared in the early phase of the disease despite severe axonal degeneration later (486). Other predictors of outcome were the patient's age, time from onset of disease (7 days or less), and the need for ventilatory support (487).

There is uniform agreement that the needle EMG findings are *more valuable* than the nerve conductions in assessing the prognosis in GBS. Three studies have reported that profuse fibrillations and positive sharp waves within the first 4 weeks of the illness, with or without nerve conduction abnormalities, are associated with a prolonged recovery time and more pronounced residual deficits (468, 482). These electrophysiological findings indicate that severe axonal degeneration has occurred. On the other hand, recovery was rapid and the quality of recovery was good in the group of patients whose electrophysiological findings were characterized by gross abnormalities in nerve conduction and an absence of fibrillation potentials during the entire course of their illness.

Serial nerve conduction studies during recovery have been undertaken by several researchers (471, 479, 480, 488). At the beginning of clinical improvement, the nerve conductions were still abnormal (489). Nerve conduction improvement was uniformly documented in all studied cases. Clinical improvement preceded electrophysiological improvement by several months. Conduction velocities usually remained abnormal at the time of complete clinical recovery and for some time thereafter (490), especially in the case of sensory and mixed nerve conductions (471, 488, 490). Analyzing nine patients from the literature (471, 480, 488) who had serial nerve conduction studies over a 1-year period, we found that clinical recovery was complete around 10 weeks after the onset of illness, whereas the nerve conduction recovery was complete only about 9 months after onset. The same analysis also showed that the maximum abnormalities in nerve conduction existed within the 8th week after the onset of the illness; the initial rapid nerve conduction recovery occurred between the 8th and 16th weeks; and this was followed by slower recovery over the next several months. McQuillen (480) and Humphrey (491) stated that the motor nerve conduction returned to normal at essentially the same time as the deep tendon reflexes.

A recent study also observed similar findings: resolution of conduction abnormalities began between weeks 6 and 10, with increased mean CMAP best reflecting functional clinical recovery (460).

In recent years, plasmapheresis has become the main mode of treatment for GBS since its effectiveness has been proven (492). It was found to be particularly effective for patients who received this treatment within 7 days of onset and for those who required mechanical ventilation. Electrophysiological studies during plasmapheresis are limited. In three patients who showed a rapid improvement with plasmapheresis, Berger et al. documented rapid improvement in the conduction block with root stimulation in the ulnar motor nerve conduction, indicating that rapid motor recovery early in the course of GBS can result from reversal of proximal conduction block (493).

Long-term follow-up studies of nerve conduction have been reported by a few researchers (480, 494, 495). An improvement in nerve conduction was documented in all cases at the final evaluation after a mean follow-up duration of 3 years (467). Most patients with GBS had normal nerve conduction studies at the follow-up examination several years after the illness. Nerve conduction abnormalities were observed in 17% (494) to 39% (467) of the clinically recovered patients. McLeod et al. (467) found no relationship between the residual clinical disability and NCV abnormalities in 18 patients at the time of final follow-up. On the other hand, Pleasure et al. (495) found a positive correlation in seven patients.

Axonal Form of GBS

Feasby et al. reported five patients with GBS who developed severe quadriplegia within 9 days of onset (496). All had very severe peripheral neuropathy with motor dysfunction greater than sensory dysfunction, inexcitable motor nerves, widespread fibrillation within 2–5 weeks of onset, and very poor recovery. Pathological studies of one patient who died revealed an acute axonal neuropathy. There was no perivascular cuffing with inflammatory cells or demyelination. In three of five cases, the spinal fluid protein was high. A major common feature distinguishing these cases from others with GBS was inexcitability of the motor nerves. Authors believe that the inexcitability of motor nerves, evidence of severe axonal degeneration, and the very poor recovery in these cases set them apart from the usual cases of GBS and that these cases constitute an *acute axonal form of GBS*. Whether these cases represent a variant of GBS or a separate disease entity remains to be settled. In the practical sense, however, it is important to *rule out other causes of acute axonal neuropathy* before one makes the diagnosis of an acute axonal form of GBS, because other axonal neuropathies can mimic GBS (497, 498).

Chronic Inflammatory Demyelinating Polyneuropathy (CIDP; Subacute Demyelinating Neuropathy; Chronic Relapsing Neuropathy)

In recent years chronic inflammatory demyelinating polyneuropathy (CIDP) has been clearly recognized as a separate entity on the basis of subacute progression of polyneuropathy, marked nerve conduction abnormalities, a high rate of relapse, and response to steroid treatment (499–502). The distinction between GBS and CIDP is shown in Table 22.16. There are two distinct groups in CIDP: monophasic and relapsing polyneuropathy. According to Oh's study, monophasic polyneuropathy was noted in 40% of patients (502). Childhood and infantile forms of CIDP have also been reported (503, 504).

The diagnosis of CIDP is based on the typical clinical features of: (*a*) subacute progression of diffuse polyneuropathy; (*b*) high spinal fluid protein level; and (*c*) marked nerve conduction abnormalities indicative of acquired demyelinating neuropathy. Diagnostic criteria for CIDP have recently been proposed (505). Four mandatory diagnostic criteria include motor-sensory neuropathy with hyporeflexia or areflexia, electrophysiological evidence of demyelination, nerve biopsy evidence of demyelination (Fig. 22.11), and the absence of cells in the spinal fluid (505). CIDP is now known to occur in association with other diseases: AIDS, dysproteinemia, and systemic lupus erythematosus.

It is important to recognize CIDP because this is one of the few polyneuropathies for which satisfactory treatment is available. According to our experience, this disorder cannot be diagnosed by clinical findings alone but requires electrophysiological

Table 22.16.
Differences Between the Guillain-Barré Syndrome and Chronic Inflammatory Demyelinating Polyneuropathy[a]

Features	Guillain-Barré Syndrome	CIDP
Onset	Acute; maximum neurological deficit in 2–3 weeks	Subacute; maximum neurological deficit in 1–12 months
Antecedent infection	Present in 70%	Absent
Cranial nerve deficit	Common	Rare
Respiratory muscle	Common	Rare
NCV	Normal or slightly slow in 50%; markedly slow in 50%	Markedly slow
Response to steroids	Not proved	Positive
Relapse	Rare	Common

[a]From Oh (692) with permission.

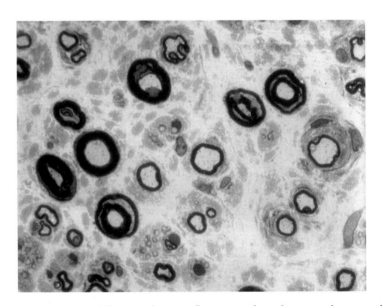

Figure 22.11. Remyelinated fibers in chronic inflammatory demyelinating polyneuropathy. About 50% of myelinated fibers are the remyelinated fibers characterized by thin myelin sheath in proportion to axon diameter. Roughly, the ratio between axon diameter and myelin thickness is 2:1. Semithin section, Toluidine blue, × 400. (From Oh SJ. Diagnostic usefulness and limitations of the sural nerve biopsy. Yonsei Medical Journal 1990;31:16.)

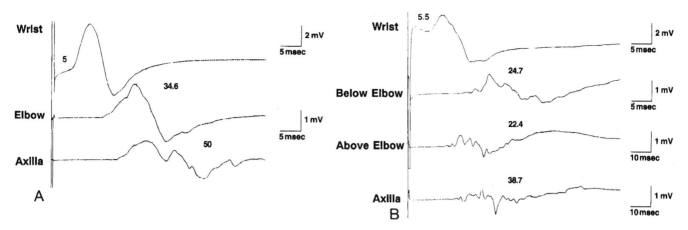

Figure 22.12. Conduction block, abnormal temporal dispersion, and nonuniform slowing of NCVs, typical of acquired demyelinating neuropathy, in CIDP. (**A**) Median nerve. (**B**) Ulnar nerve.

confirmation. The most helpful objective diagnostic finding is the typical pattern of *nonuniform demyelinating neuropathy* (Fig. 22.12).

The nerve conduction test in this disorder shows findings typical of extensive segmental demyelination. In Oh's study (502), the mean terminal latency in all tested nerves was about three times longer than normal, and the mean motor NCV in all tested nerves was less than 50% of the normal value. Sensory and mixed nerve CNAPs (with surface electrodes) were absent in almost all cases (499, 502, 506). Conduction block and/or the dispersion phenomenon were common findings. Marked slowing of the motor conduction velocity (35 m/sec in median and ulnar nerves or 30 m/sec in peroneal and posterior tibial nerves, or prolongation of the distal motor latency in median and ulnar nerves beyond 6.0 msec and in peroneal and posterior tibial nerves beyond 10.0 msec) was observed in all cases in three series (499, 502, 504), and in 22 of 23 patients in Prineas and McLeod's series (506). Ninety-three percent of cases had the slowest motor NCV (below 30 m/sec). Mean motor NCVs in CIDP were slower by 37–46% than the normal mean (507–509). Mean terminal latencies were prolonged by 43–167% of the normal mean (507, 508). Mean CMAP amplitudes were low by 52–67% of the normal mean amplitudes (508, 509). These findings are *consistent with demyelinating neuropathy*. This constency among investigators is in contrast to GBS, in which a wide spectrum of nerve conduction abnormalities is more characteristic. Dyck et al. (501) reported similar findings.

In CIDP the nerve conduction abnormalities are diffuse, involving the distal as well as the proximal segments of the nerves. The proximal segment was proportionately more impaired in 80% of cases (510). All tested nerves are affected in this disorder, though the degree of abnormality varies from nerve to nerve.

Marked abnormalities in sensory nerve conductions are noted in this disorder (488, 499, 502, 506). Sensory CNAPs were absent in the majority of patients, and a low sensory CNAP amplitude is a consistent finding (507–509). A slow sensory NCV was observed in a few exceptional cases (502, 506). Mixed nerve conduction is also markedly abnormal in this disorder (502, 506). In median and ulnar nerves, mixed nerve conduction was abnormal in all 10 cases: an absent CNAP in six and a slow NCV in four (502). Prineas and McLeod (506) were not able to record any mixed CNAPs in the peroneal nerve in any of their cases.

The F-wave and H-reflex were studied by Oh (510), who found their latencies to be either absent or markedly prolonged. Mean F-wave latency was prolonged by 48% of the normal mean (509). Thus, these late responses do not offer any additional diagnostic help. Facial nerve involvement is rare in this disorder. Electrophysiological studies show the facial nerve latency and the blink reflex to be normal in all tested cases (510). None of the patients studied had any cranial nerve involvement.

There is no correlation between the severity of disease and the motor nerve conduction abnormalities at the time of initial evaluation (506, 510). Conduction may be markedly abnormal in patients with minimal motor weakness but severe sensory impairment. Contrary to our observation, Dyck et al. (501) observed completely normal motor nerve conduction in patients with pure sensory impairment (see below). In our experience, nerve conduction abnormalities have no prognostic value, either for the monophasic group or the relapsing group.

CIDP has been treated with corticosteroids, immunosuppressives, plasma exchange, and intravenous human immunoglobulin (511, 512). Serial nerve conduction studies in a given patient reveal that the nerve conduction abnormalities generally improve during the period of clinical improvement (502, 504, 506). During treatment with corticosteroids, clinical improvement was accompanied by proportional electrophysiological improvement in two out of three cases. At the time of greatest clinical improvement, a significant improvement in distal latencies and nerve conduction velocities was observed compared with the initial values (502). However, in one-third of the patients followed, clinical improvement was not accompanied by proportional electrophysiological improvement, although no patients had worsening of nerve conduction during corticosteroid treatment.

In the monophasic group, the mean NCVs at the final evaluation were about 70% of normal mean values (502). In the relapsing group, mean NCVs were substantially abnormal, less than 50% of normal values, at final evaluation. These data may suggest the potential value of serial nerve conduction studies in the treatment of this disorder. Based on these data, we continued corticosteroid therapy in patients as long as their NCVs were substantially abnormal, regardless of their clinical status, in order to prevent relapse. None of our patients had normal nerve conduction even at their best clinical status.

Prineas and McLeod (506) observed that the conduction velocities increased during periods of clinical improvement. They stated that for the group as a whole there was poor correlation between slowing of motor NCVs in the nerves and the severity of muscle weakness. Dalakas and Engel (499) reported that although the motor NCV may improve during clinical remission, its degree is much less than that of clinical improvement, and in none of their 25 patients did it reach normal levels. With high-dose intravenous immunoglobulin treatment, Van Doorn et al. reported clinical improvement as well as insignificant improvement in the mean motor NCVs and CMAP amplitudes in the treated group compared with the untreated group (512).

Multifocal Demyelinating Neuropathy (Demyelinating Mononeuropathy Multiplex)

Multifocal demyelinating neuropathy (1) is described as a variety of CIDP. The clinical features are characterized by subacute progression of mononeuropathy multiplex (usually in the arm), eventually developing into asymmetrical sensorimotor neuropathy. CSF protein was elevated in two out of four tested cases. The key to the diagnosis is the nerve conduction study. Typically, the involved nerves show the electrophysiological characteristics of segmental demyelination, conduction block being most prominent. Two patients treated with steroids improved, whereas three untreated patients had static deficits or steady progression of symptoms.

Since then, more than 20 cases have been reported (1, 513, 514–521). Gradually the clinical and electrophysiological characteristics have emerged. The clinical features are typical of "mononeuropathy multiplex" (522) and pure motor weakness in 50% of the cases. Fasciculation was observed in 25% of the cases, and normal reflexes were elicited in 15% of the cases. Thus, sometimes these cases can mimic motor neuron disease (514, 515, 523). Spinal fluid protein was increased in one-third of the patients. Recent studies showed a high titer of GM1 antibodies in 50–80% of patients with multifocal demyelinating neuropathy (516, 524, 525). The sural nerve biopsy showed inflammatory cells in one-third and demyelination in 60% of cases. Nerve conduction abnormalities in this disorder are typical of *a nonuniform demyelinating neuropathy pattern with conduction block* in multiple nerves. It should be noted that conduction block is not present in all cases: conduction block was present in 90% of cases in the reported series and in 57% in our series (522). Conduction block was typically focal over short segments and was not confined to the usual sites of compression (1, 521). Sensory nerve conduction abnormalities (slow NCV or reduced CNAP amplitude) were observed in only one-third of patients. Many of these patients responded to immunotherapies, including steroid (1), cytoxan (516), plasma exchange (517), and intravenous gammaglobulin therapy (526).

Chronic Sensory Demyelinating Neuropathy (CSDN)

Chronic sensory demyelinating neuropathy (CSDN) has recently been reported as a sensory variant of CIDP in 10 cases (527–529). This entity is characterized by subacute or chronic progression, pure sensory neuropathy, high spinal fluid protein in the majority of cases, electrophysiological evidence of demyelination (Fig. 22.13), demyelination on sural nerve biopsy, and good response to immunotherapies in the progressive phase. Motor nerve conductions were abnormal in all cases and just as prominent as sensory nerve conduction abnormalities, although all patients had a pure sensory neuropathy. The most common abnormalities were a prolonged F-wave latency and slow motor

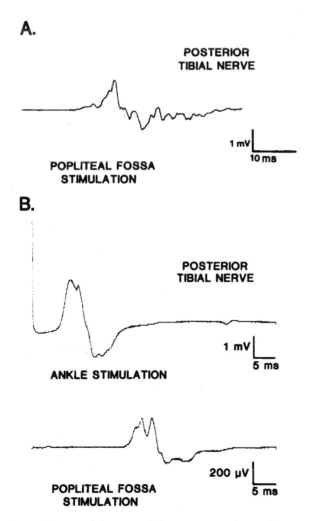

Figure 22.13. Abnormal temporal dispersion (**A**) in a CMAP with stimulation at the popliteal fossa and conduction block (**B**) in the posterior tibial nerve in a patient with chronic sensory demyelinating neuropathy. (From Oh SJ, Joy JL, Kuruoglu R. "Chronic sensory demyelinating neuropathy": chronic inflammatory demyelinating polyneuropathy presenting as a pure sensory neuropathy. J Neurol Neurosurg Psychiatry 1992;55:677.)

NCV. Electrophysiological evidence of demyelination was not widespread but was present in two or more nerves in all cases, confirming demyelinating neuropathy. Sensory nerve conduction was abnormal in all cases. The most common abnormality in sensory nerve conduction was slow NCV. Mixed nerve conduction was abnormal in most patients. The needle EMG showed chronic denervation in most cases. One patient experienced complete clinical and electrophysiological recovery with immunotherapies (577).

Fisher's Syndrome

Fisher's syndrome of acute ophthalmoplegia, ataxia, and areflexia is accepted by most authors as a variant of the Guillain-Barré syndrome (530). It is accompanied by a high CSF protein level and it has a benign course.

Guiloff studied nerve conduction in two cases with Fisher's syndrome in 1977 (531). The striking feature of these studies was the abnormality of sensory CNAPs. The motor and mixed NCVs were normal, and the H-reflex was absent. Subsequent studies confirmed the *prominent sensory nerve conduction abnormalities* in the presence of near-normal or normal motor nerve conduction (532–534). A review by Frosso and Daube showed that the sensory CNAP was either reduced or absent in the sural nerve in 70% of 20 cases, in the median nerve in 79% of 14 cases, and in the ulnar nerve in 84% of 18 cases (534–537). Reductions in sensory CNAP amplitudes far outweighed the degree of slowing. Seven patients had a moderate to severe reduction of median sensory CNAP, and eight had reduced or absent sural CNAP. The motor nerve conduction was abnormal in only 44% of 16 cases: mild slowing in 44% and low CMAP in 27% (531, 532, 534, 537). In five of seven patients in Fross and Daube's series, there was mild-to-moderate reduction of the facial CMAP amplitude without any measurable delay in conduction (534). Temporal dispersion or conduction block was not observed. Slow motor NCV to the degree of demyelination was not reported.

The blink reflex was abnormal in four of 13 tested cases (532, 534). Blink reflex R1 latencies were mildly prolonged in two patients and were absent with loss of corresponding R2 responses in two other patients in Fross and Daube's series (534). The blink reflex abnormalities were coincident with reduced facial CMAP amplitude. F-wave latency was normal in 25% of 20 cases (532, 534). Weiss and White reported a case in which slowing of 1A sensory conduction correlated directly with the degree of ataxia, without any impairment of motor or sensory nerve conduction (538).

EMG of limb muscles was relatively normal. Facial muscles were mildly abnormal in four of six patients, with fibrillations in two (534). There were more prominent changes in nine patients and fibrillation in one (532).

Thus, the pattern in Fisher syndrome seems to be more that of a *sensory axonal neuropathy or sensory neuronopathy with little electrophysiological evidence of demyelination*. These changes clearly contrast with the electrophysiological abnormalities seen in GBS with or without ophthalmoplegia. However, Weiss and White claimed that ataxia in this syndrome results from selective segmental demyelination of 1A afferent axons, and that the disorder is thus a variant of GBS (538). Gradual improvement in sensory and motor nerve conduction was documented over a 7-month period in one case (533).

Acute Sensory Neuropathy Syndrome

Sternman et al. (539) reported three patients who developed rapidly profound sensory ataxia, areflexia, and widespread sensory loss, primarily of large fiber modalities. There was no weakness. The CSF was acellular, and CSF protein was elevated in two patients. All had a severe static residual sensory deficit. No evidence of neoplastic disease has appeared during a 5-year follow-up. The nerve conduction studies showed findings typical of involvement of the dorsal root and gasserian ganglia: a slowed or absent sensory CNAP in the presence of normal motor nerve conduction.

Joy and Oh also reported four patients with sensory acute inflammatory demyelinating polyneuropathy (AIDP) who developed sensory neuropathy over a period ranging from hours to 3 weeks (540). Limb weakness was absent in all cases. Nerve conduction studies showed one or more of the following: slowing of NCV, increased temporal dispersion, conduction block, and markedly prolonged motor terminal latencies. Except for their predominant sensory manifestations, these patients resemble classic AIDP in their clinical course and electrophysiological features.

Chronic Ataxic Neuropathy

Chronic ataxic neuropathy is characterized by slow progression, distal paresthesia and sensory ataxia, normal strength, and a profound loss of proprioceptive and kinesthetic sensations (541, 542). This neuropathy is not different clinically from paraneoplastic subacute sensory neuropathy. However, carcinoma was not found in any of these patients. A serum monoclonal and polyclonal gammopathy was found in nine of 15 cases (541). Sural nerve biopsy in 13 cases showed moderate to marked loss of myelinated fibers of all diameters, with the loss particularly affecting the larger fibers. Clustering of small myelinated fibers, indicative of regeneration, was noted in three cases. These findings were secondary to the selective destruction of the dorsal root ganglion neuron. Electrophysiological studies showed the classic pattern of *"pure sensory neuronopathy"*: absent sensory CNAPs in the presence of normal needle EMG and motor nerve conduction findings (541, 542). Among nine patients with chronic ataxic neuropathy, Mamoli et al. found IgM monoclonal gammopathy of undetermined significance in four (543). Nerve biopsy showed primary axonal damage.

Steroid-Responsive Hereditary Neuropathy

Steroid-responsive hereditary neuropathy is a misnomer. It represents CIDP in patients with a preexisting hereditary motor and sensory neuropathy. In 1982, Dyck et al. reported seven patients with pes cavus and hammertoes and a positive family history of hereditary or asymptomatic neuropathy who seemed to have a progressive form of CIDP (544). These patients had high CSF protein. In two of three sural nerve biopsies, mononuclear cells were present. Motor NCVs were in the range of demyelination, at least in some nerves, and sensory CNAPs were absent or sensory NCV was reduced. In one case, abnormal temporal dispersion was observed. The most consistent finding in these cases was a good response to prednisone. In 1991, Bird and Sladky reported three children with the monophasic form of CIDP from families with dominantly inherited neuropathy (545). CSF protein was elevated, and the sural nerve biopsy showed mononuclear cells in all cases. Motor NCVs were markedly slow in two cases and minimally slow in one case. Conduction block was observed in one case. These reports suggest that CIDP can be superimposed on hereditary motor and sensory neuropathy and that steroid use is also effective in such cases. The sural nerve biopsy has been *a critical test* in documenting CIDP in these cases.

Sarcoid Neuropathy

Involvement of all parts of the nervous system is well recognized in sarcoidosis (Fig. 22.14), being observed in 5% of cases. The most frequently affected sites are the cranial nerves, particularly the 7th nerve, the meninges, and the muscles (546). Involvement of the peripheral nerves is rare, accounting for only 15% of cases with neurological involvement. All types of neuropathy have been reported—mononeuropathy, mononeuropathy multiplex, and polyneuropathy—although the most characteristic of sarcoidosis is mononeuropathy multiplex (547). Axonal degeneration was observed in Oh's case (548), and Nemni et al. (549) found axonal degeneration and segmental demyelination. According to our review (548), among seven patients in whom the actual values of NCV were available, minimal slowing (32 m/sec) of the motor NCV was reported in four cases, normal NCV in two, and moderate slowing in one (549). Sensory nerve conduction was abnormal: no potential, reduced amplitude, or mildly slow NCV in two cases (548, 549). Mixed CNAPs were absent in one case (549). Thus, all nerve

Figure 22.14. Sarcoid granuloma in sarcoid neuropathy. Noncaseating granuloma with many epitheloid cells and mononuclear inflammatory cells in the perineurial space in the upper half of figure. No granuloma or inflammatory cells are present in the perineurial space in the upper half of figure. No granuloma or inflammatory cells are present in the nerve fascicle itself in the lower half. Paraffin section, H & E, × 200. (From Oh SJ.Diagnostic usefulness and limitations of the sural nerve biopsy. Yonsei Medical Journal 1990;31:17.)

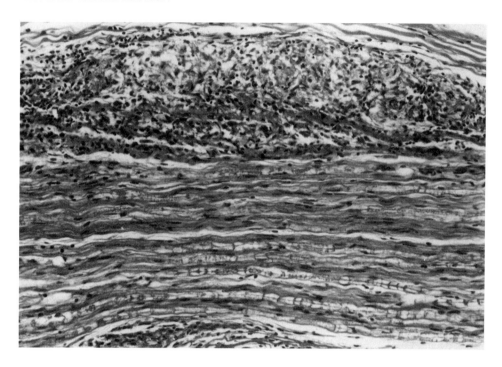

conduction findings are more consistent with *axonal degeneration,* which recent studies also confirmed (550, 551). With clinical improvement after steroid therapy, the motor, sensory, and mixed nerve conductions improved as well (549).

Neuropathies Associated with Autoantibodies

Neuropathies Associated with Anti-GM1 Antibodies

In recent years, anti-GM1 antibodies have been reported in the serum of patients with multifocal demyelinating neuropathy, sensory-motor peripheral neuropathy, motor neuropathy, and lower motor neuron syndromes (524, 552). Sadig et al. believe that these antibodies may be pathogenic because increased titers of anti-GM1 antibodies were found in particular neurologic syndromes and because clinical improvement was reported in some patients after therapeutic reduction of antibody concentrations (524). Among the various syndromes, multifocal demyelinating neuropathy seems to be most typical of neuropathies associated with anti-GM1 antibodies, a higher titer of GM1 antibodies (> 1:350) being found in 60–80% of patients with this neuropathy in one series (525) and a high titer of GM1 antibodies (> 1:800) in 50% of patients in another series (524). It should be noted that a high GM1 antibody titer has also been reported in 0% (524) to 10% (552) of patients with amyotrophic lateral sclerosis (ALS). IgM monoclonal gammopathy was found in 10–50% of patients with a high GM1 titer (524, 552). CSF protein was increased in seven of the 12 patients (524). According to Pestronk et al., this entity responds better to cyclophosphamide than to prednisone (516).

No detailed electrophysiological data were available in the aforementioned studies. However, according to summarized statements, *multifocal demyelinating neuropathy with conduction block* seems to be most typical of these neuropathies. In Kumar et al.'s series, multifocal neuropathy with conduction block was observed in 57% of patients, whereas a wide spectrum of electrophysiological abnormalities from denervation to sensorimotor neuropathy was observed in the remaining patients (524). According to Pestronk, a high titer of GM1 antibodies was found in 64% of patients with multifocal neuropathy with conduction block, which spared the sensory nerve fibers (552). In other distal and proximal lower motor neuron syndromes with a high GM1 antibody titer, the nerve conduction abnormalities of axonal neuropathy were said to be typical (552). However, no detailed data were presented.

Neuropathy Associated with Serum Antibodies to Myelin-Associated Glycoprotein (MAG)

In recent years, neuropathy associated with MAG has been reported (553–556). This neuropathy has distinct features: predominantly sensory abnormalities. IgM paraprotein, high CSF protein, and unsatisfactory response to immunotherapies (554–557). In 59% of 27 patients with neuropathy and IgM monoclonal gammopathy, antibodies to MAG were found in one series (558). The sural nerve biopsy showed demyelinating neuropathy (553–555). IgM kappa staining was demonstrated in the myelin border (555). Nerve conduction studies showed findings *typical of demyelinating neuropathy* in all cases (554–556): the motor NCV was markedly slow (554, 555); terminal latencies were markedly prolonged (554); sensory CNAPs were either absent or reduced in amplitude, but when present the sensory NCV was markedly slow (554). The blink reflex was abnormal in all of three tested cases: mildly prolonged latency in one and markedly prolonged latency in two cases (554).

Neuropathy Associated with Serum Antibodies to Sulfatide

Pestronk et al. described eight patients with a predominantly sensory polyneuropathy who had high-titer serum reactivity to sulfatide without a high-titer IgM binding to MAG (556). Two had an associated IgM paraprotein. Nerve conduction studies generally showed changes compatible with axonal disease but only minor, if any, evidence of demyelination. No other details were provided.

Neuropathy Associated with Anti-HU Antibody

The anti-HU antibody is associated with paraneoplastic syndromes connected with small-cell lung cancer. The dominant neurological syndrome associated with anti-HU antibody is *subacute sensory neuronopathy,* being observed in 86% of 14 cases (205). CSF protein was elevated in 93% of these cases, with pleocytosis in 21%. This neuropathy did not respond well to immunotherapy. Without presenting any detailed electrophysiological data, Anderson et al. reported that sensory nerve action potentials were reduced or absent, motor NCV was either normal or only mildly slow, and except in those patients with muscle weakness and wasting, the needle EMG did not show any denervation (205). These nerve conduction abnormalities are typical of the *sensory neuronopathy pattern.* A case of paraneoplastic encephalomyelitis simulating GBS was reported (559). The needle EMG showed widespread denervation with increased polyphasic MUPs and amplitude. Sensory CNAPs were not obtained. Motor NCV was slightly slowed.

Vasculitic Neuropathies

Peripheral neuropathy is common in systemic necrotizing vasculitis (Fig. 22.15). Systemic symptoms (malaise, weight loss, anorexia, and fever), multisystem involvement, and a high erythrocyte sedimentation rate (ESR) are typical of this disorder (5). Mononeuropathy multiplex is said to be most typical, but symmetrical or asymmetrical polyneuropathy is common (5); mononeuropathy is least common. Systemic necrotizing vasculitis is seen in many diseases (Table 22.17). Pathologically, vasculitic neuropathy is characterized by axonal degeneration (5, 560). Polyarteritis nodosa is a classic example of a systemic necrotizing vasculitis affecting small- and medium-sized arteries and producing systemic symptoms and multiple organ involvement. The predominantly involved organs are the peripheral nerves, kidneys, gastrointestinal tract, and liver.

Peripheral neuropathy occurs in varying frequency in association with many connective tissue diseases, ranging from 70% in polyarteritis nodosa to 1.5% in progressive systemic sclerosis (Table 22.17). Most of these are due to systemic necrotizing vasculitis.

Nerve conduction studies are *vital* to the workup of patients with systemic necrotizing vasculitis for two reasons. First, adequate nerve conduction tests can detect asymptomatic peripheral neuropathy. According to our series (5), 30–41% of patients had no

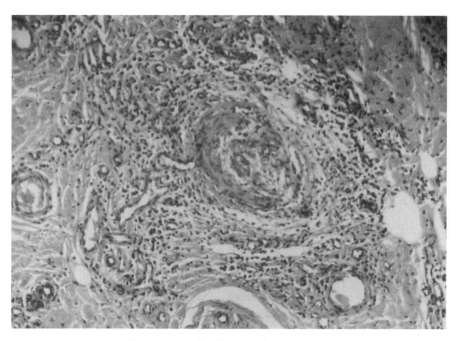

Figure 22.15. Active vasculitis. Intramural infiltration of mononuclear inflammatory cells, fibrinoid necrosis of musculorum layer, and near occlusion of vessel due to endothelial thickening are noted in an arteriole in the perineurial space. Paraffin section, H & E, × 400. (From Oh SJ. Diagnostic usefulness and limitations of the sural nerve biopsy. Yonsei Medical Journal 1990;31:7.)

Table 22.17.
Peripheral Neuropathy in the Vasculitic Syndromes[a]

Collagen Vascular Diseases	Frequency of Vasculitis (%)
Polyarteritis nodosa (697)	50–70
Churg-Strauss syndrome (698)	64
Wegener's granulomatosis	25
Lymphoid granulomatosis	15
Systemic lupus erythematosis (570)	2–18
Rheumatoid arthritis (699)	10
Hypersensitivity	10
Sjogren's syndrome (572)	9
Temporal arteritis (582)	5–14
Behcét syndrome	5
Progressive systemic sclerosis (700)	1.5
Hypereosinophilic syndrome (587)	14

[a]Unless otherwise stated, the figures are quoted from Moore and Cupps (697).

clinical signs indicative of peripheral neuropathy. Second, abnormal sural nerve conduction is a prerequisite to the demonstration of vasculitis on biopsy of this nerve. According to our experience, in all 15 patients in whom the sural nerve conduction was abnormal, vasculitic neuropathy was diagnosed by sural nerve biopsy. A later study of 47 cases showed abnormal sural nerve conduction in all cases, and the diagnosis of vasculitis was confirmed in all but one case by the sural nerve biopsy. Thus, it is recommended that abnormal sural nerve conduction be used as a guide in the nerve biopsy. This certainly will enhance the diagnostic yield of sural nerve biopsy. Nerve conduction abnormalities in vasculitic neuropathies are *typical of axonal degeneration* (Fig. 22.16) (5, 560–563).

In Hawke et al.'s series, mild to moderate slowing of motor NCV and/or reduced CMAP amplitude were most commonly observed (560). In our series, the CMAP amplitude was most severely reduced in the lower extremities, whereas in median and ulnar nerves the amplitude was more frequently normal (561). The needle EMG showed active denervation in the distal muscles of the involved limbs (562).

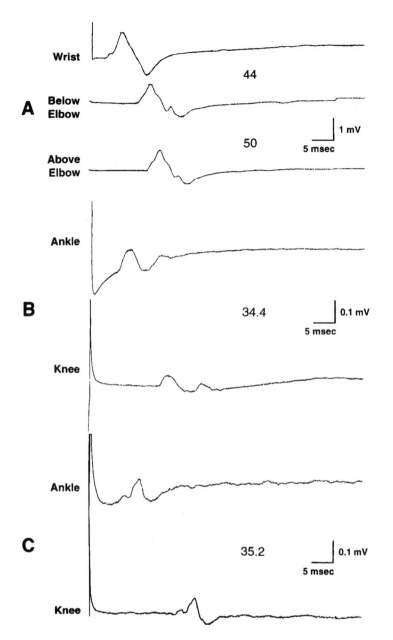

Figure 22.16.   Low CMAPs typical of axonal degeneration in vasculitis neuropathy. *A*, Ulnar nerve. *B*, Peroneal nerve. *C*, Posterior tibial nerve.

Conduction block, an electrophysiological hallmark of segmental demyelination, was rarely reported in vasculitic neuropathy. Among 65 cases, Dyck et al. reported mild focal conduction block in two cases (564). We found conduction block in one nerve in nine of 47 cases (561). In none of these cases was a multifocal conduction block observed, nor was any other electrophysiological manifestation of demyelination found. Hawke et al. observed conduction block in three patients, two of whom had mononeuritis multiplex (560). Ropert and Metral reported five cases of conduction block in one nerve in necrotizing vasculitis (565). However, their data were not conclusive in view of the extremely low distal CMAP in four cases. Jamieson et al. reported a patient with necrotizing vasculitis who showed a multifocal conduction block in the first study but classic axonal neuropathy in a later study (566). These findings suggest that conduction block may be present in a few nerves in a small number of cases and that this could be a transient phenomenon during the acute denervating stage of vasculitic neuropathy. Sensory nerve conduction was more often affected in this disorder (5). All tested sural nerves, and 70% of median and ulnar nerves showed abnormal conduction. In the sural nerve, the sensory CNAPs were absent in the majority of cases. Mixed nerve conduction over the forearm and upper arm segments of the median and ulnar nerves was abnormal in 30–40% of cases. Median and ulnar nerve motor conductions were slow in less than 8% of cases, whereas peroneal and posterior tibial nerve conductions were slow in 83% and 53% of the cases, respectively. The degree of slowing of sensory and motor NCVs was minimal (less than 35% of normal).

Churg-Strauss syndrome (allergic granulomatosis) is a variant of polyarteritis nodosa. However, unlike classic polyarteritis nodosa, it is associated with asthma, lung involvement, and peripheral eosinophilia. As in polyarteritis nodosa, peripheral neuropathy is a frequent manifestation observed in 64–69% of cases as a result of vasculitic neuropathy (567).

Vasculitic neuropathy is commonly noted in patients with long-standing rheumatoid arthritis. Milder sensory polyneuropathy and carpal tunnel syndrome are other common forms of neuropathy that may be present (568). Axonal degeneration has been well documented in patients with rheumatoid neuropathy (568).

In systemic lupus erythematosus (SLE), three distinct types of neuropathy were reported: (a) asymmetrical distal polyneuropathy, which is most common; (b) mononeuropathy or mononeuropathy multiplex; and (c) subacute or chronic demyelinating neuropathy (569, 570). In demyelinating neuropathy, the nerve conduction findings are typical of the acquired demyelinating neuropathy pattern (569). Vasculitis as the basis of nondemyelinating peripheral neuropathy is well documented in SLE (570).

In Sjögren's syndrome, symmetrical sensorimotor neuropathy is most common, followed by symmetrical sensory neuropathy (571). Trigeminal sensory neuropathy is a common manifestation in this disorder (572). Neuropathy is primarily due to vasculitic neuropathy, and the nerve conduction abnormalities represent those of vasculitic neuropathy (571). However, sensory neuronopathy caused by dorsal root ganglionitis has been described (573, 574). In this disorder, the *classic sensory neuronopathy pattern* of nerve conduction abnormalities (absent sensory CNAP with normal motor nerve conduction) was observed (571, 574–576).

In progressive systemic sclerosis, trigeminal sensory neuropathy seems to be the most common form of neuropathy, and distal polyneuropathy is rare (577). Again, vasculitis is primarily responsible for neuropathy (577).

Wegener's granulomatosis is a multisystem disease characterized by the triad of necrotizing granulomatous vasculitis in the upper and lower respiratory tracts, glomerulonephritis, and systemic small vessel vasculitis. The frequency of peripheral nerve involvement in this disease is 11–21% (578). Cranial neuropathy and polyneuropathies are most common and are caused by vasculitis (579). The nerve conduction findings in peripheral neuropathy showed widespread axonal neuropathy (580).

Temporal arteritis is easily recognized by its classic complex of fever, anemia, high sedimentation rate, muscle pain, and headache in persons over 50 years of age. The temporal artery is characteristically involved in giant cell vasculitis. Ischemic optic neuropathy is a well-known complication of temporal arteritis, occurring in 36–58% of patients (581). However, peripheral neuropathy is rare. It has been only speculated that the neuropathy is due to vasculitis. Nerve conduction data in the involved cases were typical of axonal neuropathy (582).

Lymphomatoid granulomatosis is a rare disease predominantly affecting the lungs, skin, and nervous system. Histologically, it is a necrotizing angiocentric and angiodestructive infiltrative process composed of small lymphocytes, plasma cells, histiocytes, and atypical lymphoreticular cells. The disease has been reported to progress to lymphoma in 13% of patients (583). Garcia et al. described one patient with mononeuropathy multiplex and papular anesthetic skin lesions simulating leprosy in whom vasculitic neuropathy was found in the sural nerve biopsy (585).

Hypersensitivity vasculitis refers to a large and heterogeneous group of clinical syndromes with predominantly small-vessel involvement, usually in the skin and associated with a recognizable precipitating event or exposure. Although peripheral neuropathy is rare in this disorder, vasculitis has been well documented in two patients with peripheral neuropathy (29, 586).

Hypereosinophilic syndrome, named for eosinophilia in the absence of a definable etiology, is a multisystem disorder most often affecting the heart, skin, and lungs. Among 14 patients, Chusid et al. found two (14%) who had peripheral neuropathy (587). Dorfman et al. reported three cases of subacute motor-sensory neuropathy, and in two of these the sural nerve biopsy showed probable vasculitis (588).

Eosinophilia-Myalgia Syndrome

This newly identified syndrome associated with L-tryptophan ingestion is characterized by eosinophilia, pain and tenderness of the fascia, muscles, and joints, erythema, and muscle weakness. Many patients have a florid inflammatory myopathy. Peripheral neuropathy has been reported in 27% of patients with this syndrome (589). Three different types of neuropathy were described: (*a*) neuropathy with myopathy; (*b*) painful predominantly sensory neuropathy; and (*c*) sensorimotor neuropathy (590). The sural nerve biopsy showed vasculitis with eosinophilic infiltration. Nerve conduction studies in 10 patients showed findings typical of axonal neuropathy: markedly reduced CMAP amplitude in the peroneal nerve with normal motor NCV and absent sural nerve potentials in most patients. However, two groups reported six patients with demyelinating neuropathy, although the nerve biopsy showed axonal degeneration associated with pervascular inflammatory cells (589, 591).

Neuropathy with Monoclonal Gammopathy

Neuropathy associated with malignant paraproteinemia has been well recognized for many years (Table 22.18). In recent years polyneuropathy associated with benign paraproteinemia was described. In one study, 10% of 279 patients with paraproteinemia were found to have neuropathy of unknown etiology (592). In patients with monoclonal proteins, 43% (or about 5% of all patients with idiopathic neuropathy) had a serious plasma cell disorder (592).

Thus 57% of patients with polyneuropathy and paraproteinemia have no evidence of a serious underlying plasma cell dyscrasia. This disorder was called formerly *benign monoclonal gammopathy*. However, because prolonged follow-up of these patients revealed an 11% conversion to a malignant plasma cell dyscrasia, a new designation of *"monoclonal gammopathy of undetermined significance (MGUS)"* was proposed (593).

A majority of patients with neuropathy and monoclonal gammopathy have CIDP and thus demonstrate the classic nerve conduction pattern of *demyelinating neuropathy*. An exception has been amyloid neuropathy, in which sensory features are predominant and the pattern of axonal neuropathy is typical.

Table 22.18.
Dysproteinemic Polyneuropathy

	Clinical Features	CSF Protein	Pathology	Nerve Conduction Pattern
Benign monoclonal gammopathy (MGUS)	CIDP	High	Segmental demyelination[a]	Nonuniform demyelination[a]
Amyloidosis, light-chain	Sensory-motor[b]	Normal	Axonal neuropathy; amyloid	Axonal mixed neuropathy
Multiple myeloma	Variable pattern			
Osteosclerotic myeloma	CIDP	High	Segmental demyelination	Nonuniform demyelination
Waldenström's macroglobulinemia	CIDP	High	Segmental demyelination	Nonuniform demyelination
Cryoglobulinemic neuropathy	Sensory-motor/MM	Normal	Vasculitis	Axonal mixed neuropathy
Lymphoma	CIDP/AIP	High	Segmental demyelination	Nonuniform demyelination
Angiofollicular lymph node hyperplasia	CIDP	High	Segmental demyelination	Nonuniform demyelination

[a]In IgG or IgA type, occasionally axonal degeneration is seen.
[b]Predominantly sensory.

Polyneuropathy Associated with Monoclonal Gammopathy of Undetermined Significance (MGUS)

Polyneuropathy associated with MGUS has been recently described (594, 595), and its clinical and electrophysiological characteristics have emerged (596–599). *This neuropathy typically resembles CIDP* in most patients, with distal and proximal muscle weakness, large-fiber sensory loss, and high CSF protein levels. The nerve biopsy showed demyelinating neuropathy and monoclonal IgM on the myelin sheaths of surviving myelinated nerve fibers (598). Nemni et al. described three patients in whom fiber teasing showed predominant segmental demyelination, and in other patients there was evidence of axonal degeneration (600). Nerve conduction studies showed *a classic demyelination pattern with markedly slow NCVs* in the range of 15–25 m/sec in a majority of patients (597–599). Sensory CNAPs were absent in most patients. Smith et al. stated that the CMAPs, although small, were not greatly dispersed, suggesting that surviving nerve fibers were all uniformly affected (598). Bromberg et al. did not find any significant differences in the various nerve conduction parameters between classic CIDP and CIDP associated with MGUS (599). In contrast to the majority of studies, Nemni et al.'s cases showed rather mild NCV slowing (600). Kelly stated that a minority of patients have a polyneuropathy that electrophysiologically appears to be caused primarily by axonal degeneration with distal, symmetrical involvement, low CMAP and sensory CNAP amplitudes, minimal NCV slowing, and prominent evidence of distal denervation on needle EMG (597).

Immunosuppressants have been found to have a minimal to marked beneficial effect in many patients, and plasmapheresis was effective in a few patients (601, 602), indicating that this polyneuropathy is potentially treatable.

Peripheral Neuropathy Associated with Osteosclerotic Myeloma

A distinct form of polyneuropathy associated with osteosclerotic myeloma has emerged in recent studies (603, 604). The neuropathy resembles *subacute demyelinating neuropathy or chronic inflammatory-demyelinating polyneuropathy*, with predominantly motor disability, high CSF protein, and marked nerve conduction abnormalities (603, 605). The majority of these patients had detectable levels of monoclonal M-protein (IgG or IgA and nearly always λ light chain). Some of these patients develop a dramatic POEMS syndrome (polyneuropathy, organomegaly, endocrinopathy, M-protein, and skin changes) (606). A skeletal survey showed osteosclerotic lesions in the spine, pelvic bones, and ribs. Open biopsy of suspicious bony lesions is mandatory for the diagnosis. Treatment of solitary lesions with tumoricidal irradiation usually improves the neuropathy (603, 604).

Nerve conduction studies show a *classic demyelinating neuropathy* (607). Motor NCVs are moderately slow with a mean 22 m/sec in the peroneal nerve to 34 m/sec in the median nerve in 16 patients. Terminal latencies are prolonged, with a mean of 6.2 msec in the peroneal and 4.0 msec in the ulnar nerve, and the amplitude of the CMAPs is reduced. In general, slowing of motor NCVs is proportionately greater than a reduction in the CMAP amplitude. Progressive dispersion of the CMAP is noted. An absent response is common in the peroneal nerve. Sensory CNAPs are either absent or reduced in amplitude by the surface electrode technique (603, 607). The needle EMG reveals distal and symmetrical active and chronic neurogenic changes.

Peripheral Neuropathy Associated with Typical Multiple Myeloma

Peripheral neuropathy associated with multiple myeloma can be divided into two categories: myeloma neuropathy without amyloidosis and myeloma neuropathy with amyloidosis (608). Walsh (609) found an overall incidence of peripheral neuropathy of 39% (13% clinical neuropathy and 26% electrophysiological neuropathy) among 23 subjects with multiple myeloma.

Myeloma neuropathy without amyloidosis is a *heterogeneous disorder* and bears a close resemblance to carcinomatous neuropathy (610). The basic pathological process in peripheral nerves is *axonal degeneration* (609).

Walsh (609) compared the motor and sensory conduction in 20 multiple myeloma patients and control subjects. There was a significant slowing of motor NCVs, a significant increase in latency, and a significant reduction in amplitude of the sensory CNAPs and mixed CNAPs. In sensorimotor neuropathy, motor NCV slowing is mild, with slightly low-amplitude CMAPs, and sensory CNAPs are low to absent. In sensory neuropathy, sensory CNAPs are absent and motor NCVs are normal. Kelly et al. observed similar findings (610).

Myeloma neuropathy with amyloidosis is not clinically different from nonhereditary systemic amyloidosis. Of patients with multiple myeloma and polyneuropathy, about two-thirds had amyloid neuropathy (610). Predominant sensory neuropathy, carpal tunnel syndrome, and autonomic neuropathy are common findings. Motor conduction studies reveal low-amplitude CMAPs, slight slowing of NCVs, and slight prolongation of distal latencies, with disproportionately severe involvement of the median nerve at the wrist caused by carpal tunnel syndrome. Sensory CNAPs are frequently unobtainable (610).

Neuropathy Associated with Waldenström's Macroglobulinemia

Peripheral neuropathy is a rare manifestation of macroglobulinemia (605, 611, 612). In most cases the neuropathy develops after the systemic manifestations. Sensory, sensorimotor, and motor types of neuropathy are all reported in this disorder (613). *Demyelinating neuropathy* was documented in sural nerve biopsy in two cases (614, 615).

Nerve conduction data are limited. An inability to obtain any response in the peroneal and posterior tibial nerves is a common finding in motor nerve conduction (614–616). Motor NCVs range from normal (614, 616) to markedly slow (615). Sensory CNAPs were not present in Propp et al.'s case (615), which showed marked motor conduction slowing.

Peripheral Neuropathy with Cryoglobulinemia

The incidence of clinical neuropathy in cryoglobulinemia is about 7% (617). There are two types of cryoglobulinemia: essential cryoglobulinemia and secondary cryoglobulinemia, seen in association with polyarteritis nodosa or lymphoma. In cryoglobulinemic neuropathy, *vasculitis and axonal degeneration* were documented in nerve biopsy by several investigators (618, 619).

Characteristically, the patients present with Raynaud's phenomenon, purpuric skin eruptions, and ulceration of the lower limbs. Peripheral neuropathy is predominantly sensory and asymmetrical, and is precipitated by cold weather.

Mildly slow motor NCVs and a low CMAP amplitude were observed (617, 619). Sensory CNAPs were absent in two cases, and mixed CNAPs were absent in one case (619).

Nonhereditary Amyloid Neuropathy

Nonhereditary amyloid neuropathy can be divided into two groups: primary and secondary, associated with malignant dysproteinemia. The neuropathy is sensory dominant with prominent early loss of small-fiber function followed by progressive weakness and large fiber involvement (620, 621). Dysautonomia is often severe and disabling, as is the pain associated with small fiber damage.

Clinically, electrophysiologically, and morphologically, the primary type resembles dominantly inherited amyloidosis of the lower limbs (Andrade type) with axonal degeneration of small myelinated and unmyelinated fibers (620, 622). Onset in the noninherited type, however, tends to occur at an older age, and bladder and rectal incontinence may be more delayed than in the inherited variety. Systemic manifestations include common renal insufficiency with proteinuria, abnormal protein electrophoretic patterns in the serum in about half the patients and in the urine in 90%, monoclonal proteins in approximately 90% of patients when both serum and urine are studied, and increased plasma cells on bone marrow examination in about two-thirds of the patients (623). Diagnosis depends on the histological demonstration of amyloid. Rectal biopsy may be the safest and most convenient procedure, with a 61–82% chance of identifying amyloid (623). When neuropathy is present, amyloid is found in the biopsied sural nerve.

The nerve conduction findings are consistent with *axonal degeneration* (620, 624). On the average, motor NCVs are just below the normal range. The amplitude of the CMAPs is mildly reduced, and distal latencies are prolonged in proportion to the degree of slowing of the NCV, except in the presence of a superimposed carpal tunnel syndrome. Sensory CNAPs are either absent or reduced in amplitude. Except for median nerve values in patients with carpal tunnel syndrome, the sensory NCVs are normal or minimally slow. Carpal tunnel syndrome is observed in about 20% of patients with this neuropathy (620). The nerve conduction findings in the secondary type are discussed in connection with myeloma neuropathy.

Neuropathies Associated with Infectious Diseases

AIDS Neuropathy

Peripheral neuropathy is one of the most common neurological manifestations of acquired immunodeficiency syndrome (AIDS) (Table 22.19). It may occur in as many as 20% of these patients and in all stages of AIDS infection (625). Three distinct types of peripheral neuropathy have been observed: (*a*) predominantly sensory neuropathy, the most common (626); (*b*) acute or chronic inflammatory demyelinating polyneuropathy (CIDP); and (*c*) mononeuritis multiplex (626). Less common are sensory ataxic neuropathy and polyradiculoneuropathy (627). In AIDS inflammatory neuropathy, CSF pleocytosis is the rule (627).

The pathology of the biopsied sural nerve is different among the various types of neuropathy (627). In AIDP or CIDP, the biopsied nerve showed abnormal features typical of inflammatory neuropathy: segmental demyelination and mononuclear cell infiltration (627, 628–632). In mononeuritis multiplex, the characteristic features of necrotizing vasculitis (fascicular atrophy and perineurial vasculitis) were noted in two cases (627, 632). In distal sensory painful polyneuropathy, axonal loss of myelinated and unmyelinated fibers was the key finding with or without rare inflammatory cells (627, 632). In sensory ataxic neuropathy, the sural nerve biopsy showed loss of the large myelinated fibers without any inflammatory cells, but in the dorsal root ganglia interstitial inflammatory cells were present (627). In two cases of lumbosacral polyradiculopathy, extensive necrosis, inflammatory infiltrates, focal vasculitis of spinal roots, and

Table 22.19.
Human Immunodeficiency Virus (HIV)-Associated Peripheral Neuropathies[a]

	GBS	CIDP	Mononeuropathy Multiplex	Distal Polyneuropathy	Lumbosacral Polyradiculopathy
Stage of HIV infection	Early	Early	Late	Late	Late
Frequency	Not uncommon	2nd most common	Rare	Most common	Extremely rare
Progression	Acute	Subacute/chronic	Acute/subacute	Chronic	Chronic
Clinical features	Predominantly motor, and proximal; pain uncommon.		Multifocal	Distal, symmetrical; painful	Paraplegia with sphincter involvement
CSF	High protein, lymphocyte pleocytosis		Normal	Normal/high protein	High protein/lymphocyte pleocytosis
EMG	Demyelinating neuropathy		Axonal neuropathy	Axonal neuropathy	Polyradiculopathy
Nerve biopsy	Inflammatory demyelinating neuropathy		Vasculitis	Axonal neuropathy	Inflammatory radiculopathy with CMV.
Treatment	Immunotherapies; plasmapheresis		Immunotherapies		

[a]Abbreviations: GBS, Guillain-Barré syndrome; CIDP, chronic inflammatory demyelinating polyneuropathy; CMV, cytomegalic virus.

cytomegalic virus within enlarged endoneurial and endothelial cells were documented (633, 634). In a case of sensory ataxic neuropathy, a sensory ganglionitis was documented by autopsy (635). HIV was isolated from the biopsied nerves in three cases (629, 636). In one case, a retrovirus-like particle was also found in peripheral nerve axoplasm (631).

Subclinical axonal neuropathy is present in AIDS patients. In 30 patients with AIDS without any peripheral neuropathy, there was a mean reduction in the common peroneal CMAP amplitudes of 37% and in the sural CNAP of 34% (637). Mean NCVs of both motor and sensory nerves were reduced by 1–7 m/sec, with an F-wave prolongation of 5% in the arm and 23% in the leg. Five sural nerve biopsies showed axonal neuropathy.

Electrophysiological studies in symptomatic polyneuropathy in 10 HIV-antibody patients and 10 AIDS patients showed a pattern typical of axonal neuropathy (638). In both groups, electrophysiological signs of polyneuropathy of the axonal type were present in the sural, median, and peroneal nerves, together with a greater reduction of the mean sural CNAP amplitude and greater slowing of the peroneal NCV than in patients without AIDS. These findings indicate that the electrophysiological findings are worse in AIDS patients.

Electrophysiological findings are different according to the type of neuropathy (Table 22.19). In CIDP, the classic electrophysiological manifestations of demyelinating neuropathy are present (629–632). Conduction block was a particularly helpful finding (630). In CIDP patients, the needle EMG showed the typical pattern of demyelinating neuropathy: in four of 10 patients, there was no abnormal spontaneous activity with normal MUPs (630). Fibrillations and positive sharp waves were found roughly in proportion to the severity of axonal degeneration in weak muscles in some cases. In acute GBS, Cornblath et al. reported a mixed pattern of demyelination and axonal loss in three patients (629). In mononeuropathy multiplex, electrodiagnostic studies were said to indicate a multifocal process with axonal degeneration and selective or diffuse denervation (627). However, in five patients with mononeuropathy multiplex, there was a multifocal process with axonal degeneration in three and axonal and demyelinating neuropathy in two (639). The mononeuropathy multiplex evolved into CIDP in two cases (625). This indicates that demyelinating mononeuropathy multiplex exists in some patients with mononeuropathy multiplex, although vasculitis seems to be the cause in many patients with mononeuropathy multiplex (627, 632). In distal sensory-motor symmetrical neuropathy, the classic pattern of axonal neuropathy (reduced CMAP and CNAP amplitudes with normal or nearly normal NCV) was seen in every study (626–628, 630, 632, 638, 639). The needle EMG showed denervation in distal muscles (626, 630). In one case of lumbosacral polyradiculopathy, the NCV was slightly slow in the peroneal nerve with a reduced CMAP amplitude. Needle EMG showed diffuse denervation in the leg muscles, which was out of proportion to the mildly slow NCV (634).

In distal sensorimotor polyneuropathy, the neuropathy did not change during azidothymidine (AZT) treatment (626). No improvement was documented in sural or median nerve amplitude or in NCV in seven patients with symptomatic polyneuropathy who were treated with AZT (638).

The majority of CIDP patients improve with immunotherapies including plasmapheresis and steroid (629, 630). Electrophysiological improvement has not been documented.

Inflammatory Neuropathy in HTLV I-Associated Myelopathy

The HTLV I virus, a lentivirus of the family of the human retroviruses, has recently been found to be responsible for tropical spastic paraplegia and HTLV I-associated myelopathy from Japan. Said et al. reported inflammatory demyelinating neuropathy in a patient with tropical spastic paraplegia who showed no clinical features of peripheral neuropathy (640). Motor nerve conduction in the legs was mildly slow (32–38 m/sec) with low CMAP amplitude and conduction block in the peroneal nerve. Sural nerve conduction was essentially normal.

Lyme Disease

Lyme disease is a systemic illness caused by the tick-borne spirochete *Borrelia burgdoferi.* Neuropathy occurs in 36–40% of patients with symptomatic late Lyme disease (641, 642). In Europe, the name Garin-Bujadoux or Barnwarth syndrome is used to describe the presence of a neurological triad of lymphocytic meningitis, cranial neuritis, and radiculoneuritis that follows days to weeks after erythema chronicum migrans spreading from the bitten area, the pathognomonic marker of this disease (643). In the United States, a chronic form of neuropathy has been reported (641). Sural nerve biopsy in this disorder is characterized by *perivascular collections of inflammatory cells and axonal degeneration* in a majority of cases (641, 644, 645). Neuropathy in Lyme disease can be loosely divided into acute and chronic Lyme neuropathy (646).

Although chronic Lyme neuropathy generally differs from the acute form by its time course, milder clinical presentation, and absence of cranial nerve palsy and spinal fluid pleocytosis, the acute and chronic forms of this neuropathy have several common features: (*a*) frequent radicular involvement; (*b*) frequent features of mononeuropathy multiplex; (*c*) identical nerve biopsy findings; and (*d*) a usually good response to antibiotics. Thus, it seems that acute and chronic Lyme neuropathy are closely related and have a common pathogenesis (647).

Lyme neuropathy can present in three distinct patterns: cranial neuropathy, painful radiculopathy, and peripheral neuropathy. Cranial neuropathy occurs early in the disease and can affect any cranial nerve. However, facial palsy is most common and often occurs bilaterally. Radiculopathy is usually painful and can involve the thoracic as well as cervical and lumbar areas (646). Peripheral neuropathy is characterized usually by nonpainful intermittent paresthesias and asymmetrical distribution. If some of these features are combined, then the clinical presentation is typical of mononeuropathy multiplex. Motor weakness or hyporeflexia is rare (646, 647). According to Halperin et al., sensory neuropathy is the most common form of Lyme neuropathy, followed by painful radiculopathy and Bell's palsy (647). In Barnwarth's syndrome, lymphocytic pleocytosis, often with elevated protein, is a uniform finding in the spinal fluid (643). In chronic Lyme neuropathy, a high protein is the most common abnormality in the spinal fluid (646).

Nerve conduction abnormalities in two or more nerves were found in 39% of 66 patients with Lyme disease (647). Nerve conduction abnormalities in Lyme neuropathy are characterized by a pattern typical of *axonal degeneration* (646, 647), and are summarized as follows:

1. In Barnwarth's syndrome, facial nerve latency is abnormal in most cases: in three of four tested cases, the facial nerve latency was abnormal (648). Needle EMG showed fibrillation and a reduced number of MUPs in all three cases.

2. In polyradiculopathy, the needle EMG showed denervation in paraspinal and limb muscles and normal sensory nerve conduction (643, 646). In polyradiculoneuropathy, the needle EMG showed denervation in paraspinal and limb muscles and additional sensory nerve conduction abnormality (646).

3. In sensory neuropathy, sensory conduction abnormalities are the characteristic finding: NCV is slow and CNAP amplitude is reduced. In motor nerve conduction, terminal latencies and late responses were the values most likely to be affected (647). Nerve conduction abnormalities were usually minimal and not seen in all nerves, but rather were scattered. Needle EMG was abnormal in paraspinal and limb muscles in 75% of cases (646).

4. Carpal tunnel syndrome was found clinically and electrophysiologically in 25% of 76 patients with Lyme disease in a prospective study (649). This prevalence is comparable to that described in rheumatoid arthritis, hypothyroidism, and neuropathies. Symptomatic improvement occurred following antibiotic treatment in about half the patients.

5. Despite the broad clinical spectrum of presenting manifestations, the nerve conduction and needle EMG abnormalities were surprisingly uniform in frequency and distribution, being found in both paraspinal and limb muscles.

6. Nerve conduction abnormalities also improved with antibiotic treatment (641, 647). A significant improvement was noted in sensory NCV and CNAP amplitude, terminal latencies, and F-waves (641, 647). Electrophysiological improvement was usually accompanied by clinical improvement.

Leprosy Neuropathy

Leprosy neuropathy is still the most common neuropathy in the world. It is due to infection with *Mycobacterium leprae* and occurs primarily in Asia and Africa. The cardinal symptom of leprosy is sensory loss caused by superficial neuropathy. Anesthesic depigmented skin lesions are an important finding and should be sought. Other characteristic findings are thickened nerves, trophic ulcers, mutilated digits, and Charcot's joint. In the tuberculoid form, mononeuropathy multiplex is the typical pattern, whereas asymmetrical or symmetrical polyneuropathy is most common in the lepromatous form. Motor involvement occurs in a predictable sequence as a result of nerve trunk damage to those nerves that course close to the skin surface and hence are locally cool. Nerves involved include the ulnar nerve at the elbow, the deep peroneal branch at the ankle, superficial branches of the facial nerve, and the median nerve at the wrist, more or less in that order (650). *Segmental demyelination* is the main pathology in leprosy neuropathy (651).

The best nerve conduction data are available in McLeod et al.'s study of three groups of patients (651). The nerve conduction study was helpful in four areas:

1. The test confirmed the clinical impression of neuropathy. Nerve conduction abnormalities were observed in 50% (median nerve) to 92% (sural nerve) of the clinically affected nerves.

2. The test was also useful for identifying neuropathy in the clinically unaffected nerves. Nerve conduction abnormalities were observed in 39% (posterior tibial nerve) to 77% (ulnar nerve) of clinically unaffected or unsuspected nerves. This observation indicates widespread involvement of the peripheral nerves in the disease and the value of nerve conduction studies in the early detection of leprosy.

3. This test has been used *as a guideline* for selecting patients for surgical exploration and nerve biopsy among those with enlarged nerves. Conductions were found to be abnormal in the clinically enlarged nerves of 12 of the 27 patients (44%). In nine of the 12, a pathologic diagnosis of leprosy was subsequently established. In none of the remaining three patients with abnormal conductions and in none of those with normal conduction studies has leprosy been diagnosed. It is suggested that when abnormal conduction is found in the clinically enlarged nerve of a patient at risk from the disease there is a strong probability that he has leprosy, and surgical exploration and biopsy of the nerve are indicated.

4. It is possible by electrophysiologic means to localize the segments of a nerve to which the disease is chiefly restricted. Nerve conduction studies are therefore helpful in the selection of suitable patients for the treatment of localized lesions by nerve grafting procedures.

In clinically affected nerves, the motor NCVs are minimally slow (about 12–14% below normal). The terminal latency is often prolonged and the CMAPs are temporally dispersed and decreased in amplitude. Sensory and mixed CNAPs are often difficult to obtain or else they show a reduced amplitude.

The facial nerve is commonly involved in leprosy. In patients with lagophthalmos, the facial nerve study shows either prolonged latencies or an absence of responses when recording from the orbicularis oculi muscle. Latencies to other facial muscle groups are sometimes prolonged as well (652, 653).

Improvement in the motor nerve conduction was reported in leprosy patients under sulfone treatment (654, 655). Brand (cited by Sabin and Swift (650)) studied nerve conduction on segments affected by acute neuritis, usually in the ulnar nerve at the elbow. He found that electrical stimulation of the nerve above the involved segment produced no muscle response. Upon incision of the sheath, however, the nerve immediately began to conduct impulses. During reaction with erythema nodosum leprosum, the nerves in reaction show a uniform decrease in NCVs that improves after treatment with thalidomide (656, 657).

Diphtheric Neuropathy

Diphtheria exotoxin produces segmental demyelination in animals. Diphtheric neuropathy in animals is used extensively for studying the nerve conduction of segmental demyelination.

Diphtheric neuropathy is delayed for 30–50 days after the onset of pharyngitis, though in some patients palatal or eye accommodation weakness may develop 5–12 days after infection. The CSF protein is usually high.

The nerve conduction data in human cases are limited. McDonald and Kocen (658) reported that the median motor NCV was 30 m/sec and the median sensory CNAP was absent in one case 2 weeks after the peak of neuropathy; these abnormalities returned to normal with clinical improvement. Kazemi et al. (659) studied motor conduction in diphtheria and diphtheritic myocarditis. Among 30 patients, 11 had myocarditis and nine had polyneuropathy (seven of nine had palatal paralysis alone). They found the following: (*a*) all patients with myocarditis had slow motor NCV and more pronounced slowing than patients with isolated diphtheria; (*b*) clinical polyneuropathy were usually preceded by a slow motor NCV; and (*c*) the slowest NCVs were 31 m/sec in median, 25 m/sec in ulnar, and 26 m/sec in peroneal nerves in patients with neuropathy. Kurdi and Abdul-Kader (660) studied nerve conduction in 11 patients with acute diphtheritic neuritis and bulbar palsy. Slow motor NCV and prolonged terminal latency were present in most patients within 2 weeks of the onset of the neuropathy. The NCV fell to approximately 45% of the normal mean values within 5–15 weeks after the onset of neuropathy. Nerve conduction had returned to normal within 3 months in eight patients. The authors described a striking dissociation between the time course of the clinical and electrophysiological abnormalities: Early in the illness, peripheral nerve conduction was normal in some patients despite the presence of severe weakness; later, maximum electrophysiological abnormalities were sometimes found after clinical recovery had commenced. Idiaquez reported slow motor NCV in the peroneal nerve in nine of 10 patients and slow motor NCV in the median nerve in four patients with diphtheric neuropathy (661). In four patients, the motor NCV in the peroneal nerve was in the range of demyelination (< 30 m/sec). Thus the slowest NCVs in this disorder are consistent with *segmental demyelination*.

Neuropathy Associated with Tetanus

Neuropathy has been occasionally reported in tetanus. Peripheral neuropathy was reported in 79% of 34 patients with severe tetanus (662). Clinically, this neuropathy usually occurs in the acute stage and is characterized by asymmetrical motor and sensory neuropathy, the ulnar, median, and peroneal nerves being most commonly affected. The nerve conduction study showed that motor and sensory NCVs in the affected nerves were nearly normal or mildly slow and that sensory CNAP amplitude was also reduced. The needle EMG showed active denervation process. These findings are typical of *axonal neuropathy*. Shahani et al. claimed that this neuropathy was due to the action of tetanus toxin affecting the distal parts of both sensory and motor nerves (662). Nerve conduction studies in 40 patients (clinical peripheral neuropathy in six) that was performed 11 months to 13 years after tetanus showed significantly lower motor distal latencies, slowed distal sensory NCVs, and more frequent needle EMG abnormalities (663). Authors maintained that these represented sequelae of tetanus.

Hyperexcitable Peripheral Nerve Disorders

Hyperexcitable peripheral nerve disorders are characterized by sustained muscle activity due to hyperexcitability in the distal motor axons. Hyperexcitability of the distal nerves is classically documented by the pharmacological tests: *sustained muscle activity persists after nerve block but is abolished by regional curare administration.*

Hyperexcitable peripheral nerve disorders can be associated with peripheral neuropathy (664). In these cases, there is usually clinical evidence of peripheral neuropathy in addition to sustained muscle activity. Nerve conduction is abnormal in these cases (665–667). In Warmolt et al.'s study, the nerve conduction showed mild slowing of motor NCV, absent sensory CNAPs, and repetitive discharges of CMAPs (665). Valenstein et al. and Joy found nerve conduction findings typical of demyelinating neuropathy: markedly slow NCV, conduction block, and abnormal temporal dispersion (666, 667).

There are two well-known hyperexcitable peripheral nerve disorders without clinically obvious peripheral neuropathy: *Isaacs' syndrome and cramp-fasciculation syndrome.* Isaacs' syndrome is characterized by stiffness, continuous muscle contraction, clinical improvement following phenytoin or carbamazepine therapy and continuous motor unit activity on needle EMG (668–671). On the other hand, cramp-fasciculation syndrome is characterized by cramp, fasciculation or myokymia, clinical improvement with carbamazepine therapy, and *fasciculation or myokymic discharges on the needle EMG* (664, 672, 673). Tahmoush et al. believed that the difference in these two clinical syndromes is caused by differences in hyperexcitability (673). In Isaacs' syndrome, the terminal axon is very excitable and continuously firing. In cramp-fasciculation syndrome, there is mild hyperexcitability with rare firing, which becomes more frequent after voluntary activity or nerve stimulation. This view is based on the fact that nerve stimulation in patients with both Isaacs' and cramp-fasciculation syndromes produce showers of after-discharges following the "M" (CMAP) response and show dramatic clinical improvement with carbamazepine therapy.

In Isaacs' syndrome, nerve conduction may be either normal (671) or slow (670, 674–676). Isaacs found the motor latencies to be prolonged in one patient (668). In cramp-fasciculation syndrome, the nerve conduction was either normal (664, 672, 673) or slow (672). Among Hudson et al.'s five cases, the motor NCV was slow in the posterior tibial nerve in three, and the sural nerve conduction was abnormal in two cases (672). Auger et al. observed repetitive "after-discharges" in the CMAP on stimulation of motor nerves or in the H-reflex response in six patients with cramp-fasciculation syndrome (664). We have found a similar repetitive discharge in the CMAPs, the H- and T-reflexes, and the F-waves in two cases (Fig. 20.1). *We believe that the repetitive discharges of the CMAPs are typical of cramp-fasciculation syndrome.* In Tahmoush et al.'s nine cases, supramaximal stimulation of the motor nerve at 0.5-, 1-, 2-, and 5-Hz stimulation produced showers of electrical potentials following the M-response in at least one nerve (673).

Motor Neuron Diseases

The study of motor and sensory nerve conduction is indicated in patients suspected of motor neuron disease to rule out peripheral neuropathies that can mimic motor neuron diseases. In our experience, CIDP and multifocal demyelinating neuropathy are two most common of these peripheral neuropathies. These neuropathies can be recognized by extensive nerve conduction studies and treatable with immunotherapies (1, 502).

Amyotrophic Lateral Sclerosis

The majority of motor conduction velocities fall within normal limits in patients with amyotrophic lateral sclerosis (ALS) (677). The amplitude of the CMAPs is low in some patients, in proportion to the wasting of muscles. The presence of low-amplitude CMAPs excludes nonneuromuscular causes as the basis of atrophy and is a gauge of the severity of the disease (678). Motor NCVs are slightly slowed in some patients (677, 679–681), but never fall below 70% of the lower limit of normal. This mild slowing is caused by selective loss of the larger, faster-conducting fibers with axonal degeneration after neuronal degeneration in the anterior horn. Slowing of conduction is proportional to the reduction of CMAP amplitude and to the degree of atrophy of the muscle (677). In some patients terminal latencies become prolonged as the degree of atrophy increases. When the amplitude of the CMAPs of the hypothenar muscles was less than

1 mV, the terminal latency was on the average 40% greater than normal. In a few patients terminal latency is out of proportion to slowing of NCV. This is due to multiple factors: nerve terminal sprouting, cool extremities, and technical factors associated with the very low CMAP. Without concomitant sensory nerve conduction abnormalities, this prolonged terminal latency should not be interpreted as an indication of entrapment neuropathy. Sensory nerve conduction is normal in ALS (171, 677, 679, 682). If sensory conduction is abnormal after control for age and temperature, some disorder other than ALS should be suspected (678). Ertekin (679) recorded normal mixed CNAPs from the median nerve in 15 ALS patients. Gilliatt et al. (683) recorded mixed CNAPs in the peroneal nerve in five patients with severe motor neuron disease despite a complete (or nearly complete) absence of motor fibers in the nerve. On the average, the mixed NCV was slower than in control subjects, but the reduced conduction velocities were attributed to low limb temperature. Thus, the typical nerve conduction pattern in ALS is a *pure motor neuropathy of axonal type.*

The F-wave latencies are slightly prolonged in patients with ALS (681, 684, 685) but not as prominently as in neuropathy or polyradiculopathy. The H-reflex elicited in the calf muscle is more excitable than normal in some ALS patients. The H-reflex elicited in the hand muscles by stimulation of the ulnar nerve or in the anterior tibialis muscle by stimulation of the peroneal nerve may be released from normal suppression in ALS, so that it occurs more commonly among ALS patients than among normal controls (686). Norris (687) performed an extensive H-reflex study in motor neuron diseases. In progressive muscular atrophy, the H-reflex was observed in the gastrocnemius in only seven and in opponens pollicis, hypothenar, and extensor digitorum muscles in just three of 18 patients. In ALS the H-reflex was present in the gastrocnemius in almost all cases and in the other muscles in 66–77% of 110 patients. In contrast, in patients with polyneuropathy the H-reflex was absent in the gastrocnemius in almost all cases and in other muscles in all cases. These observations indicate that *the H-reflex test can be a valuable help* in differentiating ALS from primary muscular atrophy or polyneuropathy.

Werdnig-Hoffman Disease (Infantile Spinal Muscular Atrophy)

The amplitude of the CMAPs in Werdnig-Hoffman disease is either normal or low (688, 689). Low amplitude was reported in 73% of cases (688). The motor NCV is either normal or mildly slow, the latter finding being observed in 43% of Kunz's cases (688). Sensory nerve conduction is normal (688, 690, 691).

Kugelberg-Welander's Disease (Juvenile Spinal Muscular Atrophy)

Kugelberg-Welander's disease is a benign form of motor neuron disease that may be mistaken for muscular dystrophy. Nerve conduction studies of motor and sensory fibers in this disorder are normal (689, 691). CMAPs are not as low as those in ALS and are often normal.

REFERENCES

1. Lewis RA, Sumner AJ, Brown MJ, Asbury AK. Multifocal demyelinating neuropathy with persistent conduction block. Neurology 1982;32:958–964.
2. Dyck PJ, Oviatt KF, Lambert EH. Intensive evaluation of referred unclassified neuropathies yields improved diagnosis. Ann Neurol 1981;10:222–226.
3. Buchthal F. Electrophysiological abnormalities in metabolic myopathies and neuropathies. Acta Neurol Scand 1970;46 (Suppl 43):129–171.
4. McLeod JG. Nerve conduction measurements for clinical use. Van Duijn H, Donker DNJ, Van Huffelen AC, eds. Current concepts in clinical neurophysiology. The Hague: NV Drukkerij Trio, 1977:83–98.
5. Wees SJ, Sunwoo IN, Oh SJ. Sural nerve biopsy in systemic necrotizing vasculitis. Am J Med 1981;71:525–532.
6. Bannister RG, Sears TA. The change in nerve conduction in acute idiopathic polyneuritis. J Neurol Neurosurg Psychiatry 1962;25:321–328.
7. Hopf HC, Althaus HH, Vogel P. An evaluation of the course of peripheral neuropathies based on clinical and neurographical re-examination. Eur Neurol 1973;9:90–104.
8. Kaeser HE. Das sensible Nervenaktions Potential und seine Klinishe Bedeutung. Dtsch Z Nervenheilk 1966;188:289–299.

9. Lambert EH. Diagnostic value of electrical stimulation of motor nerves. EEG Clin Neurophysiol 1962;22 (Suppl) 22:9–16.

10. Ludin HP, Lutschg J, Valsangiacomo F. Vergleichende Untersuchung orthodromer und antidromer sensibler Nervenleit geschcwindigkeiten. 2. Befunde bei polyneuropathien und bei status nach polyradikulitis. Z EEG EMG 1977b;8:180–186.

11. Buchthal F, Rosenfalck A. Sensory potentials in polyneuropathy. Brain 1971;94:241–262.

12. Clements RS. Diabetic neuropathy: new concepts of its etiology. Diabetes 1979;28:604–611.

13. Graf RJ, Halter JB, Halar E, Porte D. Nerve conduction abnormalities in untreated maturity-onset diabetes: relation to levels of fasting plasma glucose and glycosylated hemoglobin. Ann Int Med 1979;90:298–303.

14. Noel P. Sensory nerve conductions in the upper limbs at various stages of diabetic neuropathy. J Neurol Neurosurg Psychiatry 1973;36:786–796.

15. Fagerberg SE. Diabetic neuropathy: a clinical and histological study on the significance of vascular affections. Acta Med Scand 1959;164 (Suppl 354):1–97.

16. Asbury AK, Aldredge H, Herschberg R, Fisher CM. Oculomotor palsy in diabetes mellitus: a clinicopathologic study. Brain 1970;93:555–566.

17. Raff MC, Asbury AK. Ischemical mononeuropathy multiplex associated with diabetes mellitus. New Engl J Med 1968;279:17–22.

18. Raff MC, Sangalang V, Asbury AK. Ischemic mononeuropathy multiplex associated with diabetes mellitus. Arch Neurol 1968;18:487–499.

19. Clements RS. The role of abnormalities in nerve metabolism in the pathogenesis of diabetic peripheral neuropathy. Al J Med Sci 1976;13:399–404.

20. Thomas PK, Lascelles RG. The pathology of diabetic neuropathy. Q J Med 1966;35:489–509.

21. Ibrahim MM, Crosland JM, Monigsberger L, Barnes AD, Dawson-Edwards P, Newman CE. Effect of renal transplantation on uraemic neuropathy. Lancet 1974;2:739–742.

22. Sternman AB, Schaumburg HH, Asbury AK. The acute sensory neuropathy syndrome: a distinct clinical entity. Ann Neurol 1980;7:354–358.

23. Chopra JS, Hurwitz LJ, Montgomery DAD. The pathogenesis of sural nerve changes in diabetes mellitus. Brain 1968;92:391–418.

24. Behse F, Buchthal F, Carlsen F. Nerve biopsy and conduction studies in diabetic neuropathy. J Neurol Neurosurg Psychiatry 1977;40:1072–1082.

25. Said G, Slama G, Selva J. Progressive centripetal degeneration of axons in small fiber diabetic polyneuropathy. Brain 1983;106:791–807.

26. Thomas PK, Eliasson SG. Diabetic neuropathy. In: Dyck PJ, Thomas PK, Lambert EH, Bunge R, eds. Peripheral neuropathy. Vol II. Philadelphia: WB Saunders, 1984:1773–1810.

27. Dyck P. Pathology. In: Dyck PJ, Thomas PK, Asbury AK, Winegrad AJ, Porte D, eds. Diabetic neuropathy. Philadelphia: WB Saunders, 1987:223–236.

28. Abu-shakra SR, Cornblath DR, Avila O, Chaudhry V, Frimer M, Glass JD, Reim JW, Ronnett GV. Conduction block in diabetic neuropathy. Muscle Nerve 1991;14:858–862.

29. Asbury AK, Brown MJ. Clinical and pathological studies of diabetic neuropathies. In: Goto Y, Horiuchi A, Kogure K, eds. Diabetic neuropathy. Amsterdam: Excerpta Medica, 1982;50–57.

30. Lawrence DG, Locke S. Motor nerve conduction velocity in diabetes. Arch Neurol 1961;5:37–43.

31. Mayer RF. Nerve conduction studies in man. Neurology 1963;13:1021–1030.

32. Skillman TG, Johnson EW, Hamwi GJ, Driskill HJ. Motor nerve conduction velocity in diabetes mellitus. Diabetes 1961;10:46–51.

33. Downie AW, Newell DJ. Sensory nerve conduction in patients with diabetes mellitus and controls. Neurology 1961;11:876–882.

34. Lamontagne A, Buchthal F. Electrophysiological studies in diabetic neuropathy. J Neurol Neurosurg Psychiatry 1970;33:442–452.

35. Bischoff A. Diabetische Neuropathie: Pathologische Anatomie, Pathophysiologie und Pathogenese auf Grund electronenmikroskopischer Untersuchungen. Deutsche Medizineische Wochenschrift 1968;93:237–241.

36. Wiesendanger M, Bishoff A. Elektromyographische Veranderungen bei der diabetischen neuropathie. Bull Schweiz Akad Med Wiss 1962;17:233–246.

37. Gregerson G. Motor nerve function and duration of diabetes. Lancet 1964;2:733.

38. Kraft GH, Guyton JD, Huffman JD. Follow-up study of motor nerve conduction velocities in patients with diabetes mellitus. Arch Phys Med Rehabil 1970;51:207–209.

39. Gregerson G. Variation in motor conduction velocity produced by acute changes of the metabolic state in diabetic patients. Diabetologia 1968;4:273–277.

40. Gilliatt RW, Willison RG. Peripheral nerve conduction in diabetic neuropathy. J Neurol Neurosurg Psychiatry 1962;25:11–18.

41. Fraser DM, Campbell IW, Ewing DJ, Murray A, Neilson JM, Clarke BF. Peripheral autonomic nerve function in newly diagnosed diabetes mellitus. Diabetes 1977;26:546–550.

42. Ward JD, Barnes CG, Fisher DJ, Jessop JD, Baker RWR. Improvement in nerve conduction following treatment in newly diagnosed diabetics. Lancet 1971;1:428–430.

43. Ellenberg M. Diabetes neuropathy presenting as the initial clinical manifestation of diabetes. Ann Int Med 1958;49:620–631.

44. Kimura J, Yamada T, Stevland NP. Distal slowing of motor nerve conduction velocity in diabetic polyneuropathy. J Neurol Sci 1979;42:291–302.

45. Conrad B, Ashoff JC, Fischler M. Der diagnostische Wert der F-Wellen-Latenz. J Neurol 1975;210:151–159.
46. Johnson EW, Waylonis GW. Facial nerve conduction delay in patients with diabetes mellitus. Arch Phys Med Rehabil 1964;45:131–139.
47. Porter D, Graf RJ, Halter JB, Pfeifer MA, Halar E. Diabetic neuropathy and plasma glucose control. Am J Med 1981;70:195–200.
48. Graf RJ, Halter JB, Pfeifer MA, Halar E, Brozovich F, Porte D. Glycemic control nerve conduction abnormalities in non-insulin-dependent diabetic subjects. Ann Int Med 1981;94:307–311.
49. Campbell IW, Fraser DM, Ewing DJ, Baldwin VS, Harrower ABD, Murray A, Neilson JMM, Clarke BF. Peripheral and autonomic nerve function in diabetic ketoacidosis. Lancet 1976;2:167–169.
50. Service EJ, Daube JR, O'Brien PC, Dyck PJ. Effect of artificial pancreas treatment on peripheral nerve function in diabetes. Neurology 1981;31:1375–1380.
51. Tolaymat A, Roque JL, Russo LS. Improvement of diabetic peripheral neuropathy with the portable insulin infusion pump. South Med J 1982;75:185–189.
52. Pietri A, Ehle AL, Raskin P. Changes in nerve conduction velocity after six weeks of glucoregulation with portable insulin infusion pumps. Diabetes 1980;29:668–671.
53. Warmolts JR, Mendell JR, O'Dorisio TM, Cataland S. Comparison of the effects of continuous subcutaneous infusion and split-mixed injection of insulin on nerve function in type I diabetes mellitus. J Neurol Sci 1987;82:161–169.
54. Ehle AL, Raskin P. Increased nerve conduction in diabetics after a year of improved glucoregulation. J Neurol Sci 1986;74:191–197.
55. Dahl-Jørgensen K, Brinchmann-Hansen O, Hanssen KF, Ganes T, Kierulf P, Smeland E, Sandvik L, Aagenaes ø. Effect of near normoglycaemia for two years on progression of early diabetic retinopathy, nephropathy, and neuropathy: the Oslo study. Brit Med J 1986;293:1195–1199.
56. Clements RS, Vourganti B, Kuba T, Oh SJ, Darnell B. Dietary myo-inositol intake and peripheral nerve function in diabetic neuropathy. Metabolism 1979;28(Suppl 1):477–483.
57. Salway JG, Whitehead L, Finnegan JA, Karunanayaka A, Barnett D, Payne RB. Effect of myo-inositol on peripheral nerve function in diabetes. Lancet 1978;2:1282–1284.
58. Faguns J, Jameson S. Effects of aldose reductase inhibitor treatment in diabetic polyneuropathy: a clinical and neurophysiological study. J Neurol Neurosurg Psychiatry 1981;44:991–1001.
59. Gregerson G, Borsting H, Theil P. Influence of myo-inositol on human diabetic nerve and retina. Diabetologia 1977;13:397.
60. Judzewitsch RG, Jaspan JB, Polonsky KS, Weinberg CR, Halter JB, Halar E, Pfeifer MA, Vukadinovic C, Bernstein L, Schneider M, Liang KY, Gabbay KH, Rubenstein AH, Porte D. Aldose reductase inhibition improves nerve conduction velocity in diabetic patients. New Engl J Med 1983;308:119–123.
61. Jaspan J, Maselli R, Herold K, Bartkus C. Treatment of severely painful diabetic neuropathy with an aldose reductase inhibitor: relief of pain and improved somatic and autonomic nerve function. Lancet 1983;1:758–762.
62. Bassi S, Albizzati MG, Calloni E, Frattola L. Electromyographic study of diabetic and alcoholic polyneuropathic patients treated with gangliosides. Muscle Nerve 1982;5:352–356.
63. Kennedy WR, Navarro X, Coetz FC, Sutherland DER, Najarian JS. Effects of pancreatic transplantation on diabetic neuropathy. New Engl J Med 1990;322:1031–1037.
64. Solders G, Wilczek H, Gunnarsson R, Tyden G, Persson A, Groth C. Effects of combined pancreatic and renal transplantation on diabetic neuropathy: a two-year follow-up study. Lancet 1987;2:1232–1235.
65. Asbury AK. Proximal diabetic neuropathy. Ann Neurol 1977;2:179–180.
66. Subramony SH, Wilborn AJ. Diabetic proximal neuropathy. J Neurol Sci 1982;53:293–304.
67. Clements RS, DeJesus PV, Wingrad AI. Raised plasma-myoinositol levels in uremia and experimental neuropathy. Lancet 1973;1:1137–1141.
68. Williams IR, Mayer RF. Subacute proximal diabetic neuropathy. Neurology 1976;26:108–116.
69. Chokroverty S, Reyes MG, Rubino FA, Tonaki H. The syndrome of diabetic amyotrophy. Ann Neurol 1977;1:181–194.
70. Donovan WH, Sumi SM.Diabetic amyotrophy: a more diffuse process than clinically suspected. Arch Phys Med Rehabil 1976;57:397–403.
71. Bastron JA, Thomas JE. Diabetic polyradiculopathy: clinical and electromyographic findings in 105 patients. Mayo Clin Proc 1981;56:725–732.
72. Hamilton CR, Dobson HL, Marshall J. Diabetic amyotrophy. Am J Med 1963;34:775–785.
73. Ellenberg M. Diabetic neuropathic cachexia. Diabetes 1974;23:418–423.
74. Wilbourn AJ. The diabetic neuropathies. In: Brown WF, Bolton CF, eds. Clinical electromyography. Boston: Butterworth, 1987:329–364.
75. Waxman SG, Sabin TD. Diabetic truncal polyneuropathy. Arch Neurol 1981;38:46–47.
76. Stewart JD. Diabetic truncal neuropathy: topography of the sensory deficit. Ann Neurol 1980;25:233–238.
77. Boulton AMJ, Angus E, Ayyar DR. Diabetic thoracic polyradiculopathy presenting as an abdominal swelling. Br Med J 1984;1289:798–799.
78. Caldwell JW, Crane CR, Boland GL. Determinations of intercostal motor conduction time in the diagnosis of nerve root compression. Arch Phys Med Rehab 1968;49:515–518.
79. Pradhan S, Taly A: Intercostal nerve conduction study in man. J Neurol Neurosurg Psychiatry 1989;52:763–766.
80. Johnson ER, Powerl J, Caldwell J, Crane C. Intercostal nerve conduction and posterior rhizotomy in the diagnosis and treatment of thoracic radiculopathy. J Neurol Neurosurg Psychiatry 1974;37:330–332.

81. Sun SF, Streib EW. Diabetic thoraco-abdominal neuropathy: clinical and electrodiagnostic features. Ann Neurol 1981;9:75–79.

82. Kita DG, Breuer AC, Wilbourn AJ. Thoracic root pain in diabetes: the spectrum of clinical and electromyographic findings. Ann Neurol 1982;11:80–85.

83. Massey EW. Diabetic truncal mononeuropathy: electromyographic evaluation. Acta Diabetol Lat 1980;17:269–272.

84. Streib EF, Sun SF, Paustian FF, Gallagher TF, Shipp JC, Ecklund RE. Diabetic thoracic radiculopathy: electrodiagnostic study. Muscle Nerve 1986;9:548–553.

85. Riley DE, Shields RW. Diabetic amyotrophy with upper extremity involvement. Neurology 1984;34:(Suppl 1):216.

86. Child DL, Yates DAH. Radicular pain in diabetes. Rheumatol Rehab 1978;17:195–196.

87. Komini N, Nami N, Taylor HR, Hampers CL, Merrill JP. Variations in motor nerve conduction velocity in normal and uremic patients. Arch Int Med 1971;128:235–239.

88. Nielsen VK. Sensory nerve conduction studies in uremic patients. Proc Eur Dialysis Transplant Assoc 1967;4:279–284.

89. Nielsen VK. The peripheral nerve function in chronic renal failure. I. Clinical symptoms and signs. Acta Med Scand 1971;190:105–111.

90. Tenckhoff HA, Boen FS, Jefsen RH, Spiegler JH. Polyneuropathy in chronic renal insufficiency. JAMA 1965;192:1121–1124.

91. Thomas PK. Metabolic neuropathy. J R Coll Physicians Lond 1973;7:154–160.

92. Thomas PK, Hollinrake K, Lascelles RG, O'Sullivan DJ, Billoid RA, Moorhead JF, MacKenzie JC. The polyneuropathy of chronic renal failure. Brain 1971;97:761–780.

93. Dyck PJ, Johnson WJ, Lambert EH, O'Brien PC. Segmental demyelination secondary to axonal degeneration in uremic neuropathy. Mayo Clin Proc 1971;46:400–430.

94. Nielsen VK. The peripheral nerve function in chronic renal failure. V. Sensory and motor conduction velocity. Acta Med Scand 1973;194:445–454.

95. Blaggs CR, Kemble F, Taverner D. Nerve conduction velocity in relationship to the severity of renal disease. Nephron 1968;5:290–299.

96. Bolton CF. Electrophysiologic changes in uremic neuropathy after successful renal transplantation. Neurology 1976;26:152–161.

97. Guineneuc P, Ginet J. The use of the H-reflex in patients with chronic renal failure. In: Desmedt JE, ed. New developments in EMG and clinical neurophysiology, vol 2. Basel: Karger, 1973:400–403.

98. Halar EM, Brozovich FV, Milutinovic J, Inouye L, Becker VM. H-reflex latency in uremic neuropathy: correlation with NCV and clinical findings. Arch Phys Med Rehabil 1979;60:174–177.

99. Panayiotopoulos CP, Lago G. Tibial nerve H-reflex and F-studies in patients with uremic neuropathy. Muscle Nerve 1980;3:423–426.

100. Ackil AA, Shahani BT, Young RR, Rubin NE. Late response and sural conduction studies: usefulness in patients with chronic renal failure. Arch Neurol 1981;38:482–485.

101. Mitz M, Prakash AS, Melvin J, Piering W. Motor nerve conduction indicators in uremic neuropathy. Arch Phys Med Rehabil 1980;61:45–48.

102. Jebsen RH, Tenckhoff H. Comparison of motor and sensory nerve conduction velocity in early uremic polyneuropathy. Arch Phys Med Rehabil 1969;50:124–126.

103. Honet JC, Jebsen RH, Tenckhoff HA, McDonald JR. Motor nerve conduction velocity in chronic renal insufficiency. Arch Phys Med Rehabil 1966;47:647–652.

104. Cadilhac J, Dapres G, Fabre JL, Mion C. In: Desmedt JE, ed. New developments in EMG and clinical neurophysiology, vol 2. Basel: Karger, 1973:372–380.

105. Miyoshi T, Oh SJ. Proximal slowing of nerve conduction in the Guillain-Barré syndrome. EMG Clin Neurophysiol 1977;17:287–296.

106. Van der Most Vas Spijk D, Hoogland RA, Dijkstra S. Conduction velocities compared and related to degree of renal insufficiency. In: Desmedt JE, ed. New developments in EMG and clinical neurophysiology, vol 2. Basel: Karger, 1973:381–389.

107. Bolton CF. Metabolic neuropathy. In: Brown WF, Bolton CF, eds. Clinical electromyography. Boston: Butterworth, 1987:245–281.

108. Lindholm T. The influence of uraemia and electrolyte disturbances on muscle action potentials and motor nerve conduction in man. Acta Med Scand 1968; (Suppl)491:1–58.

109. Jebsen RH, Tenckhoff H, Honet JC. Natural history of uremic polyneuropathy and effects of dialysis. New Engl J Med 1967;277:327–337.

110. Nielsen VK. The peripheral nerve function in chronic renal failure. VI. The relationship between sensory and motor nerve conduction and kidney function, axotemia, age, sex, and clinical neuropathy. Acta Med Scand 1973;194:455–462.

111. Oh SJ, Clements RS, Lee YW, Diethelm AG. Rapid improvement in nerve conduction velocity following renal transplantation. Ann Neurol 1978;4:369–373.

112. Codish SD, Cress RH. Motor and sensory nerve conduction in uremic patients undergoing repeated dialysis. Arch Phys Med Rehabil 1971;52:260–263.

113. Stanley E, Brown JL, Pryor JS. Altered peripheral nerve function resulting from haemodialysis. J Neurol Neurosurg Psychiatry 1977;40:39–43.

114. Nielsen VK. The peripheral nerve function in chronic renal failure. VII. Longitudinal course during terminal renal failure and regular hemodialysis. Acta Med Scand 1974;195:155–162.

115. Teschan PE, Bourne JR, Reed RB, et al. Electrophysiological and neurobehavioral responses to therapy. The National Cooperative Dialysis Study. Kidney Int 1983;23 (Suppl 13):558–565.

116. Faller B, Marichal JF. Treatment of chronic renal failure: situation of CAPD. Int J Artif Organs 1980;9:243–244.

117. Chan MK, Bailod RA, Chuah P, et al. Three year's experience of continuous ambulatory peritoneal dialysis. Lancet 1981;1:1409–1412.

118. Rubin J, Oreopoulos DG, Gordon Blair RD, Chisholm LDJ, Meema HE, deVeber GA. Chronic peritoneal dialysis in the management of diabetics with terminal renal failure. Nephron 1977;19:265–270.

119. Tegnér R, Lindholm B. Uremic polyneuropathy: different effects of hemodialysis and continuous ambulatory periotoneal dialysis. Acta Med Scand 1985;218:409–416.

120. Lindholm B, Tegnér R, Tranaeus A, Bergström J. Progress of peripheral uremic neuropathy during continuous ambulatory peritoneal dialysis (CAPD). Trans Am Soc Artif Intern Organs 1982;28:263–268.

121. Dinapoli RP, Johnson WJ, Lambert EH. Experience with combined hemodialysis-renal transplantation program: neurologic aspects. Mayo Clin Proc 1966;41:809–820.

122. Nielsen VK. The peripheral nerve function in chronic renal failure. VIII. Recovery after renal transplantation: Clinical aspects. Acta Med Scand 1974;195:163–170.

123. Taylor N, Halar EM, Tendchoff EM, Marchioro TL, Masock AJ. Effects of renal transplantation on motor nerve conduction velocity. Arch Phys Med Rehabil 1972;53:227–231.

124. Chaumont P, Lérique J, Bigot B, Vantelon J, Zingraff J, Funk-Bretano JL. Signes électriques et électromyographiques des urémies chroniques graves après transplantation rénale. Rev Neurol 1966;115:150–153.

125. Funk-Bretano JL, Chaumont P, Vantelon J, Zingraff J. Polyneurite au cours de l'urémie chronique: évolution après transplantation rénale (10 observations personnelles). Nephron 1968;5:31–42.

126. Dobbelstein H, Altmeyer B, Edel H, Gurland HJ, Muller R, Pichelmaier H, Jabour A. Periphere Neuropathie bei chronischer Nieren-insuffiziene, bei Dauer dialysebehandlung und nach Nieren transplantation. Med Klin 1968;63:616–622.

127. Nielsen VK. The peripheral nerve function in chronic renal failure. IX. Recovery after renal transplantation: electrophysiological aspects (sensory and motor nerve conduction). Acta Med Scand 1974;195:171–180.

128. Harding AE, Fanu JL. Carpal tunnel syndrome related to antebrachial Cimino-Brescia fistula. J Neurol Neurosurg Psychiatry 1977;40:511–513.

129. Bolton CF, Driedger AA, Lindsay RM. Ischemic neuropathy in uraemic patients caused by bovine arterovenous shunt. J Neurol Neurosurg Psychiatry 1970;42:810–814.

130. Wilbourn AJ, Furlan AJ, Hulley W, Ruschhaupt W. Ischemic monomelic neuropathy. Neurology 1983;33:447–451.

131. Knezevic W, Mastaglia FL. Neuropathy associated with Brescia-Cimino arteriovenous fistulas. Arch Neurol 1984;41:1184–1186.

132. Schenck E, Dietz V. Alkoholische polyneuropathie: Elektrophysiologische und klinische Befunde bei 85 Patienten. Arch Psychiat Nervenkr 1975;220:159–170.

133. Behse F, Buchthal F. Alcoholic neuropathy: clinical, electrophysiological and biopsy findings. Ann Neurol 1977;2:95–110.

134. Walsh JC, McLeod JG. Alcoholic neuropathy: an electrophysiological and histological study. J Neurol Sci 1970;10:457–469.

135. Neundorfer B. Ein Beitrag zur Alkoholpolyneuropathie: klinisches Bild sowie elektromyographische und elektroneurographische Untersuchungsergebnisse. Fortschr Neurol Psychiatry 1972;40:270–286.

136. Tackmann W, Minkenberg R, Strenge H. Correlation of electrophysiological and quantitative histological findings in the sural nerve of man: studies in alcoholic neuropathy. J Neurol 1977;216:289–299.

137. Blackstock E, Rushwirth G, Guth D. Electrophysiological studies in alcoholism. J Neurol Neurosurg Psychiatry 1972;35:326–334.

138. Casey EB, LeQuesne PM. Electrophysiological evidence for a distal lesion in alcoholic neuropathy. J Neurol Neurosurg Psychiatry 1972;35:624–630.

139. Mawsley C, Mayer RF. Nerve conduction in alcoholic polyneuropathy. Brain 1965;88:335–356.

140. Casey EB, LeQuesne PM. Alcoholic neuropathy. In: Desmedt JE, ed., New developments in EMG and clinical neurophysiology, vol 2. Basel: Karger, 1973:279–285.

141. D'Amour ML, Shahani BT, Young RR, Bird KT. The importance of studying sural nerve conduction and the late responses in the evaluation of alcoholic subjects. Neurology 1979;29:1600–1604.

142. Takahashi K, Nakamura H. Axonal degeneration in Beriberi neuropathy. Arch Neurol 1976;33:836–841.

143. Ohnishi A, Tsuji S, Igisu H, Murai Y, Goto I, Kuroiwa Y, Tsujihata M, Takamori M: Beriberi neuropathy. Morphometric study of sural nerve. J Neurol Sci 1980;45:177–190.

144. Botez MI, Peyronnard JM, Bachevalier J, et al. Polyneuropathy and folate deficiency. Arch Neurol 1978;35:581–584.

145. Fehling C, Jagerstad M, Lindstand K et al. Folate deficiency and neurological disease. Arch Neurol 1974;30:263–265.

146. Ishii N, Nishihara Y. Pellagra among chronic alcoholics: clinical and pathological study of 20 necropsy cases. J Neurol Neurosurg Psychiatry 1981;44:209–215.

147. Taher Y, Tawfik E, El Chonemi T, Salen K, Elwan O. Peripheral nerve conduction in pellagric neuropathy. Acta Neurol Scand 1964;40:144–150.

148. Ochoa J. Isonizid neuropathy in man: quantitative electron microscope study. Brain 1970;93:831–850.

149. Ott T, Rabinowicz T, Morand B. étude clinique et histopathologique d'un cas de polynévrite survenue au cours du traitement par l'isoniazide. Revue Neurol 1959;100:103–117.

150. Schaumburg H, Kaplan J, Winderbank A, Vick N, Rasmus S, Pleasure D, Brown M: Sensory neuropathy from pyridoxin abuse. New Engl J Med 1983;309:445–448.

151. Parry GJ, Bredesen DE. Sensory neuropathy with low-dose pyridoxine. Neurology 1985;35:1466–1468.

152. Krinke G, Schaumburg HH, Spencer PS, Siter K, Thomann P, Hesse R. Pyridoxine megavitaminosis produces degeneration of peripheral sensory neurons (sensory neuropathy) in the dog. Neurotoxicology 1981;2:13–24.

153. Mayer RF. Peripheral nerve function in vitamin B$_{12}$ deficiency. Arch Neurol 1965;13:355–361.

154. Lockner D, Reisenstein P, Wennberg A, et al. Peripheral nerve function in pernicious anemia before and after treatment. Acta Haematol 1969;41:257–263.

155. Hahn A, Gilbert JJ, Brown WF. A study of the sural nerve in pernicious anemia. Can J Neurol Sci 1976;3:217.

156. McCombe PA, McLeod JG. The peripheral neuropathy of vitamin B12 deficiency. J Neurol Sci 1984;66:117–126.

157. McLeod JG, Walsh JC, Little JM. Sural nerve biopsy. Med J Aust 1969;2:1092–1096.

158. Muller DPR, Lloyd JK, Wolff OH. Vitamin E and neurological function. Lancet 1983;1:225–227.

159. Harding AE, Muller DPR, Thomas PK et al. Spinocerebellar degeneration secondary to chronic intestinal malabsorption: a vitamin E deficiency syndrome. Ann Neurol 1982;12:419–424.

160. Werlin SL, Harb JM, Swick H, et al. Neuromuscular dysfunction and ultrastructural pathology in children with chronic cholestasis and vitamin E deficiency. Ann Neurol 1983;13:291–296.

161. Weintraub MI. Hypophosphatemia mimicking acute Guillain-Barré-Strohl syndrome. JAMA 1976;235:1040–1041.

162. Yagnik P, Singh N, Burns R. Peripheral neuropathy with hypophosphatemia in a patient receiving intravenous hyperalimentation. Muscle Nerve 1962;5:562.

163. Iyer GV, Taori GM, Kapadia CR, Mathan VI, Baker SJ. Neurologic manifestations in tropical sprue. Neurology 1973;23:959–966.

164. Banerji NI, Hurwitz LJ. Neurological manifestations after gastric surgery. Acta Neurol Scand 1971;47:485–513.

165. Abaerbanel JM, Berginer VM, Osimani A, Solomon H, Charuzi I. Neurologic complications after gastric restriction surgery for morbid obesity. Neurology 1987;37:196–200.

166. Low PA, McLeod JG, Turile JR, Donnelly P, Wright RG. Peripheral neuropathy in acromegaly. Brain 1974;97:139–152.

167. Dinn JJ, Dinn E. Natural history of acromegalic peripheral neuropathy. Quart J Med New Series 1985;57:833–842.

168. Oh SJ, Sarala PK, Kuba T, Elmore R. Tarsal tunnel syndrome: electrophysiological study. Ann Neurol 1978;5:327–330.

169. Feibel JH, Campa JF. Thyrotoxic neuropathy (Basedow's paraplegia). J Neurol Neurosurg Psychiatry 1976;39:491–497.

170. Dyck PJ, Lambert EH. Polyneuropathy associated with hypothyroidism. J Neuropathol Exp Neurol 1970;29:631–658.

171. Fincham RW, Cape CA. A study of sensory nerve conduction in the upper extremities. Arch Neurol 1968;19:464–466.

172. Kaeser HE. Nerve conduction velocity measurements. In: Vinken PJ, Bruyn GW, ed. Handbook of clinical neurology, vol 7. Amsterdam: North Holland Press, 1970:116–196.

173. Schwartz MS, Mackworth-Young CG, McKeran RO. The tarsal tunnel syndrome in hypothyroidism. J Neurol Neurosurg Psychiatry 1983;46:440–442.

174. Pollard JD, McLeod JG, Honnibal A, Verheljden MA. Hypothyroid polyneuropathy. J Neurol Sci 1982;53:461–471.

175. Nemmi R, Bottacchi E, Fazio R, Mamoli A, Corbo M, Cmaerlingo M, Galardi G, Erenbough L, Canal N. Polyneuropathy in hypothyroidism: clinical, electrophysiological and morphological findings in four cases. J Neurol Neurosurg Psychiatry 1987;50:1454–1460.

176. Shirabe T, Tawara S, Terao A, Araki S. Myxedematous polyneuropathy: a slight and electronmicroscopic study of the peripheral nerve and muscle. J Neurol Neurosurg Psychiatry 1975;38:241–247.

177. Sweeney VP, Pathak MA, Asbury AK: Acute intermittent porphyria: increased ALA-synthetase activity during an acute attack. Brain 1970;93:369–380.

178. Anzil AP, Dozic S: Peripheral nerve changes in porphyric neuropathy: findings in a sural nerve biopsy. Acta Neuropathol 1978;42:121–126.

179. Maytham DV, Eales L. Electrodiagnostic findings in porphyria. S Afr Med J 1971;17:99–100.

180. Nagler W. Peripheral neuropathy in acute intermittent porphyria. Arch Phys Med 1971;51:275–284.

181. Albers JW, Robertson WC, Daube JR. Electrodiagnostic findings in acute porphyric neuropathy. Muscle Nerve 1978;1:292–296.

182. Flügel KA, Druschky KF. Electromyogram and nerve conduction in patients with acute intermittent porphyria. J Neurol 214:267–279, 1977

183. Behse F, Buchthal F. Sensory action potentials and biopsy of the sural nerve in neuropathy. Brain 1978;101:473–493.

184. Knill-Jones RP, Goodwill CJ, Dyan AD, Williams R. Peripheral neuropathy in chronic liver disease: clinical, electrodiagnostic, and nerve biopsy findings. J Neurol Neurosurg Psychiatry 1972;35:27–30.

185. Seneverathe KN, Peiris OA. Peripheral nerve function in chronic liver disease. J Neurol Neurosurg Psychiatry 1970;33:606–614.
186. Dyan AD, Williams R. Demyelinating peripheral neuropathy and liver disease. Lancet 1967;2:133–134.
187. Kardel T, Nielsen VK. Hepatic neuropathy: a clinical and electrophysiological study. Acta Neurol Scand 1974;50:503–526.
188. Thomas PK, Walker JG. Xanthomatous neuropathy in primary biliary cirrhosis. Brain 1965;88:1079–1088.
189. Charron L, Peyronnard JM, Marchand L. Sensory neuropathy associated with primary biliary cirrhosis. Arch Neurol 1980;37:84–87.
190. Ludwig J, Cyck PJ, LaRusso NF. Xanthomatous neuropathy of liver. Human Pathol 1982;13:1049–1051.
191. Danta G. Hypoglycemic peripheral neuropathy. Arch Neurol 1969;21:121–132.
192. Mulder DW, Bastron JA, Lambert EH. Hyperinsulin neuropathy. Neurology 1956;6:627–635.
193. Bolton CF, Gilbert JJ, Hahn AF, Sibbald W. Polyneuropathy in critically ill patients. J Neurol Neurosurg Psychiatry 1984;47:1223–1231.
194. Bolton CF. Electrophysiologic studies of critically ill patients. Muscle Nerve 1987;10:129–135.
195. Zochodne DW, Bolton CF, Wells GA, et al. Critical illness polyneuropathy; a complication of critical illness and multiple organ failure. Brain 1987;110:819–842.
196. Bolton C, Laverty DA, Brown JD, Witt NJ, Hahn AF, Sibbald WJ. Critically ill polyneuropathy: electrophysiological studies and differentiation from Guillain-Barré syndrome. J Neurol Neurosurg Psychiatry 1986;49:563–573.
197. Kelly JJ, Kyle RA, O'Brien PC, Dyck PJ. Prevalence of monoclonal protein in peripheral neuropathy. Neurology 1981;31:1480–1483.
198. Croft PB, Wilkinson M. The incidence of carcinomatous neuromyopathy in patients with various types of carcinoma. Brain 1965;88:427–434.
199. Dyan AD, Croft PB, Wilkinson M. Association of carcinomatous neuromyopathy with different histological types of carcinoma of the lung. Brain 1967;88:435–488.
200. Hildebrandt J, Coers C. The neuromuscular function in patients with malignant tumors. Brain 1967;90:67–82.
201. Moddly JF. Electrophysiological investigation into the neurological complications of carcinoma. Brain 1965;88:1023–1036.
202. Trojaborg W, Frantzen E, Andersen I. Peripheral neuropathy and myopathy associated with carcinoma of the lung. Brain 1969;92:71–82.
203. Croft PB, Henson RA, Urich H, Wilkinson PC. Sensory neuropathy with bronchial carcinoma: a study of four cases showing serological abnormalities. Brain 1965;88:501–514.
204. Denny-Brown, D. Primary sensory neuropathy with muscular changes associated with carcinoma. J Neurol Neurosurg Psychiatry 1948;3:237–252.
205. Anderson NE, Rosenblue MK, Graus F, Wiley RG, Posner JB. Autoantibodies in paraneoplastic syndromes associates with small-cell lung cancer. Neurology 1988;38:1391–1398.
206. Horwich, MS, Cho L, Porro RS, Posner JB. Subacute sensory neuropathy: a remote effect of carcinoma. Ann Neurol 1977;2:7–19.
207. Schaumburg HH, Spencer PS, Thomas PK. Disorders of peripheral nerves. Philadelphia: FA Davis, 1983.
208. Hawley RT, Cohen MH, Sauni H, et al. The carcinomatous neuromyopathy of oat cell lung cancer. Ann Neurol 1980;7:65–72.
209. Campbell MJ, Paty DW. Carcinomatous neuromyopathy. 1. Electrophysiological studies. J Neurol Neurosurg Psychiatry 1974;37:131–141.
210. Travainen H, Larsen A. Some features of the neuromuscular complications of pulmonary carcinoma. Ann Neurol 1977;2:495–502.
211. Croft PB, Urich H, Wilkinson M. Peripheral neuropathy of the sensoriumotor type associated with malignant disease. Brain 1967;90:31–66.
212. Rae-Grant AD, Feasby TE, Brown WF, et al. A reversible polyneuropathy associated with cancer. Neurology 1986;36(Suppl 1):8.
213. Graus F, Ferrer I, Lamarca J. Mixed carcinomatous neuropathy in patients with lung cancer and lymphoma. Acta Neurol Scand 1983;68:40–48.
214. Julien GJ, Vital C, Aupyu G et al. Guillain-Barré syndrome and Hodgkin's disease. J Neurol Sci 1980;45:23–27.
215. Lisak RP, Mitchell M, Zweiman B, et al. Guillain-Barré syndrome and Hodgkin's disease: three cases with immunological studies. Ann Neurol 1977;1:72–78.
216. Amundson DE, Goodman JC. Hodgkin's disease in association with Guillain-Barré-Strohl syndrome: case report. Milit Med 1983;148:512–513.
217. Sumi SM, Farrell DF, Knauss TA. Lymphoma ad leukemia manifested by steroid-responsive polyneuropathy. Arch Neurol 1983;40:577–582.
218. Kelly JJ. Polyneuropathies associated with malignancies and plasma cell dyscrasis. In: Brown WF, Bolton CF, eds. Clinical electromyography. Boston: Butterworth, 1987.
219. Johnson PC, Roak LA, Hamilton RH, Laguana JF. Paraneoplastic vasculitis of nerve, a remote effect of cancer. Ann Neurol 1979;5:437–444.
220. Torvik A, Berntzen AE. Necrotizing vasculitis without visceral involvement. Postmortem examination of three cases with affection of skeletal muscles and peripheral nerves. Acta Med Scand 1968;184:69–77.

221. Vincent D, Dubas F, Hauw JJ, Bodeau JP, L'Hermitte F, Buge A, Cataigne P. Nerve and muscle microvasculitis. J Neurol Neurosurg Psychiatry 1986;49:1007–1010.

222. Oh SJ, Slaughter R, Harrell L. Paraneopalstic vasculitic neuropathy: a treatable neuropathy. Muscle Nerve 1991;14:152–156.

223. Evans BK, Fagan C, Arnold T, Dropcho EJ, Oh SJ. Paraneoplastic motor neuron disease and renal cell carcinoma; improvement after nephrectomy. Neurology 1990;40:960–962.

224. Schold SC, Cho ES, Somasundaram M, Posner JB. Subacute motor neuronopathy: a remotor effect of lymphoma. Ann Neurol 1979;5:271–287.

225. Younger DS, Rowland LP, Latov N, et al. Lymphoma, motor neuron diseases, and amyotrophic lateral scolerosis. Ann Neurol 1991;29:78–86.

226. Buchannan DS, Malamud N. Motor neuron disease with renal cell carcinoma and postoperative neurologic remission. Neurology 1973;23:891–894.

227. Peacock A, Dawkins K, Rushworth G. Motor neuron disease associated with bronchial carcinoma: letter. Br Med J 1979;2:499–500.

228. Peters HA, Clatanoff DV. Spinal muscular atrophy secondary to macroglobulinemia. Neurology 1968;18:101–108.

229. Mitchell DM, Olczak SA. Remission of a syndrome indistinguishable from motor neuron disease after resection of bronchial carcinoma. Br Med J 19789;2:176.

230. Diaz-Arrastia R, Younger DS, Hair L, Inghirami G, Hays AP, Knowles DM, Odel JG, Fetell MR, Lovelace RE, Rowland LP. Neurolymphomatosis: a clinicopathologic syndrome re-emerges. Neurology 1992;42:1136–1141.

231. Gherardi R, Gaulard P, Prost C, Rocha D, Imbert M, Andre C. Rochant H, Farcet JP. T-cell lymphoma revealed by a peripheral neuropathy. Cancer 1986;58:2710–2716.

232. Kuroda Y, Nakata H, Kakigi R, Oda K, Shibasaki H, Nakashiro H. Human neurolymphomatosis by adult T-cell leukemia. Neurology 1989;39:144–146.

233. Krendel DA, Stahl RL, Chan WC. Lymphomatous polyneuropathy. Biopsy of clinically involved nerve and successful treatment. Arch Neurol 1991;48:330–332.

234. Ince PG, Shaw PJ, Fawcett PRW, Bates D. Demyelinating neuropathy due to primary IgM kappa B cell lymphoma of peripheral nerve. Neurology 1987;37:1231–1235.

235. Thomas FP, Vallejos U, Foitl DR, et al. B-cell small lymphocytic lymphoma and chronic lymphocytic leukemia with peripheral neuropathy: two cases with neuropathological findings and lymphocyte marker analysis. Acta Neuropath 1990;80:198–203.

236. Purohit DPP, Dick DJ, Perry RH et al. Solitary extranodal lymphoma of sciatic nerve. J Neurol Sci 1986;74:23–24.

237. Pillary PKL, Hardy RW Jr, Wilbourn AJ, et al. Solitary primary lymphoma of the sciatic nerve: case report. Neurosurgery 1988;23:370–376.

238. Oh SJ. Electrophysiological profile in arsenic neuropathy. J Neurol Neurosurg Psychiatry 1991;54:1103–1105.

239. Jenkins R. Inorganic arsenic intoxication and the nervous system. Brain 1966;89:479–498.

240. Donofrio P, Wilbourn A, Albers J, Rogers L, Salanga V, Greenberg H. Acute arsenic intoxication presenting as Guillain-Barré syndrome. Muscle Nerve 1987;101:14–20.

241. LeQuesne PM, McLeod JG. Peripheral neuropathy following single dose arsenic exposure: clinical course in four patients with electrophysiological and histological studies. J Neurol Sci 1977;2:437–452.

242. Murphy MJ, Lyon LW, Taylor JW. Subacute arsenic neuropathy; clinical and electrophysiological observation. J Neurol Neurosurg Psychiatry 1981;44:896–900.

243. O'Shaughnessy E, Kraft GH. Arsenic poisoning: long-term follow-up of a nonfatal case. Arch Phys Med Rehabil 1976;57:403–406.

244. Oh SJ. Abnormality in sensory nerve conduction: a distinct electrophysiological feature of arsenic polyneuropathy. EEG in Clin Neurophysiol 1980;49:21.

245. Boothby JA, DeJesus P, Rowland LP. Reversible forms of motor neuron disease. Arch Neurol 1974;31:18–23.

246. Oh SJ. Lead neuropathy: case report. Arch Phys Med Rehabil 1975;56:312–316.

247. Gombault M. Contribution à l'étude anatomique de la névrite parenchymateuse subaigue et chronique: Névrite segmentaire peri-axile. Arch Neurol 1980;1:11–38.

248. Fullerton PM. Chronic peripheral neuropathy produced by lead poisoning in guinea pigs. J Neuropathol Exp Neurol 1966;25:214–236.

249. Feldman RG, Haddow J, Kopito L, Schwachman H. Altered peripheral nerve conduction velocity: chronic lead intoxication in children. Am J Dis Child 1973;125:39–41.

250. Delwaide PJ, Chantraine A. Participation spinale dans l'intoxication saturnine: arguments électromyographiques. In: Proceedings of 6th International Congress of EEG and Clinical Neurophysiology. Vienna, 1965:643–646.

251. Simpson JA, Seaton DA, Adams JF. Response to treatment with chelating agents of anemia, chronic encephalopathy, and myelopathy due to lead poisoning. J Neurol Neurosurg Psychiatry 1964;27:536–541.

252. Yaratnam JJE, Devathasan G, Ong CN, Wong PK. Neurophysiological studies on workers exposed to lead. Br J Int Med 1985;42:173–177.

253. Seppalainen AM, Hernberg S. Sensitive technique for detecting subclinical lead neuropathy. Br J Int Med 1972;29:443–449.

254. Sessa T, Ferrari E, D'Amato CG. Velocita di conduzione nervosa nei saturnini. Folia Medica (Napoli) 1965;48:658–668.
255. Feldman RG, Hayes MKRG, Hayes JK, Younes R, Aldrich FD. Lead neuropathy in adults and children. Arch Neurol 1977;34:481–488.
256. Fiaschi AF, DeGrandis D, Ferrari F. Correlations between neurophysiological and histological findings in subclinical lead neuropathy. In: Proc 5th Internat Cong EMG Clin Neurophysiol, Rochester, 1975.
257. Cavanagh JB, Fuller NH, Johnson HRM, et al. The effects of thallium salts, with particular reference to effects of the nervous system changes. Q J Med 1974;43:293–319.
258. Limos LC, Ohnish A, Suzuki N, et al. Axonal degeneration and focal muscle fiber necrosis in human thallotoxicosis: histopathological studies of nerve and muscle. Muscle Nerve 1982;5:698–706.
259. Davis LE, Standefer JC, Kornfeld M, Abercrombie DM, Butler C. Acute thallium poisoning: toxicological and morphological studies of the nervous system. Ann Neurol 1981;10:38–44.
260. Kaeser HE, Lambert EH. Nerve function studies in experimental polyneuritis. EEG Clin Neurophysiol 1962; 22(Suppl):29–35.
261. Bank WJ, Pleasure DE, Suzuki K, Nigro M, Katz R. Thallium poisoning. Arch Neurol 1972;26:456–464.
262. Roby DS, Bennett RH, Rorke L. Thallium-induced peripheral neuropathy; clinical, electrodiagnostic and pathologic findings in four cases, and literature review. Muscle Nerve 1982;5:557.
263. Rustam H, Handi T. Methyl mercury poisoning in Iraq: a neurological study. Brain 1974;97:499–510.
264. Vroom FQ, Greer M. Mercury vapour intoxication. Brain 1972;95:305–318.
265. LeQuesne PM, Damluf SF, Rustam H. Electrophysiological studies of the peripheral nerves in patients with organic mercury poisoning. J Neurol Neurosurg Psychiatry 1974;37:333–339.
266. Windebank AJ, McCall JT, Dyck PJ. Metal neuropathy. In: Dyck PJ, Thomas PK, Lambert EH, eds. Peripheral neuropathy. Vol. II. Philadelphia: WB Saunders, 1984:2169–2179.
267. Adams CR, Ziegler DK, Lin JT. Mercury intoxication simulating amyotrophic lateral sclerosis. JAMA 1983;250:642–623.
268. Vroom FQ, Greer M. Mercury vapor intoxication. Brain 1972;95:305–318.
269. Iyer K, Goodgold J, Eberstein A, Berg P. Mercury poisoning in a dentist. Arch Neurol 1976;33:788–790.
270. Albers JW, Cavender GD, Levine SP, Langolf GD. Asymptomatic sensorimotor polyneuropathy in workers exposed to elemental mercury. Neurology 1982;32:1168–1174.
271. Goldstein NP, McCall JT, Dyck PJ. Metal neuropathy. In: Dyck PJ, Thomas PK, Lambert EH, eds. Peripheral neuropathy, vol 2. Philadelphia: WB Saunders, 1975:1227–1262.
272. Walsh JC. Gold neuropathy. Neurology 1970;20:455–458.
273. Endtz LJ. Complications nerveuses du traitement aurique. Rev Neurol 1958;99:395–410.
274. Katrak SM, Pollock M, O'Brien CP, et al. Clinical and morphological features of gold neuropathy. Brain 1980;103:671–693.
275. Mitsumoto H, Wilbourn AJ, Subramony SH. Generalized myokymia and gold therapy. Arch Neurol 1982;39:449–450.
276. Meyer M, Haecki M, Ziegler W, et al. Autonomic dysfunction and myokymia in gold neuropathy. In: Canal N, Pozza G eds. Peripheral neuropathies. Amsterdam: Elsevier/North-Holland Biomedical Press, 1978:475–480.
277. Mollman JE, Hogan M, Glover DJ, McCluskey LF. Unusual presentation of cis-platinum neuropathy. Neurology 1988;38:488–490.
278. Roelofs RI, Hrushesky W, Rogin J, Rosenberg L. Peripheral sensory neuropathy and cisplatin chemotherapy. Neurology 1984;34:934–938.
279. Riggs JE, Ashraf M, Snyder RD, Gutmann L. Propsective nerve conduction studies in cisplatin therapy. Ann Neurol 1988;23:92–94.
280. Thompson SW, Davis LE, Kornfeld M, Hilgers RD, Standefer JC. Cisplatin neuropathy, clinical, electrophysiologic, morphologic, and toxicologic studies. Cancer 1984;54:1269–1275.
281. Stuart-Harris R, Ponder BA, Wrigley PF. Tetany associated with cis-platin. Lancet 1980;2:1303.
282. Ashraf M. Cis-platin-induced hypomagnesiumia and peripheral neuropathy. Gynecol Oncol 1983;16:309–318.
283. LeQuesne PM. Neuropathy due to drugs. In: Dyck PJ, Thomas PK, Lambert EH, Bunge R, eds. Peripheral neuropathy. Philadelphia: WB Saunders, 1984:2162–2179.
284. Schaumburg HH, Spencer PS, Thomas PK. Disorders of Peripheral Nerves. Philadelphia: FA Davis, 1984:119–155.
285. Pellissier JF, Pouget J, Cros D, De Victor B, Serratrice G, Toga M. Peripheral neuropathy induced by amodarone chrlohydrate. J Neurol Sci 1984;63:251–266.
286. Jacobs JM, Costa-Jussá FR. The pathology of amiodarone neurotoxicity. II peripheral neuropathy in man. Brain 1985;108:753–769.
287. Fraser AG, McQueen INF, Watt AH, Stephens MR. Peripheral neuropathy during long-term high-dose amiodarone therapy. J Neurol Neurosurg Psychiatry 1985;48:576–578.
288. Said G. Perhexiline neuropathy: a clinicopathological study. Ann Neurol 1978;3:259–266.
289. Bouche P, Bousser MG, Peytour MA, Cathala HP. Perhexiline maleate and peripheral neuropathy. Neurology 1979;29:739–743.
290. Schaumburg HH, Spencer PS. Human toxic neuropathy due to industrial agents. In Dyck PJ, Thomas PK, Lambert EH, Bunge R, eds. Peripheral neuropathy. Philadelphia: WB Saunders; 1984:2115–2132.
291. Asbury AK, Johnson PC. Pathology of peripheral nerve. Philadelphia: WB Saunders, 1978.
292. Davenport J, Farrell DF, Sumi SM. Giant axonal neuropathy caused by industrial chemicals: neuro-axonal masses in man. Neurology 1976;21:349.

293. Korobkin R, Asbury AK, Sumner AJ, Nielsen SL. Glue-sniffing neuropathy. Arch Neurol 1975;322:158–162.

294. Oh SJ, Kim JM. Giant axonal swelling in "huffer's neuropathy." Arch Neurol 33:583–586.

295. Rasminsky M, Sears TA. Internodal conduction in undissected demyelinated nerve fibers. J Physiol 1972;227:323–350.

296. Paulson GW, Waylonis GW. Polyneuropathy due to n-hexane. Arch Int Med 1976;136:880–882.

297. Towfighi J, Gonatas NK, Pleasure D, Cooper HS, McCree L. Glue sniffer's neuropathy. Neurology 1976;26:238–243.

298. Gonzalez EG, Downey JA. Polyneuropathy in a glue sniffer. Arch Phys Med Rehabil 1972;53:333–337.

299. Goto I, Matsumura M, Inoue N, et al. Toxic polyneuropathy due to glue-sniffing. J Neurol Neurosurg Psychiatry 1974;37:848–853.

300. Ciachetti C, Albritt G, Perticoni G, Siracua A, Curradi C. Toxic polyneuropathy in shoe industry workers: a study of 122 cases. J Neurol Neurosurg Psychiatry 1976;39:1151–1161.

301. Prockop LD, Alt M, Tison J. Huffer's neuropathy. JAMA 1974;229:1083–1084.

302. Allen N, Mendell JR, Billmaier DJ, Fontaine RE, O'Neill J. Toxic neuropathy due to methyl n-butyl ketone. Arch Neurol 1975;32:209–218.

303. Fullerton PM. Electrophysiological and histological observations on peripheral nerves in acrylamide poisoning in man. J Neurol Neurosurg Psychiatry 1969;32:186–192.

304. Takahashi M, Ohara T, Hashimoto K. Electrophysiological study of nerve injuries in workers handling acrylamide. Int Arch Arbeitsmed 1971;28:1–11.

305. Tabuenca JM: Toxic-allergic syndrome caused by ingestion of rapeseed oil denatured with aniline. Lancet 1981;2:567–568.

306. Cruz Martinez A, Pérez Conde MC, Ferrer MT, Cantón R, Téllez I. Neuromuscular disorders in a new toxic syndrome: electrophysiological study—a preliminary report. Muscle Nerve 1984;7:12–22.

307. Narashashi T. Mechanism of action of tetrodotoxin and saxitoxin on excitable membranes. Fed Proc 1972;31:1124–1132.

308. Oda K, Araki K, Totoki T, Shibasaki H. Nerve conduction study of human tetrodotoxication. Neurology 1989;39:743–745.

309. Long RR, Sarfgent JC, Hammer K. Paralytic shellfish poisoning: a case report and serial electrophysiologic observations. Neurology 1990;40:1310–1312.

310. Cameron J, Flowers AE, Capra MF. Electrophysiological studies on ciguatera poisoning in man. J Neurol Sci 1991;101:93–97.

311. Ayyar DR, Mullarly WJ. Ciguatera: clinical and electrophysiologic observations. Neurology 1978;28:354.

312. Allsop JL, Martin L, Lebris H, Pollard J, Walsh J, Hodgkinson S. Les manifestations neurologiques de la ciguatera. Rev Neurol 1986;142:590–597.

313. Donat JR, Donat JF. Tick paralysis with persistent weakness and electromyographic abnormalities. Arch Neurol 1981;38:59–61.

314. Cooper BJ, Spence I. Temperature-dependent inhibition of evoked acetylcholine release in tick paralysis. Nature 1976;263:693–695.

315. Pickett JB. Neuromuscular transmission In: Sumner AJ, ed. The physiology of peripheral nerve disease. Philadelphia: WB Saunders, 1980:238–264.

316. Murnaghan MF. Site and mechanism of tick paralysis. Science 1960;131:418–419.

317. Cherington M, Snyder RD. Tick paralysis: neurophysiologic studies. New Engl Med 1968;278:95–97.

318. DeBuck FL, O'Conner S. Tick toxicosis. Pediatrics 1977;50:328–329.

319. Haller JS, Fabara JA. Tick paralysis: case report with emphasis on neurological toxicity. Am J Dis Child 1972;124:915–917.

320. Mulder DW, Lambert EH, Bastron JA, Sprague RG. The neuropathies associated with diabetes mellitus: clinical and electromyographic study of 103 unselected diabetic patients. Neurology 1961;11:275–284.

321. Swift TR, Ignacio OJ. Tick paralysis: electrophysiologic studies. Neurology 1975;25:1130–1133.

322. Morris HH. Tick paralysis: electrophysiologic measurements. South Med J 1977;70:121–122.

323. Oh SJ, Eslami N, Nishihira T, Sarala PK, et al. Electrophysiological and clinical correlation in myasthenia gravis. Ann Neurol 1982;12:348–354.

324. Dyck PJ. Inherited neuronal degeneration and atrophy affecting peripheral, motor, sensory, and autonomic neurons. In: Dyck PJ, Thomas PK, Lambert EH, eds. Peripheral neuropathy, vol 2. Philadelphia: WB Saunders, 1975:825–867.

325. Bradley WG, Madrid R, Davis CJF. The peroneal muscular atrophy syndrome. J Neurol Sci 1977;32:123–136.

326. Thomas PK, Calne DB. Motor nerve conduction velocity in peroneal muscular atrophy: evidence for genetic heterogeneity. J Neurol Neurosurg Psychiatry 1974;37:68–75.

327. Humberstone PM. Nerve conduction studies in Charcot-Marie-Tooth disease. Acta Neurol Scand 1972;48:176–190.

328. Salisachs P. Wide spectrum of motor nerve conduction velocity in Charcot-Marie-Tooth disease: an anatomicophysiological interpretation. J Neurol Sci 1974;23:25–31.

329. Buchthal F, Behse F. Peroneal muscular atrophy and related disorders. I. Clinical manifestations as related to biopsy findings, nerve conduction, and electromyography. Brain 1977;100:41–66.

330. Dyck PJ, Lambert EH. Lower motor and primary sensory neuron diseases with peroneal muscular atrophy. I. Neurologic, genetic, and electrophysiologic findings in hereditary polyneuropathies. Arch Neurol 1968;18:603–618.

331. Gilliatt RW, Thomas PK. Extreme slowing of nerve conduction in peroneal muscular atrophy. Ann Phys Med 1957;4:104–106.

332. Kimura J. F-wave velocity in central segment of the median and ulnar nerves: a study in normal and in patients with Charcot-Marie-Tooth's disease. Neurology 1974;24:539–546.

333. Kimura J, Bosch P, Lindsay GM. F-wave conduction velocity in the central segment of the peroneal and tibial nerves. Arch Phys Med Rehabil 1975;56:492–497.

334. Behse F, Buchthal F. Peroneal muscular atrophy and related disorders. II. Histological findings in sural nerves. Brain 1977;100:67–85.

335. Dyck PJ, Lambert EH, Mulder DW. Charcot-Marie-Tooth disease: nerve conduction studies of a large kinship. Neurology 1963;13:1–11.

336. Myrianthopoulous ND, Lane MH, Silverberg DH, Vincent BL. Nerve conduction and other studies in families with Charcot-Marie-Tooth disease. Brain 1964;87:589–608.

337. Dyck PJ, Lambert EH. Lower motor and primary sensory neuron diseases with peroneal muscular atrophy. II. Neurologic, genetic, and electrophysiological findings in various neuronal degenerations. Arch Neurol 1968b;18:619–625.

338. Rossi LN, Lutschg J, Vassella F. Hereditary motor sensory neuropathies in childhood. Devel Med Child Neurol 1983;25:19–31.

339. Berciano J, Combarros O, Calleja J, Polo JM, Leno C. The application of nerve conduction and clinical studies to genetic counseling in hereditary motor and sensory neuropathy type I. Muscle Nerve 1989;12:302–306.

340. Combarros O, Calleja J, Figols J, Cabellow A, Berciano J. Dominantly inherited motor and sensory neuropathy type I. Genetic, clinical, electrophysiological and pathological features in four families. J Neurol Sci 1983;61:181–191.

341. Gutmann L, Fakadej A, Riggs JE. Evolution of nerve conduction abnormalities in children with dominant hypertrophic neuropathy for the Charcot-Marie-Tooth type. Muscle Nerve 1983;6:515–519.

342. Dyck PJ. Histologic measurements and find structure of biopsied sural nerve: normal, and in peroneal muscular atrophy, hypertrophic-neuropathy, and in congenital neuropathy. Mayo Clin Proc 1966;41:742–774.

343. Roy EP, Gutmann L, Riggs JE. Longitudinal conduction studies in hereditary motor and sensory neuropathy type 1. Muscle Nerve 1989;12:52–55.

344. Dyck PJ, Karnes JL, Lambert EH. Longitudinal study of neuropathic deficits and nerve conduction abnormalities in hereditary motor and sensory neuropathy type 1. Neurology 1989;39:1302–1308.

345. Lewis RA, Sumner AJ. The electrodiagnostic distinctions between chronic familial and acquired demyelinative neuropathies. Neurology 1982;332:592–596.

346. Oh SJ. Conduction block in hereditary motor sensory neuropathy, type 1: case report. Muscle Nerve 1992;15:521–523.

347. Hoogendiijk JE, De Visser M, Bour LJ, Jennekens FGI, Ongerboer BW. Conduction block in hereditary motor and sensory neuropathy, type 1. Muscle Nerve 1992;15:520–521.

348. Oh SJ, Chang CW: Conduction block and dispersion in hereditary motor and sensory neuropathy. Muscle Nerve 1987;10:656A.

349. Oelschlager R, White HM, Neilshimke R. Roussy-Levy syndrome: report of kindred and discussion of the nosology. Acta Neurol Scand 1971;47:80–90.

350. Lapresle J, Salisachs P, Kremblin-Bicetre L. Onion bulbs in a nerve biopsy specimen from an original case of Roussy-Levy disease. Arch Neurol 1973;29:346–348.

351. Kriel RL, Cliffer KD, Berry J, Sung JH, Bland CS. Investigation of a family with hypertrophic neuropathy resembling Roussy-Levy syndrome. Neurology 1974;24:801–809.

352. Dyck PJ, Gomez EH. Segmental demyelination in Dejerine-Sottas disease: light, phase contrast, and electron microscopic studies. Mayo Clin Proc 1968;43:280–296.

353. Andermann F, Lloyd-Smith DL, Mavor H, Mathieson G. Observations on hypertrophic neuropathy of Dejerine-Sottas. Neurology 1962;12:712–724.

354. Thomas PK, Lascelles RG. Hypertrophic neuropathy. Q J Med 1967;36:223–238.

355. Gilliatt RW, Sears TA. Sensory nerve action potentials in patients with peripheral nerve lesions. J Neurol Neurosurg Psychiatry 1958;21:109–118.

356. Joosten E, Gareels F, Gabreels-Festen A, Vrensen G, Korten J, Notermans S. Electron-microscopic heterogeneity of onion-bulb neuropathies of the Dejerine-Sottas type. Acta Neuropath 1974;27:105–118.

357. Kennedy WR, Sung JH, Berry JF. A case of congenital hypomyelination neuropathy: clinical, morphological, and chemical studies. Arch Neurol 1977;34:337–345.

358. Guzzetta F, Ferriere G, Lyon G. Congenital hypomyelination polyneuropathy: pathological findings compared with polyneuropathies starting later in life. Brain 1982;105:395–416.

359. Gabreëls-Festen AWM, Joosten EMG, Gabreëls FJM. Congenital demyelinating motor and sensory neuropathy with focally folded myelin sheaths. Brain 1990;113:1629–1645.

360. Towfighi J. Congenital hypomyelination neuropathy: glial bundles in cranial and spinal nerve roots. Ann Neurol 1981;10:570–573.

361. Quinlan CD, Martin EA. Refsum's syndrome: report of three cases. J Neurol Neurosurg Psychiatry 1970;33:817–823.

362. Refsum S. Heredopathia atactica polyneuritiformis phytanic-acid storage disease, Refsum's disease: a biochemically well-defined disease with a specific dietary treatment. Arch Neurol 1981;38:605–606.

363. Lundberg A, Lijia LG, Lungerberg PE, Try K. Heredopathia atactica polyneuritiformis (Refsum's disease): experiences of dietary treatment and plasmapheresis. Europ Neurol 1972;8:309–324.

364. Oftedal SI. Motor nerve conduction velocity in Refsum's disease. EEG Clin Neurophysiol 1965;19:617.

365. Steinberg D, Mize CE, Herndon H, Fales HM, Engel WK, Vroom FQ. Phytanic acid in patients with Refsum's syndrome and response to dietary treatment. Arch Int Med 1970;125:75–87.

366. Stokke OL, Eldjain L. Biochemical and dietary aspects of Refsum's disease. In: Dyck PJ, Thomas PK, Lambert EH, eds. Peripheral neuropathy, vol 2. Philadelphia: WB Saunders, 1975:872.

367. Sahgal V, Olsen WO. Heredopathia atactica polyneuritiformis (Phytanic acid storage disease). A new case with special reference to dietary treatment. Arch Int Med 1975;135:585–587.

368. Gibberd FB, Billimoria JD, Page NGR, Retsas S. Heredopathia atactica polyneuritiformis (Refsum's disease) treated by diet and plasma-exchange. Lancet 1979;1:575–578.

369. Gibberd FB, Billimoria JD, Goldman JM, et al. Heredopathia atactica polyneuritiformis: Refsum's disease. Acta Neurol Scand 1985;72:1–17.

370. Poulos A, Pollard AC, Mitchell JD, Wise G, Mortimer G. Patterns of Refsum's disease. Arch Dis Child 1984;59:222–229.

371. Denny-Brown D. Hereditary sensory radicular neuropathy. J Neurol Neurosurg Psychiatry 1951;14:237–252.

372. Turkington RW, Stiefel JW. Sensory radicular neuropathy. Arch Neurol 1965;12:19–24.

373. Mamoli B, Pateisky K. Untersuchungen der Nervenleitgeschwindigkeit bei hereditarer sensorischer Neuropathie. Z EEG-EMG 1972;3:167–170.

374. Kuroiwa Y, Murai Y. Hereditary sensory radicular neuropathy. Neuropathy 1964;14:574–577.

375. Ohta M, Ellefson RD, Lambert EH, Dyck PJ. Hereditary sensory neuropathy, type II: clinical, electrophysiologic, histologic, and biochemical studies of a Quebec kinship. Arch Neurol 1973;29:23–37.

376. Miller RG, Nielsen SL, Sumner AJ. Hereditary sensory neuropathy and tonic pupils. Neurology 1976;26:931–935.

377. Murray TJ. Congenital sensory neuropathy. Brain 1973;96:287–294.

378. Schoene WC, Asbury AK, Astrom KE, Masters R. Hereditary sensory neuropathy: A clinical and ultrastructural study. J Neurol Sci 1970;11:463–487.

379. Nukuda H, Pollock M, Haas LF. The clinical spectrum and morphology of type II hereditary sensory neuropathy. Brain 1982;105:647–665.

380. Aguayo AJ, Nair CPV, Bray GM. Peripheral nerve abnormalities in the Riley-Day syndrome. Arch Neurol 1971;24:106–116.

381. Brown JC, Johns RJ. Nerve conduction in familial dysautonomia. JAMA 1967;201:200–203.

382. McLeod JG. An electrophysiological and pathological study of peripheral nerves in Friedreich's ataxia. J Neurol Sci 1971;12:333–349.

383. Dunn HG. Nerve conduction studies in children with Friedreich's ataxia and ataxia-telangiectosia. Devel Med Child Neurol 1973;15:324–337.

384. D'Angelo A, Di Donato S, Negri G, Beulche F, Uziel G, Boeri R. Friedreich's ataxia in northern Italy: clinical, neurophysiological and in vivo biochemical studies. Can J Neurol Sci 1980;7:359–365.

385. Bouchard JP, Barbeau A, Bouchard R, Bouchard R. Electromyography and nerve conduction studies in Friedreich's ataxia and autosomal recessive spastic ataxia of Charlevoix-Saguenay (ARSACS). Can J Neurol Sci 1979;6:185–189.

386. Peyronnard JM, Lapointe L. Bouchard JP, Lamontagene A, Lemieux B, Barbeu A. Nerve conduction studies and electromyography in Friedreich's ataxia. Can J Neurol Sci 1976;3:313–317.

387. Caruso G, Santoro L, Perretti A, Serienga L, Crisci C, Ragno M, Barbieri F, Filla A. Friedreich's ataxia: electrophysiological and histological findings. Acta Neurol Scand 1983;67:26–40.

388. Ouvrier RA, McLeod JG, Conchi TE. Friedreich's ataxia. J Neurol Sci 1982;55:137–145.

389. Oh SJ, Halsey JH. Abnormality in nerve potential in Friedreich's ataxia. Neurology 1973;23:52–54.

390. Salisachs P, Codina M, Pradas J. Motor nerve conduction velocity in patients with Friedreich's ataxia. J Neurol Sci 1975;24:331–337.

391. Desmedt JE, Noel P. Average cerebral evoked potentials in the evaluation of lesions of the sensory nerves and of the central somatosensory pathway In: Desmedt JE, ed. New developments in EMG and clinical neurophysiology, vol 2. Basel: Karger, 1973:352–371.

392. Cruz Martinez A, Barrio M, Gutierrez AM, Lopez E. Abnormalities in sensory and mixed evoked potentials in ataxia-telangiectasia. J Neurol Neurosurg Psychiatry 1977;40:44–49.

393. Aggerbeck L, McMahon JP, Schanu AM. Hypobetalipoproteinemia: clinical and biochemical description of a new kindred with Friedreich's ataxia. Neurology 1974;24:1051–1063.

394. Miller RG. The neuropathy of abetalipoproteinemia. Muscle Nerve 1980;3:181–182.

395. Tackmann W, Herdemerten S. Neurologische symptome bei der A-β-lipoproteinamie. Fortschr Neurol Psychiatry 1979;47:24–35.

396. Wichman A, Buchthal F, Pezeshkpour GH, Gree RE. Peripheral neuropathy in a-betalipoproteinemia. Neurology 1985;35:1279–1289.

397. Miller RG, Davis CJF, Illingworth DR, Bradley W. The neuropathy of abetalipoproteinemia. Neurology 30;1980:1286–1291.

398. Muller DPR, Lloyd JK, Bird AC. Long-term management of abetalipoproteinaemia. Possible role for vitamin E. Arch Dis Child 1977;52:209–214.

399. McLeod JG, Evans WA. Peripheral neuropathy in spinocerebellar degeneration. Muscle Nerve 1981;4:51–61.

400. Rossi A, Ciacci G, Federico A, Mondelli M, Rizzuto N. Sensory and motor peripheral neuropathy in olivopontocerebellar atrophy. Acta Neurol Scand 1986;73:363–371.

401. Chokrovferty S, Duvoisin RC, Sachdeo R, Sage J, Lepore F, Nicklas W. Neurophysiologic study of olivopontocerebellar atrophy with or without glutamate dehydrogenase deficiency. Neurology 1984;35:652–659.

402. Chokroverty S, Khedekar R, Derby B, et al. Pathology of olivopontocerebellar atrophy with glutamate dehydrogenase deficiency. Neurology 1984;34:1451–1455.

403. Cruz Martinez A, Ferrer MT, Fueyo E, Galdos L. Peripheral neuropathy detected on electrophysiological study as first manifestation of metachromatic leukodystrophy in infancy. J Neurol Neurosurg Psychiatry 1975;38:169–174.

404. Fullerton PM. Peripheral nerve conduction in metachromatic leukodystrophy (sulphatide lipidosis). J Neurol Neurosurg Psychiatry 1964;27:100–105.

405. Yudell A, Gomez MR, Lambert EH, Dockerty MB. The neuropathy of sulfatide lipidosis. Neurology 1967;17:103–111.

406. Clark JR, Miller RG, Vidgoff JM. Juvenile-onset metachromatic leukodystrophy: biochemical and electrophysiological studies. Neurology 1979;29:346–353.

407. Hahn AF, Gordon BA, Feleki V, Hinton GG, Gilbert JJ. A variant form of metachromatic leukodystrophy without aryl-sulfatase deficiency. Ann Neurol 1982;12:33–36.

408. Thomas PK, King RHM, Kocen RS, Brett EM. Comparative ultrastructure observations on peripheral nerve abnormalities in the late infantile, juvenile and late onset forms of metachromatic leukodystrophy. Acta Neuropathol 1977;39:237–245.

409. Lake BD. Segmental demyelination of peripheral neuropathy in Krabbe's disease. Nature 1968;217:171–172.

410. Thomas PK, Halpern JP, King RHM, Patrick D. Glactosylceramide lipidosis: novel presentation as a slowly progressive spinocerebellar degeneration. Ann Neurol 1984;16:618–620.

411. Dunn HG, Lake BD, Dolman CL, Wilson J. The neuropathy of Krabbe's infantile cerebral sclerosis. Brain 92:329–344.

412. Hogan GR, Gutmann L, Chou SM. The peripheral neuropathy of Krabbe's (globoid) leukodystrophy. Neurology 1969;19:1094–1100.

413. Lieberman JS, Oshtory M, Taylor RG. Perinatal neuropathy as an early manifestation of Krabbe's disease. Arch Neurol 1980;37:446–447.

414. Dunn HG, Dolman CL, Farrell DF, Tischler B, Hasinoff C, Wolf LI. Krabbe's leukodystrophy without globoid cells. Neurology 1976;26:1035–1041.

415. Vercruyssen A, Martin JJ, Mercelis R. Neurophysiological studies in adrenomyeloneuropathy: a report on five cases. J Neurol Sci 1982;56:327–336.

416. Griffin JW, Gorene E, Schamburg H, Engel WK, Loriaux L. A probable variant of adrenoleukodystrophy. Neurology 1977;27:1107–1113.

417. Lovelace RE, Johnson WE, Martin J. Peripheral nerve involvement and carrier detection in Palizaeus-Mezbacher's disease. Arch Phys Med Rehabil 1976;57:600.

418. Duncan C, Strub R, McGarry P, Duncan D. Peripheral nerve biopsy as an aid to diagnosis in infantile neuroaxonal dystrophy. Neurology 1970;20:1024–1034.

419. Blatt Lyon B. Peripheral nerve involvement in Batten-Spiellmeyer-Vogt's disease. J Neurol Neurosurg Psychiatry 1975;38:175–179.

420. Grumnet ML, Zimmerman AW, Lewis RA. Ultrastructure and electrodiagnosis of peripheral neuropathy in Cockayne's syndrome. Neurology 1983;33:1606–1609.

421. Ohnishi A, Mitzudome A, Murai Y. Primary segmental demyelination in the sural nerve in Cockayne's syndrome. Muscle Nerve 1987;10:163–167.

422. Argov Z, Foffer D, Eisenberg S, Zimmerman Y. Chronic demyelinating peripheral neuropathy in cerebrotendinous xanthomatosis. Ann Neurol 1986;20:89–91.

423. Katz DA, Scheinberg L, Horoupian S, Salen G. Peripheral neuropathy in cerebrotendinous xanthomatosis. Arch Neurol 1985;42:1008–1010.

424. Kuritzky A, Berginer VM, Korczyn AD. Peripheral neuropathy in cerebrotendinous xanthomatosis. Neurology 1979;29:880–881.

425. Robbins KH, Kraemer KH, Lutzner MA et al. Xeroderma pigmentosum. An inherited disease with sun sensitivity, multiple cutaneous neoplasms and abnormal DNA repair. Ann Intern Med 1974;80:221–248.

426. Thrush DC, Holti G, Bradley WG, et al. Neurological manifestations of xeroderma pigmentosum in two siblings. J Neurol Sci 1974;22:91–104.

427. Tachi N, Sasaki K, Takashi K, et al. Peripheral neuropathy in four cases of group A xeroderma pigmentosum. J Child Neurol 1988;3:114–119.

428. Thomas PK, King RHM. Peripheral nerve change in amyloid neuropathy. Brain 1974;97:395–406.

429. Dyck PJ, Lambert EH. Dissociated sensation in amyloidosis. Arch Neurol 1969;20:490–507.

430. Sales-Luis ML. Electroneurophysiological studies in amyloid polyneuropathy type. J Neurol Neurosurg Psychiatry 1978;41:847–850.

431. Mahloudji M, Teasdall RD, Adamkiewicz JJ, Hartmann WH, Lambird PA, McKusick VA. The genetic amyloidosis with particular reference to hereditary neuropathic amyloidosis, Type II (Indiana or Rukavina type). Medicine 1969;48:1–37.

432. Rukavina JG, Block WD, Jackson CE, Falls HF, Carey TH, Curtis AC. Primary systemic amyloidosis: a review and experimental, genetic and clinical study of 29 cases with particular emphasis on the familial form. Medicine 1956;35:239–334.

433. Sales Luis ML. Electrophysiological studies in familial amyloid polyneuropathy—Portuguese type. J Neurol Neurosurg Psychiatry 1978;41:847–850.

434. Boysen G, Galassi G. Kamienicka Z, et al. Familial amyloid neuropathy and corneal lattice dystrophy. J Neurol Neurosurg Psychiatry 1979;42:1020–1030.

435. Pleasure DE. A-beta-lipoproteinemia and Tangier disease. In: Dyck PJ, Thomas PK, Lambert EH, eds. Peripheral neuropathy. Philadlephia: WB Saunders, 1975; Vol. 2:928–941.

436. Spiess H, Ludin H, Kummer H. Polyneuropathie bei familiarere Analphalipoproteinotomie. Nervenarzt 1969;40:191–193.

437. Gibbles E, Schaefer HE, Schröder JM, Haupt WF, Assmann G. Severe polyneuropathy in Tangier disease mimicking syringomyelia or leprosy. Clinical, biochemical, electrophysiological, and morphological evaluation, including electron microscopy of nerve, muscle, and skin biopsies. J Neurol 1985;232:283–294.

438. Kocen RS, Lloyd JK, Lascelles PT, Fosbrooks AS, Williams D. Familial alpha-lipoprotein deficiency (Tangier disease) with neurological abnormalities. Lancet 1967;1:1341–1345.

439. Pollock M, Nukuda H, Frith RW, Simcock JP, Allpress S. Peripheral neuropathy in Tangier disease. Brain 1983;106:911–928.

440. Haas LF, Austad WI, Bergin JD. Tangier disease. Brain 1974;97:351–354.

441. Engel WK, Dorman JD, Levy RJ, Fredrickson DS. Neuropathy in Tangier disease: alpha-lipoprotein deficiency manifesting as a familial recurring neuropathy and intestinal lipid storage. Arch Neurol 1967;17:1–9.

442. Marbini A, Gemignani F, Ferrarini G, et al. Tangier disease. A case with sensorimotor distal polyneuropathy and lipid accumulation in striated muscle and vasa nervorum. Acta Neuropathol 1985;67:121–127.

443. Karpati G, Carpenter S, Eisen AA, Wolfe LS, Feindel W. Multiple peripheral nerve entrapments: an unusual phenotypical variant of the Hunter syndrome (mucopolysaccharidosis II) in a family. Arch Neurol 1974;31:418–422.

444. Miner ME, Schimke RN. Carpal tunnel syndrome in pediatric mucopolysaccharidoses. J Neurosurg 1975;43:102–103.

445. Swift TR, McDonald TF. Peripheral nerve involvement in Hunter syndrome (mucopolysaccharidosis II). Arch Neurol 1976;33:845–846.

446. Kocen RS, Thomas PK. Peripheral nerve involvement in Fabry's disease. Arch Neurol 1970;22:81–88.

447. Ohnishi A, Dyck PJ. Loss of small peripheral sensory neurons in Fabry's disease. Arch Neurol 1974;31:120–124.

448. Sheth KJ, Swick HM. Peripheral nerve conduction in Fabry disease. Ann Neurol 1980;7:319–323.

449. Lockman LA, Kennedy WR, White JG. The Chediak-Higashi syndrome: electrophysiological and electronmicroscopic observations on the peripheral neuropathy. J Pediatr 1967;70:942–951.

450. Gumbinas M, Larsen M, Mei Liu H. Peripheral neuropathy in classic Niemann-Pick disease: ultrastructure of nerves and skeletal muscles. Neurology 1975;p 25:107–113.

451. Asbury AK, Gale MK, Cox SC, Baringer JR, Berg BO. Giant axonal neuropathy: a unique case with segmental neurofilamentous masses. Acta Neuropathol (Berl) 1972;20:237–247.

452. Guazzi GC, Malandrini A, Gerli R, Federico A. Giant axonal neuropathy in 2 siblings: a generalized disorder of intermediate filaments. J Europ Neurol 1991;31:50–56.

453. Berg BO, Rosenberg SH, Asbury AK. Giant axonal neuropathy. Pediatrics 1972;49:894–899.

454. Carpenter S, Karpati G, Andermann F, Gold R. Giant axonal neuropathy: a clinically and morphologically distinct neurological disease. Arch Neurol 1974;31:312–316.

455. Igisu H, Ohia M, Tabira T, et al. Giant axonal neuropathy. Neurology 1975;25:717–721.

456. Mizuno Y, Otsuka S, Takano Y, Suzuki Y, Hosaka A, Kaga M, Segawa M. Giant axonal neuropathy. Combined central and peripheral nervous system disease. Arch Neurology 1979;36:107–108.

457. Asbury AK, Arnason BGW, Karp HR, McFarlin DE. Criteria for diagnosis of Guillain-Barré syndrome. 1978;3:565–566.

458. Lisak RP, Brown MJ. Acquired demyelinating polyneuropathies. Semin Neurol 1987;7:40–47.

459. Asbury AK, Arnason BG, Adams RD. The inflammatory lesion in idiopathic polyneuritis. Medicine (Baltimore) 1969;48:173–215.

460. Albers JW, Donofrio PD, McGonagle TK. Sequential electrodiagnostic abnormalities in acute inflammatory demyelinating polyradiculoneuropathy. Muscle Nerve 1985;8:528–539.

461. Roper AH, Wijdicks EFM, Shahani BT. Electrodiagnostic abnormalities in 113 consecutive patients with Guillain-Barré syndrome. Arch Neurol 1990;40:881–887.

462. Bradshaw DY, Jones HR. Guillain-Barré syndrome in children: clinical course, electrodiagnosis, and prognosis. Muscle Nerve 1992;15:500–506.

463. DeJesus PVL. Landry-Guillain-Barré-Stroh syndrome: neuronal disorder and clinicoelectrophysiological correlation. EMG Clin Neurophysiol 1974;14:115–132.

464. Eisen A, Humphreys P. The Guillain-Barré syndrome. Arch Neurol 1974;30:438–443.

465. Lambert EH, Mulder DW. Nerve conduction in the Guillain-Barré syndrome. EEG Clin Neurophys 1964;17 (Abstr):86.

466. Martinez-Figueroa A, Hansen S, Ballantyn JP. A quantitative electrophysiological study of acute idiopathic polyneuritis. J Neurol Neurosurg Psychiatry 1977;40:156–161.

467. McLeod JG, Walsh JC, Prineas JW, Pollard JD. Acute idiopathic polyneuritis: a clinical and electrophysiological follow-up study. J Neurol Sci 1976;27:145–162.

468. Ramon PT, Taori GM. Prognostic significance of electrodiagnostic studies in the Guillain Barré syndrome. J Neurol Neurosurg Psychiatry 1976;39:163–170.

469. Miyoshi T, Oh SJ. Proximal slowing of nerve conduction in the Guillain-Barré syndrome. EMG Clin Neurophysiol 1977;17:287–296.

470. Kimura J. Proximal versus distal slowing of motor nerve conduction velocity in the Guillain-Barré syndrome. Ann Neurol 1978;3:344–350.

471. Bergamini L, Gandiglio G, Fra L. Motor and afferent nerve conduction in the Guillain-Barré syndrome. Electromyography 1966;6:205–232.

472. Brown WF, Feasby TE. Conduction block and denervation in Guillain-Barré syndrome. Brain 1984;107:219–239.

473. Kimura J, Butzer JF. F-wave conduction velocity in the Guillain-Barré syndrome. Arch Neurol 1975;32:524–529.

474. King D, Ashby P. Conduction velocity in the proximal segments of a motor nerve in the Guillain-Barré syndrome. J Neurol Neurosurg Psychiatry 1976;39:538–544.

475. Lachman T, Shahani BT, Young RA. Late responses as aids in diagnosis in peripheral neuropathy. J Neurol Neurosurg Psychiatry 1980;43:156–162.

476. Albers JW, Kelly JJ. Acquired inflammatory demyelinating polyneuropathies: clinical and electrodiagnostic features. 1989;12:435–451.

477. Eisen A, Humphreys P. The Guillain-Barré syndrome. Arch Neurol 1974;30:438–443.

478. Kimura J. An evaluation of the facial and trigeminal nerves in polyneuropathy: electrodiagnostic study in Charcot-Marie-Tooth disease, Guillain-Barré syndrome, and diabetic neuropathy. Neurology 1971;21:745–752.

479. Baneji NK, Millar JHD. Guillain-Barré syndrome in children, with special reference to serial nerve conduction studies. Dev Med Child Neurol 1972;14:56–63.

480. McQuillen MP. Idiopathic polyneuritis: serial studies of nerve and immune functions. J Neurol Neurosurg Psychiatry 1971;34:607–615.

481. Ludin HP, Tackmann W. Sensory neurography. New York: Thieme-Stratton, Inc., 1981.

482. McLeod JG. Electrophysiological studies in the Guillain-Barré syndrome. Ann Neurol 1981;9(Suppl):20–27.

483. Cornblath DR, Mellits ED, Griffin JW, McKhann GM, Albers JW, Miller RG, Feasby TE, Quaskey SA. Motor conduction studies in Guillain-Barré syndrome. Ann Neurol 1988;23:354–359.

484. Miller RG, Peterson GW, Daube JR, Albers JW. Prognostic value of electrodiagnosis in Guillain-Barré syndrome. Muscle Nerve 1988;11:769–774.

485. Winer JB, Hughes RAC, Osmond C. A prospective study of acute idiopathic neuropathy. I. Clinical features and their prognostic value. J Neurol Neurosurg Psychiatry 1988;51:605–612.

486. Van der Meché FGA, Meulstee J, Kleyweg RP. Axonal damage in Guillain-Barré syndrome. Muscle Nerve 1991;14:997–1002.

487. McKahann GM, Gfiffin JWE, Cornblath DR, Mellits ED, Fisher RS, Quaskey SA. Plasmapheresis and Guillain-Barré syndrome: analysis of prognostic factors and the effect of plasmapheresis. Ann Neurol 1988;23:347–353.

488. Bannister RG, Sears TA. The change in nerve conduction in acute idiopathic polyneuritis. J Neurol Neurosurg Psychiatry 1962;25:321–328.

489. Hausmanowa-Petrusewicz I, Ereryk-Szajewska B, Rowinsak-Marcinska K, Jedrzejowska H. Nerve conduction in Guillain-Barré syndrome. EEG Clin Neurophysiol 1977;93 (Abstr):590.

490. Cerra D, Johnson EW. Motor conduction velocity in "idiopathic" polyneuritis. Arch Phys Med Rehabil 1961;42:159–163.

491. Humphrey JG. Motor nerve conduction studies in the Landry-Guillain-Barré syndrome: acute ascending polyneuropathy. EEG Clin Neurophysiol 1964;17(Abstr):96.

492. Guillain-Barré Syndrome Study Group. Plasmapheresis and acute Guillain-Barré syndrome. Neurology 1985;35:1096–1104.

493. Berger AR, Logigian EL, Shahani BT. Reversible proximal conduction block underlies rapid recovery in Guillain-Barré syndrome. Muscle Nerve 1988;11:1039–1042.

494. Kaeser HE. Klinische und elektromyographische Verlausuntersuchungen beim Guillain-Barré-syndrom. Schweiz Arch Neurol Neurochir Psychiatr 1964;94:278–286.

495. Pleasure DE, Lovelace RE, Duvoisin RC. The prognosis of acute polyradiculo-neuritis. Neurology 1968;18:1143–1148.

496. Feasby TE, Gilbert JJ, Brown WF, et al. An acute axonal form of Guillain-Barré polyneuropathy. Brain 1986;109:1115–1126.

497. Suggs SP, Thomas TD, Joy JL, Lopez-Mendez A, Oh SJ. Vasculitic neuropathy mimicking Guillain-Barre syndrome. Arthritis Rheumatism, 1992;35:975–978.

498. Feit H, Tindall RSA, Glasberg M. Sources of error in the diagnosis of Guillain-Barré syndrome. Muscle Nerve 1982;5:111–117.

499. Dalakas M, Engel WK. Chronic relapsing polyneuropathy: Pathogenesis and treatment. Ann Neurol 1981a;9(Suppl):134–145.

500. Dalakas MC, Hoffs S, Engel WK, Madden DL, Sever JL. CSF "monoclonal" bands in chronic relapsing polyneuropathy. Neurology 1980;30:864–867.

501. Dyck PJ, Lais AC, Ohta M, Bastron JA, Okazaki H, Groover RV. Chronic inflammatory polyradiculoneuropathy. Mayo Clin Proc 1975;50:621–736.

502. Oh SJ. Subacute demyelinating polyneuropathy responding to corticosteroid treatment. Arch Neurol 1978;35:509–516,.

503. Sladky JT, Brown MJU, Berman PH. Chronic inflammatory demyelinating polyneuropathy of infancy: a corticosteroid-responsive disorder. Ann Neurol 1986;20:76–81.

504. Colan RV, Snead OC, Oh SJ, Benton JW. Steroid-responsive polyneuropathy with subacute onset in childhood. J Pediatr 1980;97:374–377.

505. Ad Hoc Subcommittee of the AAN AIDS Task Force. Research criteria for diagnosis of chronic inflammatory demyelinating polyneuropathy (CIDP). Neurology 1991;41:617–618.

506. Prineas JW, McLeod JG. Chronic relapsing polyneuritis. J Neurol Sci 1976;27:427–428.

507. McCombe PA, Pollard JD, McLeod JG. Chronic inflammatory demyelinating polyradiculoneuropathy. Brain 1987;110:1617–1630.

508. Barohn RJ, Kissel JT, Warmolts JR, Mendell JR. Chronic inflammatory demyelinating polyradiculoneuropathy: clinical characteristics, course, and recommendations for diagnostic criteria. Arch Neurol 1989;46:878–884.

509. Albers JW. Inflammatory demyelinating polyradiculoneuropathy. In: Brown WF, Bolton CF, eds. Clinical electromyography. Boston: Butterworth, 1987:211–244.

510. Oh SJ. Subacute demyelinating neuropathy responding to corticosteroid treatment: electrophysiological findings. Muscle Nerve 1982;5:562.

511. Pollard JD. A critical review of therapies in acute and chronic inflammatory demyelinating polyneuropathy. Muscle Nerve, 1987;10:214–221.

512. Van Doorn PA, Brand A, Strengers PFW, Meulstee J, Vermeulen M. High-dose intravenous immunoglobulin treatment in chronic inflammatory demyelinating polyneuropathy;: a double-blind, placebo-controlled, crossover study. Neurology 1990;40:209–212.

513. Adams RD, Asbury AK, Michelsen JJ. Multifocal pseudohypertrophic neuropathy. Trans Am Neurol Assoc 1965;9:30–34.

514. Parry GJ, Clarke S. Multifocal acquired demyelinating neuropathy masquerading as motor neuron disease. Muscle Nerve 1988;11:103–107.

515. Chad D, Hammer K, Sargent J. Slow resolution of multifocal weakness and fasciculation: a reversible motor neuron syndrome. Neurology 1986;36:1260–1263.

516. Pestronk A, Cornblath DR, Ilyas AA, et al. A treatable multifocal motor neuropathy with antibodies to GM1 ganglioside. Ann Neurol 1988;24:73–78.

517. Van den Bergh P, Logigian EL, Kelly JJ. Motor neuropathy with multifocal conduction blocks. Muscle Nerve 1989;11:26–31.

518. Roth G, Rohr J, Magistris MR, Ochsner F. Motor neuropathy with proximal multifocal persistent conduction block, fasciculations and myokymia. Eur Neurol 1986;25:416–423.

519. Auer R, Bell R, Lee M. Neuropathy with onion bulb formations and pure motor manifestation. Can J Neurol Sci 1989;24:194–197.

520. Bradley W, Bennett R, Good P, Little B. Proximal chronic inflammatory neuropathy with multifocal conduction block. Arch Neurol 1988;45:451–455.

521. Krarup C, Stewart J, Sumner A, Pestronk A, Lipton S. A syndrome of asymmetric limb weakness with motor conduction block. Neurology 1990;40:118–127.

522. Riser E, Joy J, Oh S. Demyelinating mononeuropathy multiplex. Neurology 1988;38(Suppl 1):225.

523. Oh SJ. The "amyotrophic lateral sclerosis form" of chronic inflammatory demyelinating neuropathy. Ann Neurol 28:269, 1990

524. Sadig SA, Thomas FP, Kilidireas K, et al. The spectrum of neurologic disease associated with anti-GMS antibodies. Neurology 1990;40:1067–1072.

525. Pestronk A, Chaudhry V, Feldman EL, et al. Lower motor neuron syndromes defined by patterns of weakness, nerve conduction abnormalities, and high titers of antiglycolipid antibodies. Ann Neurol 1990;27:316–326.

526. Kaji R, Shibasaki H, Kimura J. Multifocal demyelinating motor neuropathy: cranial nerve involvement and immunoglobulin therapy. Neurology 1992;42:506–509.

527. Oh SJ, Joy JL, Sunwoo I, Kuruoglu R. A case of chronic sensory demyelinating neuropathy responding to immunotherapies. Muscle Nerve 1992;15:255–256.

528. Joy JL, Oh SJ. Sensory neuropathy as a variant of chronic inflammatory demyelinating neuropathy. Neurology 1988;38(Suppl 1):189.

529. Oh SJ, Joy JL, Kuruoglu R. "Chronic sensory demyelinating neuropathy": chronic inflammatory demyelinating polyneuropathy presenting as a pure sensory neuropathy. J Neurol Neurosurg Psychiatry (In press).

530. Fisher M. An unusual variant of acute idiopathic polyneuritis (syndrome of ophthalmoplegia, ataxia, and areflexia. N Engl J Med 1956;255:57–65.

531. Guiloff RJ. Peripheral nerve conduction in the Fisher syndrome. J Neurol Neurosurg Psychiatry 1977;40:801–807.

532. Sauron B, Bouche P, Cthala HP, Chain F, Castaigne P. Miller Fisher syndrome: clinical and electrophysiologic evidence of peripheral origin in 10 cases. Neurology 1984;34:953–956.

533. Jamel GA, MacLeod WN. Electrophysiological studies in Miller Fisher syndrome. Neurology 1984;34:685–688.

534. Fross RD, Daube JR. Neuropathy in the Miller Fisher syndrome: clinical and electrophysiological findings. Neurology 1987;37:1493–1498.

535. Rushworth O, Gallai V. A clinico-electrophysiological study of three cases of post-infective polyneuritis with severe involvement of cranial nerves. Acta Neurol (Napoli) 1979;34:351–364.
536. De Pablos C, Calleja J, Fernández F, Berciano J. Miller Fisher syndrome: an electrophysiologic case study. EMG Clin Neurophysiol 1988;28:21–23.
537. Ricker K, Hertel G. Electrophysiological findings in the syndrome of acute ocular palsy with ataxia (Fisher syndrome). J Neurol 1976;214:35–44.
538. Weiss JA, White JC. Correlation of 1A afferent conduction with the ataxis of Fisher syndrome. Muscle Nerve 1986;9:327–332.
539. Sternman AB, Schaumburg HH, Asbury AK. The acute sensory neuropathy syndrome: a distinct clinical entity. Ann Neurol 1980;7:354–358.
540. Joy LJ, Oh SJ. Predominantly sensory acute inflammatory demyelinating polyneuropathy. Muscle Nerve 1990;13:867–868.
541. Dalakas MC. Chronic idiopathic ataxic neuropathy. Ann Neurol 1986;19:545–554.
542. Kaufman MD, Hopkins LC, Jurtitz BJ. Progressive sensory neuropathy in patients without carcinoma: a disorder with distinctive clinical and electrophysiological findings. Ann Neurol 1981;9:237–242.
543. Mamoli A, Nemni R, Camerlingo M, et al. A clinical, electrophysiological, morphological and immunological study of chronic sensory neuropathy with ataxia and paraesthesia. Acta Neurol Scand 1992;85:110–115.
544. Dyck PJ, Swanson CJ, Low PA, Bartleson JD, Lambert EH. Prednisone responsive hereditary motor and sensory neuropathy. Mayo Clin Proc 1982;57:239–246.
545. Bird SJ, Sladky JT. Corticosteroid responsive dominantly inherited neuropathy in childhood. Neurology 1991;41:437–439.
546. Delaney D. Neurologic manifestations in sarcoidosis. Ann Intern Med 1977;87:336–345.
547. Matthews WB. Sarcoid neuropathy. In: Dyck PJ, Thomas PK, Lambert EH, eds. Peripheral neuropathy. Philadelphia: WB Saunders, 1975:1199–1206.
548. Oh SJ. Sarcoid polyneuropathy: a histologically proved case. Ann Neurol 1980b;7:178–180.
549. Nemni R, Galassi G, Cohen M, et al. Symmetrical sarcoid polyneuropathy: analysis of a sural nerve biopsy. Neurology 1981;31:1217–1223.
550. Galassi G, Gibertoni M, Mancini A, et al. Sarcoidosis of the peripheral nerve: clinical, electrophysiological and histological study of two cases. Eur Neurol 1984;23:459–465.
551. Zuniga G, Ropper AH, Frank J. Sarcoid peripheral neuropathy. Neurology 1991;41:1558–1561.
552. Pestronk A. Motor neuropathies, motor neuron disorders, and antiglycolipid antibodies. Muscle Nerve 1991;14:927–936.
553. Latove N, Sherman LH, Meni R et al. Plasma cell dyscrasia and peripheral neuropathy with monoclonal antibody to peripheral nerve myelin. N Engl J Med 1980;303:618–621.
554. Melmud C, Frail D, Duncan I, et al. Peripheral neuropathy with IgM kappa monoclonal immunoglobulin directed against myelin-associated glycoprotein. Neurology 1983P:33:1397–1405.
555. Hafler DA, Johnson D, Kelly JJ, Panitch H, Kyle R, Weiner H. Monoclonal gammopathy and neuropathy: myelin-associated glycoprotein reactivity and clinical characteristics. Neurology 1986;36:75–78.
556. Pestronk A, Li F, Griffin J, et al. Polyneuropathy syndromes associated with serum antibodies to sulfatide and myelin-associated glycoprotein. Neurology 1991;41:357–362.
557. Nobile-Orazio E, Baldini L, Barbieri S, et al. Treatment of patients with neuropathy and anti-MAG IgM M protein. Ann Neurol 1988;24:93–97.
558. Nobile-Orazio E, Francomano E, Daverio R, et al. Anti-myelin-associated glycoprotein IgM antibody titers in neuropathy associated with macroglobulinemia. Ann Neurol 1989;26:543–550.
559. Graus F, Elkon B, Lloberes P, et al. Neuronal antinuclear antibody (anti-Hu) in paraneoplastic encephalomyelitis simulating acute polyneuritis. Acta Neurol Scand 1987;75:249–252.
560. Hawke SHB, Davies L, Pamphlett R, Guo YP, Pollard JD, McLeod JG. Vasculitic neuropathy: a clinical and pathological study. Brain 1991;114:2175–2190.
561. Vazquez G, Oh SJ, Goyne C. Electrophysiologic findings and sural nerve biopsy in vasculitic neuropathy. Muscle Nerve 1991;14:908.
562. Bouche P, Léger JM, Travers MA, Cathala HP, Castaigne P. Peripheral neuropathy in systemic vasculitis: clinical and electrophysiological study of 22 patients. Neurology 1986;36:1598–1602.
563. Olney RK. Neuropathies in connective tissue disease. Muscle Nerve 1992;15:531–542.
564. Dyck PJ, Benstead TJ, Conn DL, Stevens JC, Windebank AJ, Low PA. Nonsystemic vasculitic neuropathy. Brain 1987;110:843–854.
565. Ropert A, Metral S. Conduction block in neuropathies with necrotizing vasculitis. Muscle Nerve 1990;13:102–105.
566. Jamieson PW, Giuliani MJ, Martinez J. Necrotizing angiopathy presenting with multifocal conduction blocks. Neurology 1991;41:442–444.
567. Oh SJ, Herrara GA, Spalding DM. Eosinophilic vasculitic neuropathy in the Churg-Strauss syndrome. Arthritis Rheumatol 1986;29:1173–1175.
568. Weller RO, Bruckner FE, Chamberlain MA. Rheumatoid neuropathy: a histological and electrophysiological study. J Neurol Neurosurg Psychiatry 1970;33:592–604.
569. Rechthand E, Cornblath DR, Stern BJ, Meyerhoff JO. Chronic demyelinating polyneuropathy in systemic lupus erythematosus. Neurology 1984;34:1375–1377.
570. McCombe PA, McLeod JG, Pollard JD, Guo YP. Peripheral sensorimotor and autonomic neuropathy

associated with systemic lupus erythematosus. Clinical, pathological and immunological features. Brain 1987;110:533–549.

571. Mellgren SI, Conn DL, Stevens C, Dyck PJ. Peripheral neuropathy in primary Sjögren's syndrome. Neurology 1989;39:390–394.

572. Kaltreider HB, Talal N. The neuropathy of Sjögren's syndrome: trigeminal nerve involvement. Ann Intern Med 1969;70:751–762.

573. Malinow K, Yannakakis GC, Glusman SM, et al. Subacute sensory neuronopathy secondary to dorsal root ganglionitis in primary Sjögren's syndrome. Ann Neurol 1986;20:535–537.

574. Griffin JW, Cornblath DR, Alexander E, et al. Ataxic sensory neuropathy and dorsal root ganglionitis associated with Sjögren's syndrome. Ann Neurol 1990;27:304–315.

575. Hankey GJ, Gubbary SS. Peripheral neuropathy associated with sicca syndrome. J Neurol Neurosurg Psychiatry 1987;50:1085–1086.

576. Kennett RP, Harding AE. Peripheral neuropathy associated with the sicca syndrome. J Neurol Neurosurg Psychiatry 1986;49:90–92.

577. Teasdall RD, Fryha RA, Shulman LE. Cranial nerve involvement in systemic sclerosis (scleroderma): a report of 10 cases. Medicine 1980;59:149–159.

578. Drachman DA. Neurological complications of Wegener's granulomatosis. Arch Neurol 1963;8:145–155.

579. Stern GN, Hoffbranch AV, Urich H. The peripheral nerves and skeletal muscles in Wegener's granulomatosis: a clinico-pathological study of four cases. Brain 1965;88:151–164.

580. Jimenez-Medina HJ, Yablon SA. Electrodiagnostic characteristics of Wegener's granulomatosis-associated peripheral neuropathy. Am J Phys Med Rehabil 1992;71:6–11.

581. Conn DL, Dyck PJ. Angiopathic neuropathy in connective tissue disease. In: Dyck PJ, Thomas PK, Lambert EH, eds. Peripheral neuropathy. Philadelphia: WB Saunders, 1984:2027–2043.

582. Caselli RJ, Daube JR, Hunder GG, Whisnant JP. Peripheral neuropathic syndrome in giant cell (temporal) arteritis. Neurology 1988;38:685–689.

583. Katzenstein AA, Carringston CB, Liebow AA. Lymphomatoid granulomatosis: a clinicopathologic study of 152 cases. Cancer 1979;43:360–373.

584. Fauci AS, Haynes BF, Costa J, Katz P, Wolff SM. Lymphomatoid granulomatosis. Prospective clinical and therapeutic experience over 10 years. New Engl J Med 1984;306:68–74.

585. Garcia CA, Hackett ER, Kirkpatrick LL. Multiple mononeuropathy in lymphomatoid granulomatosis: similarity to leprosy. Neurology 1978;28:731–733.

586. Stafford CR, Bodganoff BM, Green L, Spector HB. Mononeuropathy multiplex as a complication of amphetamine angitis. Neurology 1975;25:570–572.

587. Chusid MJ, Dale DC, West BC, Wolff SM. The hypereosinophilic syndrome: analysis of fourteen cases with review of the literature. Medicine 1975;54:1–17.

588. Dorfman LJ, Ransom BR, Forno LS, Kelts A. Neuropathy in the hypereosinophilic syndrome. Muscle Nerve 1983;6:291–298.

589. Donofrio PD, Stanton C, Miller VS, et al. Demyelinating polyneuropathy in eosinophilia-myalgia syndrome. Muscle Nerve 1991;15:796–805.

590. Smith BE, Dyck PJ. Peripheral neuropathy in the eosinophilia-myalgia syndrome associated with l-tryptophan ingestion. Neurology 1990;40:1035–1040.

591. Heiman-Patterson TD, Bird SJ, Parry GJ, et al. Peripheral neuropathy associated with eosinophilia-myalgia syndrome. Ann Neurol 1990;28:522–528.

592. Kelly JJ, Kyle RA, O'Brien PC, Dyck PJ. Prevalence of monoclonal protein in peripheral neuropathy. Neurology 1981;31:1480–1482.

593. Kyle RA. Monoclonal gammopathy of undetermined significance: natural history in 241 cases. Am J Med 1978;64:814–826.

594. Cotamin F, Singer B, Mignot R, Ecoffet M, Katatchkine M. Polyneuropathie à rechute, évoluant depuis 19 ans, associée à une gammopathie monoclonale IgG bénigne. Rev Neurol 1976;132:741–762.

595. Read DJ, Van Hegan RI, Matthews WB. Peripheral neuropathy and benign IgG paraproteinemia. J Neurol Neurosurg Psychiatry 1978;41:215–219.

596. Dalakas MC, Engel WK. Polyneuropathy with monoclonal gammopathy: studies of 11 patients. Ann Neurol 1981;10:45–52.

597. Kelly JJ. The electrodiagnostic findings in peripheral neuropathy associated with monoclonal gammopathy. Muscle Nerve 1983;6:504–509.

598. Smith IS, Kahn SN, Lacey BW, et al. Chronic demyelinating neuropathy associated with benign IgM paraproteinaemia. Brain 1983;106:169–195.

599. Bromberg MB, Feldman EL, Albers JW. Chronic inflammatory demyelinating polyradiculoneuropathy: comparison of patients with and without an associated monoclonal gammopathy. Neurology 1992;42:1157–1163.

600. Nemni R, Galassi G, Latove N, Sherman WH, Olarte MR, Hays AP. Polyneuropathy in nonmalignant IgM plasma cell dyscrasia: a morphological study. Ann Neurol 1983;14:43–54.

601. Donofrio PD, Kelly JJ. Peripheral neuropathy in monoclonal gammopathy of undetermined significance. Muscle Nerve 1989;12:1–8.

602. Kelly JJ. Peripheral neuropathies associated with monoclonal proteins: a clinical review. Muscle Nerve 1985;8:138–150.

603. Kelly JJ, Kyle RA, Miles JM, Dyck PJ. Osteosclerotic myeloma and peripheral neuropathy. Neurology 1983;33:202–210.

604. Read D, Warlow C. Peripheral neuropathy and solitary plasmacytoma. J Neurol Neurosurg Psychiatry 1978;41:177–184.

605. Iwashita H, Ohnishi A, Asada M, Kanazawa Y, Kuroiwa Y. Polyneuropathy, skin hyperpigmentation, edema, and hypertrichosis in localized osteosclerotic myeloma. Neurology 1977;27:675–682.

606. Bardwick PA, Zvaifler NJ, Gill GN, et al. Plasma cell dyscrasia with polyneuropathy, organomegaly, endocrinopathy, M-protein and skin change: the POEMS syndrome. Medicine 1980;59:311–322.

607. Kelly JJ, Kyle RA, Miles JM, Dyck PJ. Osteosclerotic myeloma and peripheral neuropathy. Neurology 1983;33:202–210.

608. Victor M, Banke BQ, Adams RD. The neuropathy of multiple myeloma. J Neurol Neurosurg Psychiatry 1958;21:73–88.

609. Walsh JC. The neuropathy of multiple myeloma: an electrophysiological and histological study. Arch Neurol 1971b;25:404–414.

610. Kelly JJ, Kyle RA, Miles JM, O'Brien PC, Dyck PJ. The spectrum of peripheral neuropathy in myeloma. Neurology 1981;31:24–31.

611. Gotham JE, Wein H, Meyer JS. Clinical studies of neuropathy due to macroglobulinemia. Can Med Assoc J 1963;89:806.

612. Latov N, Sherman WH, Nemi R, et al. Plasma-cell dyscrasia and peripheral neuropathy with a monoclonal antibody to peripheral-nerve myelin. NEJM 1980;303:618–621.

613. McLeod JG, Walsh JC. Peripheral neuropathy associated with lymphomas and other reticuloses. In: Dyck PJ, Thomas PK, Lambert EH, eds. Peripheral neuropathy. Philadelphia: WB Saunders; 1975:1314–1325.

614. Dyan AD, Lewis PD. Demyelinating neuropathy in macroglobulinemia. Neurology 1966;16.1141–1144.

615. Propp RP, Means E, Diebel R, Sherer G, Barron K. Waldenstrom's macroglobulinemia and neuropathy. Neurology 1975;25:980–988.

616. Bigner DD, Olson WN, McFarlin DE. Peripheral neuropathy: high and low molecular weight IgM and amyloidosis. Arch Neurol 1971;24:365–373.

617. Logothetis J, Kennedy WR, Ellington A, Williams RC. Cryoglobulinemic neuropathy: incidence and clinical characteristics. Arch Neurol 1968;19:389–397.

618. Chad D, Pariser K, Bradley WG, Adelman LS, Pinn VW. The pathogenesis of cryoglobulinemic neuropathy. Neurology 1982;32:725–729.

619. Cream JJ, Hern JEC, Hughes RAC, MacKenzie ILK. Mixed or immune complex cryoglobulinemia and neuropathy. J Neurol Neurosurg Psychiatry 1974;37:82–87.

620. Kelly JJ Jr, Kyle RA, O'Brien PC, Dyck PJ. The natural history of peripheral neuropathy in primary systemic amyloidosis. Ann Neurol 1979;6:1–7.

621. Trotter JL, Engel WK, Ignaszak TF. Amyloidosis with plasma cell dyscrasia: an overlooked cause of adult onset sensorimotor neuropathy. Arch Neurol 1977;34:209–214.

622. Fitting JW, Bischoff A, Regli F, DeCrousaz G. Neuropathy, amyloidosis, and monoclonal gammopathy. J Neurol Neurosurg Psychiatry 1979;42:193–202.

623. Kyle RA, Bayard ED. Amyloidosis: review of 236 cases. Medicine (Baltimore) 1975;54:271–299.

624. Melgaard B, Nielsen B. Electromyographic findings in amyloid polyneuropathy. EEG Clin Neurophysiology 1977;17:31–34.

625. Parry G. Peripheral neuropathies associated with human immunodeficiency virus infection. Ann Neurol 1988;23(suppl):S49–S53.

626. Cornblath DR, McArthur JC. Predominantly sensory neuropathy in patients with AIDS and AIDS-related complex. Neurology 1988;38:794–796.

627. Dalakas MC, Pezeschkpour G. Neuromuscular diseases associated with human immunodeficiency virus infection. Ann Neurol 1988;23(suppl):S38–S48.

628. Lipkin WI, Parry G, Kiprov D, Abrams D. Inflammatory neuropathy in homosexual men with lymphadenopathy. Neurology 1985;35:1479–1483.

629. Cornblath DR, McArthur JC, Kennedy PG, Witte AS, Griffin JW. Inflammatory demyelinating peripheral neuropathies associated with human T-cell lymphotropic virus type III infection. Ann Neurol 1987;21:32–40.

630. Miller RG, Parry GJ, Pfaeffl W, Lans W, Lippert R, Kiprov D. The spectrum of peripheral neuropathy associated with ARC and AIDS. Muscle Nerve 1988;11:857–863.

631. Bailey RD, Baltch AL, Venkatesch R, Singh JK, Bishop MB. Sensory motor neuropathy associated with AIDS. Neurology 1988;38:886–891.

632. Lange DJ, Britton CB, Younger DS, Hays AP: The neuromuscular manifestations of human immunodeficiency virus infections. Arch Neurol 1988;45:1084–1088.

633. Eidelberg D, Sotrel A, Vogel H, Walker P, Kleefield J, Crumpacker CS. Progressive polyradiculopathy in acquired immune deficiency syndrome. Neurology 1986;36:912–916.

634. Behar R, Wiley C, McTutchan A. Cytomegalovirus polyradiculoneuropathy in acquired immune deficiency syndrome. Neurology 1987;37:557–561.

635. Elder G, Dalakas MC, Pezeshkpour GH, Sever JL. Ataxic neuropathy due to ganglioneuritis after probable acute human immunodeficiency virus infection. Lancet 1986;2:1275–1276.

636. De la Monte SM, Gabuzda DN, Ho DD, Brown RH, Hedley-Whyte ET, Schooley RT, Hirsch MS, Bhan AK: Peripheral neuropathy in the acquired immunodeficiency syndrome. Ann Neurol 1988;23:485–492.

637. Fuller GN, Jacobs JM, Guiloff RJ. Subclinical peripheral nerve involvement in AIDS: an electrophysiological and pathological study. J Neurol Neurosurg Psychiatry 1991;54:318–324.

638. Smith T, Jakobsen J, Gaub J, Trojaborg W. Symptomatic polyneuropathy in human immunodeficiency virus antibody seropositive men with and without immune deficiency: a comparative electrophysiological study. J Neurol Neurosurg Psychiatry 1990;53:1056–1059.

639. So YT, Holtzman DM, Abrams DI, Olney RK. Peripheral neuropathy associated with acquired immunodeficiency syndrome. Arch Neurol 1988;45:945–948.

640. Said G, Goulon-Goeau C, Lacroix C, Feve A, Descamps H, Fouchard M. Inflammatory lesions of peripheral neuropathy with human T-lymphotropic virus type I-associated myelopathy. Ann Neurol 1988;24:275–277.

641. Halperin JJ, Litle BW, Coyle PK, Dattwyler RJ. Lyme disease: cause of treatable peripheral neuropathy. Neurology 1987;37:1700–1706.

642. Hopf HC. Peripheral neuropathy in acrodermatitis chronica atrophicans (Herxheimer). J Neurol Neurosurg Psychiatry 1975;38:452–458.

643. Pachner AR, Steere AC. The triad of neurologic manifestations of Lyme's disease: meningitis, cranial neuritis, and radiculoneuritis. Neurology 1985;35:47–53.

644. Vallat JM, Hugon J, Lubveau M, Leboutet MJ, Dumas M, Desproges-Gotteron R. Tickbite meningoradiculoneuritis: clinical, electrophysiologic, and histologic findings in 10 cases. Neurology 1987;37:749–753.

645. Camponovo F, Meier C. Neuropathy of vasculitic origin in a case of Garin-Boujadour-Bannwarth syndrome with positive borrelia antibody response. J Neurol 1986;233:69–72.

646. Logigian EL, Steere AC. Clinical and electrophysiologic findings in chronic neuropathy of Lyme disease. Neurology 1992;42:303–311.

647. Halperin J, Luft BJ. Wolkman DJ, Dattwyler RJ. Lyme neuroborreliosis. Brain 1990;113:1207–1221.

648. Wulff CH, Hansen K, Strange P, Trojaborg W. Multiple mononeuritis and radiculitis with erythema, pain, elevated CSF protein, and pleocytosis (Barnwarth's syndrome). J Neurol Neurosurg Psychiatry 1983;46:485–490.

649. Halperin JJ, Wolkman DJ, Luft BJ, Dattwyler RJ. Carpal tunnel syndrome in Lyme Borreliosis. Muscle Nerve 1989;12:397–400.

650. Sabin D, Swift TR. Leprosy. In: Dyck PJ, Thomas PK, Lambert EH, eds. Peripheral neuropathy. Philadelphia: WB Saunders, 1975:1166–1198.

651. McLeod JG, Hargrave JC, Walsh JC, Booth GC, Gye RS, Barron A. Nerve conduction studies in leprosy. Int J Leprosy 1975;43:21–31.

652. Chaco J, Magora A, Zauberman H, Landau Y. An electromyographic study of lagophthalmos in leprosy. Int J Lepr 1968;36:288–295.

653. Dastur DK, Anita NH, Divekar SC. The facial nerve in leprosy. II. Pathology, pathogenesis, electromyography, and clinical correlations. Int J Lepr 1968;34:118–138.

654. Jopling WH, Morgan-Hughes JA. Pure neural tuberculoid leprosy. Br Med J 1965;2:788–790.

655. Rosenberg RN, Lovelace RE. Mononeuritis multiplex in lepromatous leprosy. Arch Neurol 1968;19:310–314.

656. Sheskin J, Magora A, Sagher F. Motor nerve conduction studies in patients with leprosy reaction treated with thalidomide and other drugs. Int J Lepr 1969;37:359–364.

657. Sohi AS, Kandheri KC, Singh N. Motor nerve conduction studies in leprosy. Int J Dermatol 1971;10:151–155.

658. McDonald WI, Kocen RS. Diphtheric neuropathy. In: Dyck PJ, Thomas PK, Lambert EH, eds. Peripheral neuropathy, vol. 2. Philadelphia: WB Saunders; 1975:1281–1300.

659. Kazemi B, Tahernia AC, Zandia K. Motor nerve conduction in diphtheria and diphtheriomyocarditis. Arch Neurol 1973;29:104–106.

660. Kurdi A, Abdul-Kader M. Clinical and electrophysiological studies of diphtheritic neuritis in Jordan. J Neurol Surg 1979;42:243–250.

661. Idiaquez J. Autonomic dysfunction in diphtheric neuropathy. J Neurol Neurosurg Psychiatry 1992;55:159–161.

662. Shahani M, Dastur FD, Dastoor DH, et al. Neuropathy in tetanus. J Neurol Sci 1979;43:173–182.

663. Luisto M, Seppäläinen A. Electroneuromyographic sequelae of tetanus, a controlled study of 40 patients. EMG Clin Neurophysiol 1989;29:377–381.

664. Auger RG, Daube JR, Goze MR, Lambert EH. Hereditary form of sustained muscle activity of peripheral nerve origin causing generalized myokymia and muscle stiffness. Ann Neurol 1984;15:13–21.

665. Warmolts JR, Mendell JR. Neurotonia, impulse induced repetitive discharges in motor nerves in peripheral neuropathy. Ann Neurol 1980;7:245–250.

666. Valenstein E, Watson RT, Parker JI. Myokymia, muscle hypertrophy and percussion "myotonia" in chronic recurrent polyneuropathy. Neurology 1978;28:1130–1134.

667. Joy L, Allen RF, Sunwoo LN, Oh SJ, Thomas TD. Isaacs' syndrome associated with chronic inflammatory demyelinating polyneuropathy. Muscle Nerve 1990;13:868.

668. Isaacs H. A syndrome of continuous muscle fiber activity. J Neurol Neurosurg Psychiatry 1961;24:319–325.

669. Lütschg J, Jerusalem F, Ludin HP, Vassella F, Mementhaler M. The syndrome of 'continuous muscle fiber activity.' Arch Neurol 1978;35:198–205.

670. Lublin FD, Tsairis P, Streletz LJ, et al. Myokymia and impaired muscular relaxation with continuous motor unit activity. J Neurol Neurosurg Psychiatry 1979;42:557–562.

671. Welch LK, Appenzeller O, Bicknell JM. Peripheral neuropathy with myokymia, sustained muscular contraction, and continuous motor unit activity. Neurology 1972;161–169.

672. Hudson AJ, Brown WF, Gilbert JJ. The muscular pain-fasciculation syndrome. Neurology 1978;28:1105–1109.

673. Tahmoush AJ, Alonso RJ, Tahmoush GP, Heiman-Patterson TD. Cramp-fasciculation syndrome: a treatable hyperexcitable peripheral nerve disorder. Neurology 1991;41:1021–1024.

674. Wallis WE, Van Poznak V, Plum F. Generalized muscular stiffness, fasciculations and myokymia of peripheral nerve origin. Arch Neurol 1970;22:430–439.

675. Waerness E. Neuromyotonia and bronchial carcinoma. EMG Clin Neurophysiology 1974;14:527–535.

676. Irani PF, Purohit AV, Wadia NJ. The syndrome of continuous muscle fiber activity. Acta Neurol Scand 1977;55:273–288.

677. Lambert EH. Electromyography in amyotrophic lateral sclerosis. In Norris FH Jr, Kurland LT, eds. Motor neuron diseases. New York: Grune & Stratton; 1969:135–153.

678. Daube JR. EMG in motor neuron diseases. AAEE Minimonograph #18. Rochester, Minnesota: AAEE, 1982.

679. Ertekin C. Sensory and motor conduction in motor neuron disease. Acta Neurol Scand 1967;43:499–512.

680. Hausmanova-Petrusevich I, Kopec J. Possible mechanism of motor conduction velocity changes in the anterior horn cells involvement. EMG Clin Neurophysiol 1973;13:357–365.

681. Cornblath DR, Kuncle RW, Mellits ED, Quaskey SA, Clawson L, Pestronk A, Drachman DB. Nerve conduction studies in amyotrophic lateral sclerosis. Muscle Nerve 1992;15:1111–1115.

682. Jusic A, Milic S. Nerve potentials and afferent conduction velocities in the differential diagnosis of amyotrophy of the hand. J Neurol Neurosurg Psychiatry 1972;35:861–864.

683. Gilliatt RW, Goodman HV, Willison RG. The recording of lateral popliteal nerve action potentials in man. J Neurol Neurosurg Psychiatry 1961;24:305–318.

684. Albizatti MG, Bassi S, Passerini D, Crespi V. F-wave velocity in motor neuron disease. Acta Neurol Scand 1976;54:269–277.

685. Argyropoulos C, Panayiotopoulos C, Scarpalezos S. F- and M-wave conduction velocity in amyotrophic lateral sclerosis. Muscle Nerve 1978;1:479–485.

686. Teasdall RO, Park AM, Languth HW, Magladery JW. Electrophysiological studies of reflex activity in patients with lesions of the nervous system. II. Bull Johns Hopkins Hosp 1959;91:245–256.

687. Norris FH. Adult spinal motor neuron disease. In: Vinken PJ, Bruyn GW, eds. Handbook of clinical neurology, vol 22. New York: American Elsevier Publishing; 1975:1–56.

688. Kuntz NL, Gomez MR, Daube JR. EMG in spinal muscular atrophy. Neurology 1980;20:1002–1008.

689. Moosa A, Dubowitz V. Motor nerve conduction velocity in spinal muscular atrophy of childhood. Arch Dis Child 1976;51:974–977.

690. Raimbault J, Lager P. Electromyography in the diagnosis of infantile spinal amyotrophy of Werdnig-Hoffman type. Path Biol 1972;20:287–296.

691. Schwartz MS, Moosa A. Sensory nerve conduction in the spinal muscular atrophies. Dev Med Child Neurol 1977;19:50–53.

692. Oh SJ. Neuromuscular diseases. In: Todorov AB, ed. Clinical neurology. New York: Thieme-Stratton, 1983:289–306.

693. Evans OB. Polyneuropathy in childhood. Pediatrics 1979;64:96–104.

694. Nielsen VK. The peripheral nerve function in chronic renal failure. V. Sensory and motor conduction velocity. Acta Med Scand 1973;194–445.

695. McLeod JG, Walsh JC, Reye C. Electrophysiological studies in familial spastic paraplegia. J Neurol Neurosurg Psychiatry 1977;40:611–615.

696. Jedrzejowska H, Milczarek H. Recessive hereditary sensory neuropathy. J Neurol Sci 1976;29:371–387.

697. Moore PM, Cupps TR. Neurological complications of vasculitis. Ann Neurol 1983;14:155–167.

698. Chumbley LC, Harrison EG, DeRemee RA. Allergic granulomatosis and angiitis (Churg-Strauss syndrome): report and analysis of 30 cases. Mayo Clin Proc 1977;52:477–484.

699. Johnson RL, Smyth CJ, Holt GW, Lubchenco A, Valentine E. Steroid therapy and vascular lesions in rheumatoid arthritis. Arth Rheum 1959;2:224–249.

700. Gordon RM, Silverstein A. Neurologic manifestation in progressive systemic sclerosis. Arch Neurol 1970;22:126–134.

23

Traumatic Peripheral Nerve Injuries

Proper management of peripheral nerve injuries depends on accurate localization of the lesion, a precise estimate of the extent of the lesion, and careful choice of treatment. When assessing these parameters, an accurate history, careful clinical examination, and comprehensive electromyography (EMG) studies are essential. In every aspect of the management of peripheral nerve injuries, the EMG studies give the clinician valuable objective information (1). Because the needle EMG is an integral part of the evaluation, we discuss the nerve conduction abnormalities together with the needle EMG findings in this chapter.

Histological Changes after Nerve Injury

The histological changes that occur after nerve injury have been well discussed by Bradley (2) (Fig. 23.1). When a nerve is crushed, the continuity of the axon is broken. As in all cells, the distal portion of the nerve, which is separated from the neuron, gradually degenerates. In general, loss of continuity can be demonstrated in terminal branches before gross changes appear in the nerve trunk (3). Within a few days, however, changes are present in all parts of the nerve distal to the point of section.

Within 2 min. of a nerve's being crushed, there is retraction of myelin from the nodes of Ranvier and dilatation of the Schmidt-Lanterman clefts for up to 5 mm distal to the injury in all fibers. By 1 hr, the proximal and distal axoplasm adjacent to the crush develops into spirals and balls, a process that gradually spreads in both directions for up to 3 mm within the next 24 hr.

By 24 hr, axoplasmic degeneration distal to the crushed area becomes obvious, and degeneration of the myelin sheaths has begun in most of the myelinated fibers. The myelin splits at the intraperiod line, and lamellae peel off at the nodes, the Schwann cell processes expanding to cover the nodes of Ranvier. The rate of degeneration is somewhat variable; in general, it is inversely proportional to the fiber diameter.

By 48 hr, definite signs of degeneration in the myelin sheaths appear distal to the crush as the axon becomes fragmented. There is loosening of the myelin lamellae and swelling of the fibers, but still the myelin is continuous.

By the 3rd day, breakdown of myelin within the Schwann cell cytoplasm and

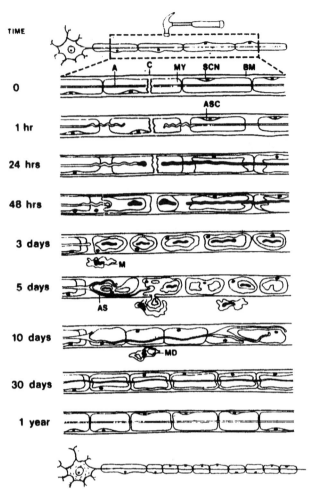

Figure 23.1. Wallerian degeneration in a myelinated nerve fiber at and below the level of a crush lesion (at various times), **A**, Axon. **C**, Connective tissue. **MY**, myelin. **SCN**, Schwann cell nucleus. **BM**, Basement membrane. **AS**, Axon sprout. **ASC**, Adjacent Schwann cell. **MD**, Myelin debris. (From Bradley WG. Disorders of peripheral nerves. Oxford: Blackwell, 1974:132.)

macrophages begins. Degeneration of the myelin sheath progresses steadily from the 3rd day.

By the 5th day, the full-blown process of myelin breakdown is occurring, with many lipid-filled macrophages within the distal nerve. This myelin breakdown is now seen as a "myelin digestion chamber" in routine histological studies. By 16 days, most of the myelin sheaths have been removed, although some myelin debris may still be seen within macrophages 3 months after nerve degeneration. In essence, fragmentation of the myelin sheaths takes place later than that of the axon in wallerian degeneration (4).

After total section, regrowth of the axon from the proximal site of discontinuity occurs if the anterior horn cell survives, and it begins to produce axoplasm. A period of 1–3 weeks is required before regeneration begins. The rate of regeneration is about 1 mm/day if recovery is to occur (4). Axon sprouts from myelinated fibers tend to grow within the tubes derived from Schwann cell basement membrane. Unmyelinated nerve fibers may grow in a haphazard fashion.

The axons gradually mature and become surrounded by Schwann cell cytoplasm and myelin. In the early phase of regeneration the nerve fibers have small axons, thin myelin sheaths, and a short internodal length. Over the next 12–24 months the axon diameter and myelin sheath thickness gradually return toward normal, although normalcy is never fully achieved. The myelin sheath remains disproportionately thin, and the short internodes persist even after the axons have attained near-normal diameters.

A number of changes occur immediately proximal to the crush, including retrograde degeneration extending back for one or two nodes, a decrease in axon diameter, and occasionally, segmental demyelination and remyelination. In the central neuron, central chromatolysis occurs as a response to the distal crush.

Time Factors for Electrophysiological Abnormalities after Nerve Injury

Successful use of EMG in managing peripheral nerve injury requires an understanding of time factors for the EMG abnormalities after nerve injury (Table 23.1; Fig. 23.2). This sequence may be divided into three stages: (*a*) the period immediately after nerve injury, when degeneration of the nerve is occurring; (*b*) the period of denervation after degeneration of the nerve is completed; and (*c*) the period of reinnervation. To avoid confusion, only the time factors related to total section of a nerve are discussed.

Immediately after nerve injury, there will be no motor unit potential (MUP) with voluntary contraction, no compound muscle action potential (CMAP) response to stimulation of the nerve proximal to injury, and no compound nerve action potential (CNAP) in the injured segment. However, it is important to remember that the distal

Table 23.1.
Time Factors for Electrophysiological Abnormalities in Severed Peripheral Nerves

Time After Injury	Motor Nerve Conduction	Sensory or Mixed Nerve Conduction	Needle EMG/Strength-Duration Curve
Immediate	No response to stimulation of the nerve proximal to injury	Absence of CNAP across the injured segment	Absence of MUP with voluntary control
1–3 days	Normal response distally	Normal response distally	
	Diminished nerve excitability	Progressive decline in CNAP amplitude	
	Progressive decline in CMAP amplitude	No change in NCV	
	No or minimal change in NCV		
4–5 days	Absence of any CMAP response to stimulation over the distal segment	Further decline in the CNAP amplitude	
6–10 days		Absence of CNAP	Denervation strength duration curve in the muscle
8–14 days			Positive sharp waves
14–21 days			Spontaneous fibrillation

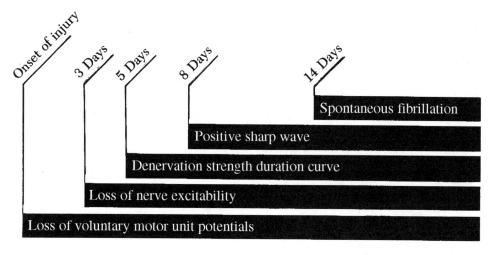

Figure 23.2. Time factors following total nerve section. Immediately after injury there is loss of voluntary motor unit potential, even though the distal portion of the nerve maintains its excitability for 3–5 days. After this, the excitability of the nerve diminishes and only the muscle fibers remain excitable. The denervation strength duration curve occurs 5–10 days after injury. Positive sharp waves appear 8–14 days after injury, and spontaneous fibrillation occurs within 2–3 weeks after injury.

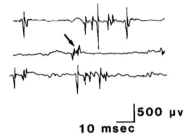

Figure 23.3. Motor unit potentials on minimal contraction during regeneration. The *arrow* indicates small polyphasic MUPs (reinnervation potentials). (From Oh SJ. Electromyographic studies in peripheral nerve injuries. South Med J 1976;69:179.)

portion of the nerve maintains its electrical excitability for 3–5 days, after which the nerve becomes inexcitable and the conduction ceases. Gilliatt and Hjorth (5) emphasized that failure of neuromuscular transmission precedes loss of conduction in the nerve trunk during wallerian degeneration. They showed advanced degeneration in the terminal branches of intramuscular nerve fibers, whereas the same fibers in the nerve trunk showed only minimal abnormalities. In the nerve examined electrophysiologically, the CNAPs were present after the muscle response to nerve stimulation had disappeared. Thus, *the earliest evidence of degeneration of the nerve is failure of the nerve to respond to electrical stimulation below the site of the injury.* The quantitative measurement of electrical excitability is called the nerve excitability test (see Chapter 11).

During the first 3–5 days, several electrophysiological changes occur in the distal segment. The two most prominent changes are: (*a*) a gradual decrease in nerve excitability, requiring increasing intensity and duration of stimulus; and (*b*) a gradual decrease in the amplitude of the CMAPs and CNAPs. Slowing of the motor and sensory nerve conduction velocities (NCVs) is only minimal during this period, after which nerve excitability is lost abruptly (5, 6). These electrophysiological changes are caused by the gradual degeneration and fragmentation of the axon in the distal segment and a steep fall in the amount of acetylcholine in the severed nerve trunk (4).

The motor end-plate retains its full excitability for a further 5–10 days, during which time the last fragment of axis cylinder in the motor end-plate disappears (4). The excitability of the end-plate then diminishes, so that only the muscle fibers remain excitable. Thus, the denervation strength-duration curve occurs.

The earliest significant objective evidence of denervation is a transient appearance of positive sharp waves after insertion or movement of the needle electrode (7). Positive sharp waves appear 8–14 days after injury and spontaneous fibrillation potentials within 2–4 weeks after injury, appearing first in the muscles just distal to the injury.

More distant muscles show fibrillation at a later date. Weddell and associates (8) reported that spontaneous fibrillations appear in limb muscle 16–18 days after injury, in facial muscles within 12–14 days, and in the sacrospinalis muscle 10–12 days after injury. Abnormal spontaneous potentials persist in partially denervated muscle for many years. If the muscle is completely denervated and becomes atrophic, they usually disappear in about 1 year (7).

During regeneration of a nerve, which usually occurs 1–3 weeks after injury, both the strength-duration curve and the needle EMG give advance information of recovery before there is any visible sign of voluntary contraction. The first evidence of reinnervation provided by the strength-duration curve is the appearance of a kink or discontinuity in a curve which previously was of the denervated type (9). A discontinuity in the curve may be demonstrated 2–4 months before clinical evidence of recovery. *The first EMG sign of reinnervation is the appearance of small and highly polyphasic potentials (reinnervation potentials)* (Fig. 23.3) 2 months before clinical evidence of recovery (10).

Nerve Conduction Changes During Wallerian Degeneration

Since Rosenblueth and Dempsey (11) studied the NCV during the course of wallerian degeneration in cats in 1939, many experimental data have been gathered for animal nerves but few for human nerves (Table 23.2). A summary of these data follows.

1. *There is considerable variation among different species in the time to conduction failure distal to the nerve section.* For motor nerve conduction, this time ranged from 24–36 hr in the rabbit to 96–144 hr in the baboon (Fig. 23.4), to 120–192 hr in human subjects (Fig. 23.5). For sensory conduction, this time ranged from 71–78 hr in the rabbit to 120–216 hr in baboons (Fig. 23.4) and to 185–240 hr in human subjects (Fig. 23.6). This finding indicates that data from lower mammals cannot be transferred directly to man. There is a suggestion that the time to conduction failure is longer in primates and humans. In human subjects, Gilliatt and Taylor (3) succeeded in recording muscle responses 4–7 days after severance of the facial nerve in seven patients, and Landau (12) obtained muscle twitch 3–5 days after section of the ulnar and median nerves. Wilbourn studied serially the CMAP response in a patient with 99% infarction of the

Table 23.2.
Time to Conduction Failure Distal to Nerve Section

Study	Species/Nerve	Time to Failure (hr)
In vitro compound nerve conduction		
Levenson and Rosenbluth (37)	Frog sciatic	912–984
Rosenblueth and Dempsey (11)	Cat sciatic	71–101
Erlanger and Schoepfle (38)	Dog phrenic	96
Gutmann and Holubar (6)	Rabbit peroneal	71–78
	Rat peroneal	79–81
	Guinea pig sciatic	72–101
Sensory nerve conduction		
Gilliatt and Hjorth (5)	Baboon peroneal	120–216
Wilbourn (13)	Human ulnar	192
Pilling (15)	Human digital	185,
	Human radial	240
Chaudhry and Cornblath (14)	Human sural	240
Motor nerve conduction		
Levenson and Rosenbluth (39)	Frog sciatic	144–168
Lisak et al. (40)	Cat sciatic	69–79
Gutmann and Holubar (6)	Rabbit peroneal	30–32
Kaeser and Lambert (16)	Guinea pig sciatic	40–45
Miledi and Slater (41)	Rat sciatic	24–36
Gilliatt and Hjorth (5)	Baboon peroneal	96–144
Landau (12)	Human median/ulnar[a]	85–128
Gilliatt and Taylor (3)	Facial	120–192
Wilbourn (13)	Human ulnar	120[b]
Chaudhry (14)	Human ulnar/median	192

[a]This is not the CMAP recording but is based on observation of muscle twitch.
[b]This was not a complete transection. There was 99% injury of the nerve on the basis of the CMAP amplitude.

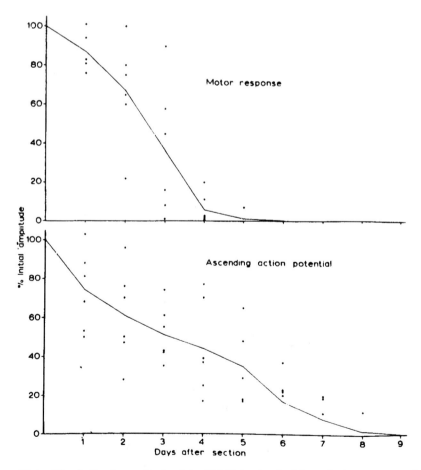

Figure 23.4. The decline in amplitude of the CMAP *(top)* and of the orthodromic CNAP *(bottom)* after nerve section in the baboon. Mean values for the six nerves are shown by the *continuous lines.* (From Gilliatt RW, Hjorth R. Nerve conduction during wallerian degeneration in the baboon. J Neurol Neurosurg Psychiatry 1972;35:337.)

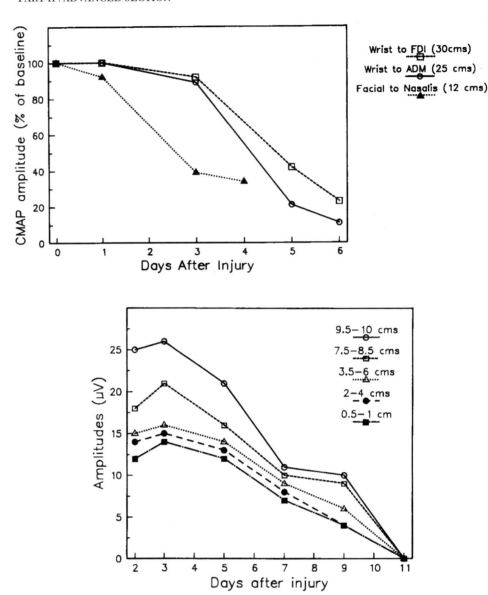

Figure 23.5. Correlation of the length of the distal stump and wallerian degeneration in motor nerves. The facial nerve with a shorter distal stump (12 cm) shows earlier and greater percent reduction in compound muscle action potential (CMAP) amplitude at days 1 to 4, when compared with a longer ulnar nerve with a distal stump length of 25 cm. (From Chaudhry V, Cornblath DR. Wallerian degeneration in human nerves. Muscle Nerve 1992;15:692.)

Figure 23.6. Sequential sensory nerve action potential amplitude recorded from the ankle with stimulation at different distances from the biopsy site in a human patient. Days 5 and 7 show greater reduction at distal stimulation sites from biopsy (9.5–10 cm away) than at proximal stimulation sites (0.5–4 cm from biopsy site). Days 9 and 11 show similar reduction at all sites. (From Chaudhry V, Cornblath DR. Wallerian degeneration in human nerves. Muscle Nerve 1992;15:689.)

ulnar nerve and observed that 75–90% of the amplitude decline occurred between days 2 and 5 (13). After that, the CMAP was stabilized. Digital sensory potentials were unchanged through day 5, then progressively declined in the amplitude, and disappeared on day 9. Chaudhry reported 50% reduction of the CMAP amplitude at 3 and 5 days after the injury and no response by day 9 (14). On the other hand, sensory CNAP amplitudes were reduced by 50% by 7 days after injury, and the response was absent by day 11 (14). Pilling found a 40–50% decline of the sensory CNAP in the digital nerve at 115–192 hr after the cut and no sensory CNAP at 185–240 hr in two cases (15).

2. *Neuromuscular transmission fails before conduction in the nerve fails. Comparing motor conduction to sensory conduction, it is clear that the sensory conduction is preserved longer than motor conduction before the conduction fails (Figs. 23.4–23.6).* This phenomenon has also been observed in human nerves (13, 14). These data have some practical importance in that the recording of the CNAPs in the absence of a motor response should not be interpreted as a "partial lesion" because the CNAPs persist a few days longer (2–3 days in the baboon (5) and 2–4 days in humans (13, 14)) than the motor response.

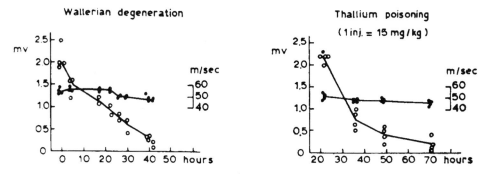

Figure 23.7. Motor NCV (●) and amplitude of the CMAP (○) during wallerian degeneration. (From Kaeser HE. Nerve conduction velocity measurements. In: PJ Vinken, GW Bruyn, eds. Handbook of clinical neurology, vol 7. Amsterdam: North Holland, 1972:154. Originally quoted from Kaeser HE, Lambert EH. Nerve function studies in experimental polyneuritis. EEG Clin Neurophysiol (Suppl) 1962;22:29–35)

3. *Little change in sensory or motor NCVs occurs in nerve fibers as they degenerate (Fig. 23.7).* A fall in NCV of the order of 10% was described by Gutmann and Holubar (6) and by Kaeser and Lambert (16), but from the results of Gilliatt and Hjorth (5) it seems that in many cases the motor and sensory NCVs remain normal until conduction ceases altogether. In the human facial nerve, Gilliatt and Taylor (3) did not observe any latency change. Wilbourn observed no change in the latency or NCV in the sensory nerve conduction or in the motor nerve conduction with first dorsal interosseous recording but found a 20% slowing in the motor NCV with hypothenar recording in a case of ulnar nerve injury (13). Pilling did not find any change in the sensory NCV in the digital nerves after the cut while the CNAP was recordable (15).

4. *There is a gradual decrease in nerve excitability, requiring an increase in the intensity and duration of the stimulus.* This was demonstrated in cats (11) and in human facial nerves (3). Eventually, the nerve became inexcitable.

5. *A steep decline in amplitude of the CMAPs and the CNAPs occurs until conduction ceases altogether (5, 6, 16). The decline in the amplitude was much steeper in the CMAPs than in the CNAPs (5)* because of the longer preservation of conduction in the nerve trunk (Fig. 23.4). A similar phenomenon was observed in human nerves (13, 14).

6. *There is a length-dependent relationship in the time to conduction failure of the nerve.* Sensory and motor nerves with shorter distal stumps showed earlier loss of amplitudes than did those with longer distal stumps (14). This finding has some clinical implication. For example, after injury at the axilla or in the thigh, the CMAP may not start to decline until 7–9 days later. In essence, the nerve conduction changes during wallerian degeneration show all the characteristic findings observed in axonal degeneration.

Minor nerve conduction changes also occur in the portion of nerve proximal to the transection. The nerve remains excitable (6). However, the amplitude of the CNAPs was reduced by 50% 6 months after nerve section, and the mixed NCV fell by 30%. Using the rabbit peroneal nerve, Cragg and Thomas (17) found a mild (10–20%) reduction in maximal NCV proximal to the site of a nerve crush. The reduction was seen 50–100 days after the crush and had usually disappeared after 200 days. These functional changes were attributed to a reduction in the diameter of the largest myelinated fibers (18). Skorpil (19) measured the conduction velocity of the proximal part of the ulnar nerve after traumatic transection at the elbow. Conduction was decreased to 55 m/sec compared with 60 m/sec on the opposite side (20). Gilliatt and Hjorth (5) observed about 30% reduction in motor NCV in the forearm and upper arm segments proximal to the nerve suture at the wrist. It is interesting that this reduction was not confined to the portion of the nerve immediately proximal to the lesion. The anatomical basis for this phenomenon is uncertain.

Nerve Conduction Under Regeneration

There is a technical difficulty in measuring conduction velocity during the early stages of regeneration. At this time the electrical threshold of the regenerating fibers is so high

Table 23.3.
Nerve Conduction in Regenerated Nerve Fibers

Study	Species/Nerves	Type of Injury	Time After Injury	Conduction Velocity (% of normal)	Other Studies
Motor Nerve Conduction					Increase of Terminal Latency (% of Normal)
Hodes et al. (35)	Human ulnar	Suture	42 mo	50–60	50%
Struppler and Huckauf (42)	Human ulnar	Suture	17 yr	71–96	43–50%
Tallis et al. (22)	Human median, ulnar	Autologous nerve graft	2.5 yr	40–85	
Donoso et al. (48)	Human median, ulnar	Suture	40–55 mo	91	
Sensory Nerve Conduction					Reduction of Amplitude (% of Normal)
Muheim (43)	Human digital	Suture	2–8 yr		CNAP present in 60% of cases
Ballantyne and Campbell (21)	Human median, ulnar	Surgical repair	53 mo	70–80	10–40%; CNAP absent before 10 mo
Tallis et al. (22)	Human median, ulnar	Autologous nerve graft	2.5 yr	7–68	7–46%; CNAP present in 44%
Almquist and Eeg-Olofson (23)	Human median, ulnar	Suture	5 yr	62	
Buchthal and Kuhl (25)	Children	Suture	13–16 mo	65–75	7–68%
	Adult	Suture	40 mo	75	7–46%
Donoso et al. (48)	Human median, ulnar	Suture	40–55 mo		CNAP present in 75% of cases
Hallin et al. (47)	Human median	Suture	5 yr	80–95	CNAP present in all cases
In Vitro Compound Nerve Conduction					
Berry et al. (44)	Cats	Section, suture	446 days	80	
Sanders and Whitteridge (45)	Rabbits	Crush	400–500 days	100	
Erlanger and Schoepfle (38)	Cats	Section, suture	343 days	60–80	
Jacobson and Guth (46)	Rats	Crush	56 days	75	
Cragg and Thomas (17)	Rabbits	Crush	480 days	75	

that they are unlikely to be excited by an electrode on the skin. One way of avoiding this difficulty is by stimulating the nerve proximal to the site of injury. When this is done with recording electrodes over an appropriate muscle, CMAPs that have a latency more than 10 times the normal value may be recorded (5).

As noted in Table 23.3, the NCVs in the regenerated nerve do not reach normal values even after full regeneration. These findings are summarized as follows:

1. For motor conduction, fewer than 50% of transected nerves showed a motor response before 10 months after suture (20). After 10–20 months, however, a motor response was obtainable in 90% of nerves. The NCV reached about 75% of normal 2 years after the suture. Further improvement in the NCV thereafter is extremely slow. Steady improvement in terminal latency parallels the improvement in the motor NCV.

2. Compared with motor conduction, electrophysiological recovery in sensory nerve fibers was poor (20). Sensory CNAPs were often absent for 10–12 months after the suture. Ballantyne and Campbell (21) were not able to record the sensory CNAPs with surface electrodes before 10 months after suture. Two years after the suture, the sensory CNAPs were recordable in 20–44% of cases (20, 22). When the sensory CNAPs were recordable, the amplitude of the CNAPs was greatly reduced (to 30% of normal) with no tendency to larger potentials during a prolonged follow-up, and the sensory NCVs ranged from 65–80% of normal (21).

3. Often the mixed CNAPs were unobtainable less than 10 months after the suture (21). When the potentials were obtainable, the amplitude was extremely small (40% of normal), and the mixed NCVs showed a moderate reduction compared with normal controls (91%) (21). There was no tendency to significant improvement in NCVs with the passage of time. In contrast to the sensory CNAPs, the amplitude of the mixed CNAPs showed a progressive rise during the follow-up period.

The slow NCV in the regenerated nerve fiber is due to the disproportionately thin myelin sheath and the short internodes that persist even after the axons have attained near-normal diameters.

Almquist and Eeg-Olofson (23) examined 19 patients between the ages of 10 and 35 years with lesions of the median and ulnar nerves that had been sutured at least 5 years earlier. The orthodromic NCV was between 22 and 48 m/sec. The two-point discrimination was also measured. These authors stressed that two-point discrimination is more useful than measurement of the NCV in the assessment of clinical function. Ludin and Tackmann (24) claimed that the best way to assess regeneration is to measure the sensory NCV using near-nerve electrodes and an electronic averager. In fact, Buchthal and Kuhl (25) were able to record the sensory CNAPs across the suture line after a delay of 3–4 months corresponding to a growth rate of 1.5–2.0 mm/day. From early in the course of regeneration the sensory potential was dispersed in 40 components. They claimed that the cumulative amplitude shows a better relationship to the number of regenerated fibers and a better correlation with the reestablishment of touch sensation. The measurement of somatosensory evoked potentials has also proved to be a valuable supplementary aid in the assessment of regeneration in cases where no CNAPs can be recorded over the nerve trunk (see Chapter 19).

Electrophysiological Changes in Relation to the Severity of Nerve Injury

The most commonly accepted classification of nerve injuries is that of Seddon (26): neurapraxia, axonotmesis, and neurotmesis (Table 23.4; Fig. 23.8). Although admitting that his classification is only a rough approximation, simple enough to be workable, Seddon found that many nerve injuries can be fitted without difficulty into these three classes or into certain fairly obvious combinations of them. To avoid confusion, the electrophysiological changes related to the complete and pure forms of the three types of nerve injury are discussed below (Table 23.5).

Neurapraxia

Neurapraxia is associated predominantly with motor paresis caused by focal and selective segmental demyelination of the large fibers without any interruption of axons. The result is a local block in conductivity, so that conduction across the block is slowed or stopped; but above and below the block conduction is quite normal, as is the excitability threshold of the nerve. If the block is complete, the nerve will be inexcitable in the region of the block. Thus, all the characteristic findings of segmental demyelination (see

Table 23.4.
Pathological and Clinical Features According to the Degree of Nerve Injury

Feature	Neurapraxia	Axonotmesis	Neurotmesis
Pathology			
Anatomical continuity	Preserved	Preserved	May be lost
Essential damage	Selective segmental-demyelination of larger fibers; no degeneration of axons	Damage of axon; neural tube preserved	Damage of axon and neural tube
Clinical manifestation			
Motor paralysis	Complete	Complete	Complete
Muscle atrophy	Very little	Progressive	Progressive
Sensory paralysis	Usually much sparing	Complete	Complete
Autonomic paralysis	Usually much sparing	Complete	Complete
Recovery			
Surgical repair	Not necessary	Not necessary	Essential
Rate of recovery	Rapid: days or weeks	1–2 mm/day	1–2 mm/day after repair
March of recovery	No order	According to order of innervation	According to order of innervation
Quality	Perfect	Perfect	Always imperfect
Common causes	Transiet traction	Traction	Glass and knife cut
	Transient compression	Chronic compression	Missiles
	Transient ischemia	Fracture	Severe traction
		Ischemia	

^aModified from Seddon (26)

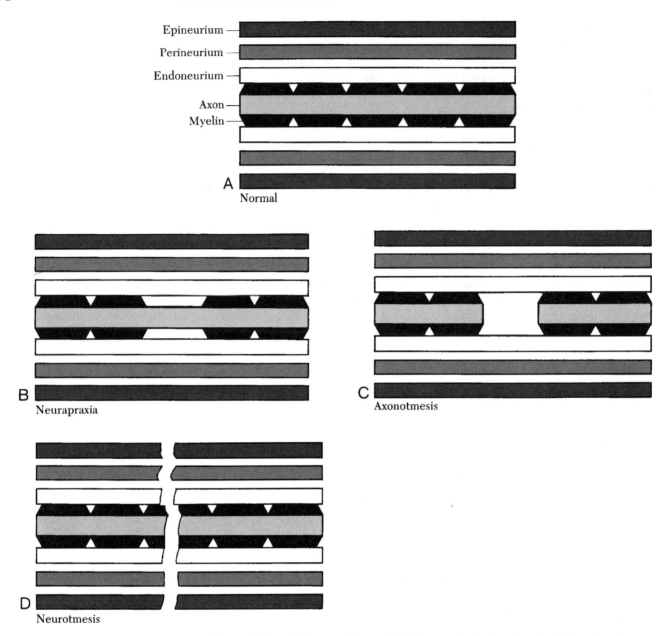

Figure 23.8. **A**, Diagrams of normals. **B**, Neurapraxia. **C**, Axonotmesis. **D**, Neurotmesis.

Chapter 20) are found across the lesion. In motor nerve conduction, an unequivocal slow motor NCV, a conduction block, and the abnormal temporal dispersion are observed over the injured segment. In sensory nerve conduction over the injured segment, the NCV is slow and the amplitude reduced or absent with the surface electrode technique. Conduction block and dispersion phenomenon may be observed with the near-nerve needle technique. The motor and sensory nerve conduction distal to the injury is completely normal. The needle EMG shows absent MUPs on maximal recruitment but does not show fibrillation or positive sharp waves. During the recovery phase, the nerve conduction abnormalities across the lesion improve and the number of MUPs during recruitment increases. Recovery is complete within days or weeks, and the quality of recovery is good. The best example of neurapraxia is acute compression neuropathy (see Chapter 21), e.g., Saturday night palsy or tourniquet palsy. As a traumatic lesion, this condition may be seen in patients with transient traction, compression, and ischemia. On many occasions, some axonal damage is combined with neurapraxia. Even Seddon (26) admits that "pure" neurapraxis (like pure axonotmesis) is a lesion that can be produced only in the laboratory.

Table 23.5.
Electrophysiological Changes According to the Degree of Nerve Injury

Injury	Neurapraxia	Axonotmesis	Neurotmesis
Initial postinjury period (0–5 days)			
Nerve conduction across the lesion	Absent	Absent	Absent
Nerve conduction distal to the lesion	Normal NCV	Normal NCV	Normal NCV
	Amplitude ↓	Amplitude ↓	Amplitude ↓
Fibrillation/PSW[a]	Absent	Absent	Absent
MUPs on recruitment	Absent	Absent	Absent
During denervation period (5–21 days)			
Nerve conduction across the lesion	Absent	Absent	Absent
Nerve conduction distal to the lesion	Normal	Absent	Absent
Fibrillation/PSW	Absent	Present	Present
MUPs on recruitment	Absent	Absent	Absent
During regeneration period			
Nerve conduction across the lesion	Conduction ↑	Conduction ↑	Absent
Nerve conduction distal to the lesion	Normal	Amplitude ↑	Absent
		Conduction ↑	
Fibrillation/PSW	Absent	↓	Present
MUPs on recruitment	↑	"Reinnervation potential"; MUP ↑	Absent

[a]PSW, positive sharp waves. ↓ Decreasing. ↑ Increasing.

In clinical practice it is important to recognize the "relatively" neurapraxic cases because of the *good prognostic implication*. Dissociated paralysis, predominantly motor, focal nerve conduction abnormalities indicative of segmental demyelination, preservation of nerve conduction distal to the lesion, and absence of fibrillation and positive sharp waves are pathognomonic findings in these cases.

Axonotmesis

Axonotmesis is characterized by total interruption of the axons and their myelin sheaths, but the rest of the nerve (its neural tube—endoneurium, perineurium, and epineurium) is preserved. This is *classic wallerian degeneration,* but regeneration occurs spontaneously and is of excellent quality because the intact endoneurial tubes guide the outgoing streams of axoplasm to their proper peripheral connections. The best examples of this lesion are stretching, traction, prolonged compression, and fractures. Nerve crush in the experimental animal typifies the changes that follow axonotmesis.

Neurotmesis

Neurotmesis is the most serious form of nerve injury and describes the state of a nerve that has either been completely severed or is so seriously disorganized by scar tissue that spontaneous regeneration is impossible. The neural tube is lost so that it cannot direct the axonal sprouts to their proper peripheral connections. This term, according to Seddon (26), is more inclusive because it embraces lesions in which the nerve preserves an appearance of continuity but is, in fact, totally destroyed over a longer or shorter distance. The best examples of this injury are laceration of the extremity by glass or knife, severe traction injuries, and gunshot wounds. Recovery is poor, and the quality of recovery is always imperfect. Surgical treatment is essential in this group of patients.

Neurotmesis and axonotmesis are clinically and electrophysiologically indistinguishable except in their behavior during the recovery period (24, 26). The classic findings observed during the degeneration phase of wallerian degeneration are observed in axonotmesis and neurotmesis. Motor and sensory nerve conduction is lost distal to the lesion. Fibrillation and positive sharp waves are prominent. The MUPs are completely absent. However, during the "regeneration period," when spontaneous recovery could occur, the electrophysiological findings are different between axonotmesis and neurotmesis (Table 23.5). In axonotmesis, *electrophysiological evidence of "reinnervation" is present.* This consists of: (*a*) the return of nerve excitability followed by a gradual increase in the amplitude of the CMAPs and CNAPs; (*b*) reduction of the amount of fibrillation and positive sharp waves; and (*c*) the appearance of "reinnervation potentials" followed by a gradual increase of MUPs on recruitment. In contrast, with neurotmesis the electrophysiological findings seen during the denervation period persist throughout the "regeneration period," indicating that reinnervation has not occurred. Motor and sensory nerve conduction is absent in the nerve distal to the lesion. Fibrillation and positive sharp waves are prominent. There is no MUP on recruitment.

Sunderland (27) classified nerve injuries according to five degrees, as follows:

- Degree 1—neurapraxia;
- Degree 2—axonotmesis; and
- Degree 3—damage to the axon and endoneurium but preservation of the perineurium and fascicular architecture of the nerve. Regeneration is less complete than in degree 2, but is still relatively effective.
- Degree 4—damage to the axon, endoneurium, and perineurium, though the nerve remains macroscopically intact. Regeneration is poorly oriented and less effective; and
- Degree 5—complete anatomical section of the nerve.

Sunderland's degrees 3–5 are included in Seddon's term neurotmesis.

In practice, it is difficult to place nerve injuries into these classifications. From our experience, pure neurapraxia is rare in traumatic nerve injury and is rarely examined in the EMG laboratory. A majority of partial nerve lesions (the presence of partial clinical and electrophysiological function of the nerve distally) fit best under "partial axonotmesis." In contrast, the majority of complete nerve lesions belong under either complete axonotmesis or neurotmesis. *Follow-up evaluation* differentiates only between complete axonotmesis and neurotmesis.

Value of EMG Studies in Peripheral Nerve Injury

In the early stage (1 week) after nerve injury, the nerve excitability test and strength duration curve give particularly useful information (28). NCV measurements must be interpreted with caution at this stage because normal or near-normal NCV may be obtained for several days after a nerve lesion. At this time, the attenuated amplitude of the CMAP or CNAP is of more value than the NCV. The only value of the needle EMG is for detecting minimal residual innervation, which may not be evident on clinical examination (7). The presence of a few MUPs in a severe nerve injury indicates that at least a few nerve fibers are still intact. Unfortunately, the nerve excitability test and strength duration curve require a subjective evaluation of the response. Because of this technical difficulty and additional disadvantages, these tests are rarely used in the modern EMG laboratory. One exception is the beneficial use of nerve excitability tests in the management of Bell's palsy (see Chapter 21). Abnormal nerve excitability is detected as early as the 3rd day after nerve injury. This principle is used in testing facial nerves in Bell's palsy.

Because the definite objective evidence of denervation—spontaneous fibrillation and positive sharp waves—appears within 8–14 days after injury, *the ideal time for the diagnosis of nerve injury is during the 3rd or 4th week after injury.* At this time, the full-blown nerve conduction and needle EMG abnormalities are observed in the involved nerve.

Differentiating Nerve Injury from Hysteria

EMG studies are of great value in the occasional instance when the clinician has difficulty deciding whether weakness in an extremity is caused by a peripheral nerve injury or is a conversion reaction. In the hysterical patient, motor and sensory conduction studies give normal results. With the needle EMG, fibrillation and positive sharp waves are absent, and the configuration of MUPs is normal. Because the EMG pattern on maximal contraction requires full cooperation of the patient, observation of this pattern is not very helpful. Occasionally in hysterical patients, irregular bursts of grouped MUPs are observed on maximal contraction because of the lack of sustained contraction.

Localizing the Site of Injury

To localize the lesion, all the resources of nerve conduction studies (NCS) and the needle EMG must be mobilized. A few general rules are helpful in localizing the lesion. When a root avulsion, radiculopathy, or traumatic myelopathy is suspected, paraspinal muscles are studied by needle EMG. Under these conditions, the paraspinal needle EMG study shows fibrillation and positive sharp waves. The orthodromic sensory nerve conduction study is essential to distinguish between root avulsion and plexus lesions. If a sensory CNAP can be elicited despite the loss of sensory function, the lesion lies proximal to the dorsal root ganglion, as noted in root avulsion. The absence of a sensory CNAP indicates a lesion distal to the dorsal root ganglion. With injuries of the brachial or lumbosacral plexus, the needle EMG must be done to pinpoint the lesion at the various levels of the plexus because the nerve conduction study of this segment is not available. For localizing a peripheral nerve lesion, the segmental NCS across the lesion is particularly rewarding. The nerve conduction tests should also include study of the distal segment to assess the degree of wallerian degeneration. When the segmental nerve conduction study is not available, the needle EMG study is valuable for localizing the nerve injury.

Estimating the Extent of Injury

Once the site is determined, the clinician is interested in the extent of injury. Partial nerve injury is usually treated nonsurgically, whereas surgery is considered in cases of complete nerve injury (29). To measure the extent of injury, needle EMG as well as nerve conduction studies should be done. With partial injury, the needle EMG shows minimal fibrillations and positive sharp waves, a considerable number of MUPs with an increased proportion of polyphasic MUPs, and a reduced recruitment of MUPs on maximal contraction; nerve conduction studies show a slow motor NCV, with decreased amplitude of the CMAP and an absent CNAP, or slow sensory NCV (30). With complete nerve injury, one observes failure to elicit any CMAPs with supramaximal stimulus, an absence of CNAPs, and numerous fibrillations and positive sharp waves, with no MUP on maximal attempt at contraction on the needle EMG.

With a complete nerve lesion (absence of any clinical and electrophysiological function of the nerve), for obvious reasons, the clinician is interested in two questions: (*a*) whether the lesion is axonotmesis or neurotmesis; and (*b*) whether there is continuity or discontinuity. A nerve that has been completely sectioned or lacerated or that is classified as having neurotmesis must be repaired surgically. Unfortunately, present-day EMG techniques cannot provide this information during the denervation period because there is *no electrophysiological parameter* that can distinguish between axonotmesis and neurotmesis and between continuity and discontinuity of a damaged nerve. As discussed earlier, axonotmesis can be differentiated from neurotmesis by the electrophysiological responses only during the "regeneration period." *The question of continuity or discontinuity of the nerve cannot be answered satisfactorily even during the "regeneration period,"* because in neurotmesis a lesion in "apparent continuity" may not show any electrophysiological improvement.

Following the Progression of Degeneration or Regeneration

Serial EMG examinations are critically important in patients with severe nerve injury. Although there are divergent opinions regarding the best timing for surgical exploration and repair of severe peripheral nerve injury, there seems to be common agreement on two points. First, the sooner the surgical repair is done, the greater is the chance for good recovery. Peripheral nerve suture between 3 weeks and 3 months after injury is followed by satisfactory recovery of function in 60% of cases. When suturing is done 3–15 months after injury, the rate of satisfactory recovery is 30% (31). According to Millesi, the results of nerve repair performed within 6 months of injury were better than those of nerves sutured after more than 6 months: the rate of satisfactory improvement was 85% when the repair was performed within 6 months, and 47% when the repair was performed after 6–12 months (32). Second, the rate of satisfactory improvement is poor when suturing is done more than 1 year after injury. Millesi reported a 43% improvement rate (32). Davis did not recommend surgical repair more than 1 year after injury because the denervation process in muscles and nerves is irreversible after this period (31). We recommend that surgical exploration be carried out if there is no evidence of clinical and electrophysiological improvement within 4 weeks after the first EMG study (ideally about 8 weeks after injury). This timing is based on the work of Kline and DeJonge (33), whose experimental evidence documented the appearance of the CNAP in the explored nerve by the 10th week after suture and the 6th week after partial crush in primate subjects. They further demonstrated, by an in vivo study of the CNAP, that nerve action potentials could be recorded weeks before EMG evidence of distal reinnervation and that needle EMG evidence of reinnervation always was accompanied by positive recording of a CNAP, but the converse was not always true (33).

Serial EMG studies are helpful in the follow-up of patients with partial nerve injury or with surgical repair. EMG study is recommended 8 weeks after surgical repair to assess the degree of regeneration. NCV studies are not helpful during the early stages of regeneration because no CMAP can be recorded until reinnervation of the muscle has begun. For many months after clinical recovery has been apparent, conduction velocity shows marked slowing (28). On the other hand, *the needle EMG is very helpful in evaluating regeneration.* When reinnervation begins, there may be a reduction in the amount of fibrillation. However, *the earliest positive evidence of reinnervation is the appearance of "reinnervation potentials"* (7). Reinnervation potentials appear about 2 months before clinical evidence of improvement (10). About 3 weeks later, complex, frequently polyphasic potentials of longer duration appear. These potentials are most easily recorded from the vicinity of the motor point and, in later stages, are succeeded by polyphasic potentials of much greater amplitude and duration. As more segments of the muscle undergo reinnervation, the number of motor units recruited during voluntary contraction increases until, if recovery is complete, an interference pattern is evident on maximal effort. Some small polyphasic potentials may be present even after complete functional recovery. Thus, appearance of a few "reinnervation potentials" is a source of encouragement to the patient and is a justification for continued conservative treatment, although it is no guarantee that good functional recovery of the muscle will occur (34).

To assess the recovery or residual of a lesion, a final EMG examination 18 months after partial injury or repair is probably appropriate. One study showed that maximal improvement of sensory and motor function was apparent at 15 months and that no significant change occurred in nerve conduction beyond 15 months after suture (21). When nerve injury is partial, the conduction velocity eventually may return to normal, but after nerve section and suture some degree of slowing of NCV (about 20% decrease) is likely to be permanent (35), as discussed previously.

Neurolysis Versus Neurorrhaphy

During surgical exploration, conduction study directly on the exposed nerve can render valuable help to the surgeon. This subject is further discussed in Chapter 16. A nerve that is completely cut presents no question in surgical management—it must be sutured. On the other hand, nerves that have been crushed, stretched, contused, or partially lacerated present a real problem. The management of these lesions in continuity has been improved by the in vivo recording of CNAPs from the surface of peripheral nerves (36). In general, if a CNAP can be evoked through the area of injury and recorded distally, careful neurolysis is carried out, leaving the nerve intact. However, if a CNAP cannot be recorded distal to an area of injury, the lesion is resected and neurorrhaphy is done. Thus, recording a CNAP provides an objective measurement of injury, as well as identifies the area of injury.

This in vivo technique provides objective, early evaluation of "reinnervation" before maturation (which is evident by EMG study) and makes possible earlier surgical exploration without potential damage to the surviving or regenerating nerve fibers.

Medicolegal Problems

The usefulness of the EMG study in medicolegal problems is based upon two fundamental principles: (a) the actual time at which fibrillation and positive sharp waves appear; and (b) the precise location from which these potentials are recorded (30). If medicolegal implications exist, it is important to have *a complete EMG study within the first 5 days*. This recommendation is based on an observation that transient positive sharp waves and fibrillation may occur as early as 5 days after nerve injury (28). Detection of fibrillation and positive sharp waves within this period is strong evidence of a previous injury predating the alleged present injury. The basic principle of location is based on finding these potentials in the muscle group only beyond the point where the nerve is injured or compressed. Thus, if these abnormal potentials are found in the muscle innervated by other nerves or in the muscle proximal to the injury, the findings are not consistent with the alleged injury. Further, the "time and location" principle is also demonstrated to be helpful, in a negative way, in evaluating hysterical paralysis or malingering.

REFERENCES

1. Oh SJ. Electromyographic studies in peripheral nerve injuries. South Med J 1976;69:177–182.
2. Bradley WG. Disorders of peripheral nerves. Oxford: Blackwell, 1974.
3. Gilliatt RW, Taylor JC. Electrical changes following section of the facial nerve. Proc R Soc Med 1959;52:1080–1083.
4. Gutmann E. Histology of degeneration and regeneration. In: Licht S, ed. Electrodiagnosis and electromyography. New Haven, CT: E Licht, 1971:113–133.
5. Gilliatt RW, Hjorth R. Nerve conduction during wallerian degeneration in the baboon. J Neurol Neurosurg Psychiatry 1972;35:335–341.
6. Gutmann E, Holubar J. The degeneration of peripheral nerve fibers. J Neurol Neurosurg Psychiatry 1950;13:89–105.
7. Lambert EH. Electromyography and electrical stimulation of peripheral nerve and muscles: In: Clinical examination in neurology. 3rd ed. Philadelphia: WB Saunders 1971:271–299.
8. Weddell G, Feinstein B, Pattle RE. The electrical activity of voluntary muscle in man under normal and pathological conditions. Brain 1944;67:178–257.
9. Wynn Parry CB. Techniques of neuromuscular stimulation and their clinical application. In: Walton JN, ed. Disorders of voluntary muscles. Edinburgh: Churchill, 1969:763–784.
10. Goodgold J, Eberstein A. Electrodiagnosis of neuromuscular diseases. Baltimore: Williams & Wilkins, 1972:175–178.
11. Rosenblueth A, Dempsey EW. A study of wallerian degeneration. Amer J Physiol 1939;207:507–528.
12. Landau WM. The duration of neuromuscular function after nerve section in man. J Neurosurg 1953;10:64–68.
13. Wilbourn AJ. Serial conduction studies in human nerve during wallerian degeneration. EEG Clin Neurophysiol 1977;43:616.
14. Chaudhry V, Cornblath DR. Wallerian degeneration in human nerves. Muscle Nerve 1992;15:687–693.
15. Pilling JB. Nerve conduction during wallerian degeneration in man. Muscle Nerve 1978;1:81.
16. Kaeser HE, Lambert EH. Nerve function studies in experimental polyneuritis. EEG Clin Neurophysiol (Suppl) 1962;22:29–35.
17. Cragg BG, Thomas PK. Changes in conduction velocity and fiber size proximal to peripheral nerve lesions. J Physiol (Lond) 1961;157:315–327.
18. Gilliatt RW. Recent advances in the pathophysiology of nerve conduction. In: Desmedt JE, ed. New developments in EMG and clinical neurophysiology. Basel: Karger, 1972:2–18.
19. Skorpil V. Conduction velocity of human nerve structures. Rozpr Cesk Akad Ved 1965. Cited by Kaeser (20).
20. Kaeser HE. Nerve conduction velocity measurements. In: Vinken PJ, Bruyn GW, eds. Handbook of clinical neurology, vol. 7. Amsterdam: North Holland, 1972:116–196.

21. Ballantyne JP, Campbell MJ. Electrophysiological study after surgical repair of sectioned human peripheral nerves. J Neurol Neurosurg Psychiatry 1973;36:797–805.
22. Tallis R, Staniforth P, Fisher TR. Neurophysiological studies of autogenous sural nerve grafts. J Neurol Neurosurg Psychiatry 1978;41:677–683.
23. Almquist E, Eeg-Olofson O. Sensory nerve conduction velocity and two-point discrimination in sutured nerves. J Bone Joint Surg 1970;51A:791–796.
24. Ludin HP, Tackmann W. Sensory neurography. New York: Thieme-Stratton, 1981.
25. Buchthal F, Kuhl U. Nerve conduction, tactile sensibility, and the electromyogram after suture of compression of peripheral nerves: longitudinal study in man. J Neurol Neurosurg Psychiatry 1979;42:436–451.
26. Seddon H. Surgical disorders of the peripheral nerves, 2nd ed. Edinburgh: Churchill Livingstone, 1975.
27. Sunderland S. Nerves and nerve injuries, 2nd ed. Edinburgh: Churchill Livingstone, 1978.
28. Lenman JAR, Ritchie AE. Clinical electromyography. Philadelphia: JB Lippincott, 1970:84–87.
29. Brown HA, Brown BA. Treatment of peripheral nerve injuries. Rev Surg 1967;24:1–8.
30. Marinacci AA. Applied electromyography. Philadelphia: Lea & Febiger, 1968.
31. Davis RA. Management of peripheral nerve injuries. Postgrad Med 1965;38:509–514.
32. Millesi H. Interfascicular nerve grafting. Orthop Clin North Am 1981;12:287–301.
33. Kline DG, DeJonge BR. Evoked potentials to evaluate peripheral nerve injuries. Surg Gynecol Obstet 1968;127:1239–1248.
34. Howard FM. The electromyogram and conduction velocity studies in peripheral nerve trauma. Clin Neurosurg 1970;17:63–76.
35. Hodes R, Larrabee MC, German W. The human electromyogram in response to nerve stimulation and the conduction velocity of motor axons. Arch Neurol Psychiatry 1948;60:340–365.
36. Vanderark GD, Meyer GA, Kline DG, Kempe LG. Peripheral nerve injuries studied by evoked potential recordings. Milit Med 1970;135:90–94.
37. Levenson D, Rosenbluth J. Electrophysiologic changes accompanying wallerian degeneration in frog sciatic nerve. Brain Research 1990;523:230–236.
38. Erlanger J, Schoepfle GM. A study of nerve degeneration and regeneration. Am J Physiol 1946;147:550–581.
39. Levenson D, Rosenbluth J. Electrophysiologic changes accompanying wallerian degeneration in frog sciatic nerve. Brain Research 1990;523:230–236.
40. Lisak K, Dempsey EW, Rosenblueth A. The failure of transmission of motor nerve impulses in the course of wallerian degeneration. Amer J Physiol 1939;128:45–56.
41. Miledi R, Slater CR. On the degeneration of rat neuromuscular junctions after nerve section. J Physiol (Lond) 1970;207:507–528.
42. Struppler A, Huckauf H. Propagation velocity in regenerated motor nerve fibers. EEG Clin Neurophysiol Suppl 1962;22:58–60.
43. Muheim G. Vergleichende Beurteilung verschiedener Untersuchungsmethoden nach Finger-nerven Durchtrennung. Schweiz Med Wochenschr 1969;99:1176–1184.
44. Berry CM, Grundfest H, Hinsey JC. The electrical activity of regenerating nerves in the cat. J Neurophysiol 1944;7:103–115.
45. Sanders FK, Whitteridge D. Conduction velocity and myelin thickness in regenerating nerve fibers. J Physiol (Lond) 1946;105:152–174.
46. Jacobson S, Guth L. An electrophysiological study of the early stage of peripheral nerve regeneration. Exp Neurol 1965;11:48–60.
47. Hallin RG, Siesenfeld, Lungnegård H. Neurophysiological studies of peripheral nerve functions after neural regeneration following nerve suture in man. Int Rehab Med 1981;3:187–192.
48. Donoso RS, Ballantyne JP, Hansen S. Regeneration of sutured human peripheral nerves: an electrophysiological study. J Neurol Neurosurg Psychiatry 1979;42:97–107.

Index

Page numbers followed by "t" denote tables; those followed by "f" denote figures.

688   INDEX

Index of Method Authors